ECHOCARDIOGRAPHY IN CARDIAC INTERVENTIONS

Developments in Cardiovascular Medicine

VOLUME 96

ECHOCARDIOGRAPHY IN CARDIAC INTERVENTIONS

Edited by

IVO CIKES, M.D.
Institute of Cardiovascular Disease
University of Zagreb,
Zagreb, Yugoslavia

KLUWER ACADEMIC PUBLISHERS
DORDRECHT / BOSTON / LONDON

Library of Congress Cataloging in Publication Data

Echocardiography in cardiac interventions.

   (Developments in cardiovascular medicine)
   Includes index.
   1. Heart--Interventional radiology. 2. Echocardiography. I. Cikes, I. II. Series. [DNLM: 1. Echocardiography. 2. Heart Diseases--diagnosis.
W1 DE997VME / WG 141.5.E2 I613]
RD589.35.I55E27 1989   617'.412   88-26847

ISBN-13: 978-94-010-6897-0   e-ISBN-13: 978-94-009-0907-6
DOI: 10.1007/978-94-009-0907-6

Published by Kluwer Academic Publishers,
P.O. Box 17, 3300 AA Dordrecht, The Netherlands

Kluwer Academic Publishers incorporates
the publishing programmes of
D. Reidel, Martinus Nijhoff, Dr W. Junk and MTP Press.

Sold and distributed in the U.S.A. and Canada
by Kluwer Academic Publishers,
101 Philip Drive, Norwell, MA 02061, U.S.A.

In all other countries, sold and distributed
by Kluwer Academic Publishers Group,
P.O. Box 322, 3300 AH Dordrecht, The Netherlands.

printed on acid free paper

This book is dedicated to
Nada and Maja

Contents

Preface xi
List of contributors xiii

1. INTRACARDIAC INTERVENTIONS 1

1.1. Intracardiac echocardiography
D. A. Conetta 3
1.2. Endomyocardial biopsy of the left ventricle guided by echocardiography
H. Egeblad & S. A. Mortensen 19
1.3. Echocardiographic guidance of endomyocardial biopsy of the
right ventricle
G. A. Williams 31
1.4. Two-dimensional echocardiographic-assisted balloon atrial
septostomy
J. B. Seward 41
1.5. Color flow Doppler guiding of atrial septostomy
S. Kyo & R. Omoto 49
1.6. Echocardiography in transseptal cardiac catheterization
I. Kronzon & E. Glassman 57
1.7. Percutaneous transvenous mitral commissurotomy guided
and assessed by echocardiography
K. Inoue & C. Chen 67
1.8. Cardiac catheterization guided by ultrasound
I. Cikes, B. Breyer, K. Chandrasekaran, P. J. Pearson,
J. B. Seward & A. J. Tajik 77
1.9. Ultrasonically marked pacing system
B. Ferek-Petric, I. Cikes, B. Breyer, K. Chandrasekaran &
A. J. Tajik 89
1.10. Transcatheter laser angioplasty and related techniques guided
by echocardiography
W. J. Bommer, G. Lee, M. C. Chan, R. I. Low & D. T. Mason 99

1.11. Echocardiographic assessment of coronary venous retroperfusion
S. Kar & J. Areeda   117

2. INTRAPERICARDIAL INTERVENTIONS   131

2.1. Pericardiocentesis guided by ultrasound
I. Cikes, A. Ernst, J. A. Callahan & M. E. Goldman   133

3. CONTRAST ECHOCARDIOGRAPHY   147

3.1. Contrast echocardiography
*J. Roelandt, C. Tirtaman, W. B. Vletter, F. J. ten Cate,
D. Romdoni, W. J. Gussenhoven & H. Rijsterborgh*   149
3.2. New echocardiographic contrast agents
R. S. Meltzer, X. Feng, M. Nanna & R. Gramiak   179
3.3. Myocardial perfusion study by contrast echocardiography
E. Corday & I. Hajduczki   191

4. TRANSESOPHAGEAL ECHOCARDIOGRAPHY   207

4.1. Transesophageal echocardiography – technique and standard views
M. Schlüter, B. A. Langenstein & P. Hanrath   209
4.2. Transesophageal echocardiography – an overview of applications
B. Shively & N. B. Schiller   227
4.3. Transesophageal echocardiographic imaging of the thoracic aorta in aortic dissection
*R. Erbel, S. Mohr-Kahaly, M. Drexler, N. Wittlich,
N. Börner & J. Meyer*   249
4.4. Detection of cardiac and extracardiac masses by transesophageal echocardiography
*W. G. Daniel, U. Nellessen, A. Mügge, E. Schröder &
P. R. Lichtlen*   261
4.5. Diagnosis of infective endocarditis by transesophageal echocardiography
W. G. Daniel, A. Mügge & P. R. Lichtlen   273

4.6. Detection of prosthetic valve malfunction by transesophageal echocardiography
    W. G. Daniel, U. Nellessen, A. Mügge, E. Schröder, D. Hausmann & P. R. Lichtlen   281
4.7. Transesophageal Doppler color flow mapping: initial experience
    N. P. de Bruijn, F. M. Clements & J. A. Kisslo   291

5. INTRAOPERATIVE ECHOCARDIOGRAPHY   299

5.1. Intraoperative evaluation of valvular disease
    M. E. Goldman, T. Guarino & B. P. Mindich   301
5.2. Intraoperative echocardiography in valvular heart disease – quantitative study of left ventricular properties
    H. M. Spotnitz, M. L. Antunes, M. B. Clark, C. Y. H. Wong & R. C. Robbins   313
5.3. Intraoperative two-dimensional echocardiography in congenital heart disease
    W. J. Gussenhoven, L. A. van Herwerden, H. K. The, E. Bos, J. Roelandt, M. A. Taams, M. Witsenburg & N. Bom   331
5.4. Intraoperative two-dimensional echocardiography for guiding surgical correction in subvalvular aortic obstruction
    L. A. van Herwerden, W. J. Gussenhoven, O. A. Schippers, E. Bos & F. J. ten Cate   343
5.5. Intraoperative assessment of left ventricular performance
    M. N. Kotler   351
5.6 Intraoperative contrast echocardiography can directly assess myocardial perfusion
    M. E. Goldman, T. Guarino & B. P. Mindich   363
5.7. Intraoperative epicardial echocardiography in recognizing acute myocardial ischemia
    K. Chandrasekaran, J. F. Greenleaf, J. B. Seward & J.A. Tajik   367

6. DOPPLER ECHOCARDIOGRAPHY IN INTERVENTIONS

6.1. Intraoperative color flow Doppler imaging in valvular heart disease
    R. Omoto, S. Takamoto, S. Kyo, M. Matsumura & Y. Yokote   381

6.2. Doppler for guiding and flow measurement in coronary artery surgery
H. Engedal, K. Matre & L. Segadal 395

6.3. Color flow evaluation of coronary anastomosis
S. Kyo, R. Omoto, S. Takamoto & M. Matsumura 407

6.4. Intraoperative Doppler color flow mapping in dissecting aneurysm of the aorta
S. Takamoto & R. Omoto 415

6.5. Doppler monitoring of cardiac output using an implantable aortic transducer
L. Segadal, K. Matre & H. Engedal 423

6.6. Doppler echocardiography and cardiac pacing
G. J. Perry & N. C. Nanda 431

6.7. Duplex scanning in arterial and venous disease
D. C. Taylor, G. L. Moneta & D. E. Strandness 449

6.8. Doppler techniques for intraoperative arterial assessment
R. E. Zierler 463

6.9. Doppler guiding of venous and arterial puncture
T. Shine & M. Nugent 473

7. STRESS ECHOCARDIOGRAPHY 481

7.1. Exercise echocardiography
W. F. Armstrong 483

7.2. Stress echocardiography with transesophageal atrial pacing
S. Iliceto & P. Rizzon 495

7.3. Stress Doppler echocardiography
S. M. Teague & J. A. Heinsimer 509

8. CARDIOVASCULAR DRUG INTERVENTIONS 521

8.1. Echocardiography in the assessment of cardiovascular drug interventions
B. Clarke & D. Gibson 523

Index of Subjects 541

Preface

This monograph represents an attempt to collect the methods developed within the past decade in which echocardiography was being used to guide or to assess the results of some cardiovascular interventions or to overcome the imaging limitations of transthoracic approaches. I have entitled this book Echocardiography in Cardiac Interventions, although I am aware that this title is not entirely applicable to all the included methods. In these interventive procedures echocardiography preserves its noninvasive nature, and by combining it with invasive procedures, they become more accurate, safer and less invasive.

The book is divided into 8 sections and 42 chapters written by many authorities in the field. When such comprehensive contributions from many authors are used, some overlapping cannot be avoided.

I would like to express my appreciation to the individual contributors for their dedication and cooperation in preparing this book. I am indebted to Dr. A. J. Tajik from the Mayo Clinic, who created a pleasant milieu for preparing the book during my sabbatical year at the Mayo Clinic.

It is hoped that the reader will derive from this book a sense of where and how the ultrasound can be used in cardiovascular interventions today and what new approaches might be forthcoming.

Ivo Cikes

List of contributors

M. L. Antunes, M.D., Department of Surgery, Columbia University College of Physicians and Surgeons, New York, New York, USA.

J. Areeda, Cedars-Sinai Medical Center, Los Angeles, California, USA.

W. F. Armstrong, M.D., Wishard Memorial Hospital, Krannert Institute of Cardiology and Indiana University School of Medicine, Indianapolis, Indiana, USA.

W. J. Bommer, M.D., University of California, Davis, California, USA.

N. Börner, M.D., II. Medical Clinic, Johannes Gutenberg-University Mainz, Federal Republic Germany.

N. Bom, Ph.D., Thoraxcenter, Erasmus University Rotterdam and the Interuniversity Cardiology Institute, The Netherlands.

E. Bos, M.D., Thoraxcenter, Erasmus University Rotterdam and the Interuniversity Cardiology Institute, The Netherlands.

B. Breyer, Ph.D., Medical Physics Department, University Gynaecological Hospital, Zagreb, Yugoslavia.

N. P. de Bruijn, M.D., Department of Anesthesiology, Duke University Medical Center, Durham, North Carolina, USA.

F. J. ten Cate, M.D., Thoraxcenter, Erasmus University Rotterdam and the Interuniversity Cardiology Institute, The Netherlands.

M. C. Chan, M.D., Western Heart Institute, San Fransisco, California, USA.

K. Chandrasekaran, M.D., Department of Cardiology, Mayo Clinic, Rochester, Minnesota, USA.

C. Chen, M.D., Guangdong Provincial Cardiovascular Institute, Guangzhou, People's Republic of China.

I. Cikes, M.D., Institute of Cardiovascular Diseases, School of Medicine, University of Zagreb, Zagreb, Yugoslavia.

M. B. Clark, M.D., Department of Surgery, Columbia University College of Physicians and Surgeons, New York, New York, USA.

B. Clarke, M.D., Southampton General Hospital, Shirley, Southampton, United Kingdom.

F. M. Clements, M.D., Department of Cardiology, Duke University Medical Center, Durham, North Carolina, USA.

D. A. Conetta, M.D., University of Florida College of Medicine, Jacksonville, Florida, USA.

E. Corday, M.D., Cedars-Sinai Medical Center, Los Angeles, California, USA.

W. G. Daniel, Department of Cardiology, Hannover Medical School, Hannover, Federal Republic Germany.

M. Drexler, II. Medical Clinic, Johannes Gutenberg-University Mainz, Federal Republic Germany.

H. Egeblad, Medical Department B, The Rigshospital, University Hospital of Copenhagen, Copenhagen, Denmark.

H. Engedal, M.D., Department of Surgery, Haukeland Hospital, University of Bergen, Norway.

R. Erbel, M.D., II. Medical Clinic, Johannes Gutenberg-University Mainz, Federal Republic Germany.

A. Ernst, M.D., Institute of Cardiovascular Diseases, School of Medicine, University of Zagreb, Zagreb, Yugoslavia.

X. Feng, M.D., Department of Medicine, University of Rochester, Rochester, New York, USA.

B. Ferek-Petric, E.E., Department of Surgery, School of Medicine, University of Zagreb, Zagreb, Yugoslavia.

D. Gibson, M.D., Department of Cardiology, Brompton Hospital, London, United Kingdom.

E. Glassman, M.D., Department of Medicine, New York University Medical Center, New York, USA.

M. E. Goldman, M.D., Division of Cardiology, Department of Medicine, Mount-Sinai Medical Center, New York, New York, USA.

R. Gramiak, M.D., Departmenbt of Radiology, university of Rochester, Rochester, New York, USA.

J. F. Greenleaf, Ph.D., Department of Physiology and Biophysics, Mayo Clinic and Mayo Foundation, Rochester, Minnesota, USA.

T. Guarino, RN, Division of Cardiology, Department of Medicine, New York, New York, USA.

W. J. Gussenhoven, M.D., Thoraxcenter, Erasmus University Rotterdam and the Interuniversity Cardiology Institute, The Netherlands.

I. Hajduczki, M.D., Department of Cardiology, Cedars-Sinai Medical Center, Los Angeles, California, USA.

P. Hanrath, M.D., 2nd Department of Medicine, General Hospital St. Georg, Hamburg, Federal Republic Germany.

D. Hausmann, M.D., Department of Cardiology, Hannover Medical School, Hannover, Federal Republic Germany.

J. A. Heinsimer, M.D., Noninvasive Cardiac Laboratory, Harper Hospital, Wayne State University, Detroit, Michigan, USA.

L. A. van Herwerden, M.D., Thoraxcenter, Erasmus University Rotterdam and the Interuniversity Cardiology Institute, The Netherlands.

S. Iliceto, M.D., Division of Cardiology, University of Bari, Italy.

K. Inoue, M.D., Department of Thoracic Surgery, Kochi Municipal Hospital, Kochi, Japan.

S. Kar, M.D., Department of Medicine, Cedars-Sinai Medical Center, Los Angeles, California, USA.

J. A. Kisslo, M.D., Department of Medicine, Duke University Medical Center, Durham, North Carolina, USA.

M. N. Kotler, M.D., Division of Cardiovascular Diseases, Albert Einstein Medical Center, Temple University School of Medicine, Philadelphia, Pennsilvania, USA.

I. Kronzon, M.D., Department of Medicine, New York University Medical Center, New York, New York, USA.

S. Kyo, M.D., Department of Surgery, Saitama Medical School, Saitama, Japan.

B. A. Langenstein, M.D., Department of Cardiology, University Hospital Eppendorf, Hamburg, Federal Republic Germany.

G. Lee, M.D., Northern California Heart and Lung Institute, Concord, California, USA.

P. R. Lichtlen, M.D., Department of Cardiology, Hannover Medical School, Hannover, Federal Republic Germany.

R. I. Low, M.D., Diagnostic and Interventional Cardiology Consultants, Sacramento, California, USA.

D. T. Mason, M.D., Western Heart Institute, San Francisco, California, USA.

K. Matre, M.D., Department of Surgery, Haukeland Hospital, University of Bergen, Norway.

M. Matsumura, M.D., Department of Surgery, Saitama Medical School, Saitama, Japan.

R. S. Meltzer, M.D., Ph.D., Department of Medicine, University of Rochester Medical Center, Rochester, New York, USA.

J. Meyer, M.D., II. Medical Clinic, Johannes Gutenberg-University Mainz, Federal Republic Germany.

B. P. Mindich, M.D., Division of Cardiothoracic Surgery, St. Luke's/Roosevelt Hospital Center, New York, New York, USA.

S. Mohr-Kahaly, M.D., II. Medical Clinic, Johannes Gutenberg-University Mainz, Federal Republic Germany.

G. L. Moneta, M.D., Department of Surgery, University of Washington, School of Medicine, Seattle, Washington, USA.

S. A. Mortensen, M.D., Department of Cardiology and Internal Medicine B, Central Hospital, Hillerød, Denmark.

A. Mügge, M.D., Department of Cardiology, Hannover Medical School, Hannover, Federal Republic Germany.

N. C. Nanda, M.D., Division of Cardiovascular Diseases, University of Alabama at Birmingham, Birmingham, Alabama, USA.

M. Nanna, M.D., Department of Medicine, University of Rochester, Rochester, New York, USA.

U. Nellessen, M.D., Department of Cardiology, Hannover Medical School, Hannover, Federal Republic Germany.

M. Nugent, M.D., Department of Anesthesiology, Mayo Clinic, Rochester, Minnesota, USA.

R. Omoto, M.D., Department of Surgery, Saitama Medical School, Saitama, Japan.

P. J. Pearson, Mayo Medical School, Rochester, Minnesota, USA.

G. J. Perry, M.D., Division of Cardiovascular Disease, University of Alabama at Birmingham, Birmingham, Alabama, USA.

H. Rijsterborgh, M.D., Thoraxcenter, Erasmus University Rotterdam and the Interuniversity Cardiology Institute, The Netherlands.

P. Rizzon, M.D., Division of Cardiology, University of Bari, Italy.

R. C. Robbins, M.D., Department of Surgery, Columbia University College of Physicians and Surgeons, New York, New York, USA.

J. Roelandt, M.D., Thoraxcenter, Erasmus University Rotterdam and the Interuniversity Cardiology Institute, The Netherlands.

D. Romdoni, M.D., Thoraxcenter, Erasmus University Rotterdam and the Interuniversity Cardiology Institute, The Netherlands.

N. B. Schiller, M.D., University of California, San Francisco, Moffitt Hospital, San Francisco, California, USA.

O. A. Schippers, M.D., Thoraxcenter, Erasmus University Rotterdam and the Interuniversity Cardiology Institute, The Netherlands.

M. Schlüter, Ph.D., Department of Cardiology, University Hospital Eppendorf, Hamburg, Federal Republic Germany.

E. Schroder, M.D., Department of Cardiology, Hannover Medical School, Hannover, Federal Republic Germany.

L. Segadal, M.D., Department of Surgery, Haukeland Hospital University of Bergen, Norway.

J. B. Seward, M.D., Department of Cardiology, Mayo Clinic, Rochester, Minnesota, USA.

T. Shine, M.D., Department of Anesthesiology, Mayo Clinic, Jacksonville, Florida, USA.

B. Shively, M.D., University of California, San Francisco, Moffitt Hospital, San Francisco, California USA.

H. M. Spotnitz, M.D., Department of Surgery, Columbia University College of Physicians and Surgeons, New York, New York, USA.

D. M. Strandness, M.D., Department of Surgery, University of Washington, School of Medicine, Seattle, Washington, USA.

M. A. Taams, M.D., Thoraxcenter University Rotterdam and the Interuniversity Cardiology Institute, The Netherlands.

J. A. Tajik, M.D., Department of Cardiology, Mayo Clinic, Rochester, Minnesota, USA.

S. Takamoto, M.D., Division of Cardiovascular Surgery, Showa General Hospital, Kodaira, Tokyo, Japan.

David C. Taylor, M.D., Department of Surgery, University of Washington, School of Medicine, Seattle, Washington, USA.

S. M. Teague, M.D., Echocardiographic Laboratory, University of Oklahoma Health Sciences Center, Oklahoma City, Oklahoma, USA.

H. K. The, M.D., Thoraxcenter, Erasmus University Rotterdam and the Interuniversity Cardiology Institute, The Netherlands.

C. Tirtaman, M.D., Academic Hospital Rotterdam-Dijkzigt, The Netherlands.

W. B. Vletter, Thoraxcenter, Erasmus University Rotterdam and the Interuniversity Cardiology Institute, The Netherlands.

G. A. Williams, M.D., V.A. Cardiology Section, Saint Louis University, St. Louis, Missouri, USA.

M. Witsenburg, M.D., Thoraxcenter, Erasmus University Rotterdam and the Interuniversity Cardiology Institute, The Netherlands.

N. Wittlich, M.D., II. Medical Clinic, Johannes Guttenberg-University Mainz, Federal Republic Germany.

C. Y. H. Wong, M.D., Department of Surgery, Columbia University College of Physicians and Surgeons, New York, New York, USA.

Y. Yokote, M.D., Department of Surgery, Saitama Medical School, Saitama, Japan.

R. Zierler, M.D., Department of Surgery, Seattle VA Medical Center, Seattle, Washington, USA.

PART 1: Intracardiac Interventions

1.1. Intracardiac echocardiography

DONALD A. CONETTA

Introduction

The development of intracardiac echocardiography began in 1960 when Cieszynksi [1] used an ultrasonic catheter to record reflected sound from canine cardiac chambers and pulmonary artery. In 1962, Kimoto et al. [2] studied 8 patients with 5 and 10 MHz, 5 mm (diameter) piezo-electric crystals mounted on stainless steel pipes introduced into the right atrium via jugular and femoral veins. An ASD was identified from an A-Mode display in this first human study. In 1968, Carleton et al. [3] attached a 2.25 MHz, 8 mm, cylindrical crystal to 8 French catheters. These radially emitting, (non-directional beam) transducers were positioned against the interventricular septa of canine right ventricles. These A-Mode recordings of the left ventricular (LV) posterior wall were the first used to estimate changes in LV cavity diameter during changes of heart rate, preload and afterload. They concluded that the echocardiographic (echo) measurements were accurate and reflected changes expected with the physiologic alterations. Manoli [4] and Brundage et al. [5] used 3 mm, spherical, non directional, catheter-tip transducers in animal left ventricles to measure dimension changes during the cardiac cycle. The transducers, introduced via the femoral artery, recorded the strongest echoes from LV structures with the greatest area normal to the crystal's surface. Manoli reported a 4.1% difference between echo estimated and dye dilution LV stroke volume and Brundage good correlations of echo and sonomicrometer LV short (mean r = 0.82) and long axis (mean r = 0.92) dimension measurements. This method assumed stability of crystal position (on the LV long axis) throughout the cardiac cycle. Transducer motion associated with rotation about and shortening of the LV long axis during systole in fact may have led to imaging of different myocardial segments during the cycle (*infra vide*).

In 1970, Eggleston et al. [6] studied canine anesthetized LVs with a transducer system consisting of four, 10 MHz crystals mounted 90 degrees apart on a catheter-tip. The system, introduced via the carotid artery, was mechanically rotated during sequential excitation of the crystals for 8 seconds of recording. A-Mode dimension measurements were acquired during in 24

I. Cikes (ed.), *Echocardiography in Cardiac Interventions*, 3–18, 1989.

periods during each R-R interval. Signal processing included a signal mixer for integration, external echo transducers to track catheter-tip motion and a computer to organize, synthesize and store dimension data. The output was 24 'frames' of a reconstructed 2-dimensional, LV short axis endocardial border for an average cardiac cycle. However, inaccurate prediction of crystal motion, requirement of a constant R-R interval, and inability to provide continuous, real time images were major limitations. A cylindrical transducer with 32 radially arranged (0.35 mm wide), 5.6 MHz crystals on a 9 French catheter (tip) was designed by Bom [7]. The crystals of this transducer were excited circumferentially (similar to a radar sweep). This excitation pattern allowed recording of 150 frames/second and had a potential to provide real time images. However, only *in vitro* testing was reported, and the author also noted that transducer motion might well limit image quality.

This brief historical review underscores the evolution of crystal and catheter design, and documents the feasibility of A-Mode (right and left heart) intracardiac echocardiography. However, data from these studies cannot be directly related to conventional M-Mode or 2-D echocardiograms. The echo beams could not be directed, LV wall excursion was not corrected for transducer motion and wall thickness changes could not be determined. While the multi-crystal system might provide averaged, LV short axis area data, it was limited by transducer motion, and the lack of continuous, real time recording of changes in LV dimensions and wall thickness.

M-Mode intracardiac echocardiography

Our interest in intracardiac echocardiography was stimulated by experiments requiring simultaneous, continuous M-Mode echo and LV hemodynamic measurements. The high incidence of chronic pulmonary disease in our patient population resulted in limited quality external M-Mode recordings. Therefore, we designed a catheter-mounted, directional, single crystal transducer to provide continuous M-Mode recordings of LV dimensions and wall motion [8]. The 3.5 and 5 MHz transducers consisted of lead zirconate crystals (Aerotech Laboratories, Lewiston, PA) enclosed in cylindrical stainless steel housings with a 2.0×13 mm window, to expose the emitting surface (Fig. 1A). The transducer was bonded proximally to a 9 French, thin-walled catheter segment (USCI Billerica, MA, and Cordis, Miami, FL). Flexible, sealed, tapered catheter tips (2, 5 or 7 cm) were bonded to the distal end of the transducer housing. A coaxial cable within the proximal catheter lumen connected the crystal to a 3.3. micro henry tuning element and a microdot connector (Fig. 1B). The transducer was interfaced to a Smith-

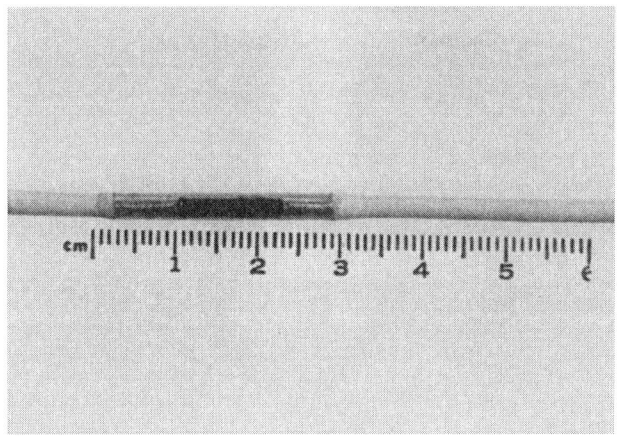

Fig. 1A. Enlarged view of the transducer section of the catheter-probe.

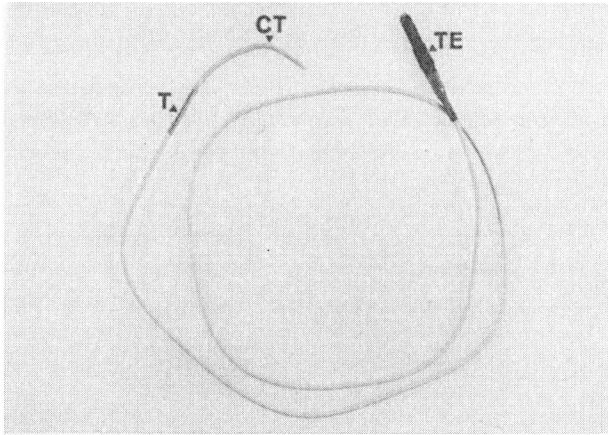

Fig. 1B. Catheter-mounted echocardiographic probe. T = Transducer Element, CT = Stabilizing Catheter Tip, TE = Tuning Element.

Kline 20A Ultrasonograph by extension cable and recordings were made by strip chart.

After informed consent, the catheter-mounted ultrasonic transducer (catheterprobe) was introduced via brachial or the femoral venous access to the right heart of patients undergoing routine catheterization. Under fluoroscopic guidance, the catheterprobe was positioned with its distal tip in the pulmonary artery. The proximal end of the catheter was connected to the ultrasonoscope and while monitoring the echo, the catheter was rotated so that the crystal imaged the aorta and/or left atrium. It was then pulled back,

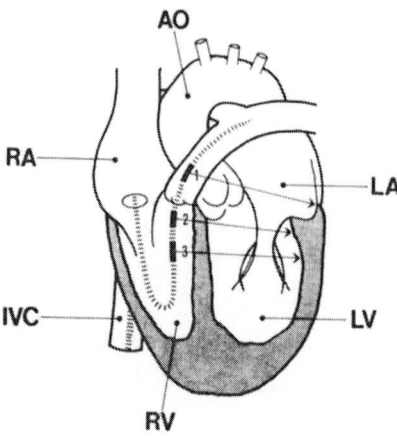

Fig. 2A. Graphic presentation of the catheter-probe positioned in the right ventricular outflow tract during a pull back scan. The catheter is indicated by dash lines, transducer by solid bars, and beam direction by arrows. Three crystal positions are indicated which coincide with the continuous echo scan presented in 2B.

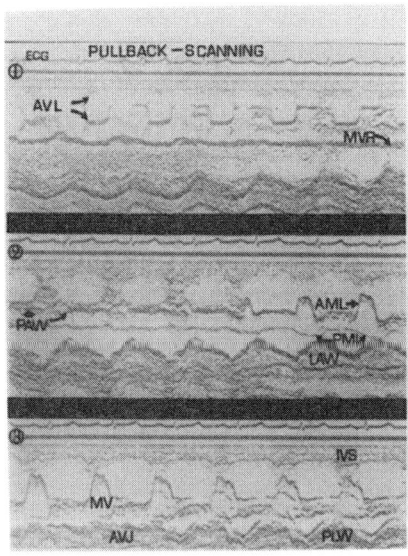

Fig. 2B. Echocardiographic recording made during catheter pull back to position the crystal. AVL = Aortic Valve Leaflets, MVR = Mitral Valve Ring, PAW = Posterior Aortic Wall, AML = Anterior Mitral Leaflet, PML = Posterior Mitral Leaflet, LAW = Left Atrial Wall, MV = Mitral Valve, AVJ = Atrial Ventricular Junction, IVS = Interventricular Septum, PLW = Posterior Left Ventricular Wall. Reproduced with permission from Catheterization and Cardiovascular Diagnosis.

scanning the mitral valve annulus, mitral valve leaflets and positioned to obtain the best image of the LV cavity (Fig. 2). The LV image was verified by recording contrast echoes of LV injections of saline, indocyanine green dye and angiographic contrast. Transducer position was stabilized by the distal catheter-tip in the pulmonary artery. No complications were encountered while studying patients with the catheter-probe continuously for periods of 20 minutes to 1.5 hours.

In an initial feasibility study, the left atrium, mitral valve, and LV walls were imaged in 12 of 12, and the aortic root and valve in 6 of 12 patients. Simultaneous LV dimension and hemodynamic changes were documented in 5 patients by simultaneous intracardiac echo and aortic pressure recordings made during valsava maneuver (Fig. 3).

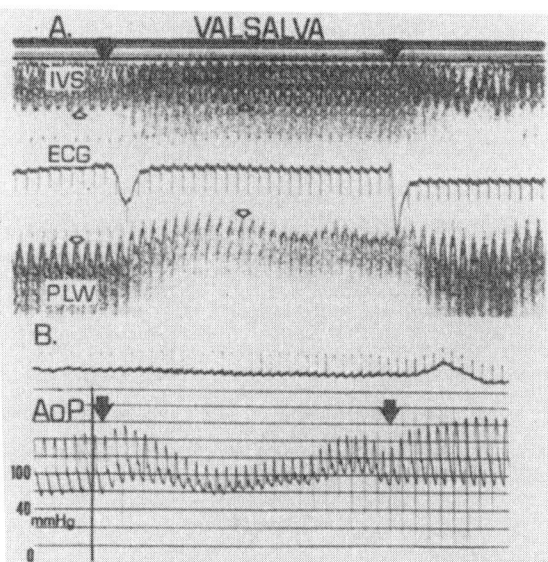

Fig. 3. Simultaneous echocardiographic recording (Panel A) and aortic pressure recording (Panel B) during a valsalva maneuver (paper speed 10 mm/second). Solid arrows at left mark the onset of strain, those at right mark the peak fall in aortic pressure (Phase III). Note the pronounced changes in systolic left ventricular cavity dimension (open arrows) and during the strain phase as compared to those during control at the extreme left. Reproduced with permission from Catheterization and Cardiovascular Diagnosis.

Intracardiac — external echo comparisons

A second study group of 22 patients had intracardiac and external echoes on the same day to compare measurements made from each. Three to six beats from each internal and external echo were digitized. The data analyzed by

Table 1A. Comparison of intracardiac and external echocardiographic parameter measurements.

Echo method	Cavity dimensions		Wall thickness				Wall motion		Shortening Fraction	Dimensional changes	
			Systolic		Diastolic					dD/dT/D	
	EDD (mm)	ESD (mm)	IVS (mm)	PW (mm)	IVS (mm)	PW (mm)	E_s (mm)	E_{pw} (mm)	SF (%)	Max Sec^{-1}	Min Sec^{-1}
Intracardiac	47.8±8.5	32.5±9.5	14.9±2.5	17.4±3.1	10.6±2.1	10.8±2.4	5.0±4.4	12.2±4.2	32.9±8.1	2.9±1.5	−2.0±2.4
External	48.6±9.3	33.3±9.0	14.8±2.4	16.8±3.4	10.7±2.0	10.2±2.2	6.7±2.8	10.5±3.5	32.0±8.4	2.7±1.0	−2.0±1.0

Table 1B. Intracardiac – External echo parameter differences.

	EDD	ESD	IVS	PW	IVS	PW	E_s	E_{pw}	SF	Max	Min
	−0.8±4.2	−0.8±5.4	−0.2±2.3	0.6±1.2	−0.1±1.6	0.8±1.4	−1.7±3.5	2.0±3.0	0.9±6.8	0.3±.9	1.0±.9
P.	N.S.	N.S.	N.S.	N.S.	N.S.	N.S.	<.05	<.07	N.S.	N.S.	N.S.
N.	22	22	20	22	21	22	19	21	22	9	9

Note: All parameter values are expressed as mean ± 1 S.D.

EDD	=	End Diastolic Diameter
ESD	=	End Systolic Diameter
IVS	=	Septal Thickness
PW	=	Posterior Wall Thickness
E_s	=	Septal Excursion
E_{pw}	=	Posterior Wall Excursion
dD/dT/D Max	=	Peak Diastolic L.V. Dimension Change
dD/dT/D Min	=	Peak Systolic L.V. Dimension Change
N	=	Number of Patients
P	=	Probability Value

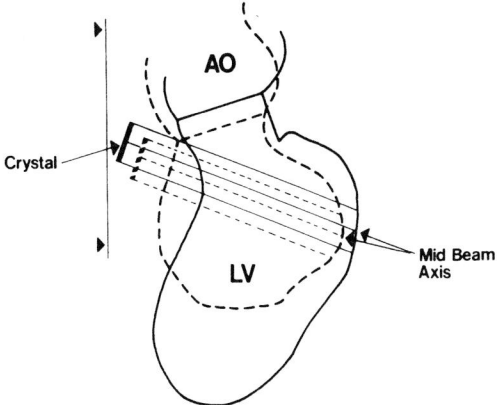

Fig. 4A. Superimposed tracings of the left ventricle at end systole (dashed lines) and end diastole made from selected cineangiographic frames (left anterior oblique projection). Solid arrows and line denote position of anterior chest wall markers. The position of the radiopaque crystal in the right ventricular outflow tract is shown in diastole (solid bar) and systole (hatched bar). Echo beam direction is indicated by the solid and dashed lines emanating from the bars.

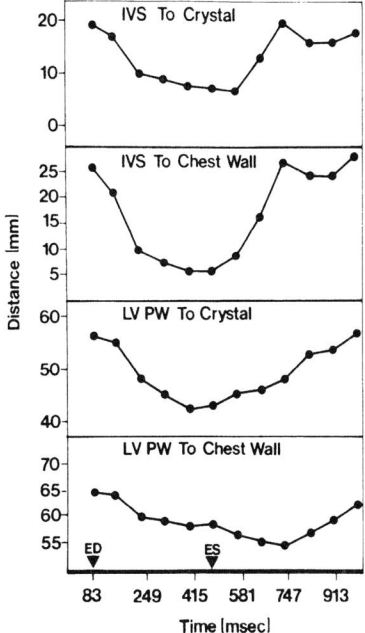

Fig. 4B. Graphic presentation of crystal and left ventricular wall motion shown as distance measurements between the indicated structures, taken from the cine tracings (4A) (every 83 msec) during a single cardiac cycle. IVS = Interventricular Septum, LVPW = Left Ventricular Posterior Wall, ED = End Diastolic Frame, ES = End Systolic Frame.

computer, provided measurements of LV cavity dimensions, wall thicknesses, wall excursions, shortening fraction, and normalized rates of dimension change. Group mean parameter values and mean internal-external measurement differences were computed. Differences were tested for significance by paired t test. The results (Table 1) revealed similar mean values of cavity dimensions, wall thicknesses, fractional shortening, and normalized peak rates of dimension change. Differences between these internal and external measurements were smal and not statistically significant. On the other hand, there was a clear under estimation $(1.7 \pm 3.5$ mm) of septal (IVS) and an exaggeration $(2.0 \pm 3$ mm) of posterior wall (PW) excursion by intracardiac echo. The latter differences were a consequence of recording of *relative* wall motion. As can be seen in Fig. 4A the transducer crystal moved posteriorly, and the LV moved anteriorly relative to the chest wall during systole. The plots of these motions (Fig. 4B) reveal a reduction of IVS and exaggeration of PW excursion, measured as changes of distance between each wall and the crystal, rather than distance changes to the stationary chest wall (standard reference point for external M-Mode echoes).

Thus, while the tip of the catheter-probe stabilized the crystal position along the LV long axis allowing accurate recording of mid-ventricular cavity dimensions, its anterior-posterior motion only allowed recording of relative wall motion. Figure 5 reveals that the error in wall excursion was not constant, i.e. IVS motion could be relatively flat, normal or paradoxical depending upon transducer motion in a given heart.

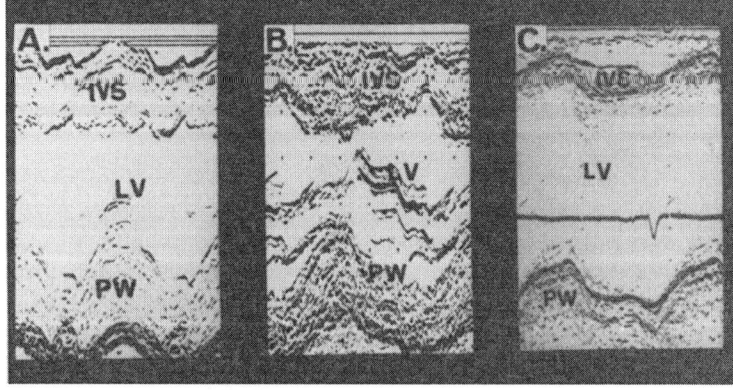

Fig. 5. Panel A shows flattened, Panel B shows normal, and Panel C shows paradoxic septal motion recorded in different hearts using the intracardiac technique. IVS = Interventricular Septum, LV = Left Ventricle, PW = Posterior Wall.

Intracardiac studies during interventions

Left ventricular contrast injections and atrial pacing during catheterization were situations in which the catheter-probe could be used to continuously monitor LV dimension changes. Figure 6 shows a recording made during routine left ventriculography. During a control recording, the patient asked to take a 'small breath in and stop breathing' (first set of arrows), instead performed a valsalva maneuver (decrease in LV dimension, end of Panel A). In Panel B, the onset of injection (large arrow) and the contrast effect of dissolved gas was demonstrated. A further decrease of cavity dimension (smaller arrows, Panel B) occurred with the onset of ventricular tachycardia. A partial re-expansion of the cavity occurs with prolonged filling during the post extra systolic beat (last arrow). In Panel C, the contrast effect lasted through beat 11; however, only 8 beats were visualized radiographically (arrows-beat 10 show a return to control diastolic dimension with an increased SF). Panel D, recorded 2 minutes after injection with a diastolic dimension greater than control, suggested a prolonged effect of LV contrast

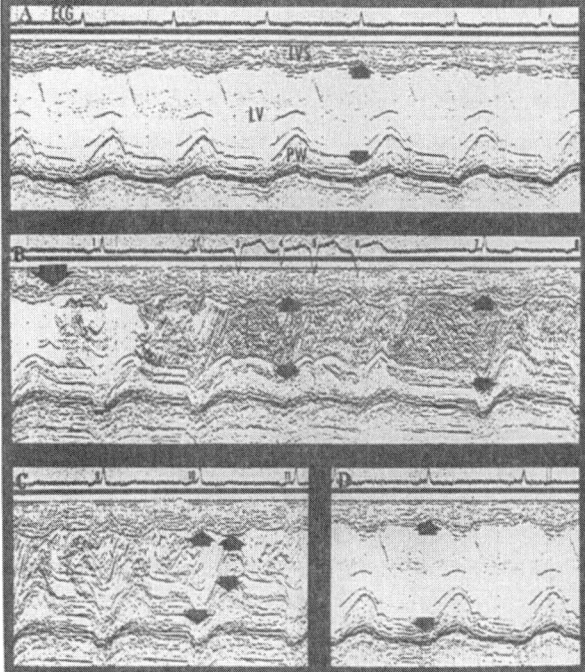

Fig. 6. Shows intracardiac echocardiogram of left ventricular contrast angiography in Panels A, B, and C, as well as, delayed contrast effect in Panel D. For details, see text. ECG = Electrocardiogram, IVS = Interventricular Septum, LV = Left Ventricle, PW = Posterior Wall.

12

media. Subsequently, we studied 8 consecutive patients prior to, during, 2 and 5 minutes after LV contrast injections. A subset of 5 patients were also observed before, during, and after equivolumic injection of saline to control for simple volume related dimension changes. The results (Table 2A) revealed significant increases of left ventricular end diastolic pressure (EDP) 2 and stroke work index (SWI) (calculated from echo estimated stroke volume) 2 and 5 minutes post contrast injection. These findings resulted in a positive LV function slope (calculated as Δ SWI/Δ EDP) [9] at both 2 and 5 minutes. The echo correlates of these findings in Table 2B revealed increased end diastolic dimension (EDD) and shortening fraction (SF) 2 and 5 minutes post injection, suggesting that angiographic contrast media increased preload and LV function without affecting heart rate or afterload. No significant changes were noted after saline injection, suggesting the contrast effect was

Table 2A. Parameter changes observed after L.V. contrast angiography. Hemodynamic parameters.

Experimental period	HR (BPM)	MLVSP (mmHg)	LVEDP (mmHg)	SWI gm · m/m^2	Δ SWI/Δ EDP
Control	74.4 ± 13.3	119.1 ± 20.0	10.9 ± 5.8	33.9 ± 14.0	
2 minutes post angiography	74.9 ± 14.1 (NS)	124.6 ± 23.5 (NS)	16.5 ± 6.9 (p < .024)	48.1 ± 15.6 (p < .024)	4.3 ± 4.9
5 minutes post angiography	74.5 ± 12.5 (NS)	126.9 ± 20.5 (NS)	14.8 ± 8.0 (NS)	48.1 ± 15.1 (p < .024)	4.9 ± 3.7

Table 2B. Echocardiographic parameters.

	EDD (mm)	ESD (mm)	SF (%)
Control	49.1 ± 12.4	35.0 ± 13.6	26.4 ± 8.6
2 minutes post angiography	51.3 ± 11.7 (p < .054)	35.0 ± 14.1 (NS)	30.5 ± 10.8 (p < .016)
5 minutes post angiography	52.7 ± 12.5 (p < .054)	35.4 ± 15.5 (NS)	31.3 ± 10.8 (p < .016)

( ) denotes p values for experimental data compared to control using Wilcoxon Signed Rank Sum Test.

HR	= Heart Rate	MLVSP	= Mean Left Ventricular Systolic Pressure
SWI	= Stroke Work Index	LVEDP	= Left Ventricular End Diastolic Pressure
EDD	= End Diastolic Dimension	Δ SWI/Δ EDP	= Left Ventricular Function Slope
ESD	= End Systolic Dimension	SF	= Shortening Fraction

not directly related to volume increases with injection. Our findings were similar to those reported previously by Cohn et al. [9] and Brundage et al. [10], who studied the hemodynamic responses to LV contrast injections, and found increases in the LV function slope, (Δ SWI/Δ EDP) in patients with normal LV function. Thus, intracardiac echo was able to detect pharmacologic contrast effects described previously by means of hemodynamics and cineangiography.

Figure 7 is an example of an intracardiac echo recorded during atrial pacing stress in a patient with coronary artery disease. Panel A, recorded during a control period, showed slightly decreased SF with an increased

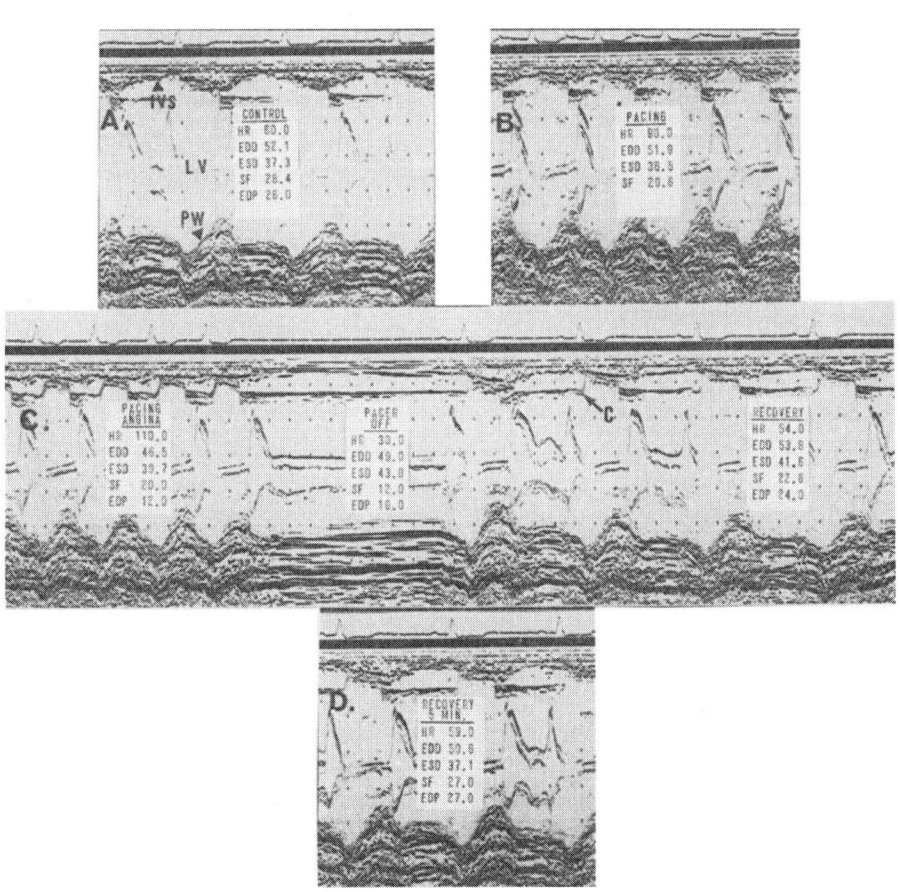

Fig. 7. Shows selected recordings from an intracardiac echocardiogram during atrial pacing stress. Panel A control, Panel B pacing at 90 BPM without angin, Panel C pacing at 110 BPM with angina, termination and early recovery. Panel D recovery 5 minutes after termination of pacing. For detailed explanation, see text. IVS = Interventricular Septum, LV = Left Ventricle, PW = Posterior Wall, C = Left Ventricular Catheter.

EDP. Parameter measurements made during pacing at 90 BPM (Panel B) without angina were essentially unchanged. Panel C, with a decreased EDD, increased ESD, and decreased SF during pacing with angina suggested ischemic LV dysfunction despite the decreased EDP. On the beat prior to termination of pacing, the slightly increased EDP, and increased EDD and ESD, and decreasing the SF suggest progressive LV dysfunction. After a period of sinus arrest (3rd post pacing beat) the EDD was back to control with a slightly increased ESD and depressed SF. The ischemic changes in ESD and SF were directly related to the diminished IVS excursion (compared to control). Five minutes after termination of pacing all parameter values recovered to baseline. In this example intracardiac echo helped document ischemic LV dysfunction when the conventional criteria of ischemia i.e., elevation in EDP and ST segment depression were absent.

In summary, these studies demonstrate that intracardiac echo can provide images, quite similar to those obtained from standard external M-Mode examinations, but only relative wall motion can be recorded. However, by using the patient as his own control, changes in wall motion may be detected. Recordings made during valsalva maneuver, contrast angiography and atrial pacing, suggested that the intracardiac technique could be used to observe and measure physiologic, pharmacologic, and pathophysiologic related dimension changes.

Special clinical applications

Glassman et al. [11] studied 20 patients with a cylindrically shaped, (0.2 mm in length × 0.5 mm in diameter) 7.5 MHz transducer, mounted on a thin, flexible, coaxial cable during cardiac catheterization (Fig. 8). The transducers introduced by passing them through the lumen of 8 French catheters prepositioned in the right heart were pulsed by Echoline 20A or Picker EDC Echo View Ultrasonographs. The authors were able to image right and left heart structures. A special application of this technique was used to guide trans-septal punctures during catheterization. With the transducer positioned at the tip of a trans-septal needle, the right atrium was scanned as the needle was moved from the superior to the inferior right atrium. The simultaneous loss of aortic contour and appearance of the left atrial image occurred as the needle tip entered the fossa ovalis (See Fig. 9). The complication of aortic puncture was avoided in the 10 patients using this technique.

Stephens et al. [12] using a transducer design similar to that of Glassman measured pericardial thickness adjacent to the right atrium and right ventricle. They studied 15 patients with intracardiac echo and myocardial biopsy in whom catheterization data did not differentiate constrictive pericarditis

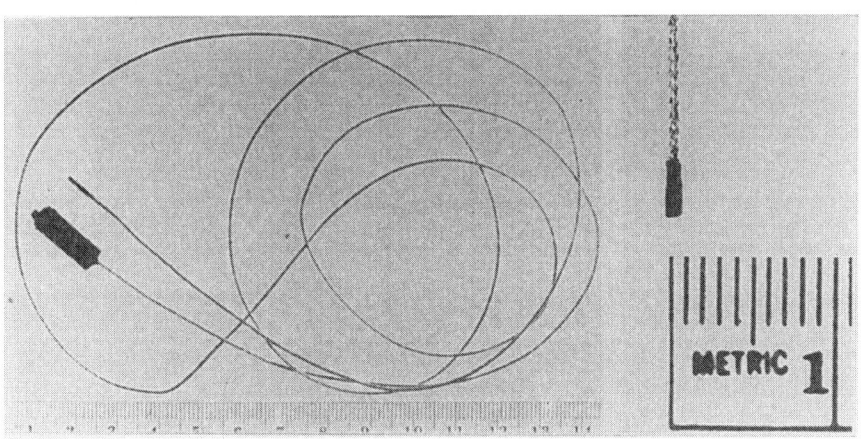

Fig. 8. Left, miniaturized transducer used by Glassman et al attached to a coaxial cable, which terminates in the standard microdot connector. Right, closeup view of the transducer. Reproduced with permission from the American Journal Cardiology and Dr. Glassman.

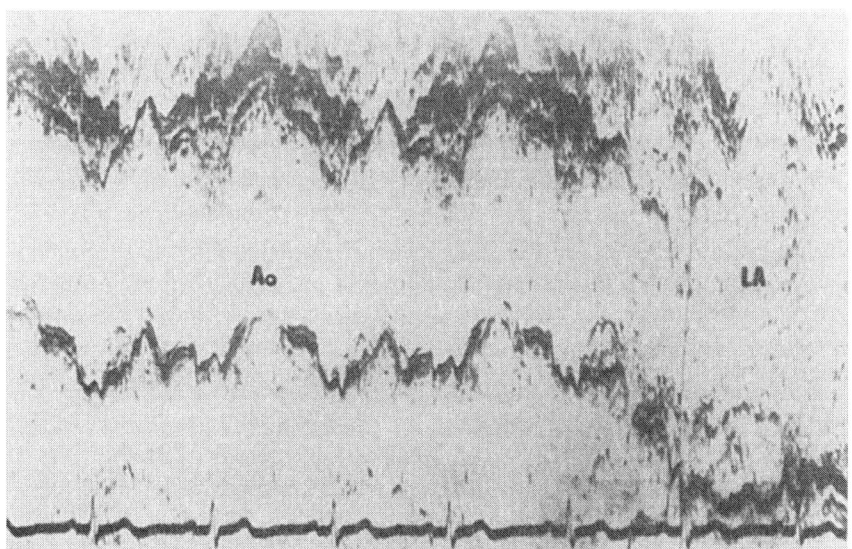

Fig. 9. A recording obtained using the transducer shown in Fig. 8, in a trans-septal needle positioned in the right atrium. As the needle is moved from superior to inferior sites, the aorta (AO) and the left atrium (LA) are consecutively visualized. The sudden loss of aortic contour and appearance of left atrium occur as the needle tip enters the fossa ovalis. Reproduced with permission from the American Journal of Cardiology and Dr. Glassman.

from restrictive cardiomyopathy. In the 7 patients with a pericardial thickness greater than 3 mm, constriction was documented at surgery or autopsy. The remaing 8 patients had thicknesses less than 1.4 mm and all had biopsy evidence of myocardial disease. The authors concluded that in selected cases, intracardiac echo and myocardial biopsy, could differentiate constrictive pericarditis from restrictive cardiomyopathy.

Limitations of the method

Intracardiac echocardiography is an invasive procedure that requires fluoroscopic guidance of catheters (and x-ray exposure). Introduction via brachial vein, with a large catheter diameter relative to that of the vein and the acute angle of the turns through which the catheter passed, were factors which increased resistance to catheter advancement during transducer positioning. Some of these problems were overcome by using a femoral vein sheath for introduction. However, difficulty in catheter advancement through the tricuspid valve, into the pulmonary artery encountered by this approach increased fluoroscopy time. Differences in size and configuration of right hearts, allowed different degrees of crystal stabilization and observation of only relative wall motion. Many of the problems related to crystal placement noted above were bypassed by Glassman and Stephens; however, their method sacrificed some image quality (a smaller crystal surface area) and had less ability to stabilize the crystal during LV studies.

Several physical limitations of ultrasonic transducers were noted including a diminished resolution at the proximal edge of the near field. A 3-dimensional mathematical model developed by Lockwood and Willette [13] is felt to represent the contours of the sound wave front emanating from a rectangular transducer [14]. The predicted amplitude difference between pressure maxima and minima make the very near field an irregular wave front and decrease its resolution. Empirically, we noted that with the crystal touching the IVS, that the first 3–5 mm of the recording were free of echoes. This limitation could decrease the accuracy of measurements of thin structures, e.g. a great vessel wall or atrial septum abutting the crystal. Our crystals, and those used by Glassman, were driven by ultrasonoscopes employing band pass filters allowing the return of only selected MHz frequencies. However, only poor quality images were recorded when the transducers were driven by newer commercially available ultrasonoscopes without filters, because of poor impedence matching. Finally, each of the catheter systems discussed contained small piezo-electric crystals which radiate sound more like a point source than the cylindrical, cohesive, easily directed beam of external transducers. Thus to record images, intracardiac transducers must exclude all but a few reflected echoes and can interrogate only a small segment of an imaged chamber.

Even with these limitations there still may be selected instances in which intracardiac echocardiography has an advantage over the standard M-Mode technique. These circumstances have involved the use of ultrasound imaging at catheterization during fluoroscopy, when x-ray exposure to the echo technician and the lack of reproducible images using hand held external transducers can be significant problems. The special applications of Glassman et al and Stephens et al have clearly been shown to be clinically useful.

Acknowledgements

I would like to thank Donna Singleton and Siony Loy for manuscript preparation and Suzanne Hendricks for graphic illustrations. This work in part was supported by a grant-in-aid from the Florida Affiliate of the American Heart Association.

References

1. Cieszynski M: Intracardiac method of ultrasonic heart structure investigation. Archiwum Immunologii i Terapii Doswiadczalnej 8: 55 I, 1960.
2. Kimoto S, Omoto R, Tsunemoto M, Muroi T, Atsumi K, Uchida R: Ultrasonic tomography of the liver and detection of heart atrial septal defect with the aid of ultrasonic intravenous probes. Ultrasonics 2: 82–86, 1964.
3. Carleton RA, Clark JG: Measurement of left ventricular diameter in the dog by cardiac catheterization. Validation and physiologic meaningfulness of an ultrasonic technique. Circulation Research 22: 545–558, 1968.
4. Manoli SH: An intraventricular ultrasound method for measurement of left ventricular dimensions. IEEE Trans of Bio Med Eng 21: 333–335, 1974.
5. Brundage BH, Peeters GA, Tyberg JV: A catheter-tip echo transducer for continuous measurement of left ventricular internal dimensions. J Clin Res, 27: 69A, (abs), 1979.
6. Eggleton RC, Townsend C, Herrick J, Templeton G, Mitchell JH: Ultrasonic visualization of left ventricular dynamics. IEEE Trans Sonics and Ultrasonics, SU-17: 143–153, 1970.
7. Bom N: *New Concepts In Echocardiography*, 'Catheter Tip Ultrasonic Scanner.' 44–55, H.E. Stenfert; Krosser NV ED., Leiden, 1972.
8. Conetta DA, Christie LG, Pepine CJ, Nichols WW, Conti CR: Intracardiac M-echocardiography for continuous left ventricular monitoring: Method and potential application. Cath and Cardiovasc Diag 5: 135–143, 1979.
9. Cohn PF, Horn AR, Teicholz LE, Kreulen TH, Herman MV, Gorlin R: Effects of angiographic contrast medium on left ventricular function in coronary artery disease: Comparison with static and dynamic exercise. Am J of Cardiol, 32: 21–26, 1973.
10. Brundage, BH, Farr JE: Comparison of contrast medium and atrial pacing as tests of ventricular function in coronary artery disease. Brit HJ, 40: 250–255, 1978.
11. Glassman E and Kronzon I: Transvenous intracardiac echocardiography. Am J Cardiol, 47: 1255–1259, 1981.

12. Stephens DD, Palacios IF, Parillo JE, Aretz T, Block PC, Weyman AE: Differentiation of constrictive pericarditis from restrictive cardiomyopathy by combined intracardiac echocardiography and trans venous endomyocardial biopsy. Circulation, Supp IV: IV-25, (abs), 1981.
13. Lockwood JC, Willette JG: High speed method for computing the exact solution for pressure variations in the near field of a baffled piston. J Acoust Soc Amer, 53: 735–741, 1973.
14. Wells PT, Ed: *Bio Medical Ultrasonics*, Chapter 2 'Radiation'. New York: Academic Press, 31–33, 1977.

1.2. Endomyocardial biopsy of the left ventricle guided by echocardiography

HENRIK EGEBLAD & SVEND A. MORTENSEN

Ultrasonic guidance has improved precision and increased safety of biopsies from most organs [1–3]. Myocardial biopsies from the ventricles were earlier provided by percutaneous needle technique [4, 5]. Ultrasonic guidance of needle biopsy from the myocardium has only been used in a minority of patients (Fig. 1), whereas ultrasonically guided puncture of the pericardium [6] has gained widespread employment. Today, percutaneous transthoracic needle biopsy of the myocardium is replaced by endomyocardial biopsy by means of catheter introduced bioptomes [7–9]. Endomyocardial biopsy permits acquisition of multiple tissue samples from different regions of the ventricles. The samples contain endocardium, they are greater than in needle biopsies, and endomyocardial biopsy is associated with fewer complications [5, 8, 9]. Monitoring of endomyocardial biopsy is performed by fluoroscopy, pressure measurement, palpation with the bioptome, and recording of surface and intracardiac ECG. Visualization of the bioptome by two-dimensional echocardiography is also possible [10–17]. Our experience with echocardiography during left ventricular endomyocardial biopsy is presented in this chapter.

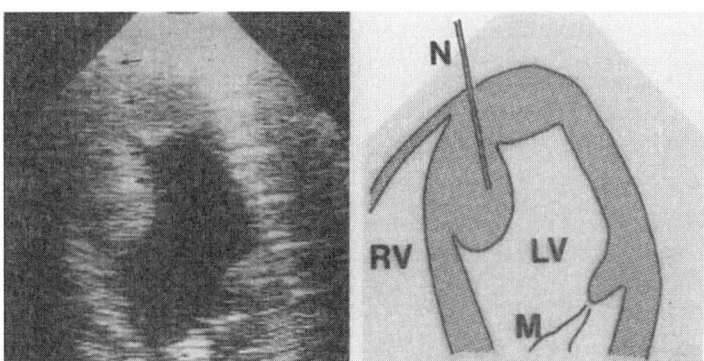

Fig. 1. Ultrasonically guided percutaneous transthoracic needle biopsy (arrows) of malignant tumor in the septum and apex of the left ventricle. The condition of the patient did not permit invasive procedures. Apical view reproduced by courtesy of Per Lindgren, Chief of Ultrasonic Laboratory, Department of Diagnostic Radiology, University Hospital, S-75014, Uppsala, Sweden. LV, left ventricle; M, mitral valve apparatus: N, Needle: RV, right ventricle.

I. Cikes (ed.), *Echocardiography in Cardiac Interventions*, 19–29, 1989.
© 1989 *Kluwer Academic Publishers*.

Indications

Dilated cardiomyopathy, as a clincal and echocardiographic picture, may conceal a variety of myocardial diseases. Inflammatory heart disease, sarcoidosis and collagenoses may, however, be revealed by endomyocardial biopsy [14,18–21]. Thus, in patients suspected of dilated cardiomyopathy, biopsy may sometimes modify the treatment crucially. In case of increased thickness of the myocardium, biopsy can be used to differentiate between myocardial hypertrophy and infiltration, and the nature of the infiltration can be determined [22–24]. Biopsy is also useful for the demonstration of more rare conditions with a restrictive pathophysiology such as Löffler's endocarditis and endomyocardial fibrosis [25]. Finally, endomyocardial biopsy is valuable when anthracycline cardiotoxicity is suspected [26]. Heart transplantation is not yet performed in our country; postoperative monitoring generally includes serial right ventricular biopsy [27].

Primary myocardial diseases can often be adequately evaluated by biopsy of either ventricle. However, pathological anatomical studies have shown great topographic variation in the individual heart [8, 28]. Samples from more than one location (preferably 5) seem to be necessary in order to obtain representative material [28]. Therefore, the combination of right and left ventricular biopsy is standard in our institution. Complications do not seem to occur more frequently in left ventricular endomyocardial biopsy than in biopsy from the right ventricle [8, 9].

Contraindications

A stable condition without overt heart failure should be obtained before left ventricular biopsy. The examination is omitted in the presence of mobile or protruding thrombi [29], in case of recent systemic arterial embolism, and in patients with posterior or inferior aneurysm.

Methods

M-mode and two-dimensional echocardiography are performed a few days before biopsy. A tentative diagnosis and information of the severity of the disease are obtained. Aneurysms, possible thrombi, and regions with particular impairment of the wall motion or thin walled scar tissue are identified.

Invasive procedure

Heart catheterization from the groin including pressure recording, determination of cardiac output, left ventricular cineangiography, and coronary arteriography is carried out immediately before biopsy. In left ventricular endomyocardial biopsy, the arterial catheter is replaced by a long sheath (Cook[R]). The sheath is guided during fluoroscopy to the left ventricle by means of a 7.5 F pigtail catheter introduced through the sheath. With a stable and satisfactory position of the sheath, the pigtail catheter is replaced by King's bioptome (KeyMed[R]). The bioptome is advanced through the sheath (Fig. 2), and the jaws are opened immediately after leaving the sheath. Wall contact is primarily recorded by ectopic activity in the ECG but may in some cases be revealed on the X-ray monitor as a slight bending of the bioptome. The jaws of the bioptome are subsequently closed for sampling and the bioptome is rapidly withdrawn. A slight resistance, as confirmation of direct wall contact, is usually felt when a tissue sample is excised.

Echocardiographic monitoring of the sampling

The sheath is positioned apically but at least 2 cm from the border of the fluoroscopic silhouette of the heart (Fig. 2). By echocardiography, the tip of the sheath is identified by means of parasternal or more apically located

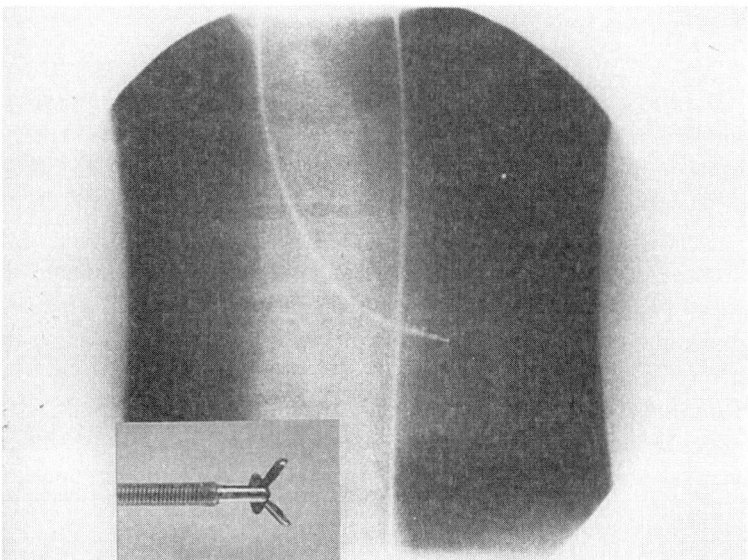

Fig. 2. Fluoroscopic presentation of sheath and bioptome in aorta and left ventricle. The macroscopic appearance of the opened forceps is inserted in the lower left corner.

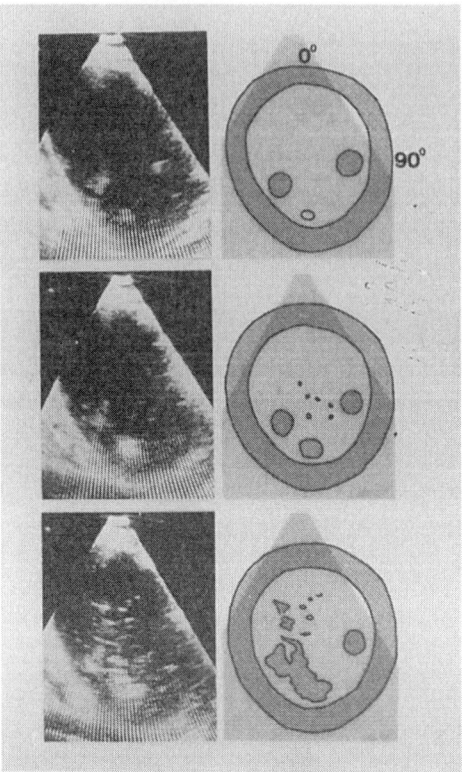

Fig. 3. Short axis view. Top: Sheath positioned between the papillary muscles at 180°. Middle and bottom: Tip of sheath documented by injection of isotonic glucose.

short axis views. In equivocal cases, the localization can be improved by injection of isotonic glucose (Fig. 3). The level of the tip can be classified as either apical (beyond the papillary muscles), at the level of the papillary muscles, or posterior to the papillary muscles. The position in the short axis view is recorded by dividing the short axis view of the left ventricle in 360° with 0° at the top and the anterolateral papillary muscle approximately at 90° (Fig. 3). In general, no significant displacement of the sheath takes place during introduction of the bioptome, but echocardiography is repeated for confirmation of the position.

Before sampling, the transducer is rotated to obtain an oblique scanning plane determined by the direction of the peripheral 3–5 cm of the sheath and bioptome (Fig. 4). During sample recording the echocardiographer is wearing a lead glove because of the fluoroscopy.

Echocardiography permits visualization of the myocardial contact of the bioptome in the left ventricle with a high success rate. The tissue sampling was recorded in all of 80 consecutive left ventricular biopsies (95–100% with

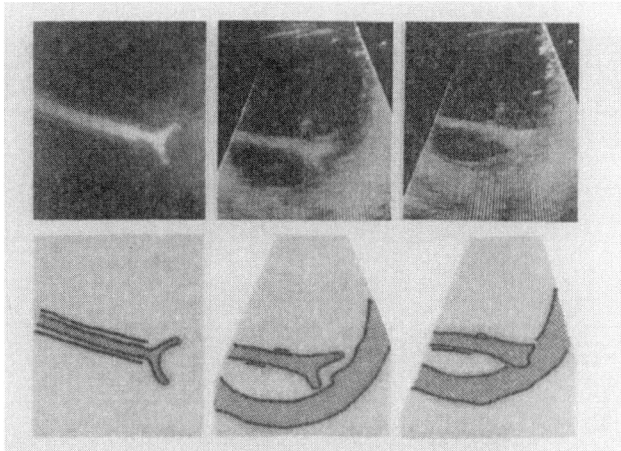

Fig. 4. Endomyocardial biopsy by means of King's bioptome. Left: The sheath is clearly seen on X-ray. Middle and right: The myocardial contact of the bioptome can be imaged by echocardiography (oblique parasternal view).

95% confidence limits), performed in 20 of our patients. Other studies have confirmed the feasibility of echocardiographic monitoring of left ventricular biopsy [10, 11, 13].

In one of our patients, the radiological orientation was severely impeded because of metastases in the lungs and anterior mediastinum. The examination was performed because of suspected adriamycin cardiotoxicity. Multiple left ventricular endomyocardial biopsies were obtained exclusively by means of echocardiographic monitoring.

The myocardial contact of the forceps cannot be imaged by fluoroscopy (Fig. 4). However, fluoroscopy seems to be superior to echocardiography for visualization of the position of the bioptome in relation to the sheath (Fig. 4). In order to avoid myocardial perforation, it is important to open the forceps when the tip of the instrument is leaving the sheath. By fluoroscopy it is also easier to observe the entire peripheral loop of the bioptome from aorta to the left ventricle (Fig. 2). For these reasons, the operator doing the biopsy pays much attention to the X-ray monitor during sampling. We do not think that echocardiography immediately will replace fluoroscopy for monitoring of the sampling.

Location of the biopsy site

Simultaneous echocardiography and fluoroscopy during biopsy is inconvenient. The lead glove renders the ultrasound examination extremely

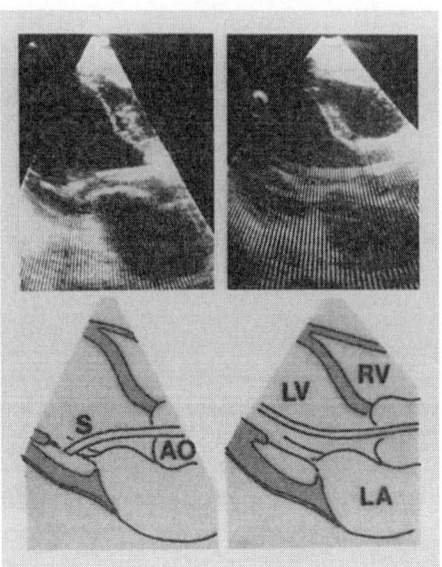

Fig. 5. Long axis view. Left: Sheath (S) positioned inappropriately close to the mitral valve apparatus. Right: Corrected position towards the inferior wall. AO, aorta; LA, left atrium; LV, left ventricle; RV, right ventricle.

awkward, and sometimes it may be time-consuming to position the transducer without concealing the tip of the bioptome on the X-ray monitor. However, alternating echocardiography and fluoroscopy before sampling may give valuable information. The biopsy site can be identified by the position and direction of the bioptome before the biopsy as significant displacement does not take place during sampling (Fig. 4). Echocardiography can improve positioning of the bioptome free of possible mural thrombi, thin walled scar tissue or the mitral valve apparatus (Fig. 5). However, corrections are hardly necessary in more than 5–10% of the positions selected by fluoroscopy [12]. It might prove of greater importance that echocardiographic guidance can be used to identify the location of the biopsy site and to obtain selective biopsies from regions with particularly impaired wall motion [14].

In 27 left ventricular biopsies, performed in five consecutive patients, the location of the biopsy site as determined by combined fluoroscopy and catheter palpation was compared with the position as defined by echocardiography. There was only one discrepancy regarding the left ventricular level of biopsy. However, the difference between the methods in localization of the bioptome in the short axis view varied from 0° to 90° with a mean difference of 32° [12]. Using echocardiography, the biopsy site can be determined in relation to the papillary muscles and the circular framework of the left ventricle. Assuming that the echocardiographic localization of the biopsy site is true, the data showed that a considerable error can be expected when the position is determined by fluoroscopy and palpation.

Limitations

The biopsy sites in our initial examinations were selected by means of fluoroscopy. Echocardiography showed that they all were located inferiorly [12]. A second series of patients were studied to delineate the area available for biopsy. Gentle exploration with numerous repositions of the sheath by means of the pigtail catheter were performed in 10 consecutive patients. Fifty-two left ventricular biopsies were carried out during guidance both by fluoroscopy and echocardiography. Biopsy from the posterior wall of the upper third of the ventricle was omitted in order to avoid damage on the mitral valve and chordae. Otherwise it was attempted to obtain biopsies from the entire wall of the ventricle. The number of biopsies provided from the individual parts of the ventricle is shown in Fig. 6. It appears that the sheath

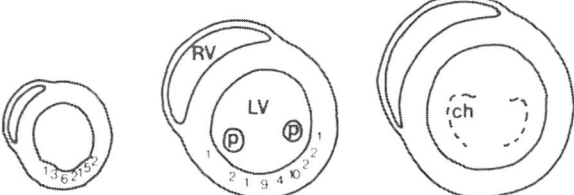

Fig. 6. Number of biopsies obtained from individual regions of the left ventricle (LV) in 10 consecutive patients (see text). Apical third of the ventricle depicted to the left. ch, mitral valve chordae; p, papillary muscles; RV, right ventricle.

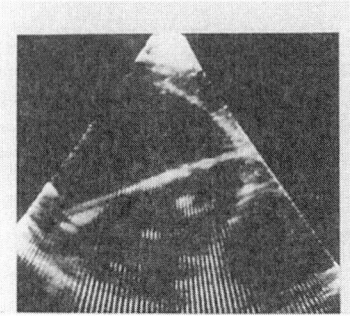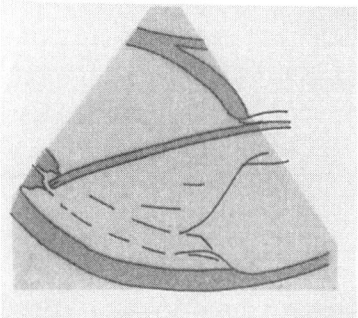

Fig. 7. Long axis view in a patient suspected of dilated cardiomyopathy; biopsy demonstrated sarcoidosis. Sheath and bioptome visualized from aorta to the lower part of the posterior wall which exhibited particularly reduced wall motion.

and bioptome tends to aim inferiorly. This feature of the bioptome is also illustrated in Fig. 7. The direction of the relatively stiff instrument is mainly determined by the direction of the ascending aorta. A quantitative analysis showed that only 21(7–35)% of the left ventricular area selected for biopsy could be reached with the bioptome. Biopsies from the anterior wall and anterior part of the septum and lateral wall cannot be expected although this impression sometimes may occur when the X-ray monitor is watched.

Morphological variation, serial examinations

Repeated biopsies are used after heart transplantation. This approach might also prove useful for monitoring of drug intervention in inflammatory or infiltrative myocardial diseases. However, morphological variation manifest itself within the region which can be reached with the bioptome. Interpretation of a morphological change during treatment may therefore depend on the reproducibility of the biopsy site.

A quantitative morphological analysis was performed in 10 consecutive patients. The myocardial fibre diameter, nucleus diameter, their ratio, and the volume fraction of collagen were measured. Data from the two endomyocardial samples obtained farthest away from each other were compared. The mean value of the difference between the morphometric variables was 12–50%. It was reduced to 7–13% when two biopsies from the same echocardiographic site were compared. These preliminary data indicate that an improved monitoring of medical intervention may be obtained by serial biopsies guided by echocardiography.

The morphological variation within the field of biopsy makes it essential to obtain multiple biopsies from different locations. Echocardiography is superior to fluoroscopy to confirm a difference between sampling regions. In our experience a new biopsy site as determined by fluoroscopy is frequently demonstrated by echocardiography to be identical with a region from which biopsy already is obtained.

Complications

Extension of an invasive heart examination may lead to complications. Monitoring of the tissue sampling by two-dimensional echocardiography delays each biopsy by approximately one min. Identification of the site selected for biopsy takes 5–10 sec. Three mobile polypoid clots appeared in our initial series of 20 patients. Echocardiographic monitoring of the tissue sampling was performed in these patients. The clots were related to the inferior wall of the left ventricle [30]. One clot occurred after angiography, two following biopsy. It is unclear whether the clots were formed in the catheters or occurred locally due to endothelial damage. In one of the patients, embolization of the mobile tail of the clot was directly observed by echocardiography, but clinical signs of embolism did not occur. The extended examination procedure may indirectly have caused the formation of the clots. It is also possible that echocardiography merely revealed a defect of the invasive procedure. Clots have not been demonstrated after establishment of continuous flush of the sheath with heparin solution.

The risk of myocardial perforation, fragmentation of thrombi and mitral valve injury may be reduced by means of echocardiography, but this potential of the technique has not been proved.

Conclusion

In endomyocardial biopsy of the left ventricle, monitoring of the tissue sampling is possible by two-dimensional echocardiography. However, the technique is more inconvenient than fluoroscopy, and it extends the procedure. At the present technical stage, echocardiographic monitoring of the sampling can only be recommended when fluoroscopy is impracticable. In contrast, echocardiography is superior to fluoroscopy for accurate definition of the biopsy site, and this employment of echocardiography does not result in significant delay. It has been demonstrated by echocardiography that the anterior wall cannot be reached with the bioptome. A considerable topographic variation of the morphology may be present in the remaining part of the ventricle. However, echocardiography can be used to ensure that the field of sampling has been utilized to full extent. Inappropriate positions can be avoided, selective biopsies from regions with poor mechanical function can be obtained, and the location of the biopsy can be reproduced in serial examinations.

Acknowledgement

We are greatful to Dr. Ulrik Baandrup, University Institute of Pathology, Municipal Hospital Aarhus, DK-8000 Aarhus C, Denmark. Ulrik Baandrup performed all histologic examinations and the quantitative morphometry.

28

References

1. Holm HH, Kristensen JK, Rasmussen SN, Northeved A, Barlebo H: Ultrasound as a guide in percutaneous puncture technique. Ultrasonics 10: 83–6, 1972.
2. Holm HH, Kristensen JK: Interventional ultrasound. Munksgaard, Copenhagen, 1985.
3. Lindgren PG: Ultrasonically guided punctures. A modified technique. Radiology 137: 235–7, 1980.
4. Sutton DC, Sutton GC: Needle biopsy of the human ventricular myocardium: Review of 54 consecutive cases. Am Heart J 60: 364–70, 1960.
5. Shirey EK, Hawk WA, Mukerji D, Effler DB: Percutaneous myocardial biopsy of the left ventricle. Experience in 198 patients. Circulation 46: 112–22, 1972.
6. Pedersen JF: Multitransducer scanning in pericardial effusion. Diagnosis and aid in puncture. J Clin Ultrasound 2: 244 (Abstract), 1974.
7. Richardson PJ: Biopsy of the human heart. J. Biomed Eng 9: 353–5, 1974.
8. Brooksby AB, Jenkins BS, Coltart DJ, Webb-Peploe MM, Davies MJ: Left-ventricular endomyocardial biopsy. Lancet 2: 1222–5, 1974.
9. Mason JW: Techniques for right and left ventricular endomyocardial biopsy. Am J Cardiol 41: 887–92, 1978.
10. William GA, Habermehl KK, Kaintz RP: Clinical utility of 2D echocardiography in myocardial biopsy, 1982. Circulation 66 (suppl II): II-8 (Abstract).
11. French JW, Popp RL, Pitlick PT: Cardiac localization of transvascular bioptome using 2-dimensional echocardiography. Am J Cardiol 51: 219–23, 1983.
12. Mortensen SA, Egeblad H: Endomyocardial biopsy guided by cross-sectional echocardiography. Br Heart J 50: 246–51, 1983.
13. Alberti E, Klugman S, Medugno G, Pinamonti B, Salvi A, Camerini F: Two-dimensional echocardiography during endomyocardial biopsy. Eur J Cardiol 4 (Suppl E): 21 (Abstract), 1983.
14. Mortensen SA, Baandrup U, Egeblad H: Cardiac sarcoidosis mimicking dilated cardiomyopathy. J Cardiovasc Ultrasonogr 3: 277–80, 1984.
15. Pierard L, ElAllaf D, D'Orio V, Demoulin JC, Carlier J: Two-dimensional echocardiographic guiding of endomyocardial biopsy. Chest 85: 759–62, 1984.
16. Williams GA, Kaintz RP, Habermehl KK, Nelson JG, Kennedy HL: Clinical experience with two-dimensional echocardiography to guide endomyocardial biopsy. Clin Cardiol 8: 137–40, 1985.
17. Strachovsky G, Zeldis SM, Katz S, McNulty-Mackey M: Two-dimensional echocardiographic monitoring during percutaneous endomyocardial biopsy. J Am Coll Cardiol 6: 609–11, 1985.
18. Olsen EGJ: Endomyocardial biopsy. Br Heart J 40: 95–8, 1978.
19. Mortensen SA, Hansen BF, Bundgaard A: Eosinophilia and myocardial ischemia secondary to polyarteritis. A discussion of pathogenesis on the basis of a case history Acta Cardiol 38: 237–45, 1983.
20. Zee-Cheng CS, Tsai CC, Palmer DC, Codd JE, Pennington DG, Williams GA: High incidence of myocarditis by endomyocardial biopsy in patients with idiopathic congestive cardiomyopathy. J Am Coll Cardiol 3: 63–70, 1984.
21. Ansari A, Larson PH, Bates HD: Cardiovascular manifestations of systemic lupus erythematosus: Current perspective. Prog Cardiovasc Dis 27: 421–34, 1985.
22. Schroeder JS, Billingham ME, Rider AK: Cardiac amyloidosis. Diagnosis by transvenous endomyocardial biopsy. Am J Med 59: 269–73, 1975.
23. Hanley PC, Shub C, Seward JB, Wold LE: Intracavitary cardiac melanoma diagnosed by endomyocardial left ventricular biopsy. Chest 84: 195–8, 1983.

24. Werbel GB, Skom JH, Mehlman D, Michaelis LL: Metastatic squamous cell carcinoma to the heart. Unsual cause of angina decubitus and cardiac murmur. Chest 88: 468–9, 1985.
25. Davies MJ, Spry CJF, Sapsford R, Olsen EGJ, dePerez G, Oakley CM, Goodwin JF: Cardiovascular features of 11 patients with eosinophilic endomyocardial disease. Quart J Med 52: 23–39, 1983.
26. Mortensen SA, Olsen HS, Baandrup U: Chronic anthracycline cardiotoxicity: haemodynamic and histopathological manifestations suggesting a restrictive endomyocardial disease. Br Heart J 55: 274–82, 1986.
27. Baumgartner WA, Reitz BA, Bieber CP, Oyer PE, Shumway NE, Stinson EB: Current expectations in cardiac transplantation. J Thor Cardiovasc Surg 75: 525–30, 1978.
28. Baandrup U, Florio RA, Olsen EGJ: Do endomyocardial biopsies represent the morphology of the rest of the myocardium? A quantitative light microscopic study of single versus multiple biopsies with the King's bioptome. Eur Heart J 3: 171–8, 1982.
29. Frandsen EH, Egeblad H, Mortensen SA: Transience of left ventricular thrombus. Br Heart J 49: 193–4, 1983.
30. Egeblad H: Intracardiac thrombus – systemic arterial embolism. Contribution of echocardiography. Acta Med Scand suppl 730, 1988.

1.3. Echocardiographic guidance of endomyocardial biopsy of the right ventricle

GEORGE A. WILLIAMS

Endomyocardial biopsy was first reported as an investigative tool in 1962 [1]. At that time it was a radical procedure, performed retrogradely from the femoral artery or vein to the left or right ventricle under flouroscopic control at cardiac catheterization. Although it provided new information about the ultrastructure of the living heart, it was disappointing when used to evaluate myocardial diseases, and, as a result, remained a little used technique until the mid 1970's. The advent of heart transplant as a therapeutic procedure and the need for anatomic diagnosis of anthracycline drug toxicity [2, 3] made endomyocardial biopsy clinically useful. In 1974, the introduction of the Caves-Schultz forceps [4] allowed the relatively easy use of the internal jugular vein for approaching the lower pressure right ventricle. Both left and right ventricular endomyocardial biopsy have until recently remained procedures which are performed under flouroscopy in the cardiac catheterization laboratory. However the ability to use an alternate imaging technique can allow biopsy to be routinely performed in other areas of the hospital, with little risk to the patient.

Echocardiographic technique

Two dimensional echocardiography has been used to guide right ventricular biopsy with varying success [5, 9]. The utility of echocardiography depends on the aproach to the heart, the ventricle being biopsied, the echocardiographic view used, and the body habitus of the patient.

Approach to the heart. Right ventricular endomyocardial biopsy is routinely performed through a superior approach from the internal jugular vein, or through the inferior vena cava from a femoral approach. When the bioptome is introduced from the superior vena cava, its arc of rotation within the heart occurs in a plane similar to that obtained in the apical four chamber view. The bioptome tip is oriented inferiorly and apically, and medial angulation toward the right ventricular free wall moves the tip both medially and upward. Rotation of the bioptome laterally toward the right ventricular

I. Cikes (ed.), *Echocardiography in Cardiac Interventions*, 31–40, 1989.

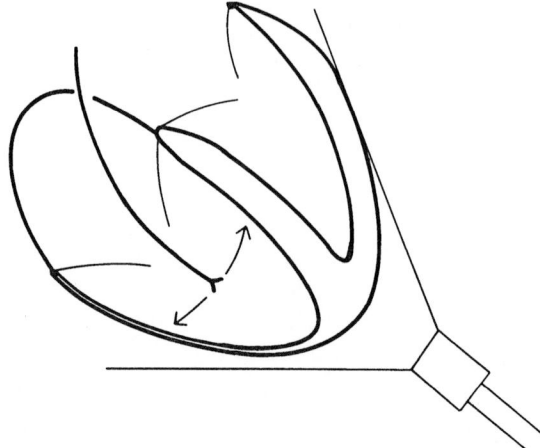

Fig. 1. Schematic view of the heart in the four chamber view, with the transducer at the left ventricular apex. The bioptome has been inserted from the internal jugular approach. The open tip of the bioptome remains in the field of view throughout its rotation within the left ventricle (arrows).

septum again produces both a lateral and superior motion (Fig. 1). The femoral approach, however, does not lend itself as well to echocardiographic imaging in one plane. The bioptome tends to be oriented superiorly in the ventricle, and is more difficult to image. Unless the forceps is within a curved sheath, the tip lies near the right ventricular outflow tract. The longer femoral forceps are more flexible than the jugular forceps, and rotation of the bioptome produces less predictable intracardiac motion.

Ventricle biopsied. The majority of biopsies are presently taken from the right ventricle. Although early reports [10] noted an unacceptably high incidence of wall perforation during right ventricular biopsy, the overall experience reveals an incidence of 1% or less with only rare episodes of tamponade [11].

Left ventricular biopsy has been considered for several reasons. First, the left ventricular wall is thicker, and, therefore less easy to perforate. Since the majority of myocardial tissue is in the left ventricle, evaluation for localized disease may be better performed from the left ventricle. The major drawback to left ventricular biopsy has been the necessity to enter the high pressure arterial system, requiring longer observation after the procedure than for a venous approach. As a result, less experience is available for left ventricular biopsy guided by echocardiography than for right ventricular procedures.

Echocardiographic view. A variety of echocardiographic views have been investigated for utility during endomyocardial biopsy [7, 9]. The most consistantly useful views are the apical four chamber view, subcostal four chamber, and parasternal short axis views. The apical four chamber view is the one most consistently helpful for right ventricular biopsy. As noted above, the bioptome jaws tend to move in arc along the four chamber plane. The tip can be visualized in the right atrium and guided through the tricuspid valve. With inferior angulation of the transducer, the jaws can be localized within the right ventricular cavity, and placed along the septum, free wall, or apex.

The subcostal four chamber view can be utilized similarly to that from the apex. The transducer is placed in the right subxiphoid area, and the forceps can be visualized from right atrium to ventricular apex. In patients with chest deformity, the subcostal approach may be the only window available to the echocardiographer.

Parasternal short axis views have also been used to localize the bioptome [6, 9]. This window seems especially helpful in left ventricular biopsy. The forceps were localized within the left ventricle and guided toward the inferior septal area. The short axis view, however, does not provide as good base-apex localization as do the apical or subcostal windows.

Body habitus. As with all echocardiographic procedures the available windows are determined by the habitus of the patient. Markedly obese patients may not be visualized from any window, due to the physical depth of their heart and secondary deformity of thoracic and abdominal structures. Lack of penetration limits the use of parasternal or apical windows, and the combined protruding abdominal wall and visceral weight elevating the diaphragm may make the heart inaccessable from the subcostal window.

Patients with chronic lung disease, on the other hand, are often impossible to interrogate from the thoracic windows, but easily visualized from the subxiphoid approach. Although the lung mass often obscures the usual windows, the heart becomes more vertically oriented, producing almost a true four chamber view from below the diaphragm.

Biopsy technique

Insertion of the bioptome. At Saint Louis University, 95% of all biopsies are done from the internal jugular approach. A 7 or 8F arterial sheath is placed in the vein to allow repeated venous access with a minimum blood loss. The bioptome used is a modified 50 cm. endoscopic forceps (Storz 10329L), the distal 20 cm. of which are curved more gently than the Caves-Schultz forcep. Both this bioptome and the Caves-Schultz forceps have been successfully used. The bioptome is placed into the sheath with the tip oriented laterally to

34

the patient. As the forceps is advanced it is rotated anteriorly (counterclockwise) to avoid the coronary sinus.

Echocardiographic localization. The echo is performed from a modified apical or subcostal parasternal view. The transducer is moved medially from the usual window to encompass the entire right ventricle and atrium, cutting off most of the left ventricle. Cephalad angulation of the transducer will visualize the bioptome as it enters the right atrium. The tip can then be guided through the tricuspid valve annulus by gentle rotation. The forceps can be followed in its course through the ventricle and manipulated to the selected biopsy site (Fig. 2).

The technique for left heart biopsy is similar. A sheath placed through the aortic valve can be localized within the left ventricle and the bioptome seen leaving the sheath and advancing to the myocardium. In using this technique, however, Mortenson and Egeblad [7] did not use echocardiographic guidance to manipulate the catheter. Although they used long and short axis as well as apical views, the final transducer planes were also oriented according to catheter position.

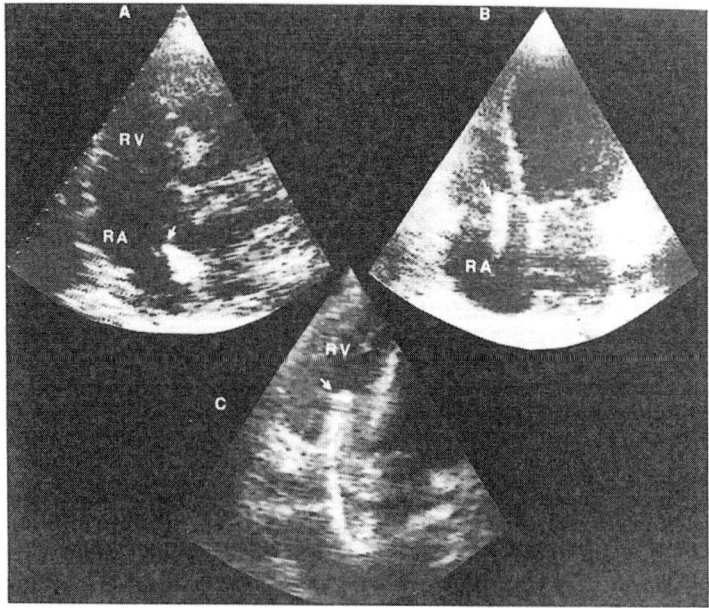

Fig. 2. Echocardiographic guidance of the bioptome into the right ventricle. A. The bioptome is in the high right atrium, with the tip (arrow) approaching the tricuspid valve annulus. B. The tip of the bioptome (arrow) is now slightly through the tricuspid annulus, within the left ventricle. C. The tip (arrow) has been guided to the mid right ventricle and lies next to the interventricular septum.

Biopsy technique. Echocardiography allows visualization of the forceps and the ventricular walls. Because of this ability, the biopsy technique has been modified from that of Mason, et al. [11]. Instead of advancing the forceps to the wall prior to opening the jaws, the bioptome is opened just prior to contact. The closed jaws of the bioptome have a relatively sharp profile, whereas the opened jaws have a more flat surface contacting the endocardium. Although the likelihood of perforating the wall is small, it may be reduced by not advancing a closed tip until contact is made. Once the jaws contact the myocardium, they are closed and withdrawn in the usual manner.

Results

Echocardiographically guided biopsy was first reported to be a feasable procedure in 1982, [5] when 25 patients were reported who had endomyocardial biopsy using a combination of radiography and echo, or echocardiography alone for forceps guidence. Shortly thereafter, a similar technique was found to give additive information in children [6]. Seven children underwent 12 biopsies; 1 left ventricular, and 11 right ventricular biopsies were performed. In all cases, the forceps could be localized in the cardiac chambers. The apical four chamber view was used for the right ventricular biopsies, while long and short axis views were best for the left ventricle. The authors observed that while flouroscopy gave information about the general position of the forceps within the cardiac shadow, echocardiography provided intra-cardiac localization. Importantly, they also noted that despite adequate appearing bioptome position on flouroscopy, echocardiography revealed improper forceps position in over 50% of their cases.

They also felt that echocardiography offered the potential for improved positioning in patients with distorted ventricles, and for less radiation exposure using a combination of echo and flouroscopy.

Experience with echocardiography has not been uniformly successful, however. In 1983, Mortensen and Egeblad evaluated echocardiography and flouroscopy in 10 patients undergoing left heart (28 biopsies), and right heart (34 biopsies) [7]. Their technique involved placing a sheath in the ventricle from the femoral artery or vein flouroscopically. The forceps was then advanced until it protruded from the sheath on radiography. At that point, the forceps was opened, advanced until resistance was met, and the sample taken. Although only 18% of right ventricular biopsies were seen by echo, one patient had malposition within the right ventricle recognized first by echocardiography and confirmed by radiographic contrast injection. The authors of this study felt that echo localization of the forceps tip was superior to radiography during left ventricular biopsy, but that right ventricular biopsy was not as useful due to the small percentage of successful studies. In addition they felt that echocardiography was useful only as an adjunct to radiography.

This study makes two major points: first, that the bioptome is not in a good plane for echocardiographic localization when the femoral vein approach is the right ventricle is used, and second, that radiologic guidance is necessary when the femoral approach is used for biopsy of either ventricle. Considering the safety of flouroscopic guidance alone, echocardiography adds little when using this approach.

In 1985, the experience at Saint Louis University was reviewed [8]. Echocardiographic guidance of the bioptome was begun in 1979, initially as an adjunct to flouroscopy. The internal jugular approach was used exclusively. In 17 patients, the bioptome was placed in the right atrium under flouroscopic control, and a combination of echocardiography and flouroscopy was used to position the forceps in the ventricle. As was shown in the earlier studies, the intracardiac localization afforded by echo was superior to that from radiography alone. After 39 combined procedures in the 17 patients, biopsy was performed using echocardiographic guidance alone, initially in the cardiac catheterization laboratory, and then in the special procedure/electrophysiology suite attached to the coronary intensive care unit. By November, 1983, 139 procedures had been performed with echocardiographic guidance alone.

At the present time, echocardiographic guidance of the bioptome is used exclusively at Saint Louis University when the internal jugular approach is used, accounting for approximately 95% of biopsies. Over 560 procedures have been performed using echocardiography alone. Due to the ease of performing biopsies in this manner, they are done in several locations. Routine biopsies for transplant follow-up, evaluation of cardiomyopathy, and anthracycline toxicities are performed in the electrophysiology laboratory. Patients who are immediately post heart transplant, and those who are too ill to easily move due to respirators or indwelling catheters are biopsied in their bed in the intensive care unit.

Echocardiographic guidance has been successful in 99% of cases. Two patients were not visualized with this technique. Both were obese (236 and 270 pounds respectively) and standby flouroscopy was required to complete the procedure. The biopsies are completely done in 20 minutes or less, unless difficulties are encountered placing the venous sheath, and the patients are discharged from the hospital after 30 minutes of post biopsy observation.

In the majority of cases, the bioptome is first visualized in the right atrium. It is then guided through the tricuspid valve echocardiographically. 'Hanging up' of the bioptome on the tricuspid annulus is easily recognized, and corrected for by adjusting the curve of the bioptome. Using intracardiac localization as described above, samples are then taken from four to six areas. The entire right ventricle is sampled, including the right ventricular free wall (Fig. 3). Despite the fragility of the free wall, only two perforations have occurred. Both were recognized immediately by echo (Fig. 4). In both cases, the patient was undergoing a severe rejection episode, and the tissue obtained was extremely friable. This incidence of 0.4% compares favorably with the results using radiographic guidance.

The bioptome, being metal, produces strong echoes, requiring lowering of the machine amplification to avoid reverberation artifact. With proper gain settings, the bioptome produces little artifact, and the ventricular walls are clearly seen. Opening the jaws of the bioptome produces a characteristic broadening of the echo at the tip. Rotation of the bioptome then allows sampling at any point within the right ventricle, with the tip remaining in the echocardiographic plane.

Further experience with echo guided biopsy was reviewed in 1985 [9]. In this study, the effect of various transducer positions was studied. All biopsies were performed from the internal jugular approach. In 83% of the patients, the bioptome could be localized in the four chamber plane, making this the most useful view, similar to the results from Saint Louis University. The subcostal view was useful in 34% of cases. The long axis view was successful in 17% of patients. Two patients were not visualized: both had an increased A-P diameter of the thorax. In two others, the subcostal view was the only useful

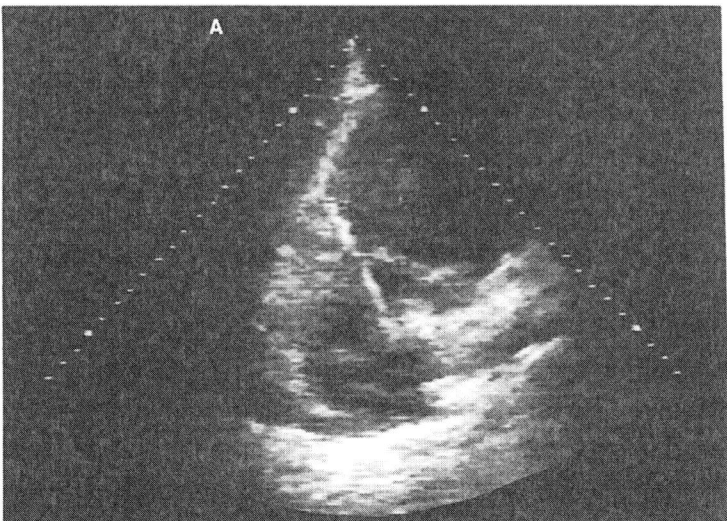

Fig. 3. Biopsy of several sites within the right ventricle:
A. Biopsy of the basal right ventricular free wall. Biopsy of this site has proven safe despite the thin structure at this point.

38

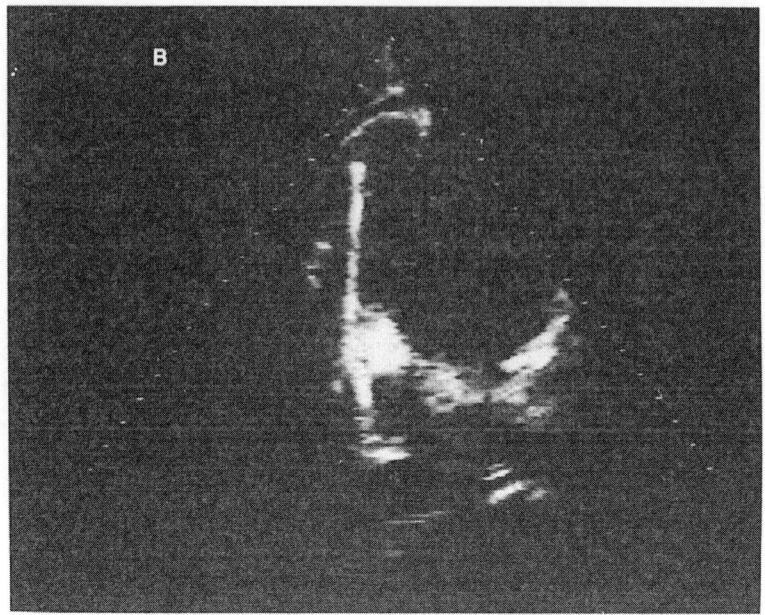

Fig. 3. Biopsy of several sites within the right ventricle:
B. Sampling at the distal right ventricular wall/apex. Biopsies at this site frequently appear adequately positioned under fluoroscopic control.

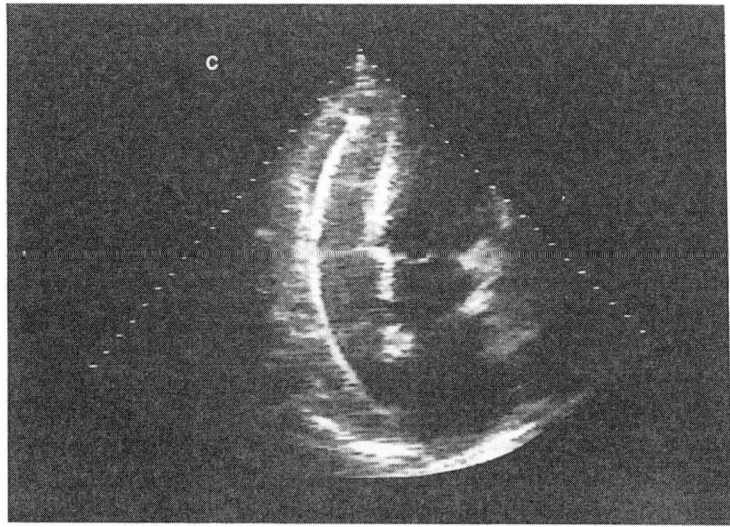

Fig. 3. Biopsy of several sites within the right ventricle:
C. Biopsy of the distal interventricular septum at the right ventricular apex.

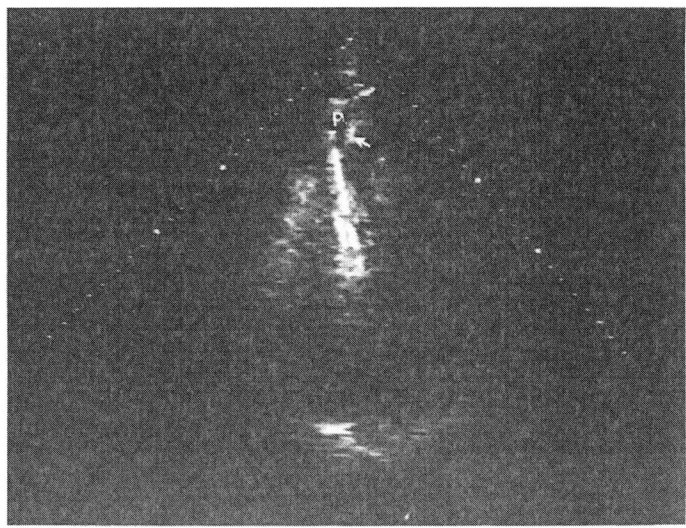

Fig. 4. Perforation of the right ventricular free wall. This complication can be immediately recognized by echocardiography, but has occurred only rarely (see text). Arrow: right ventricular wall. P: Pericardial space. The tip of the bioptome is at the base of the 'P', clearly external to the myocardium.

view. The overall success rate was 91%. When echo localization was compared to flouroscopy, the bioptome was not positioned appropriately in 18% of cases which appeared adequate by flouroscopy. Changes in position of the tip of the bioptome related to opening the jaws were recognized by echo but not by flouro. Finally, a septal perforation was clearly seen only by echocardiography. This study suggests that complications occur more frequently than recognized when using radiography alone, and confirm that echocardiography can be useful in the majority of patients undergoing right ventricular biopsy.

In summary, echocardiographic bioptome guidance is a feasable technique for left ventricular biopsy, and for right ventricle biopsy performed from the internal jugular approach. It can adequately localize bioptome position, and may be more sensitive than radiography in recognizing malposition of the forceps. Complications from the procedure are recognized immediately, alerting the physician to the need for more careful monitoring. Used alone, echocardiographic bioptome localization allows right ventricular biopsy to be performed outside of the cardiac catheterization laboratory, in any setting where electrocardiographic and hemodynamic monitoring is available. It allows recent cardiac transplant patients to remain in the intensive care unit instead of being transferred to the catheterization laboratory, and has simplified the evaluation of extremely ill patients. The right ventricle can be

40

more extensively sampled with little or no increase in risk. As more patients undergo evaluation for myocardial disease and the number of patients undergoing cardiac transplantation rises, endomyocardial biopsy will become a more routine procedure. Echocardiography is a safe and effective guidance technique which, when used in the appropriate setting, is a useful alternative to radiography.

References

1. Sakakibara S, Konno S: Endomyocardial Biopsy. Jap. Heart J 3: 537, 1962.
2. Bristow MR, Mason JW, Billingham ME, Daniels JR: Dose effect and structure-funtion relationships in doxorubricin cardiomyopathy. Am. Heart J. 102: 709, 1981.
3. Bristow MR, Mason JW, Billingham ME, Daniels JR: Doxorubicin cardiomyopathy: evaluation byphonocadiography, endomyocardial biopsy, and cardiac catheterization. Ann. Intern. Med. 88: 168, 1978.
4. Caves PK, Schultz WP, Dong E Jr., Stinson EB, Shumway NE: New instrument for transvenous cardiac biopsy. Am. J. Cardiol. 33: 274, 1974.
5. Williams GA, Kaintz RP, Habermehl KK: Clinical utility of two dimensional echocardiography in endomyocardial biopsy. Circulation 66: II (Abst.), 1982.
6. French JW, Popp RL, Pitlick PT: Cardiac localization of transvenous bioptome using 2-dimensional echocardiography. Am. J. Cardiol. 51: 219, 1983.
7. Mortensen SA, Egeblad H: Endomyocardial biopsyguided by cross sectional echocardiography. Br. Heart J., 50: 246, 1983.
8. Williams GA, Kaintz RP, Habermehl KK, Nelson JG, Kennedy HL: Clinical experience with two dimensional echocardiography to guide endomyocardial biopsy. Clin. Cardiol., 8: 137, 1985.
9. Strachovsky G, Zeldis SM, Katz S, McNulty-Mackey M: Two dimensional echocardiographic monitoring during percutaneous endomyocardial biopsy. J. Am. Coll. Cardiol. 6: 609, 1985.
10. Kober G, Kunkel B, Becker HJ, Bussman WD, Kaltenbach M: Technical aspects, experiences and complications of right and left ventricular endomyocardial biopsy. In Cardiomyopathy and Endomyocardial Biopsy. Kaltenbach M, Loojen F, Olsen EG, Eds, Springer-Verlag, Berlin, 40, 1978.
11. Mason JW: Technique for right and left ventricular endomyocardial Biopsy. Am J Cardiol 41: 887, 1978.

1.4. Two-dimensional echocardiographic-assisted balloon atrial septostomy

JAMES B. SEWARD

Summary

Two-dimensional echocardiography can detect congenital cardiac lesions accurately and expeditiously. This noninvasive examination also can assist in the performance of catheter therapy techniques such as balloon atrial septostomy, transseptal catheterization, and blade septostomy. Confident visualization of the catheter and surrounding anatomy greatly enhances the safety of the procedure. The result can be determined more accurately by direct visualization of the atrial septal defect and the flail valve of the fossa ovalis that are produced. Use of two-dimensional echocardiography has greatly enhanced the management, safety, and appreciation of result of percutaneous catheter atrial septostomy.

Introduction

Balloon atrial septostomy has revolutionized the management of cyanotic congenital heart disease [1, 2]. The creation of an intra-atrial communication permits mixing at atrial level and thus increasing arterial blood oxygen saturation and changing a critical situation into a manageable 'palliated' congenital cardiac lesion. However, several complications have been reported in association with this catheter procedure [1, 3–7]. Classically used in patients with complete transposition of the great arteries, this technique has been applied in any case in which the pulmonary arterial and systemic arterial beds are anatomically separated, as with tricuspid and mitral atresia, pulmonary atresia with intact ventricular septum, or total anomalous pulmonary venous return. Balloon atrial septostomy became the first widely used interventional catheter procedure. More recently, to extend the septostomy procedure, Park et al. [8] developed a catheter-blade technique for assisting septostomy of a thickened atrial septum not amenable to conventional balloon septostomy.

The introduction of high-resolution two-dimensional echocardiography has had a most dramatic impact on the imaging of congenital cardiac lesions.

I. Cikes (ed.), *Echocardiography in Cardiac Interventions*, 41–48, 1989.
© 1989 *Kluwer Academic Publishers*.

Such techniques have substantially changed the indication for cardiac catheterization, particularly in newborn and young children [9–12]. The vivid detail of internal cardiac anatomy that is provided is superior to that of other currently available techniques, including angiography [13]. Echocardiography can be performed at the bedside and has none of the risks of catheterization. In the logical extension of technology, this new imaging modality has impacted on procedures heretofore performed in the catheterization laboratory, such as balloon septostomy [14–17].

Echocardiography-assisted atrial septostomy initially began in the catheterization laboratory, permitting precise placement of the catheter and balloon within the cardiac chambers and avoidance of surrounding vital structures. The advantage was immediate appreciation of catheter position and anatomic confirmation without contrast angiography. Use of contrast echocardiography in conjunction with the procedure permits estimation of the relative degree of right-to-left shunt before and after septostomy [17].

From the catheterization laboratory, investigators moved echocardiography-assisted atrial septostomy to the bedside [13]. First, detailed two-dimensional echocardiographic anatomic assessment is utilized to recognize and to characterize cardiac anatomy [18]. If clinically indicated, atrial septostomy can be performed at the same time, usually in the neonatal intensive care unit. Because no additional imaging apparatus is needed, the procedure can be performed at the bedside. The approach expedites management decisions and does not require transport of a critically ill newborn or introduction of unfamiliar personnel into an unstable situation.

Technique

Ultrasound instrument

A two-dimensional echocardiographic instrument fitted with a high-resolution transducer is needed. A range of transducer types and frequencies are available (5-MHz near focus, 7.5-MHz, and 10-MHz are the most ideal neonatal transducer frequencies). Video image recording assists in documentation and slow-motion assessment of events.

Contrast echocardiography

Injection of small amounts of isotonic saline will suffice to provide ultrasound contrast in the newborn [17]. Injection of 0.5 to 1.0 ml of agitated saline into the inferior vena cava or a peripheral vein before and after the septostomy procedure can assist in visual quantification of the right-to-left shunt produced by the septostomy.

Procedure

Entry

A subcostal transducer position is best for imaging. First, during the *entry phase* of the study, the inferior vena cava, right atrium, and atrial septum are imaged simultaneously (Fig. 1). The long-axis sagittal view of the venae cavae is obtained by putting the transducer in a right paravertebral orientation. With this view or a comparable one, the catheter can be advanced up the inferior vena cava to the right atrium. Manipulation of the catheter across the atrial septum is visualized by using a similar view and often facilitating it by medial tilt of the transducer to provide better visualization of the fossa ovalis.

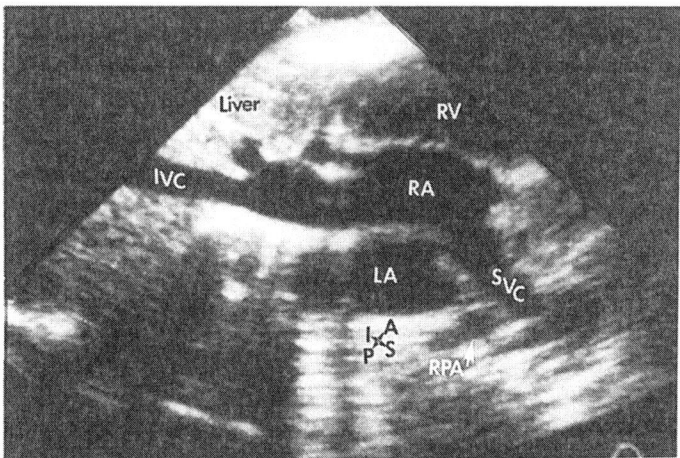

Fig. 1. Subcostal long-axis view with simultaneous visualization of the inferior (*IVC*) and superior (*SVC*) vena cava. The ultrasound beam is in a paravertebral orientation. Confident visualization of the advancing catheter is facilitated. Slight medial tilt of the transducer will image the fossa ovalis. This view also can be utilized during the pullback maneuver to follow the position of the balloon. *RA*, right atrium; *LA*, left atrium; *RV*, right ventricle; *RPA*, right pulmonary artery; *I*, inferior; *A*, anterior; *S*, superior; *P*, posterior. (From Seward JB, Tajik AJ, Edwards WD, Hagler DJ [eds]. In press. Comprehensive Two-Dimensional Echocardiographic Atlas of Congenital Heart Disease: Anatomic Correlations. New York, Springer-Verlag, chapter 2. By permission of the publisher.)

Inflation

Once the catheter tip is in the left atrial cavity, a subcostal four-chamber projection of a heart is utilized during the *inflation phase* of the balloon septostomy (Fig. 2). The four-chamber view allows confident simultaneous visualization of the left ventricle, mitral valve, pulmonary veins, atrial septum, and atrial cavities. Filling the balloon with a small amount of fluid will best assist visualization of the catheter tip and permit avoidance of inappropriate positioning and further inflation of the balloon.

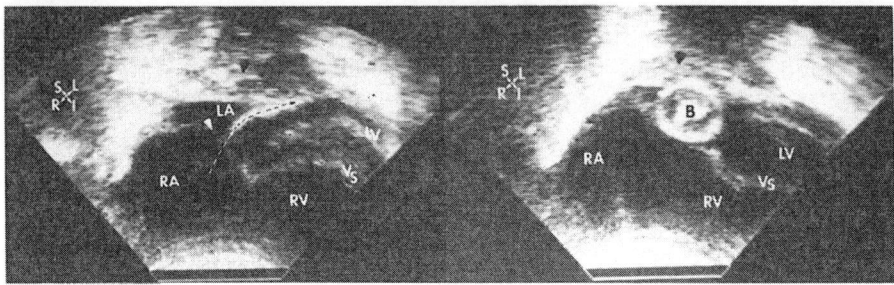

Fig. 2. Subcostal four-chamber view of atrial septum. *Left*, Catheter (*broken line and arrowhead*) is visualized crossing the plane of the atrial septum (*white arrowhead*). *Right*, The balloon (*B*) has been partially inflated and positioned to approximate the atrial septum. The balloon is approximately equal in size to the fossa ovalis. *LA*, left atrium; *RA*, right atrium; *VS*, ventricular septum; *LV*, left ventricle; *RV*, right ventricle; *S*, superior; *L*, left; *R*, right; *I*, inferior.

Pullback

It is important for the operator to observe the inflation of the balloon continuously. The enlarging balloon can be approximated to the fossa ovalis. The first inflation and pullback is best performed when the balloon is inflated to the approximate diameter of the fossa ovalis (Fig. 2). During the pullback, it is best to visualize the inferior vena cava and atrial septum with a subcostal long-axis projection (Fig. 1). Occasionally, the balloon transiently leaves the field of view because of distortion of the heart and surrounding anatomy during the pullback. Repeated inflations and pullbacks are monitored for size of balloon relative to size of left atrium and change in heart function.

Relationship of balloon size to left atrium

Size. Usually, for effective septostomy the balloon ultimately must nearly equal the size of the left atrial cavity in the newborn (Fig. 3).

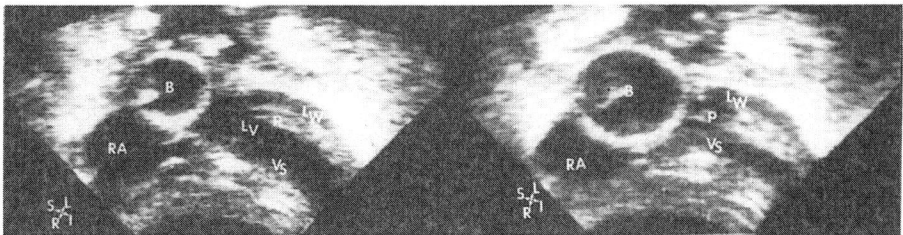

Fig. 3. Subcostal four-chamber view. *Left,* Inflation of the balloon to slightly larger than the fossa ovalis. Note that size of left ventricle is normal. *Right,* With excessive inflation, left atrial inflow and mitral valve are occluded. Note that left ventricle cavity is nearly obliterated. The infant's heart rate slowed transiently. This potentially dangerous situation was quickly relieved by slight deflation of the balloon. *LW,* lateral wall; *P,* papillary muscle; *B,* balloon; *RA,* right atrium; *LV,* left ventricle; *VS,* ventricular septum; *S,* superior; *L,* left; *R,* right; *I,* inferior. (*Right,* From Currie PJ, Seward JB, Hagler DJ, Tajik AJ: Two-dimensional/Doppler echocardiography and its relationship to cardiac catherization for diagnosis and management of congenital heart disease. Cardiovasc Clin 17 No. 1: 301–322, 1986. By permission of FA Davis Company.)

Change in cardiac function. Simultaneous two-dimensional (2-D) echocardiographic monitoring of the balloon inflation allows immediate recognition of changing cardiac hemodynamics. At full balloon inflation, the left atrial cavity may appear nearly obliterated. Excessive inflation results in inflow occlusion, secondary decrease in left ventricular volume, and slowing of the heart rate (Fig. 3). Impending compromise can be relieved by slight balloon deflation.

Result

Adequacy of balloon septostomy is best appreciated by 2-D echocardiographic inspection of the atrial septum. The size of the resultant defect and the flail appearance of the valve of the fossa ovalis are important details (Fig. 4). My associates and I have found that the operator tends to stop short of an adequate septostomy if echocardiographic visualization is not utilized. An insufficient septostomy often appears as a mere stretching of the orifice of the fossa ovalis whereas an adequate septostomy consistently shows a torn flail valve of the fossa ovalis.

Right-to-left shunt can be documented with contrast echocardiography (Fig. 5). Injection of small amounts of saline into a central or peripheral vein at the start of the procedure and at completion can yield a qualitative appreciation of the amount of shunt. More recently, color-flow imaging has been used to assess degree of right-to-left shunting.

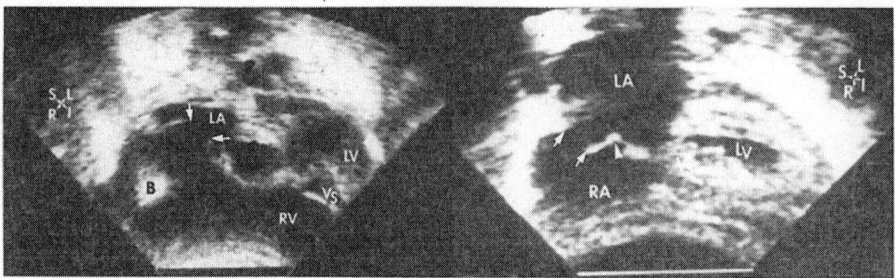

Fig. 4. Subcostal four-chamber views in two patients after successful echocardiography-assisted balloon atrial septostomy. In each, a large atrial septal defect (*small arrows*) occupying the fossa ovalis is evident. The flail edges of the membrane of the valve of the fossa ovalis undulate between left atrium (*LA*) and right atrium. In one patient (*Right*), there was a hinge point (*arrowhead*) at the lower limbus of the flail membrane. *B*, balloon; *LV*, left ventricle; *RA*, right atrium; *RV*, right ventricle; *VS*, ventricular septum; *S*, superior; *L*, left; *R*, right; *I*, inferior.

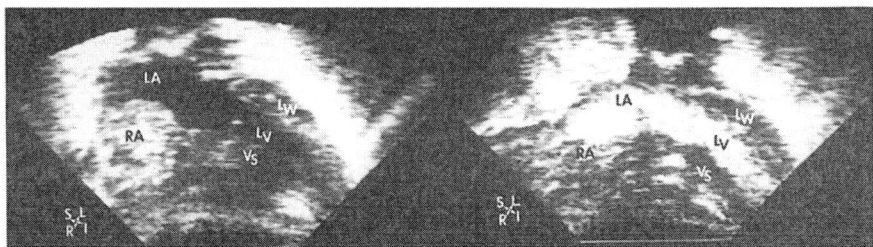

Fig. 5. Subcostal four-chamber view. *Left*, Before septostomy. Opacification of the right atrial (*RA*) cavity is seen after rapid intravenous injection of saline. In this ductal-dependent newborn, there was a negligible amount of shunt at atrial level. *Right*, After septostomy. After a venous injection of saline, there is dense opacification of the left atrium (*LA*) and left ventricle (*LV*). This pattern coincided with improved arterial saturation and the 2-D echocardiographic appearance of a large atrial septal defect. *LW*, lateral wall; *VS*, ventricular septum; *S*, superior; *L*, left; *R*, right; *I*, inferior.

Related techniques

In transseptal catheterization and blade atrial septostomy (Fig. 6), 2-D echocardiographic imaging techniques can be utilized to direct the safe performance of procedures designed to gain access to the left atrium. Visualization of the atrial septum is particularly helpful when the heart or the plane of the atrial septum is in an unusual orientation. The transseptal needle or catheter-blade can be accurately positioned along the plane of the atrial septum. The actual perforation or laceration of the septum can be monitored continuously which decreases the chance of complications. In the event of a complication such as tamponade, recognition and treatment can be facilitated by immediate echocardiographic examination and assisted treatment [19].

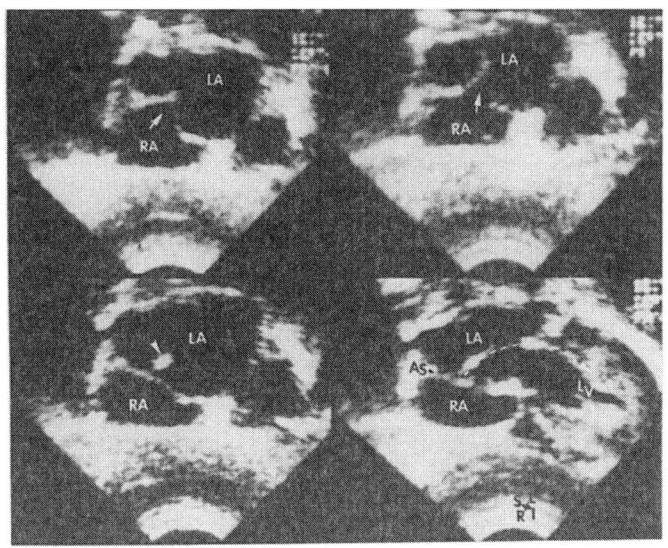

Fig. 6. Subcostal four-chamber visualization of the atrial septum in 2-D echocardiography-assisted transseptal catheterization. *Upper,* Increasing distortion of atrial septum (*arrow*) by the transseptal needle. *Lower Left,* With perforation of the atrial septum, the dilating sheath is visible in the left atrial cavity (*arrowhead*) adjacent to the left atrial septum. *Lower Right,* Catheter (*broken line and arrowhead*) is across atrial septum and positioned in left ventricular (*LV*) cavity. *LA,* left atrium; *RA,* right ventricle; *AS,* atrial septum; *S,* superior; *L,* left; *R,* right; *I,* inferior. (From Currie PJ, Seward JB, Hagler DJ, Tajik AJ: Two-dimensional/Doppler echocardiography and its relationship to cardiac catheterization for diagnosis and management of congenital heart disease. Cardiovasc Clin 17 No. 1: 301–322, 1986. By permission of FA Davis Company.)

References

1. Rashkind WJ, Miller WW: Creation of an atrial septal defect without thoracotomy: a palliative approach to complete transposition of the great arteries. JAMA 196: 991–992, 1966.
2. Hurwitz RA, Girod DA: Percutaneous balloon atrial septostomy in infants with transposition of the great arteries. Am Heart J 91: 618–622, 1976.
3. Rashkind WJ: The complications of balloon atrioseptostomy. J Pediatr 76: 649–650, 1970.
4. Hawker RE, Celermajer JM, Cartmill TB, Bowdler JD: Thrombosis of the inferior vena cava following balloon septostomy in transposition of the great arteries. Am Heart J 82: 593–595, 1971.
5. Ellison RC, Plauth WH Jr, Gazzaniga AB, Fyler DC: Inability to deflate catheter balloon: a complication of balloon atrial septostomy. J. Pediatr 76: 604–606.
6. Vogel JHK: Balloon embolization during atrial septostomy. Circulation 42: 155–156, 1970.
7. Blanchard WB, Knauf DG, Victoria BE: Interatrial groove tear: an unusual complication of balloon atrial septostomy. Pediatr Cardiol 4: 149–150, 1983.

8. Park SC, Neches WH, Mullins CE, Girod DA, Olley PM, Falkowski G, Garibjan VA, Mathews RA, Fricker FJ, Beerman LB, Lenox CC, Zuberbuhler JR: Blade atrial septostomy: collaborative study. Circulation 66: 258–266, 1982.

9. Rice MJ, Seward JB, Hagler DJ, Mair DD, Feldt RH, Puga FJ, Danielson GK, Edwards WD, Tajik AJ: Impact of 2-dimensional echocardiography on the management of distressed newborns in whom cardiac disease is suspected. Am J Cardiol 51: 288–292, 1983.

10. Stark J, Smallhorn J, Huhta J, de Leval M, Macartney FJ, Rees PG, Taylor JFN: Surgery for congenital heart defects diagnosed with cross-sectional echocardiography. Circulation 68 Suppl 2: 129–138, 1983.

11. Leung MP, Mok CK, Lau KC, Lo R, Yeung CY: The role of cross sectional echocardiography and pulsed Doppler ultrasound in the management of neonates in whom congenital heart disease is suspected: a prospective study. Br Heart J 56: 73–82, 1986.

12. Alboliras ET, Seward JB, Driscoll DJ, Hagler DJ: Impact of two-dimensional echocardiography in the care of children 2 years old or younger with heart disease (1975 versus 1985) (abstract). Circulation 74 Suppl 2: 379, 1986.

13. Seward JB, Tajik AJ, Hagler DJ, Edwards WD: Internal cardiac crux: two-dimensional echocardiography of normal and congenitally abnormal hearts. Ultrasound Med Biol 10: 735–745, 1984.

14. Perry LW, Ruckman RN, Galioto FM Jr, Shapiro SR, Potter BM, Scott LP III: Echocardiographically assisted balloon atrial septostomy. Pediatrics 70: 403–408, 1982.

15. Allan LD, Leanage R, Wainwright R, Joseph MC, Tynan M: 1982. Balloon atrial septostomy under two dimensional echocardiographic control. Br Heart J 47: 41–43, 1982.

16. Lin AE, Di Sessa TG, Williams RG: Balloon and blade atrial septostomy facilitated by two-dimensional echocardiography. Am J Cardiol 57: 273–277, 1986.

17. Currie PJ, Seward JB, Hagler DJ, Tajik AJ: Two-dimensional/Doppler echocardiography and its relationship to cardiac catheterization and for diagnosis and management of congenital heart disease. Cardiovasc Clin 17 No. 1: 301–322, 1986.

18. Callahan JA, Seward JB, Tajik AJ, Holmes DR Jr, Smith HC, Reeder GS, Miller FA Jr: Pericardiocentesis assisted by two-dimensional echocardiography. J Thorac Cardiovasc Surg 85: 877–879, 1983.

19. Seward JB, Tajik AJ, Hagler DJ: Contrast echocardiography in the assessment of cyanotic and complex congenital heart disease: peripheral venous, invasive, and unique applications. In: Contrast Echocardiography. Edited by RS Meltzer, J. Roelandt. The Netherlands: Martinus Nijhoff Publishers BV, pp 235–277, 1982.

1.5. Color flow Doppler guiding of atrial septostomy

SHUNEI KYO & RYOZO OMOTO

Introduction

In a significant number of the patients with severe cyanotic congenital heart disease and a critical cardio-respiratory failure, an adequate interatrial opening is essential for survival in their early stages of life [1]. In such critical patients, quick establishment of diagnosis is required to determine proper therapeutic managements for their survival. Cardiac catheterization was considered to be the standard means of diagnosing most congenital heart disease in the past, however, angiography entails the use of radiation and contrast medium and is associated with morbidity and mortality [2]. Color Flow Mapping real-time, two-dimensional Doppler Echocardiography (2-D Doppler) has become as a tool for the diagnosis in congenital heart disease with definitive anatomic and intracardiac blood flow information [3,4]. Therefore, it also has potential use in directing medical or surgical management and in changing the indications for cardiac catheterization. In our institution, there has been a shift toward the non-invasive technique either to supplement or to replace cardiac catheterization in selected situations, particularly in critically ill infants [5].

Balloon atrial septostomy is an accepted method for palliation of certain types of congenital heart disease. However, malposition of the balloon may lead to cardiac perforation, avulsion of an atrioventricular valve, or laceration of the systemic or pulmonary veins. Therefore, recently balloon atrioseptostomy has been performed with the assistance of two-dimensional echocardiography in the catheterization laboratory or at the bed side in the intensive care unit or neontal unit [6,7,8]. However, even after creation of a sizable atrial septal defect, a significant hypoxemia occasionally persists after the procedure [9]. Therefore, evaluation of the shunt flow, which can contribute to the intracardiac mixing of arterial and venous blood flow through the atrial septal defect during the procedure, and follow up of intracardiac blood flow dynamics are indispensable in such critically ill patients [10].

The purpose of this study is to evaluate the clinical usefulness of Color Flow Mapping Doppler Echocardiography in diagnosis and treatment of the

I. Cikes (ed.), *Echocardiography in Cardiac Interventions*, 49–56, 1989.
© 1989 *Kluwer Academic Publishers*.

patients with critical cyanotic congenital heart disease, and its usefulness as a tool for echo-guiding of balloon atrial septostomy.

Materials and methods

After introduction of real-time two-dimensional Doppler echocardiography in September 1982, we evaluated 52 patients with cyanotic congenital heart disease under one-year-old by 2-D Doppler. For these patients 2-D Doppler examination was performed immediately after admission either in the echo laboratory or at the bedside. By 2-D Doppler examination, abnormalities in cardiac anatomical structure and intracardiac flow hemodynamics of patients could be fully evaluated within twenty minutes without any sedation.

In 12 cases, an emergency balloon atrial septostomy was performed with the assistance of 2-D Doppler monitoring in the cardiac catheterization laboratory, in the intensive care unit, or in the operating room where a cardiorespiratory support system is fully equiped.

The average age of nine cases was 19.10 days (2–44 day) and the average body weight was 3291 g (2390–4450 g) at the time when balloon atrial septostomy was performed. Six of twelve cases were already in shock condition at the time of addmission which required endotracheal intubation and/or mechanical ventilation support by respirator (Table 1).

According to the 2-D Doppler evaluation of cardiac structure and hemodynamics, intravenous prostaglandine E1 administration was started immediately, if indicated. Also a balloon atrial septostomy was prepared as a sequence of therapeutic management, depending the on 2-D Doppler diagnosis.

Before a balloon atrial septostomy contrast echocardiogram was taken by gas (carbon dioxyside), a mixed saline was injected through the venous line in the lower extremity to check the atrio-vena caval connection. With 2-D Doppler assistance, a Miller balloon catheter (Edwards Laboratory) was easily introduced into the left atrium through the small interatrial opening (IAO) in a short time. According to the sizes of IAO and both atrial cavities the balloon was inflated to an appropriate size. Then a balloon atrial septostomy was performed until an adequate size of IAO and an adequate blood flow mixing through the IAO was determined by 2-D Doppler evaluation. Immediately after the BAS hemodynamic improvement of the patients was evaluated and followed up by 2-D Doppler at least once a week during hospitalization and at least once every two months at the outpatient clinic. Full catheterization was also performed at appropriate timing after the BAS. A second balloon atrial septostomy was performed in two patients with

Table 1. Materials.

	1st BAS	(2nd BAS)
d-TGA (type 1)	8 pts	(3 pts)
d-TGA (type 2)	1 pt	
Pulmonary atresia	1 pt	
Tricuspid atresia	2 pts	
	12 pts	(3 pts)
(1) 1st BAS		
Age	2–44 days	(19 ± 13 days)
Male : Female	6 : 6	
Body Weight	2390–4450 g	(3291 ± 685 g)
Shock on admission (Mechanical ventilation)	6 cases	
(2) 2nd BAS		
Age	2–7 months	(3.7 ± 2.4 months)

d-transposition of great arteries at 2 and 7 months after the first septostomy, owing to the re-narrowing of the interatrial opening (Table 1).

The Miller balloon atrioseptostomy catheter (Edwards Laboratory) and the Blade atrioseptostomy catheter (Cook Incorporated) were used for balloon and/or balde atrioseptostomy. Color flow mapping 2-D Doppler echocardiograms were obtained using Aloka XA-54 (prototype: 2.5, 3.0, and 3.5 MHz), Aloka SSD 880 (commercial type: 2.5 and 3.5 MHz), and Aloka XA-340 (prototype: 5.0 and 7.5 MHz) especially for premature infants.

Results

The 2-D Doppler examination on admission demonstrated the size of interatrial opening smaller than 2 mm in diameter in 7 of 12 patients and only a small shunt flow through the opening. In five cases a moderate size of interatrial opening was observed, however, the shunt flow through it in these cases was judged not to be satisfactory by 2-D Doppler. In 10 of 12 cases a shunt flow through the ductus arteriosus was observed which was markedly increased in 2-D Doppler examination after the administration of prostaglandin E1.

Evaluation of the associated intracardiac abnormalities is important for patient management before and after balloon atrial septostomy. Figure 1 demonstrates the case with transposition of great arteries with a large atrial

52

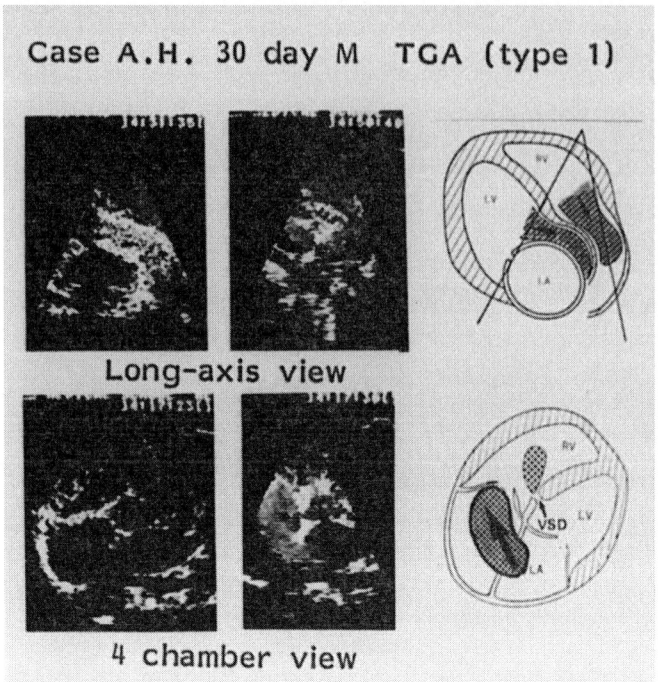

Case A.H. 30 day M TGA (type 1)

Long-axis view

4 chamber view

Fig. 1. 2-D Doppler images in d-transposition of great arteries (TGA). The parasternal long-axis view demonstrates the parallel orientation of the great vessels: The flow in the pulmonary artery is depicted with mosaic pattern. The apical four-chamber view shows a satisfactory size of the interatrial opening and the shunt flow through it, and a small ventricular septal defect. LA = left atrium; LV = left ventricle; RV = right ventricle; VSD = ventricular septal defect.

septal defect, a small ventricular septal defect, and a moderate pulmonary valvular stenosis. With the 2-D Doppler echocardiogram all three intracardiac abnormalities were easily and quickly illustrated, thus this patient was judged to have a satisfactory intracardiac shunt flow for survival. Table 2 shows all the associated abnormalities detected by the 2-D Doppler examination on admission. With 2-D echo monitoring, we can easily recognize the position of the balloon and the location of the catheter tip in the cardiac cavity.

A representative 2-D Doppler image which demonstrate the effects of BAS is shown in Fig. 2. In this 10-day-old female case of transposition of great arteries, the size of interatrial opening was enlarged to about 10 mm in diameter after balloon atrial septostomy and the 2-D Doppler examination after the procedure shows that the shunt flow through it was markedly increased; also a reversed direction of shunt flow can be seen at the end of diastole.

In one case of transposition of great arteries on which the second balloon

Table 2. 2-D Doppler Observation on Admission.

	Case	Diag.	IAO	PDA	VSD	PS
1.	O.K.	d-TGA	small	+	−	−
2.	F.U.	d-TGA	small	+	small	−
3.	A.H.	d-TGA	moderate	+	small	+
4.	I.K.	d-TGA	small	+	−	−
5.	Y.G.	d-TGA	moderate	+	−	−
6.	N.R.	d-TGA	small	+	−	−
7.	Y.Y.	PA	small	+	−	−
8.	T.K.	TA	moderate	−	+	+
9.	S.Y.	TA	moderate	+	−	−
10.	A.T.	d-TGA	small	−	+	−
11.	U.R.	d-TGA + Ao interuption	small	+	+	−
12.	N.R.	d-TGA	moderate	+	−	−

IAO: interatrial opening
small: IAO size < 2 mm
moderate: IAO size 2 mm–5 mm

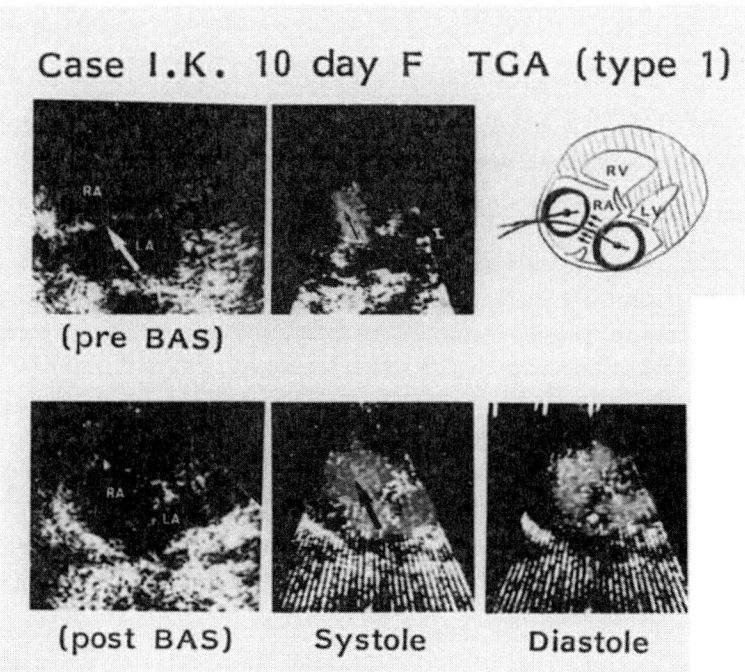

Fig. 2. The 2-D Doppler images of flow through the interatrial opening in a representative case of balloon atrial septostomy. Note the marked increase of the size of interatrial opening and the flow through it after balloon atrial septostomy.

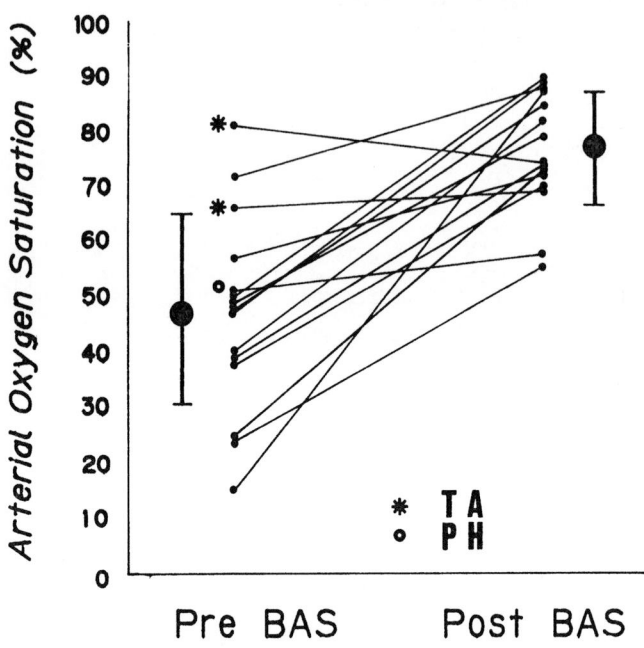

Fig. 3. Effect of balloon and/or atrial septostomy on the arterial oxygen saturation in 12 cases studied including two cases of second balloon atrial septostomy. The arterial oxygen saturation did not change in two cases of tricuspid atresia with intact ventricular septum (TA) and in one case of d-transposition of the great arteries with advanced pulmonary hypertension.

and blade atrial septostomy was performed at 7 months after the initial septostomy, neither evidence of an increase of the shunt flow in the 2-D Doppler nor an increase of arterial oxygen saturation was obtained even after obtaining significant size of interatrial opening, (open circle in Fig. 3). Cardiac catheterization following the second septostomy revealed markedly advanced pulmonary hypertension in this case.

The average oxygen saturation before balloon atrial septostomy, excluding two cases of tricuspid atresia, was 46.8 ± 17.5% and that after balloon atrial septostomy was 76.5 ± 10.7% (Fig. 3). In two cases with tricuspid atresia, the arterial oxigen saturation did not change after septostomy as shown by the star mark in Fig. 3.

Discussion

The infant with d-transposition of great arteries, tricuspid atresia or pulmonary atresia with intact ventricular septum is often seriously ill with hypoxia, acidosis, and heart failure, which require mechanical ventilatory support on admission. Because it is not always possible to obtain complete hemodynamic data and to establish the correct diagnosis in the initial cardiac catheterization, and because the radiographic contrast material may depress cardiac, respiratory, and renal function in critically ill patients, it seems to be reasonable to direct medical and surgical management on the basis of the non-invasive technique to supplement or to replace cardiac catheterization [5]. In this study we demonstrated 12 cases of successful performance of balloon atrial septostomy, depending only on 2-D Doppler diagnosis without hemodynamic information given by cardiac catheterization. The balloon atrial septostomy assisted by two-dimensional echocardiography is a technique that minimizes the risk of the procedure which makes it available to use in the patient with complex congenital heart disease with abnormalities in cardiac position, situations which in the past would require thoracotomy and Blalock-Hanlon atrial septostomy [6, 7, 8]. As a substitute surgical palliation to Blalock-Hanlon septostomy, a balloon catheter can be easily introduced into the left atrium, guided by echocardiography and balloon atrial septostomy can be safely performed even directly through the right atrial wall with a small right thoracotomy as we have already reported [5]. Another advantage of echocardiographically assisted balloon atrial septostomy using 2-D Doppler is that the effect of the procedure can be evaluated immediately not only by the size of the created interatrial opening, but also by the adequacy of the shunt flow, which contributes to the intracardiac mixing of the arterial and venous blood flow, although it is qualitative. This technique is also useful for the early detection of re-narrowing of the created interatrial opening in the follow up. Thus, the use of two-dimensional Doppler echocardiography to determine the indication for atrial septostomy, and its use as a guide in performing balloon and/or blade atrial septostomy should significantly contribute to the speed, efficacy, and safety of the procedure [8].

References

1. Rashkind WJ: Transcatheter treatment of congenital heart disease. Circulation 67: 711–716, 1983.
2. Rice MJ, Seward JB, Hagler DJ, Mair DD, Feldt RH, Puga FJ, Danielson GK, Edwards WD, Tajik AJ: Impact of 2-dimensional echocardiography on the management of distressed newborns in whom cardiac disease is suspected. Am J Cardiol 51: 288–292, 1983.

3. Kyo S: Congenital Heart Disease. In: Omoto R, ed. Color atlas of real-time two-dimensional Doppler echocardiography. Tokyo: Shindan-to Chiryo Co., Ltd, 81–134, 1984.

4. Omoto R, Yokote Y, Takamoto S, Kyo S, Ueda K. Asano H, Namekawa K, Kasai C, Kondo Y, Koyano A: The development of real-time two-dimensional Doppler echocardiography and its clinical significance in acquired valvular diseases. With special Reference to the evaluation of valvular regurgitation. Jap Heart J 25: 325–340, 1984.

5. Kyo S, Takamoto S, Takanawa E, Matsumura M, Yokote Y, Omoto R: Does color flow mapping Doppler echocardiography allow the catheterization laboratory to be bypassed in surgery in congenital heart disease? In: Roelandt J, ed. Color Doppler flow imaging and other advances in Doppler echocardiography. Dordrecht: Martinus Nijhoff Publishers, 107–121, 1986.

6. Bullaboy CA, Jennings RB, Johnson DH, Fulcher CW: Bedside balloon atrial septostomy using echocardiographic monitoring. Am J Cardiol 53: 971, 1984.

7. Perry LW, Ruckman RN, Galioto Jr. FM, Shapiro SR, Potter BM, Scott III LP: Echocardiographically assisted balloon atrial septostomy. Pediatrics 70: 403–408, 1982.

8. Allen LD, Leanage R, Weinwright R, Joseph MC, Tynan M: Balloon atrial septostomy under two dimensional echocardiographic control. Br Heart J 47: 41–43, 1982.

9. Henry CG, Goldring D, Hartmann AF Weldon CS, Strauss AW: Treatment of d-transposition of the great arteries: Management of hypoxemia after balloon atrial septostomy. Am J Cardiol 47: 299–306, 1981.

10. Kyo S, Omoto R, Takamoto S, Yokote Y, Takanawa E: Echo guide balloon atrioseptostomy by color flow mapping real-time two-dimensional Doppler echo. J Am Coll Cardiol 5: 453, 1985 (Abstract).

1.6. Echocardiography in transseptal cardiac catheterization

ITZHAK KRONZON & EPHRAIM GLASSMAN

In selected patients, transseptal cardiac catheterization is the technique of choice for evaluation of left atrial and left ventricular anatomy and hemo-dynamics [1–3]. Although in many instances the measurement of left atrial pressure has been replaced by that of pulmonary wedge pressure, the latter is not always accurate and may be impossible to record (e.g. severe pulmonary hypertension). Left atrial catheterization is the reference standard for measuring left atrial pressure and mitral valve gradient and for approaching the left ventricle in an antegrade direction when the retrograde technique is difficult or hazardous. This situation may occur in patients with severe, cal-cific aortic stenosis or a prosthetic aortic valve. The technique is not used in every cardiac catheterization laboratory because of the need for special skill, experience and equipment. In the Cardiac Catheterization Laboratory of New York University Medical Center more than 3000 transseptal catheteri-zations were performed between 1969 and 1985. Table I summarizes the indications for transseptal catheterization. Table II summarizes the contra-indications for such procedure. In experienced hands, complications are relatively rare. The most ominous complication is perforation of the intra-pericardial structures, which may lead to cardiac tamponade. Although the operator tries to puncture the interatrial septum at the fossa ovalis, puncture of the aorta, right ventricular wall, right atrial wall, coronary sinus and even the left atrial free wall has been described [1]. In conditions that cause signifi-cant chamber enlargement, especially right atrial enlargement or aortic root dilatation, the anatomic relation of the cardiac chambers may vary, and the identification of the exact point for the interatrial septal puncture may become difficult.

Methods

In our laboratory, transseptal cardiac catheterization is performed using the right femoral vein. As previously described [1], after transcutaneous punc-ture of the vein, a wire is passed to the right atrium and a polyethylene catheter was advanced over the wire. The wire is removed and a Ross needle

I. Cikes (ed.), *Echocardiography in Cardiac Interventions*, 57–65, 1989.

Table 1. Indications for Transseptal Catheterization.

	Remarks
1) Evaluation of Mitral Stenosis	Transseptal cathetarization (TSC) indicated mainly when pulmonary wedge pressure is unobtainable, or considered inadequate or inaccurate.
2) Evaluation of a Prosthetic Mitral Valve	idem
3) Evaluation of Aortic Stenosis	TSC is indicated mainly when the valve is calcified (risk of calcium embolization by 'poking' the valve during attempts to cross it) or when it is difficult, dangerous or impossible to cross a damaged, infected or stenosed valve.
4) Evaluation of a Prosthetic Aortic Valve	TSC is indicated mainly when retrograde approach to the LV may be impossible or may interfere with the prosthetic valve function.
5) Evaluation of LV Outflow Obstruction (Subaortic Stenosis, IHSS)	TSC permits accurate measurement of the LV *inflow* tract pressure. Retrograde catheterization is used to measure LV outflow pressures.
6) Left Atrial (and/or Left Ventricular) Angiography	TSC is indicated especially when the approach to the LV in a retrograde way is impossible or dangerous (e.g. LV clot, aortic dissection). This technique is an alternative to the levophase of PA angiography.
7) Evaluation of Cor Triatriatum	Demonstration of pressure gradient between the pulmonary capillary wedge pressure and the left atrium (entered by TSC).
8) Evaluation of Pulmonary Venous Obstruction	idem
9) Left atrial – Femoral Artery Bypass	A possible technique for temporary LV bypass during acute stage of left ventricular injury.
10) Percutaneous Balloon Mitral Valvuloplasty	Antegrade approach to a stenosed mitral valve for balloon dilatation.

is advanced to the tip of the catheter. The needle and catheter are manipulated into the fossa ovalis under fluoroscopy. The interatrial septum is punctured with the needle and, after the location of the needle tip in the left atrium is confirmed by pressure recordings and sampling of blood, the catheter is advanced over the needle into the left atrium. During the procedure pressure and fluoroscopic monitoring of the transseptal catheter and needle are constantly performed.

Table 2. Contraindications of Transseptal Catheterization.

	Remarks
1) Left agrial Mass (myxoma, other tumors, clot)	Risk of embolization
2) Recent (0–12 month) history of arterial embolization	Risk of embolization, especially if the source may be in in the left atrium
3) Severe chest or back deformation (e.g. severe kyposcoliosis)	Inability to pass the TS needle
4) Occluded inferior vena cava	Inability to pass the TS catheter
5) Defective coagulation mechanism	Risk of hemopericardium
6) Change in anatomic relations of the inter-atrial septum	Very large RA, ascending aortic aneurysm
7) Inexperienced operator	

In addition, in each patient, cardiac catheterization also includes right-sided catheterization (through the femoral vein) as well as retrograde left-sided catheterization (through the femoral artery).

M-Mode echocardiography

This study should be performed in conjunction with two dimensional evaluation for screening candidates for transseptal catheterization. The anatomy of the valves, chamber size, wall motion and thickness may clarify the indications for transseptal catheterization. Findings that are a contraindication to transseptal catheterization (e.g. LA myxoma) or findings that may complicate the procedure (i.e. dilated aortic root) may also be disclosed. Special attention is paid to the presence and size of pericardial effusion. In the case of unsuccessful puncture, repeat echocardiography is indicated to detect any new effusion and signs of pericardial tamponade. However, routine M-mode echocardiography is not useful *during* the transseptal catheterization procedure. Although the catheter can sometimes be identified, its tip cannot be recognized with certainty. The relation between the tip of the transseptal needle, the interatrial septum and the adjacent cavities and structures cannot be accurately observed.

Transvenous intracardiac M-mode echocardiography

In order to improve the ability to monitor the distance between the needle tip and the interatrial septum and adjacent structures we investigated the use of a

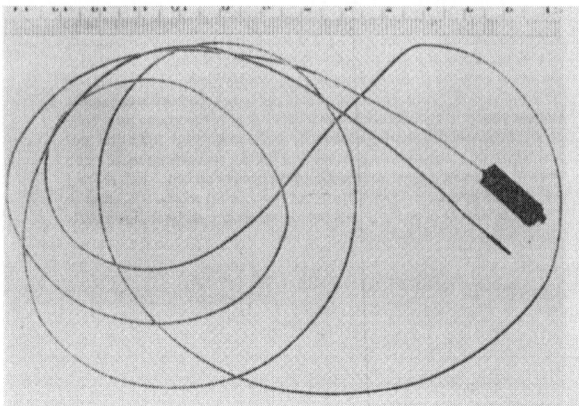

Fig. 1A. The transducer attached to a coaxial cable, which terminates in a standard, microdot connector.

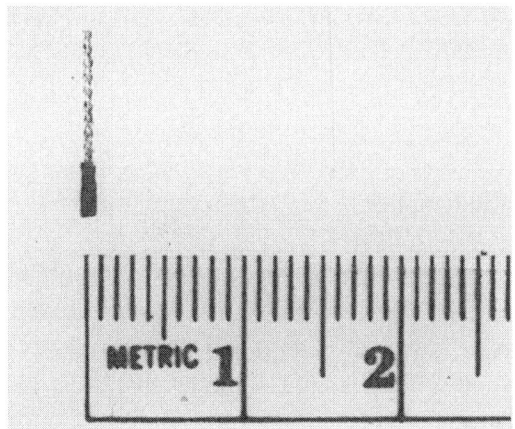

Fig. 1B. Close-up view of the transducer. Reproduced from Glassman and Kronzon [4] with permission.

small 5–7.5 mHz, M-mode echocardiographic transducer (diamter 0.5–0.75 mm, thickness 0.2 cm). The transducer capacitance ranges between 20 and 60 picofarads. It is mounted on a gold coaxial cable, 125 cm long and 1 mm in diameter which terminates in a miniature microdot connector. The entire cable and connector has a capacitance of 100 picofarads. The transducer and the cable are capable of passing through a 17 gauge transseptal needle (Fig. 1).

The possibility of increasing the safety of transseptal catheterization using the intracardiac echogram was explored in 10 patients. Figure 2 was obtained

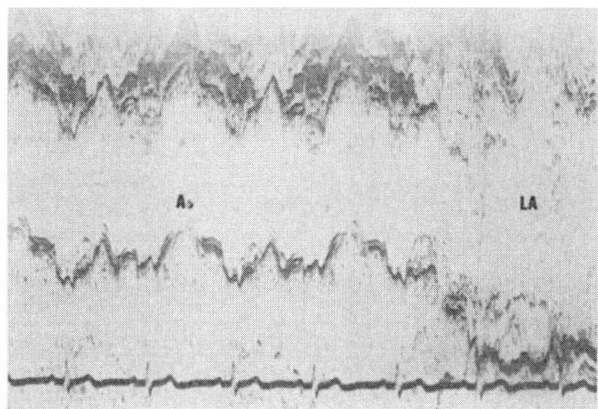

Fig. 2. Recording obtained using a small transducer in a transseptal needle positioned against the interatrial septum. As the needle is moved from the superior to inferior sites, the aorta (AO) and left atrium (LA) are consecutively visualized. The sudden loss of the aortic contour and simultaneous appearance of the left atrium occur as the needle tip enters the fossa ovalis. This loss is helpful in positioning the needle for septal puncture. Reproduced, with permission from Glassman and Kronzon [5].

with the transducer placed at the tip of a transseptal needle positioned relatively high in the right atrium and directed medially and posteriorly. The echocardiographic beam outlines the aorta. As the needle is withdrawn inferiorly, the aortic cavity is replaced by that of the left atrium. Puncture of the septum at this point will permit passage of the catheter into the left atrium and avoidance of the aorta. In each of the 10 patients studied septal puncture at the site indicated by combined fluoroscopic observation and echocardiographic localization yielded a satisfactory result.

Two dimensional echocardiography *(Figs. 3–5)*

This technique provides real time, high resolution images of cardiac chambers and structures. For the reasons mentioned under M-mode Echocardiography, it is recommended for screening and follow up, before and, when necessary, after transseptal catheterization.

We performed two dimensional echocardiography on 32 patients (18 women, 14 men; aged 28 to 78 years), who underwent diagnostic cardiac catheterization which required the transseptal technique. Ten patients had severe aortic stenosis, eight had mitral valve disease, six had prosthetic mitral valves, three had previous mitral valvuloplasty, three had prosthetic aortic valves, and two had idiopathic hypertrophic subaortic stenosis.

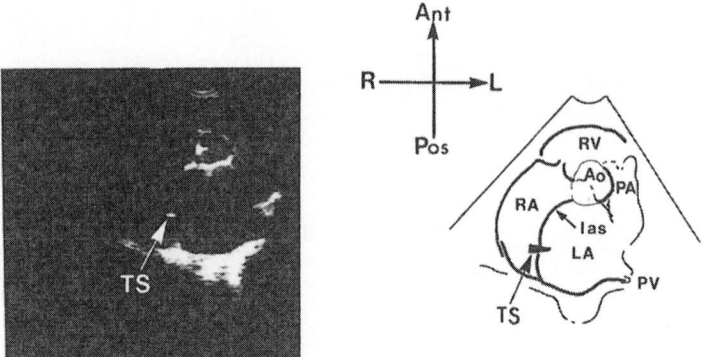

Fig. 3. Short axis view just before puncture. The tip of the transseptal (TS) needle is noted in the right atrium (RA), just near the atrial septum.

Long axis, short axis and apical four chamber views were obtained and recorded on videotape for further analysis. During flushing of the Ross needle before and after the puncture, the presence and location of interatrial microcavitation were ascertained (Fig. 5). In each patient the site of the inter-atrial septal puncture was made on the basis of fluoroscopy and not from the echocardiographic findings. The latter were used as supplementary data and for future reference.

Transseptal puncture was successful in 31 of the 32 patients. In one patient, puncture of the aortic root was detected and the needle was im-mediately withdrawn. The left atrium was entered in another attempt and no complications ensued.

The long axis view does not show the right atrium and, therefore, does not provide useful information about catheter position. The subxiphoid evalua-tion of the interatrial septum, considered by many to be the best view for visualization of this structure, is not used because it interfers with the sterile drapes. Therefore, this study was limited to the apical four chamber and the short-axis views.

Adequate short axis views with visualization of both atria and interatrial septum were obtained in 23 of the 32 patients. In each patient, the catheter and the needle were clearly visualized. Becuase the interatrial septum is posterior and to the right of the root of the aorta, these two structures can be clearly separated. In each successful puncture, the needle tip could be seen penetrating the middle third of the septum (Fig. 3). Contrast echocardiog-raphy performed during flushing of the needle confirmed its location in the right atrium before the puncture and in the left atrium after the puncture. The short-axis view was not informative in the patient who had aortic root puncture.

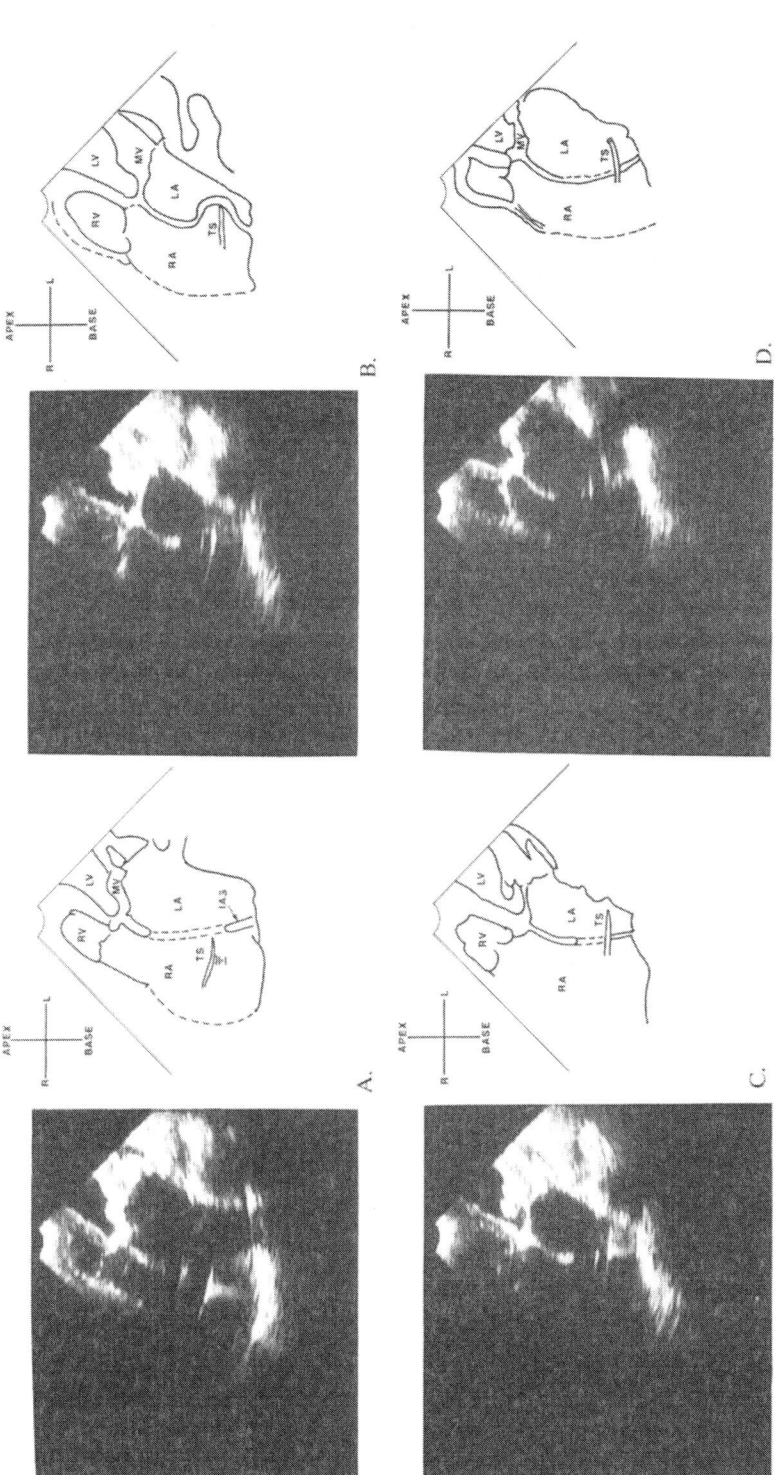

Figs. 4A–D. **Four chamber view during transseptal catheterization in a patient with dilated atria and calcific mitral stenosis.** A. The Brockenbrough transseptal (TS) catheter with the Ross needle in the right atrium (RA) near the puncture site. Note the dense needle echo with the reverberations behind it. B. Just before the puncture, the interatrial septum (IAS) bulges toward the left atrium (LA). C. Immediately after the puncture, the interatrial septum snaps back to its original position. The tip of the Ross needle is now in the left atrium. D. The catheter was advanced to the left atrium, and the needle withdrawn. Note the visualization of the catheter and its lumen in the left atrium.

Abbreviations: L = left atrium, LV = left ventricle, MV = mitral valve, R = right, RA = right, RV = right ventricle.

Reproduced with permission from Kronzon, et al. [5].

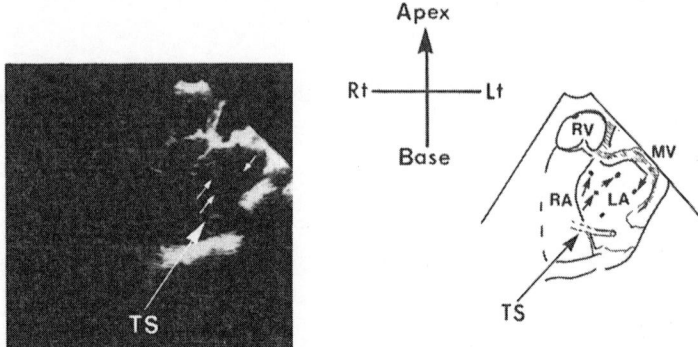

Fig. 5. After transseptal puncture, during catheter flushing, microbubbles (small arrows) are noted in the left atrium (LA). The transseptal catheter is marked with a large arrow (TS).

The four chamber apical view provided good visualization of all cardiac chambers in 28 of the 32 patients (Fig. 4). In each patient, the location of the interatrial septum and its relation to the needle and transseptal catheter could be clearly visualized. In four patients, continuous recording were obtained during the transeptal puncture. The apical approach enabled us to avoid the placement of the echocardiographer's hand in the fluoroscopic field. In each of these patients, just before the puncture, the septum bulged toward the left atrium before the needle punctured it and then snapped back to its original position (Fig. 4B and 4C). The location of the puncture in each patient was in the basilar part of the interatrial septum. In the patient with aortic puncture, it appeared that the position of the catheter was in a more apical part of the interatrial septum. Because of its inability to delineate the entire interatrial septum, the so-called five chamber view was not routinely used.

Limitation of the technique

Although the catheter and the transseptal needle are almost always visualized, poor quality echocardiograms prevented the demonstration of the relation between the needle tip and the inter-atrial septum in 9 of 32 patients (27%) of the patients studied in the short axis view, and in 5 of 32 patients (15%) of patients studied in the four chamber view. The interatrial septum could not be visualized in either view in 2 of 32 patients (6%). In many patients the evaluation of the apical four chamber view required tilting of the patient to the left, while the transseptal catheter and needle were in position. Since most studies were done on a tilt table, this was not a major problem, however, this may prove more difficult and possibly dangerous on fixed tables with C arms.

Certain technical problems exist which make visualization of the need tip uncertain. The metal creates multiple reverberations and also transmits sound with a faster velocity than tissues. Both of these may create distortion of the needle image. Most importantly, one can never be certain whether the tip of the needle is definitely visualized. A further limitation arises due to the fact that the image is two dimensional and the tip os three dimensional. Consequently, the tip may be in a difficult plane than is being imaged rendering identification impossible. Further developments, including the use of a needle tip echo transmitter, as described by Cikes [6], may solve this problem.

Summary

We have demonstrated that it is possible to monitor the location of the needle in relation to the interatrial septum and other intracardiac structures during puncture of the interatrial septum. More experience is required to determine the accuracy, pitfalls and the exact sensitivity of this technique for positioning the needle tip during interatrial septal puncture. At present, this procedure should be performed under fluoroscopic quidance with pressure monitoring, and the echocardiographic observations are not an alternative to the traditional technique. However, in the future, this technique may improve the safety of transseptal catheterization and decrease its complications.

References

1. Conti CR: Percutaneous approach and transseptal catheterization. In Grossman W. ed. cardiac catheterization and Angiography. Philadelphia: Lea & Febiger, 34: 40, 1974.
2. Brackenbrough EC, Braunwald E: A new technique for left ventricular angiography and transseptal left heart catheterization. Am J Cardiol 6: 1002, 1960.
3. Ross J Jr: Considerations regarding the technique for transseptal left heart catheterization. Circulation 34: 391, 1966.
4. Glassman E, Kronzon I: Transvenous intracardiac echocardiography. Am J Cardiol 47: 1255–1259, 1981.
5. Kronzon I, Glassman E, Cohen M, Winer HE: Use of two dimensional echocardiography during transseptal cardiac catheterization. JACC 4: 425–428, 1984.
6. Cikes I, Breyer B, Ernst A: Cardiac catheterization guided by ultrasound (Abstract). JACC 3: 565, 1984.

1.7. Percutaneous transvenous mitral commissurotomy guided and assessed by echocardiography

KANJI INOUE & CHUANRONG CHEN

We have developed a procedure of percutaneous transveneous mitral commissurotomy (PTMC) using a specially devised balloon catheter [1]. The balloon has an unique shape and construction that ensures not only its proper placement into the affected mitral valves but also the generation of sufficient expansile force to separate fused commissures in a well-controlled manner, as will be described below.

Since its first introduction, this procedure has been applied to 38 patients thus far with significant clinical improvements in all but a few cases who had rigid leaflets and/or extremely severe calcifications, which hampered effective opening of stenotic valves.

With further refinements in the device itself, for example, percutaneous insertion, as well as ancillary technical maneuvers incorporated during those applications, PTMC has now become a dependable treatment for mild to severe mitral stenosis that can be readily performed by any experienced hand.

In the actual procedure of PTMC, 2D-Echocardiography and X-ray fluoroscopy serve important aids at various stages. First, 2D-Echocardiography is used to assess valve conditions, on which basis patients are selected for PTMC. Second, the balloon placement can be guided by monitoring with 2D-Echocardiography and X-ray fluoroscopy, which should be particularly helpful in initial trials, though not necessarily required after sufficient experience. Third, the effect of PTMC is evaluated by 2D-Echocardiographic measurement of the mitral valve orifice area as well as by a pressure measurement of the mitral valve gradient. This article outlines the whole procedure of PTMC along with its typical clinical applications, with stress on how those monitoring aids are practically used.

There have been other trials of percutaneous mitral commissurotomy by using a balloon similar to the conventional angioplasty balloon [2–7].

2D-Echocardiographic guidance of balloon placement

Figures 1, 2 and 3 show the balloon catheter developed for PTMC and its use.

I. Cikes (ed.), *Echocardiography in Cardiac Interventions*, 67–76, 1989.

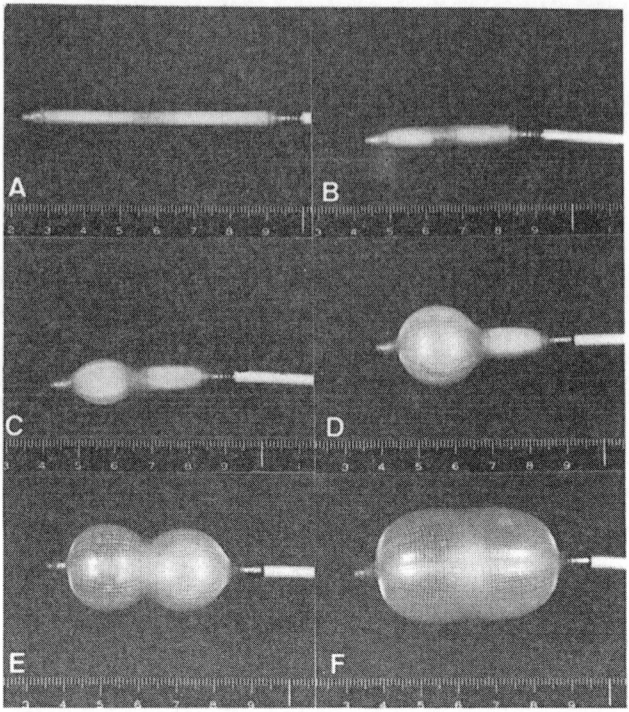

Fig. 1. A new balloon catheter. At deflation, the balloon section is slenderized (5 mm in diameter) by stretching so as to be inserted percutaneously (A, B). The shape of the balloon changes from (C) to (F) depending on the extent of inflation. The diameter of the inflated balloon is adjustable from 26 mm to 29 mm with an internal pressure of over 1.5 kg/cm^2 by which most fused commissures can be divided.

Some modifications added to the prototype balloon catheter [1]. When the balloon catheter is inserted in the left atrium, X-ray fluoroscopy is moved from antero-posterior projection to right anterior oblique projection, and a 2D-Echocardiographic transducer is placed in the third or fourth intercostal space at the left sternal border to record the mitral valve in the long axis view. 2D-Echocardiographic monitoring demonstrates the position of the balloon catheter in relation to the mitral orifice. For example, in the case of the giant left atrium, the balloon catheter tends to be directed toward the posterior wall of the left atrium, that is, in the opposite direction to the mitral orifice postitioned anteriorly, which makes it difficult to insert the balloon into the mitral orifice. These difficulties are overcome by using stylet with curvature more anterior. In one case, these difficulties were overcome by repeating the septal puncture at a point lower than the initial puncture.

Figure 4 shows sequential frames obtained from 2D-Echocardiographic monitoring illustrating the balloon catheter inserted through the mitral

Transvenous Mitral Commissurotomy

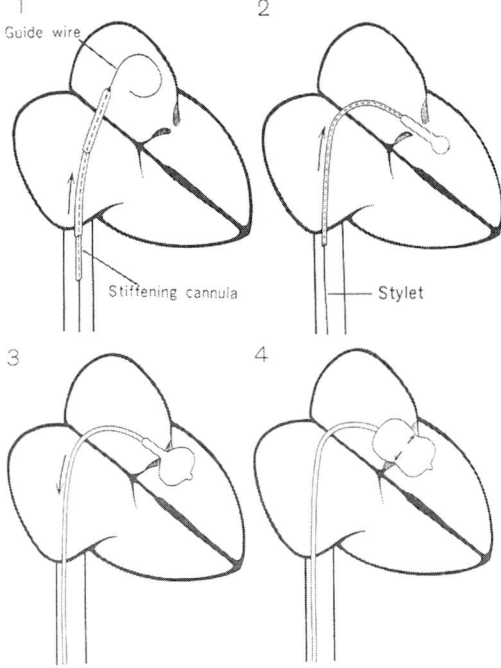

Fig. 2. Manipulation of the balloon catheter.

1. A special guide wire is percutaneously inserted into the left atrium by using the transseptal catheter technique. A 16F-dilater is inserted over the guide wire to dilate the puncture holes of the groin and the atrial septum. The balloon catheter, with a stiffening cannula inserted, is percutaneously inserted over the guide wire and pushed into the left atrium.

2. Then the guide wire and the stiffening cannula are exchanged for a curved stylet to direct the balloon toward the mitral orifice.

At that time, the tip of the balloon is slightly inflated with carbon dioxide gas in the same way as a direct flow balloon-tip catheter. (See Fig. 1-C).

3. Once inserted in the left ventricle, the distal half of the balloon is inflated with the diluted contrast medium. It is pulled until some resistance is felt, to bring it into contact with the mitral valve.

4. With further infusion, the balloon is inflated to full extent across the mitral orifice and thereby separates the fused commissures.

orifice, and subsequent dilating manipulation. The echo from the deflated balloon in the left ventricle is clearly shown in Fig. 4A. When the distal portion of the balloon is inflated, the echo reflects from its only side near the transducer. Fig. 4B and 4C show the distally inflated balloon placed in the cavity of the left ventricle and attached to the anterior mitral leaflet. After proper balloon placement is confirmed by the echocardiographic monitoring above mentioned, the balloon is inflated fully in place.

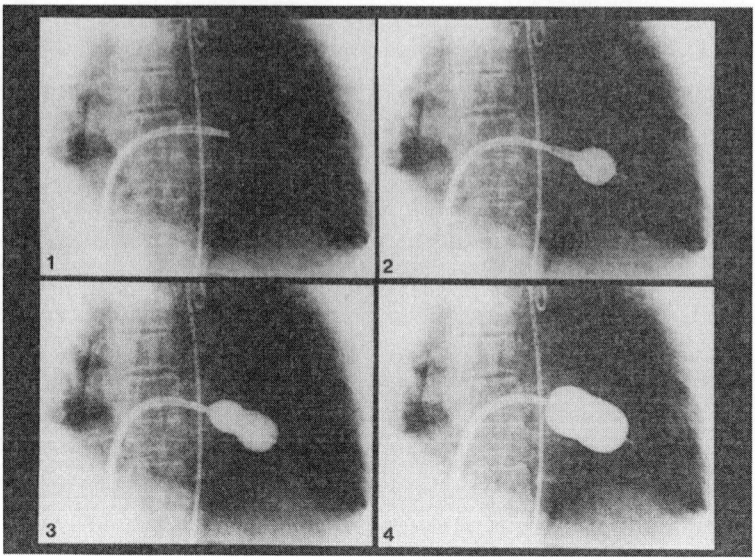

Fig. 3. Sequential frames from cineangiography obtained during balloon mitral commissurotomy. 1, The deflated balloon positioned in the left ventricle. 2, The distally inflated balloon attached to the mitral orifice. 3, and 4, Inflation and full inflation across the mitral orifice.

2D-Echocardiographic monitoring for PTMC was carried out in five patients early in the series of PTMC. The results showed that the new balloon catheter was easily and properly placed across the mitral valve and its position was maintained during dilatation, by the changes of balloon shape. On the basis of these studies, the subsequent PTMC procedure has been successfully performed with manual sensing without 2D-Echocardiographic monitoring. However, it is still advisable to use the 2D-Echocardiographic monitoring during initial trials of PTMC until enough experience is gained.

2D-Echocardiographic assessment of mitral stenosis

It is well established that 2D-Echocardiography is a reliable method for assessment of mitral stenosis [8–12]. We selected the patients by means of 2D-Echocardiography, assessing the pliability of the valve, calcification, subvalvular lesions and mitral valve orifice area.

Two-dimensional mitral valve echocardiography was recorded in the standard manner of long axis and short axis view. The long axis view was

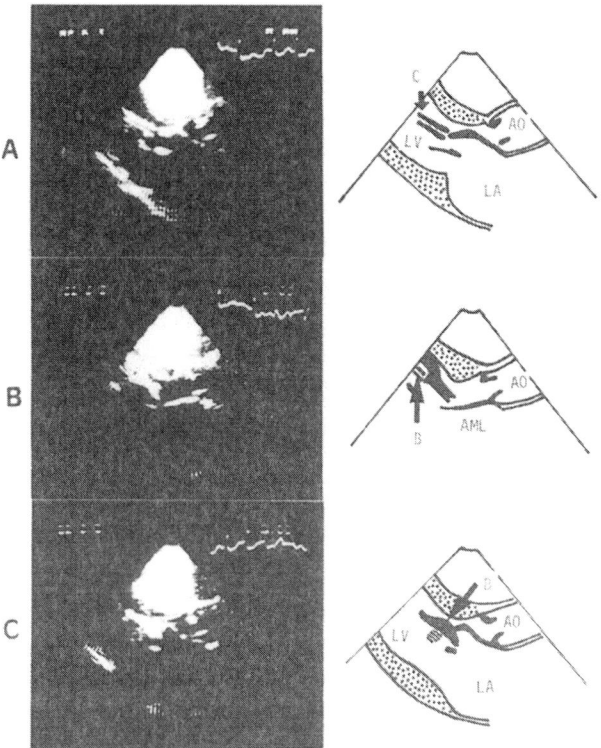

Fig. 4. Sequential frames from two-dimensional echocardiography in the parasternal long-axis view obtained during PTMC. A, Echo originating from the deflated balloon (arrow) positioned in the left ventricle. B, The distally inflated balloon (arrow) in the left ventricle. C, The distally inflated balloon (arrow) attached to the mitral orifice. Ao – Aorta, LV – Left ventricle, LA – Left atrium, AMC – Anterior mitral leaflet.

obtained in the direction at the scan along the long axis of the left ventricle at the mid portion of the anterior leaflet, and at the posterior mitral commissure of necessary. It was difficult to obtain the long axis view at the anterior commisure in most cases. Pliability of the anterior leaflet is judged by the dome formation of the echo from the anterior leaflet in the long axis view. Severe subvalvular lesions (fusion and shortening of chordae) are judged by a mass formation of echo from the free edge and subvalvular apparatus in the long axis view. The mitral valve orifice area was measured by planimetry of the internal margin of the echos from the structure on the short axis view. Calcification and its localization was suggested by a considerably dense echo in the long and short axis view.

Balloon mitral commissurotomy under direct vision in comparing the intra-operative finding with 2D-Echocardiographic assessment of mitral valve before and after the operation

The capacity of the balloon to separate fused commissures was evaluated by using it under direct vision as an auxiliary means of open mitral commissurotomy. These manipulations were conducted on eight patients with Sellers type I and type II mitral stenosis (Table I). These patients had 2D-Echocardiography before and after the operation.

Preoperative evaluation of mitral stenosis by 2D-Echocardiography was roughly concordant with intraoperative findings. Patient 7 had pliable leaflets but small nodular calcifications at the whole tip of the leaflets. Preoperative echocardiography of this patient showed pliable leaflets but a significant thickening of the tip of leaflet in the long axis view (Fig. 5). The fusion of both commissures in this patient was so tough as to be resistant to the balloon commissurotomy with usual pressure. After repeated dilatation with much higher pressure, the posterior commissure was separated by 50% of the total fusion but the posterior leaflet was ruptured about 5 mm with the fused anterior commissure unaffected. Mild regurgitation was found by flushing saline through the left ventricular vent. Therefore, in the dilating manipulation of PTMC, if the waist of the balloon due to restricted mitral orifice

Table 1. Extent of commissural separation achieved by using the balloon catheter under direct vision.

Case No.	Body weight (kg)	Patho-logical severity*	Diameter of mitral orifice (mm)		Extent of separation (%)		Diameter of balloon (mm)
			Pre-dilatation	Post-dilatation	Anterior commissure	Posterior commissure	
1	41	I	9	26	75	50	25×20*
2	38	II	9	26	0	100	25×20*
3	59	II	18	26	100	25	25×20*
4	66	II	14	27	100	50	28×20*
5	49	II	18	29	100	100	27+
6	42	II	8	27	50	100	26+
7	55	II	14	26	–	50	29+
8	61	II	20	26	100	0	26+

* Longer diameter and shorter diameter in cross section of the pillow-shaped balloon at inflation.
+ Diameter in cross section of the barrel-shaped balloon at inflation.
* Classification of Sellers, in which patholigical changes of the mitral valve are classified into three groups from the pliable valve to the rigid one as types I, II and III (13).

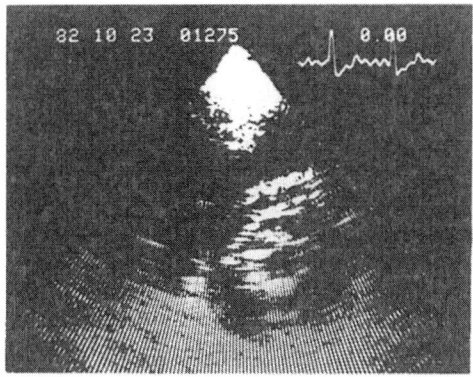

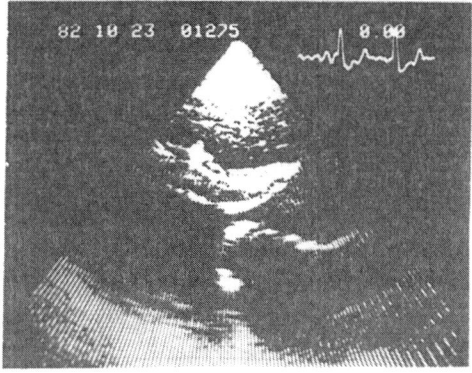

Fig. 5. 2D-Echocardiograms obtained from patient 7 showing a pliable leaflet but significant thickening of the tip of the leaflet in the long axis view. (Bottom).

remains unchanged even at full inflation with usual pressure, further dilatation by using the balloon with extremely high pressure might result in rupture of the leaflets. In the remaining seven patients, the fused commissures were separated correctly along their natural lines without any injury to the leaflets or tearing of the chordae.

At least one of the two commissures was adequately separated in each patient. The degree of separation in the other commissure ranged from negligible to complete depending on the severity of the lesion. There were severe subvalvular fusions and/or localized calcification at the unseparated commissure in patients 2, 3 and 8 (Fig. 6). If a further attempt is made to open such valves by using a balloon of wider diameter, the attachments of the already opened commissure may be torn without the other undivided commissure being affected, leading to regurgitation. Therefore when transvenous mitral commissurotomy is performed, the balloon should be inflated stepwise toward its maximal size, and after each step of dilatation, the effect should be evaluated by means of pressure measurement, 2D-Echocardiog-

74

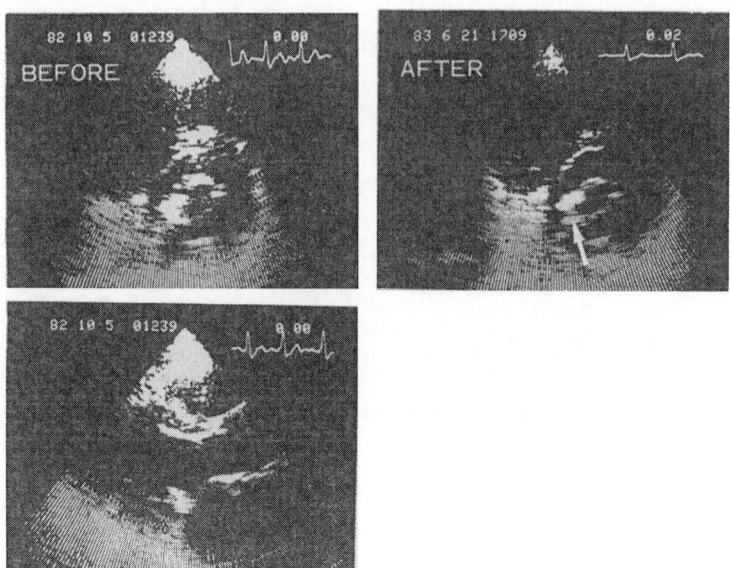

Fig. 6. 2D-Echocardiograms obtained before and after the open mitral commissurotomy in patient 8. Severe calcifications localized at the posterior commissure are shown in the short axis view (top, left), and severe subvalvular lesions at the same commissure in the long axis view. The anterior commissure was completely separated by the intraoperative balloon dilatation but the posterior commissure was unaffected.

The sharp incision was added in the posterior commissure and its subvalvular fusion. 2D-Echocardiogram in the short axis view after the operation shows a good opening of the anterior commissure divided by the balloon, but a slit-like opening (arrow) of the posterior commissure divided by sharp incision (top, right).

raphy and auscultation to detect a heart murmur. In this way, the degree of resultant regurgitation would be minimized, even if it should occur.

2D-Echocardiographic assessment of PTMC

From June, 1982 to September 1986, 38 patients underwent PTMC in Japan and in the People's Republic of China. All the patients had 2D-Echocardiography before and after the procedure as well as pressure measurement. The patients early in the clinical series of PTMC had mitral stenosis of various severity from a pliable valve to rigid one. The balloon sizes used for the early series ranged wide, from 22.5 to 28 mm in diameter.

In this preliminary study, the results were evaluated in morphology and hemodynamic function by using 2D-Echocardiography and catheterization. PTMC appeared to be an effective method for the patients with pliable valves but less significant for the patients with rigid and/or widely calcified valves.

After the preliminary clinical studies, 19 patients underwent PTMC from November, 1985 to June, 1986 at Guangdong, People's Republic of China. Most of these patients had mitral stenosis with pliable leaflets, no significant calcifications and no severe subvalvular lesions. The balloon size used for this series was between 26 and 29 mm. The summary of the results of PTMC in the series is as follows. Mitral valve orifice area was 1.32 ± 0.32 and 2.11 ± 0.41 cm pre- and post-PTMC (P 0.001) by 2D-Echocardiographic evaluation, mean left atrial pressure measured 20.33 ± 6.91 and 6.81 ± 4.34 mmHg (P 0.001). Mitral valve gradient was 16.97 ± 6.40 and 3.04 ± 3.40 mmHg (P 0.001), pulmonary systolic pressure was $46.95 \pm 19,56$ and 27.70 ± 12.17 mmHg (P 0.001) and cardiac capacity changed from class II or III to class I, except for one who changed from class III to class II. One patient had mild mitral requrgitation after PTMC. All patients had significant clinical improvement during following period.

Conclusions

The applicability of transvenous mitral commissurotomy depends on the condition of the valve, which can be conveniently evaluated by 2D-Echocardiography. We have carefully investigated this problem on the basis of our clinical experience of balloon commissurotomy performed either under direct vision or transvenously, and also by taking into account published information on closed, open and percutaneous mitral commissurotomy [2–7, 14–18].

Pliable valves without significant calcification nor severe subvalvular fusions are suitable for PTMC. Pliable valves with calcified lesions localized at one commissure and/or with subvalvular fusions at the same commissure are almost always suitable for the procedure. However, the results may not be as good as for the cases mentioned above. For rigid and/or widely calcified valves, PTMC would be less effective, theoretically. However, some examples have shown that significant clinical improvement could be obtained even in such cases as encountered in this and other institutes [6–7]. Therefore, it would be worthwhile to try PTMC in those cases with sufficient cautions.

As the size of balloon has to be adjusted for each patient, 2D-Echocardiography is very useful to this end. The analysis provides clues to the valve condition, which is a crucial factor for balloon selection. As an example, for a valve with calcification or severe subvalvular lesion in one commissure, a relatively small balloon should be used so as to separate the other commissure selectively to the most appropriate extents.

References

1. Inoue K, Owaki T, Nakamura T, Kitamura F, Miyamoto N: Clinical application of transvenous mitral commmissurotomy by a new balloon catheter. J Thorac Cardiovasc Surg 87: 394–402, 1984.
2. Lock JE, Khalilullah M, Shrivastava S, Bahl V, Keane JF: Percutaneous catheter commissurotomy in rheumatic mitral stenosis. N Engl J Med 313: 1515–1518, 1985.
3. Babic UU, Pejcic P, Djurisic Z, Vucinic M, Grujicic SM: Percutaneous transarterial balloon valvuloplasty for mitral valve stenosis. Am J Cardiol 57: 1101–1104, 1986.
4. Zaibag MA, Ribeiro PA, Kasab SA, Fagih MRA: Percutaneous double-balloon mitral valvotomy for rheumatic mitral-valve stenosis. Lancet 5: 757–761, 1986.
5. Kveselis DA, Rocchini AP, Beekman R, Snider AR, Crowley D, Dick M, Rosenthal A: Balloon angioplasty for congenital and rheumatic mitral stenosis. Am J Cardiol 57: 348–350, 1986.
6. Mckay RG, Lock JE, Keane JF, Safian RD, Aroesty JM, Grossman W: Percutaneous mitral valvuloplasty in an adult patient with calcific rheumatic mitral stenosis. J Am Coll Cardiol 7: 1410–1415, 1986.
7. Palacios IF, Lock JE, Keane JF, Block PC: Percutaneous transvenous balloon valvotomy in a patient with severe calcific mitral stenosis. J Am Coll Cardiol 7: 1416–1419, 1986.
8. Henry WL, Griffith JM, Michaelis LL, McIntosh CL, Morrow AG, Epstein SE: Measurement of mitral orifice area in patients with mitral valve disease by real-time, two-dimensional echocardiography. Circulation 51: 827–831, 1975.
9. Nichol PM, Gilbert BW, Kisslo JA: Two dimensional echocardiographic assessment of mitral stenosis. Circulation 55: 120–128, 1977.
10. Martin RP, Rakowski H, Kleiman JH, Beaver W, London E, Popp RL: Reliability and reproducibility of two dimensional echocardiographic measurement of the stenotic mitral valve orifice area. Am J Cardiol 43: 560–568, 1979.
11. Heger JJ, Wann LS, Weyman AE, Dillon JC, Feigenbaum H: Long-term changes in mitral valve area after successful mitral commissurotomy. Circulation 59: 443–448, 1979.
12. Okamura K, Fukuda I, Maeta H, Mitsui T, Hori M: Two-Dimensional Echocardiographic evaluation of the severity of mitral stenosis with reference to the prediction for mitral valve commissurotomy or replacement. Clin. Cardiol. 9: 99–105, 1986.
13. Sellors TH, Bedford DE, Somerville W: Valvotomy in the treatment of mitral stenosis. Br Med J2: 1059–1067, 1953.
14. Ellis LB, Singh JB, Morales DD, Harken DE: Fifteen-to-twenty-year study of one thousand patients undergoing closed mitral valvuloplasty. Circulation 48: 357–364, 1973.
15. Mullin EM, Glancy DL, Higgs LM, Epstein SE: 1972, Current results of operation for mitral stenosis. Clinical and hemodynamic assessments in 124 consecutive patients treated by closed commissurotomy, open comissurotomy, or valve replacement. Circulation 46: 298–308, 1972.
16. Ankeney JL: Indications for closed or open-heart surgery for mitral stenosis. Review of 152 operated cases. Ann Thorac Surg 3: 389–405: 1967.
17. Harken DE, Ellis LB, Ware PF, Norman LR: 1948, The surgical treatment of mitral stenosis. I. Valvuloplasty. N Eng J Med 239: 801–809, 1948.
18. Hanlon R, Kaiser GC, Mudd JG, Willman VL: 1968, Closed mitral commissurotomy for mitral stenosis. Ann Surg 167: 796–800, 1968.

1.8. Cardiac catheterization guided by ultrasound

I. CIKES, B. BREYER, K. CHANDRASEKARAN, P. J. PEARSON,
J. B. SEWARD & A. J. TAJIK

Currently used cardiac catheterization under x-ray guidance is still a procedure with risks due to ionizing radiation and the potential toxic effects of
iodine contrast agent [1, 2]. Further disadvantages of the method include:
changes of basic hemodynamics due to injection of the large volume of
iodine contrast, lack of intracardiac anatomic details and spatial orientation,
and the relatively high cost of x-ray equipment, space, installation and
maintenance. Having acknowledged echocardiography as the method which
can overcome the above-mentioned disadvantages of x-ray guidance of
cardiac catheterization, the idea of ultrasonic guidance of cardiac catheterization seemed very promising.

The portions of the flexible catheter which are in the scanning plane can
be ultrasonically imaged within the cardiac cavities due to their different
acoustic impedance. In order to perform the safe and precise guidance of
cardiac catheterization, it is essential to identify the catheter tip. As illustrated in Fig. 1 each point at which the flexible catheter enters or leaves the
scanning plane can be potentially misinterpreted as the tip. Some cardiac
structures such as papillary muscles, trabeculae, parts of the valvular

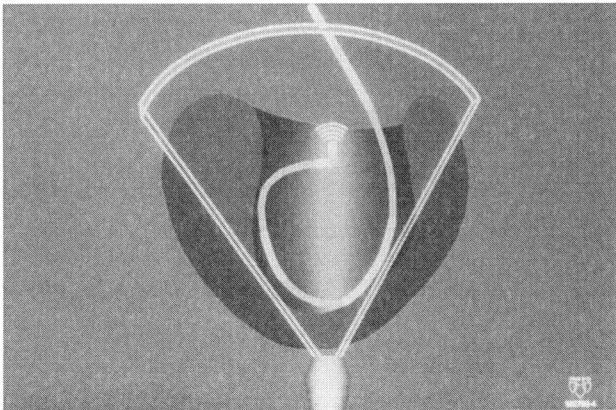

Fig. 1. Difficulties in ultrasonic imaging of the flexible catheter and identification of the
catheter tip. Each point where the catheter is leaving or entering the scanning plane can be
potentially misinterpreted as the tip. This can be avoided by marking the catheter tip.

I. Cikes (ed.), *Echocardiography in Cardiac Interventions,* 77–88, 1989.
© 1989 *Kluwer Academic Publishers.*

apparatus, can also be sources of misinterpretation of the catheter tip. Other possible problems may be phantom or spurious echoes. All these make conventional echocardiographic guidance of catheters impractical and inappropriate.

We have evaluated several methods of ultrasonic identification of the catheter tip. Injection of the contrast through the catheter has proved to be an unreliable method as the catheter tip during injection usually moves out of the scanning plane whereby part the catheter can be misinterpreted as the tip. Marking the catheter tip with a material of different acoustic properties (i.e. metal insertion), acting as a passive reflector, was promising in our in vitro experiments, but unsatisfactory in vivo. This is because of the numerous echoes from the already-mentioned cardiac structures or spurious echoes which obscure the image of the tip reflector.

The basic problem is to detect whether the marked tip of the catheter is within the echocardiographic scanning plane, and if it is, to show this as an unambiguous mark on the echocardiographic image.

The problem of the ultrasonic identification of the catheter tip was ultimately overcome by mounting a miniature cylindrical piezoelectric transducer near the tip of the catheter [3–16]. The transducer is connected via built-in electrical conductors running along the catheter to the localization electronic circuit. The marker transducer is mounted flush with the catheter surface, it is cylindrical in shape, of dimensions fitting the catheter used. Its inner lumen is in line with the catheter lumen to allow blood sampling. It is covered with a waterproof membrane of a thickness (0.1 mm) much less than the wavelength of ultrasound used (Fig. 2).

The catheter transducer can act in active, passive or transponder mode [5, 11–16].

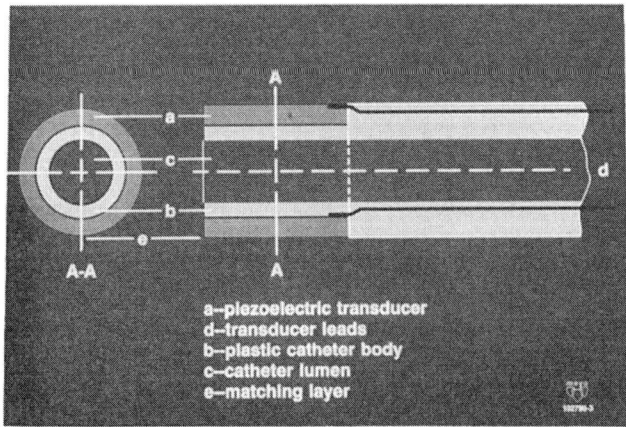

Fig. 2. Ultrasonically marked catheter tip in longitudinal and sagittal sections.

Active localization system. In the active system an external pulse generator connected to the catheter transducer induces ultrasonic pulses which are picked up by the scanner transducer. These appear on 2-dimensional echocardiographic image as a bright line, always crossing the catheter transducer. Although this system is simple and independent of the scanner, its main disadvantages are the introduction of relatively high voltages (up to 5 V) into the heart (necessitating special safety insulation) and the lack of depth resolution.

Passive localization system. This system consists of an echoscope, an ultrasonically marked catheter and a specialized electronic circuit (Fig. 3). If the marker transducer on the catheter tip is within the scanning plane, it is triggered by ultrasound pulses from the scanner transducer and the generated signal is used as a timing signal. It is amplified and taken to a time doubler circuit. The time doubler circuit doubles the time elapsed between the transmission from the scanning transducer and reception by the marker transducer. This procedure then generates a signal at the correct moment to add a characteristic electronic signal to the real-time imaging signal, which appears as a recognizable blinking mark in the ultrasonic image. The mark indicates the location of the marker transducer, namely the catheter tip. The time doubling is necessary to account for the round trip of ultrasonic signals which compose an ultrasonic image. A well-defined blinking marker adjacent to the catheter tip can be seen on 2D-echocardiographic image. It can be easily differentiated from the cardiac structures and is visible at any gain setting. Figure 4 represents a simplified block scheme of operating the passive localization system.

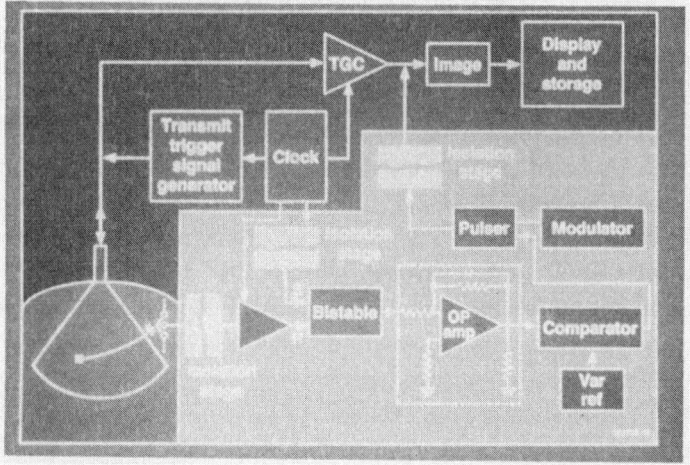

Fig. 3. Block diagram of the components of the passive marking system.

80

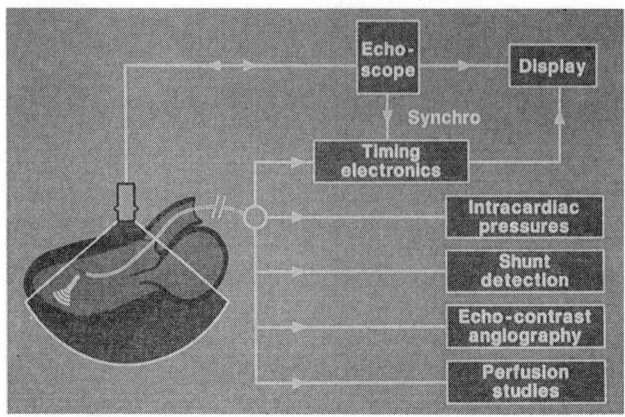

Fig. 4. Simplified block diagram of operating the passive localization system.

The passive system has advantages in that it does not introduce electrical pulses into the heart, it has the best marker properties and a good axial and lateral resolution. Unlike in the case of the transponder, with the passive system the added signal can be of any polarity or form. It can be made black or white or look like any character, which may be important if more than one marker transducer is required (i.e. in electrophysiologic procedures). The disadvantage of the passive system is scanner dependance such that the localization electronics input and output must be designed specifically for each different scanner.

Transponder localization system. A transponder is a pulse train generator triggered by signals from the marker transducer, if the marked part of the catheter is within the ultrasonic scanning plane (Fig. 5). When an ultrasonic pulse reaches the marker transducer, the electrical pulse thus induced in it triggers a pulse generator whose output is taken back to the same marker transducer. The marker transducer now becomes an ultrasound transmitter producing a visible signal, marking its position in the echographic image on the screen. It is essential that the reaction time of the pulse generation be short (in our case 40 ms) in order to generate a mark on the screen adjacent to the marked position of the catheter.

The transponder is not dependent on the type of scanner and it is not galvanically connected to it. However, the signals from a transponder appear on the scanner screen in the same shade of gray as the signals from cardiac structures. Fortunately, this pose no significant practical problems.

Of the three localizing systems inicially tested only the transponder and the passive system proved practically applicable [5].

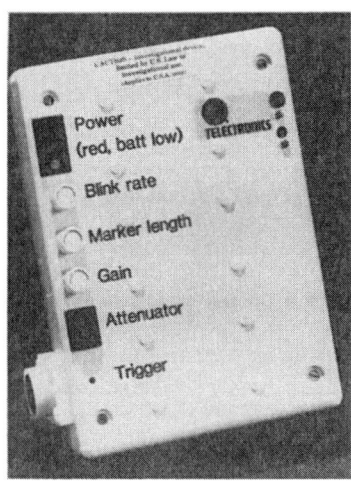

Fig. 5. Transponder box with the marker controls.

Catheter directivity. The measured directivity function of our practical ultra-sonically-marked cardiac cathether is shown in Fig. 6. This effective directivity function is fairly even, without peaks or dips, and contains sensitivity reductions along the marker transducer axis (which coincides with the catheter long axis). This sensitivity reduction (dip) at 90° is between 13 and 16bdB. There is a nearly blind cone along the catheter axis at −90° of less than ± 10° [10].

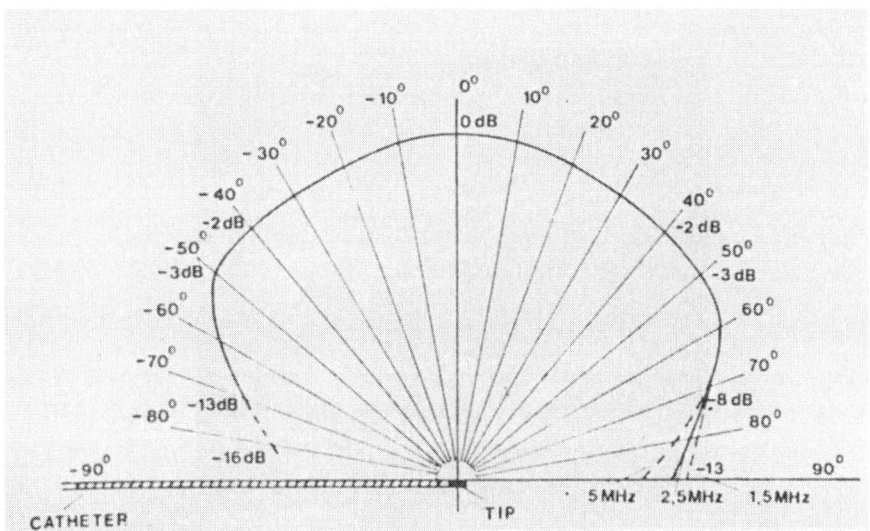

Fig. 6. Ultrasonically marked catheter directivity diagram at 1.5, 2.5 and 5 MHz pulsed ultrasound.

82

Efficacy testing

In 1983 the prototype of the ultrasonically-marked catheter and pacing lead with associated marking electronics was designed in the Echocardiographic

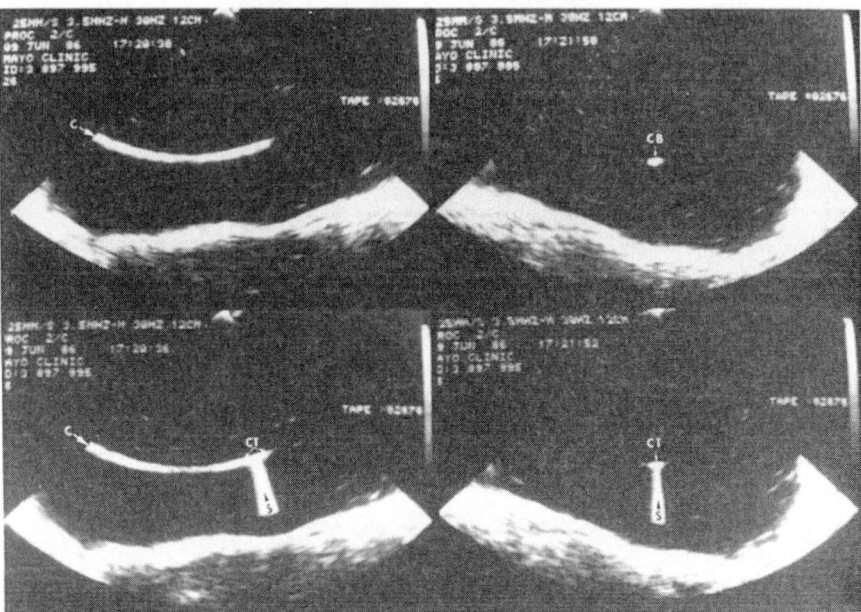

Fig. 7. Long and short axis sections of the nonmarked catheter in the water bath (above). Confident identification of the catheter tip is not possible. Ultrasonically marked catheter in the same sections with blinking signal at the catheter tip (CT). C: catheter, CB: catheter body.

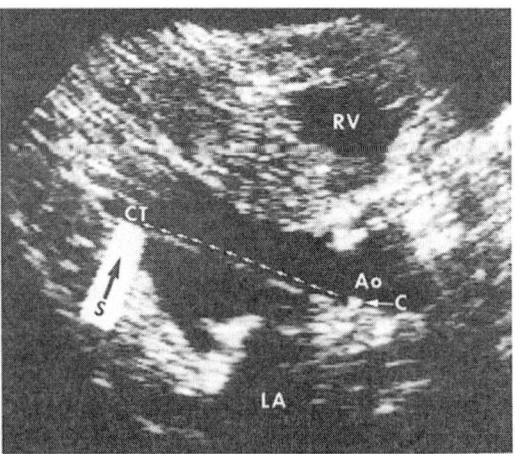

Fig. 8. Cadaveric heart with ultrasonically marked catheter (C) in left ventricular cavity. Its tip (CT) is in apical portion as indicated by flashing signal (S). RV: right ventricle, Ao: aorta, LA: left atrium.

laboratory of the Institute of Cardiovascular Disease, University of Zagreb, Yugoslavia. Later, the marked catheters were manufactured by Argon Corporation, Texas (1984) and from 1986, by Telectronics Inc., Englewood, Colorado. Telectronics Inc. is manufacturing the transponder electronics and recently designed the first small portable ultrasonic scanner with an incorporated PC board for marking cardiac catheters and pacing leads.

The efficacy of the prototype system was tested in a water bath, in cadaveric hearts and in beating dog hearts [3–16]. The study started in Zagreb was continued at the Mayo Clinic, Rochester, USA in 1986 and 1987. During the study, catheters and marking electronics were optimized and with the last version, a well-defined flashing marker indicating the catheter tip was obtained in all instances in vitro and in vivo (Figs. 7–10). The experiments in vivo showed that the flashing signal at catheter tip allows its easy positioning on selected points within cardiac cavities. The rate of successful catheter

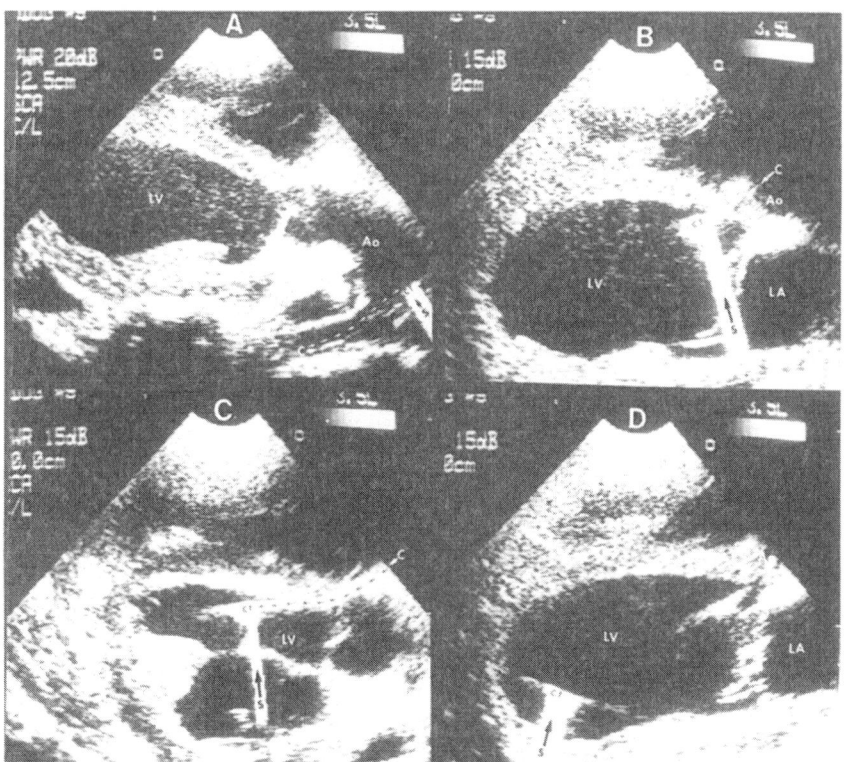

Fig. 9. Sequential frames showing the introduction of ultrasonically marked catheters (C) into left ventricular cavity (LV) of a transplanted canine heart. Catheter was introduced from femoral artery in aortic arch (A), left ventricular outflow tract (B), midventricular (C) and apical portions (D) of left ventricle. S: blinking signal, CT catheter tip, LA: left atrium, Ao: aorta.

84

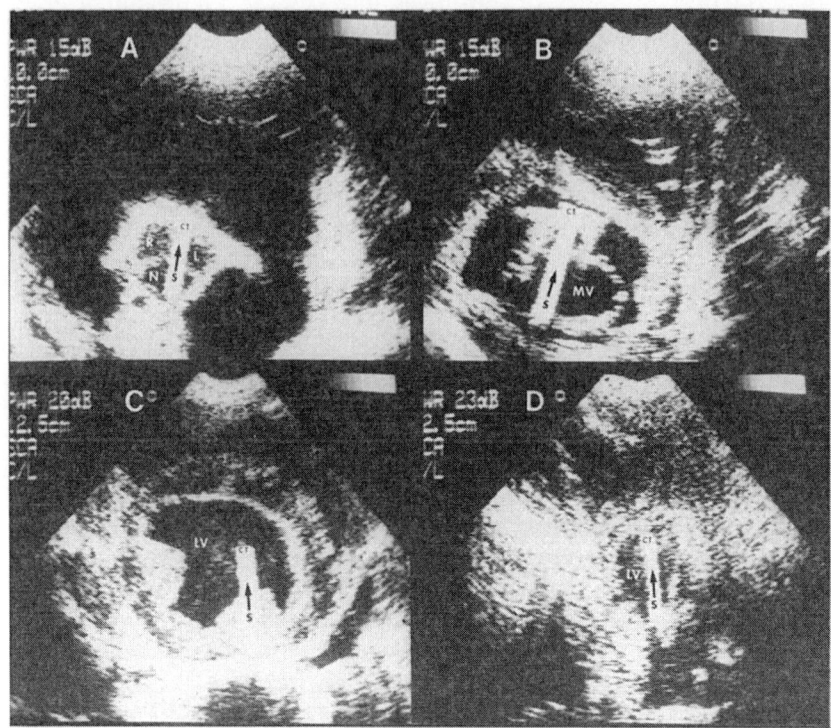

Fig. 10. Visualization of the ultrasonically marked catheter tip (CT) at short axis sections of the canine heart on the level of aortic valve (A). Left ventricular outflow tract (B), papillary muscles (C) and left ventricular apex (D) of the canine heart. R: right coronary cusp, L: left coronary cusp, N: noncoronary cusp, MV: mitral valve orifice, S: flashing signal.

positioning was significantly improved with experience. A small human pilot study done in Institute of Cardiovascular Disease in Zagreb also showed the feasibility of echocardiographic guidance of ultrasonically marked catheters within the human cardiac cavities [7,10] (Figs. 11, 12). Except for sampling the blood for oxymetry, and recording the intracardiac pressures, ultrasonically marked catheters can be used for selective echo-contrast angiography and myocardial perfusion studies (Fig. 13).

Occasionally a spurious mark can be generated on 2D-echocardiographic image. It is caused by retriggering by strong posterior echoes. This phenomenon should not create practical difficulties, since it disappears first at sensitivity reduction because an echo, appearing later, is normally smaller than the direct pulse impinging on the marker transducer.

Using our ultrasonically marked temporary pacing catheters and transponder electronics, Landzberg and coauthors [17] from Schiller's laboratory in San Francisco proved the feasibility of the method in precise localizing of the catheter tip within the right atrium, by comparing its echo-position with

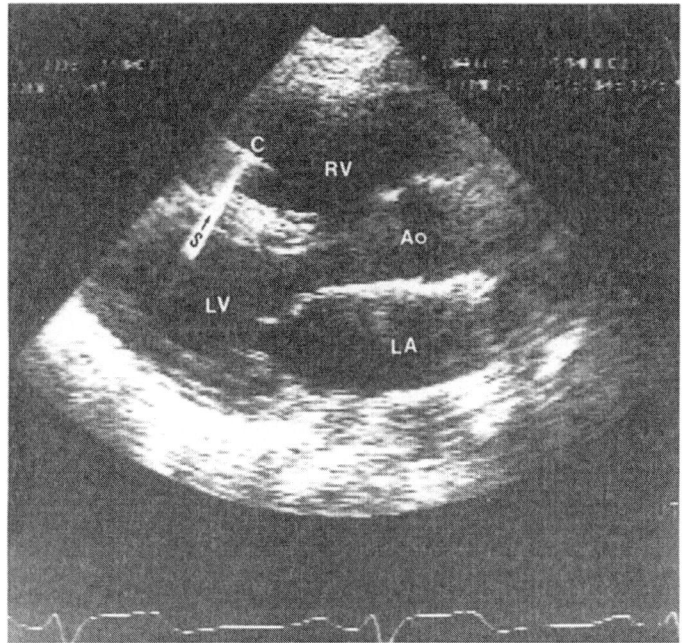

Fig. 11. In a patient with atrial septal defect, the tip of ultrasonically marked catheter (C) is in apical portion of right ventricle (RV). Although very small part of the catheter is visualized, its tip is confidently identified by flashing signal (S). LV: left ventricle, Ao: aorta, LA: left atrium.

the lesions produced by radiofrequency energy delivered at the distal electrode.

Although this method is not suitable for imaging of the coronary arteries, some data on myocardial perfusion could be obtained especially if a more appropriate echo-contrast agent could be developed. We were able to follow the ultrasonically marked catheter in the main coronary arteries (Fig. 13). As a result the idea of its possible application in intracoronary interventions is raised.

For proper use of the ultrasonically marked system one should be aware that the localization accuracy depends on proper scanner and localization electronics settings. In practice, the routine procedure is as follows:

1. A good 2-D echocardiographic image of desired section of the heart is obtained.

2. The ultrasonically marked catheter is introduced with the transponder switched to high sensitivity. In this way, the localization mark is easily obtained on the screen, but with reduced accuracy.

3. Once the mark on the screen indicates that the tip of the pacing lead is near its intended position, the transponder triggering sensitivity is reduced. In this way the localization accuracy is improved. If the localization

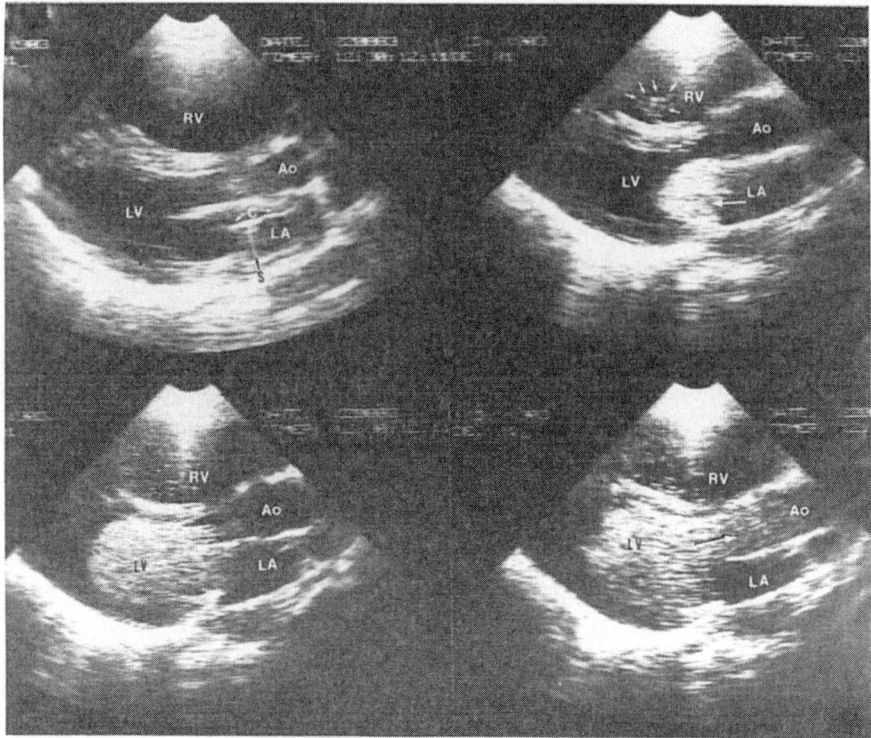

Fig. 12. Cardiac catheterization with ultrasonically marked catheter (C) in a patient with atrial septal defect. Under echo-guidance the catheter was introduced into the left atrium (LA) through ASD. Selective echo contrast angiography was performed and showed opacification of the mitral orifice and early appearance of the contrast in RV (small white arrows) indicating left to right shunt at the atrial level. Below: left ventricular (LV) angiography in diastole (left) and systolic ejection into the aorta (right). S: flashing signal, AO: aorta.

mark now disappears from the visualized section of interest, but appears in a nearby section (this is checked by tilting the scanning probe), then the catheter must be repositioned to the intended position. Controlling the sensitivity of the localization electronics (transponder or passive) is a one-knob operation.

In comparison with the conventional x-ray guided cardiac catheterization, ultrasonic guidance has the following advantages: patients and laboratory personnel are not exposed to x-ray; the potential toxic and volume effects of iodine contrast can be overcome with selective echo-contrast angiography; myocardial perfusion studies could be performed using echo-contrast; instead of catheter guidance in fluoroscopic heart shadow by this method catheter is guided in tomographic sections of the heart with detailed intra-cardiac anatomy. In addition, the equipment is about ten times less expensive,

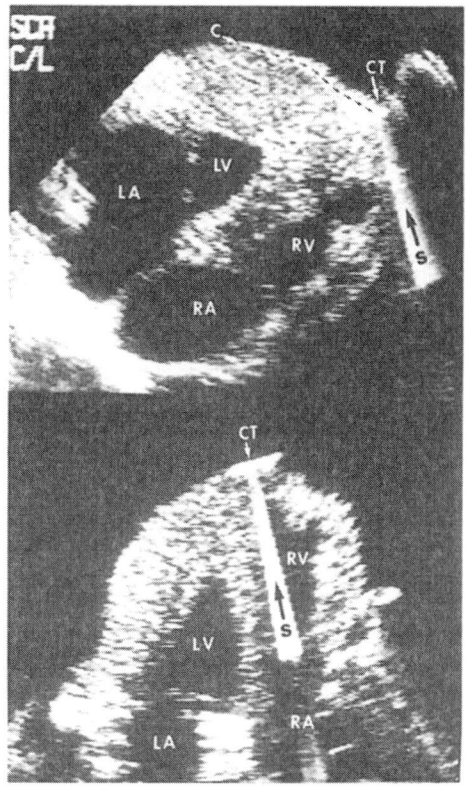

Fig. 13. Ultrasonically marked catheter (C) in left anterior descending canine coronary artery in long axis (above) and short axis (below). CT: catheter tip, S: blinking signal, LA: left atrium, LV: left ventricle, RA: right atrium, RV: right ventricle.

and the cost of the added technology to the basic echoscape is relatively small.

The disadvantages of this method lie in the impracticability of the imaging of coronary arteries morphology and in the difficulties of breaking established habits and switching to new technology.

Future directions

To make the ultrasonic guidance of cardiac catheterization fully applicable, other types of catheter in routine use should be ultrasonically marked. This is particularly desirable for catheters used in interventions (transseptal puncture, atrial septostomy, valvulotomy). Further possible applications of the method are in endomyocardial biopsy, pericardiocentesis, pacemaker lead introduction and follow-up, endocardial mapping and electrophysiologic interventions (see Chapter 1.9.).

88

References

1. Reuter FG: Physician and patient exposure during cardiac catheterization. Circulation 58: 134, 1978.
2. Shehadi WH, Toniolo G: Adverse reactions to contrast media: A report from the Committee of Safety of Contrast Media of The International Society of Radiology. Radiology 137: 299, 1980.
3. Cikes I: Interventional echocardiography. Fifth symposium on echocardiography (abstr), Rotterdam, p. 38, 1983.
4. Cikes I, Breyer B: Complete cardiac catheterization guided by ultrasound. Eur Heart J, 4 (suppl E): 21, 1983.
5. Breyer B, Cikes I: Ultrasonically marked catheter – a method for positive echographic catheter position identification. Med Biol Eng Comp 22: 268, 1984.
6. Cikes I, Breyer B, Ernst A, Custovic F: Cardiac catheterization guided by ultrasound. J Am Coll Cardiol (abstr) 3: 564, 1984.
7. Cikes I, Breyer B, Ernst A, Custovic F: Cardiac catheterization with ultrasonically marked catheters. J Am Coll Cardiol (abstr) 5: 387, 1985.
8. Cikes I, Breyer B, Ernst A, Custovic F: Interventional echocardiography. In: Interventional Ultrasound, Holm HH, Kristensen JK, Eds. Munskgaard International Publishers, Copenhagen, pp. 160–168, 1985.
9. Breyer B, Cikes I: Imaging of ultrasonically marked catheters and pacemaker electrodes. In: Proceedings of the Fourth Meeting of the World Federation for Ultrasound in Medicine and Biology, RW Gill, MJ Dadd, eds., Pergamon Press, Sydney, p. 553, 1985.
10. Cikes I, Breyer B, Ferek-Petric B, Malcic I, Sesto M, Goldner V: Echocardiographic guidance of ultrasonically marked cardiac catheters and pacing leads. In: Proceedings of the Fourth Meeting of the World Federation for Ultrasound in Medicine and Biology, RW Gill, MJ Dadd, eds., Pergamon Press, Sydney, p. 399, 1985.
11. Breyer B, Cikes I, Ferek-Petric B: Ultrasonical marking of catheter. In Recent Advances in Ultrasound Diagnosis 5, Kurjak A, Kossoff G, eds., Elsevier Science Publ, Amsterdam/New York, pp. 95–101, 1986.
12. Cikes I, Breyer B, Ferek-Petric B: Progress in interventional echocardiography. In Recent Advances in Ultrasound Diagnosis 5, Kurjak A, Kossoff G, Eds., Elsevier Science Publ, Amsterdam/New York, pp. 53–64, 1986.
13. Cikes I, Breyer B: Echocardiographic aid during heart catheterization. In Proceedings of 5th International Congress on Echocardiography, Rome, 1986, Dagianti A, Feigenbaum H, Eds, pp. 72–75
14. Cikes I, Breyer B: Cardiac ultrasonically marked catheter, U.S. Patent No 4, 697.595, October 6, 1987.
15. Breyer B, Cikes I, Ferek-Petric B: Ultrasonically marked lead, U.S. Patent No 4, 706.681, November 17, 1987.
16. Landzberg JS, Franklin JO, Langberg JJ, Herre JM, Schiller NB: Echo guided transponder catheter placement in the right atrium. Circulation, 76:IV-192, 1987.

1.9. Ultrasonically marked pacing system

B. FEREK-PETRIC, I. CIKES, B. BREYER, K. CHANDRASEKARAN
& A. J. TAJIK

In order to circumvent the x-ray guidance of a pacing lead implantation and to improve the pacing system follow-up, we have designed an ultrasonically marked pacing system. This development was based on our previous experience with the ultrasonically marked cardiac catheter (see Chapter 1.8.). In comparison to 'blind' fluoroscopic guidance one can expect easier and more precise positioning and follow-up of ultrasonically marked pacing lead tip under direct vision.

A miniature piezoelectric transducer was mounted near the distal electrode of the pacing lead. The marker transducer electrode (fired-on silver or similar) is conductively glued or, preferably, soldered to the thin electrical conductors which connect it along the catheter to an outside electrical connector at the other end of the lead. When the transducer on the lead tip is in the scanning plane it is energized by ultrasound beams from the transducer of the routine echoscope. Thus, generated high frequency pulses are conducted via built-in electrical conductors along the pacing lead to the localization electronic circuit [1–12] (Figs. 1, 2).

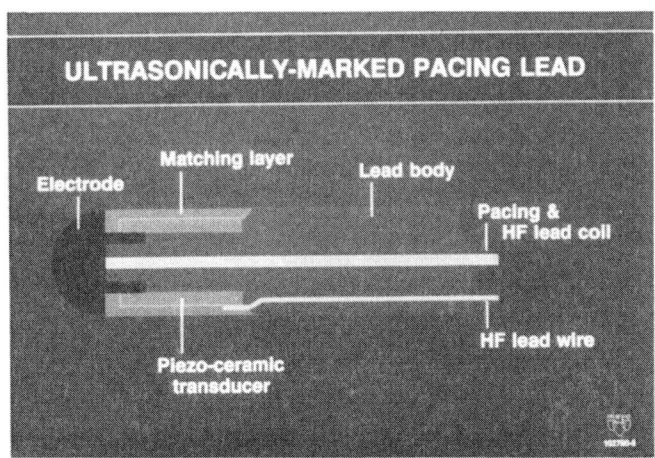

Fig. 1. Ultrasonically marked pacing lead tip.

I. Cikes (ed.), *Echocardiography in Cardiac Interventions*, 89–98, 1989.
© 1989 *Kluwer Academic Publishers.*

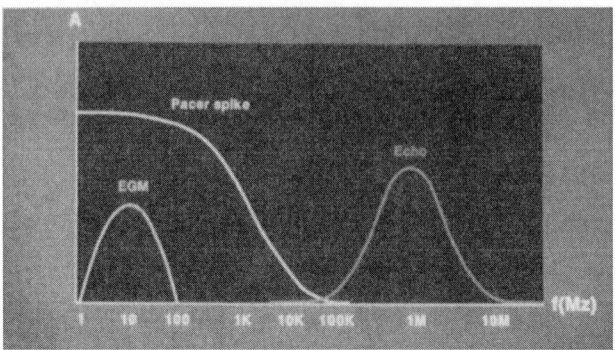

Fig. 2. High frequency pulses from microtransducer at the lead tip do not interfere with low frequency pulses from pacer spike. This makes the construction of ultrasonically marked lead possible.

External temporary pacemaker

An external temporary pacemaker has been designed with either a passive marking system or a transponder marking system as described in Chapter 1.8. The transponder system was incorporated within the commercially available battery powered external pacemaker. The passive system was incorporated within the commercially available echocardiographic scanner having the safety isolation which prevents the harzardous electric microshock. These pulses are used for generation of a clearly visible flashing marker on the two-dimensional real-time images of the heart. The flashing marker always points to the transducer on the lead tip allowing its easy positioning within cardiac cavities. Figure 3 represents a simplified block

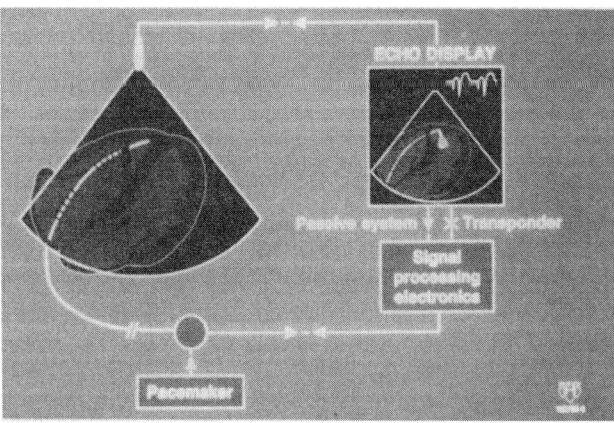

Fig. 3. Block diagram of the components of an ultrasonically marked external temporary pacing system.

diagram of the ultrasonically marked pacing system for temporary pacing. Except for the marking of the two-dimensional echocardiographic image, the operator can also use the intracardiac electrogram displayed within the same image. In contrast to fluoroscopic imaging of the catheter shadow within the shadow of the heart, here one can see the pacing lead tip, as indicated by flushing signal, within a good spatial anatomy of the heart and the close contact of the electrode to the endocardium.

The prototype of the ultrasonically marked pacing system was tested in vitro and in beating dog hearts [1–11]. It was shown that the blinking marker adjacent to the pacing lead tip was visible in all instances. The system allows precise electrode placement at the desired position in right heart cavities under ultrasonic guidance. Apart from lead introduction, the follow-up of its position, the dislocation and microflotation of the lead as well as myocardial perforation could be diagnosed by echocardiography (Figs. 4–6). The advantages of ultrasonic guidance over 'blind' x-ray guidance in temporary pacing include: avoidance of x-ray hazards, direct visual control of the procedure, direct visualization of electrode-endocardium contact, the procedure is time saving, the use of portable inexpensive scanner can make the transvenous temporary pacing a real emergency method.

The implantable pacemaker

Except for the marking of the pacing lead, this system requires a special pacemaker comprising high frequency circuits (Fig. 7). After permanent

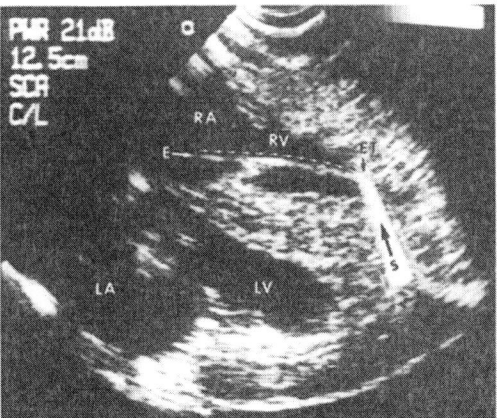

Fig. 4. Ultrasonically marked pacing electrode (E) in apical portion of canine right ventricle (RV). Electrode tip (ET) is in close contact with endocardium. Flashing signal indicates the position of the electrode tip.

92

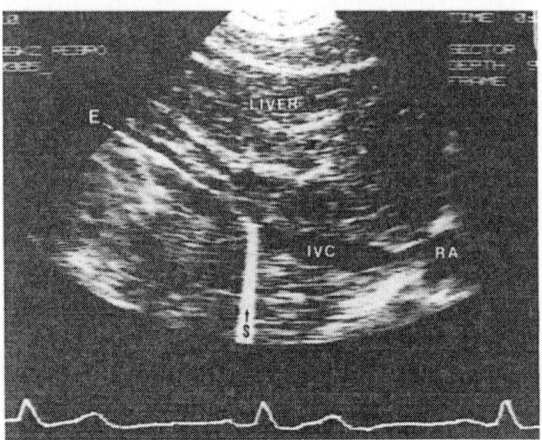

Fig. 5. Ultrasonically marked temporary pacing lead (E) in human inferior vena cava (IVC), inserted through femoral vein, before entering the right atrium (RA).

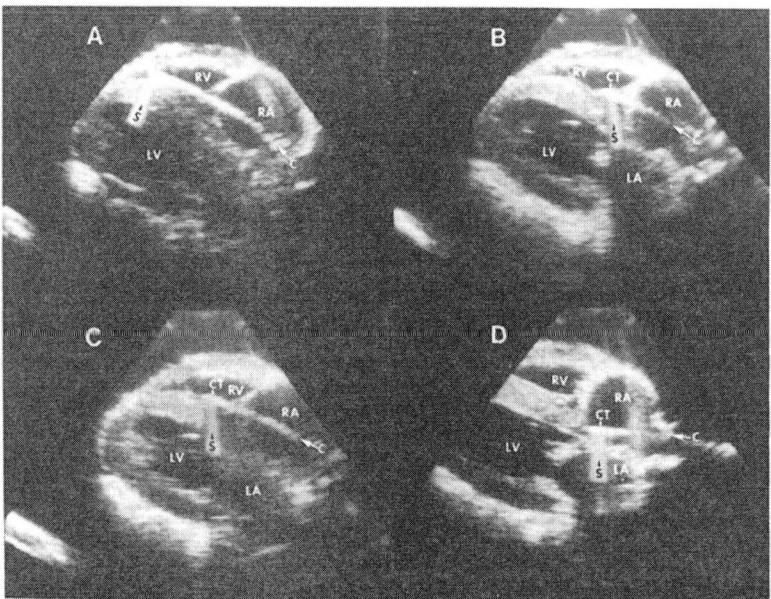

Fig. 6. Sequential frames from canine heart showing the positioning of ultrasonically marked temporary pacing catheter (C) from right ventricular (RV) apex to His bundle position at the base of anterior tricuspid leaflet (A–D). CT: electrode tip, LV: left ventricle, LA: left atrium, RA: right atirum, S: flashing signal.

93

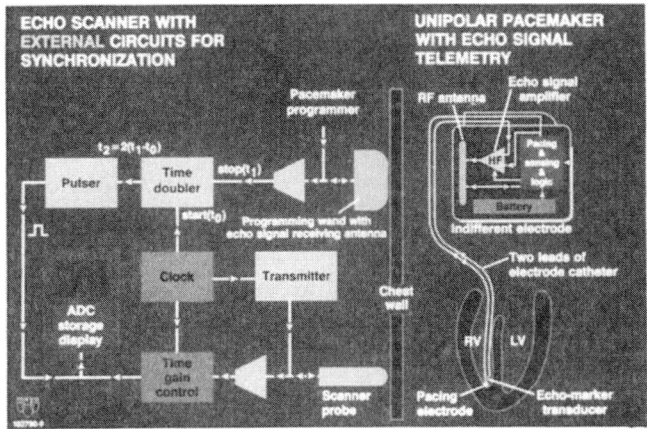

Fig. 7. Block diagram of the implantable ultrasonically marked pacing system. It consists of ultrasonically marked pacing lead, performed pacing batery with high frequency circuits and antena for telemetry of high frequency signals.

implantation it can provide the marking function by means of the telemetry of the high frequency signals. Except for the marking of the lead tip, this high frequency circuits provide the means for detection of a lead fracture [7, 8, 11, 12].

The implantable pacemaker can only be provided by the passive marking electronics (see Chapter 1.8.), which does not significantly increase the battery drain current. Besides the echocardiographic guidance of the transvenous lead implantation, the system provides additional follow-up methods. A simplified block diagram of a permanent unipolar pacing system is shown in Fig. 8.

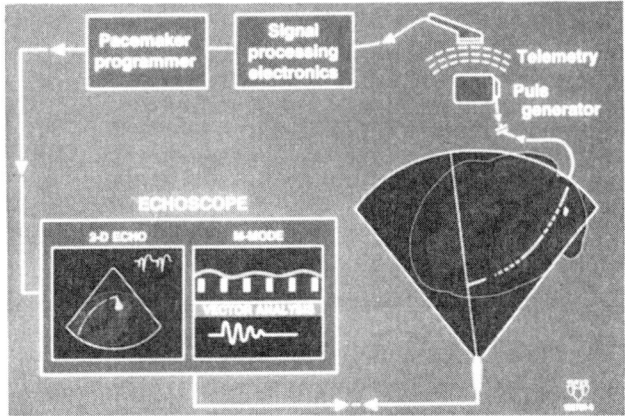

Fig. 8. A simplified block diagram of the implantable unipolar ultrasonically marked pacing system.

Follow-up methods of the ultrasonically marked pacing system

Currently-used methods for detection of a lead conductor or insulation fracture include: ECG analysis, x-ray diascopy, spike vector and waveform analysis, telemetry of the lead impedance and the inhibition threshold measurement [13]. Although these methods proved to be very useful in a pacemaker clinic, the small insulation cracks as well as the early phase of the lead wire fracture cannot be reliably detected [14]. In order to prevent the sudden loss of capture, it is essential to design a permanent pacing system which can accurately evaluate the lead condition, thus enabling the prediction of a fracture.

An ultrasonically marked lead comprises a piezoelectric transducer electrically connected to the pacing electrode as shown in Fig. 1. There are two lead wires in unipolar configuration: one for the pacing-sensing signal and the high frequency signal (connected to the electrode), and another one for the high frequency signal (connected to the marker transducer). Several methods of follow-up are possible, which cannot be done with the conventional pacing system:

1. Marking in 2-D echocardiographic image,
2. Marking in M-mode echocardiographic image,
3. High frequency vector detection,
4. Spike-marker differential diagnosis,
5. Lead impedance measurement by high frequency signal.

Marking in 2-D echocardiographic image. The marker in 2-D image enables the exact positioning of the lead tip within the right heart. The movement as well as the position of the lead tip relative to the endocardium can be visualized. Therefore the myocardial perforation as well as the electrode microdisplacement can be diagnosed.

Marking in M-mode echocardiography image. More accurate diagnosis is obtained by means of the marker in M-mode image. The marker in M-mode image is obtained by adjusting the M-mode cursor on the marker in 2-D image. Figure 9 demonstrates markers in 2-D as well as in M-mode image of an ultrasonically marked lead in a water bath connected to the transponder marking system. If the lead is connected to the passive electronic marking system, the marker appears as the brightest line within the M-mode image. If the marker in 2-D image moves within the line determined by the M-mode cursor, the marker in M-mode image appears consistently. The distance of the lead tip marker transducer from the endocardial wall as well as the variation of distance during the cardiac cycle can be visualized and measured

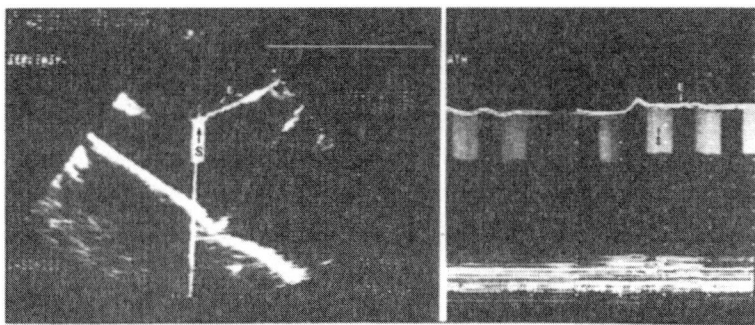

Fig. 9. Marking of ultrasonically marked electrode (E) in 2-D echocardiographic image in water bath (left) and marker in M-mode image (right), obtained by adjusting the M-mode cursor on the marker in 2-D image. M-mode is superior over 2-D technique in visualization of a small dislocation of the electrode (microflotation).

within the range of the echocardiographic scanner resolution. Therefore, the electrode stability can be precisely estimated and the initial phase of myocardial perforation can be diagnosed. Having better time resolution M-mode echocardiography is superior over 2-D technique in visualization of such a small dislocation of the electrode.

High frequency vector detection. It is a noninvasive method for insulation break detection. A unipolar ultrasonically marked lead and a pacing system are shown in Fig. 10. It is assumed that an ultrasonically marked lead comprises lead conductors designed as the coaxial bipolar lead conductors. The central lead wire is a pacing and high frequency conductor, and the outer lead wire is a high frequency conductor. Normally, only the pacing spike vector V_p

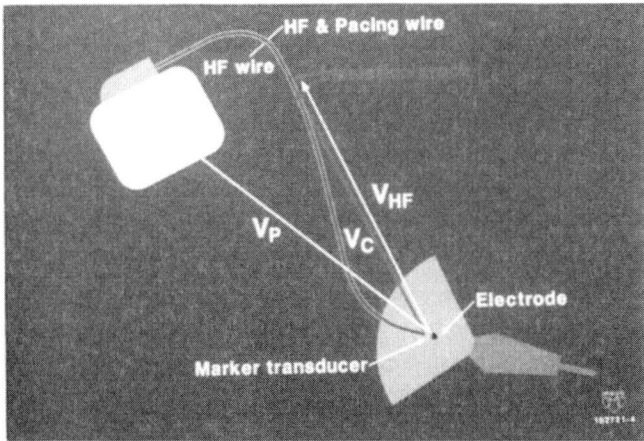

Fig. 10. High frequency vector detection for diagnosis of insulation break.

can be detected by an oscilloscope. In the case of insulation break, the vector V_c will be superimposed on the vector V_{p^*}. The vector V_{p^*} is the one with the same orientation as the vector V_p, but has a decreased magnitude. It is possible to detect the resultant vector of vector V_{p^*} and V_c which does not have to be significantly different in magnitude and orientation, in comparison with vector V_p [15,16]. In our system, the high frequency signal exists on lead wires whenever an external ultrasonic transmitter probe energizes the marker transducer. When the insulation is good, there is no measurable high frequency signal on the body surface. In the case of insulation break, a high frequency vector V_{hf} occurs. This high frequency signal is not hazardous to the patient.

Spike-marker differential diagnosis. Whenever the external probe energizes the marker transducer, a marker occurs in 2-D image. This marker is switched-of by every pacing spike due to the transient saturation of a high frequency amplifier. Therefore, the marker is blinking in rhythm of cardiac pacing. There are several possible malfunctions of the pacing system which cause the marking disturbance, thus enabling the spike-marker differential diagnosis of the malfunction.

If the pacing spike disappears and the marker does not blink, there is no pacemaker output. If there is a normal pacing spike and the marker disappears, several malfunctions can be suspected: high frequency circuits failure, significant insulation break (large V_{hf} occurred), fracture of the outer high frequency lead wire, and shortcircuit for high frequency signal through insulation break between two lead wires. If the pacing spike and the marker disappear, there is a complete lead fracture.

Lead impedance measurement by high frequency signal. Currently-used systems for telemetry of the lead impedance measure the impedance by means of the pacing spike signal. The value of impedance depends on the pacemaker output, the electrode-tissue interface and the tissue conductivity. In our system, there is a high frequency signal source at the lead tip. Normally, the high frequency signal is transmitted only through lead wires and thus there is no influence of body tissue on this transmission. The high frequency signal transmission is more susceptible on the capacitance variation (insulation cracks) than the low frequency signal.

In our system, the lead impedance measurement is done by means of the high frequency internal source impedance measurement. The high frequency equivalent circuit of the ultrasonically marked lead and possible lead failures is shown in Fig. 11. The equivalent circuit is connected to the impedance measurement circuit that is a part of an implantable pacemaker.

The high frequency source i.e. the marker transducer is 'grounded'

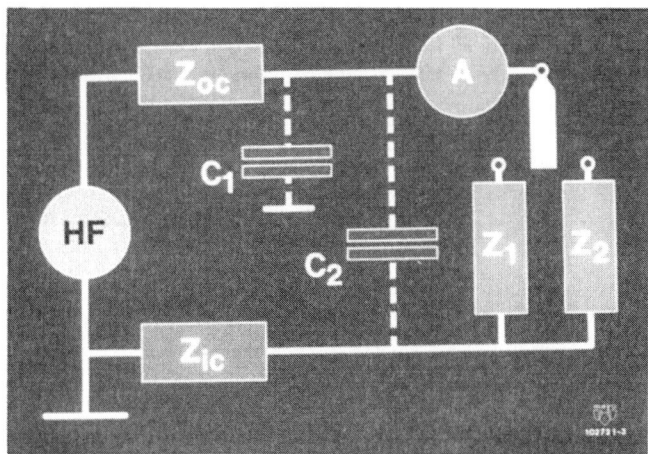

Fig. 11. Diagram showing a lead impedance measurement by high frequency signal.

through pacing electrode to the body. The output signal of the high frequency source is very variable and its amplitude depends on the external ultrasonic probe position and output. If the high frequency source is loaded, the high frequency current flowing through the load can be measured. If two different loads Z_1 and Z_2 are alternatively switched much faster than the source output change, two currents I_1 and I_2 respectively can be measured. The internal source impedance i.e. lead impedance ZL is calculated by the equation:

$$ZL = \frac{I_2 \times Z_2 - I_1 \times Z_1}{I_1 - I_2}$$

If the insulation break occurs, the capacitance C_1 between the outer conductor and the body will change the impedance ZL. If the insulation break between two conductors occurs, the capacitance C_2 will change the impedance ZL. The increase of impedance Z_{oc} and Z_{ic} (i.e. fracture) will also be accurately measured. The measured impedance also depends on the frequency of the external ultrasonic probe which energizes the marker transducer.

References

1. Cikes I: Interventional echocardiography. Fifth symposium on echocardiography (abstr), Rotterdam, p. 38, 1983.
2. Cikes I, Ferek B, Breyer B: Clinical usefulness of ultrasonically marked pacing electrodes, Eur Heart J abstr. 5: 304, 1984.
3. Breyer B, Cikes I: Ultrasonically marked catheter – a method for positive echographic catheter position identification. Med Biol Eng Comp 22: 268, 1984.

98

4. Breyer B, Cikes I: Imaging of ultrasonically marked catheters and pacemaker electrodes. In: Proceedings of the Fourth Meeting of the World Federation for Ultrasound in Medicine and Biology, RW Gill, MJ Dadd, eds., Pergamon Press, Sydney, p. 553, 1985.

5. Cikes I, Breyer B, Ferek-Petric B, Malcic I, Sesto M, Goldner V: Echocardiographic guidance of ultrasonically marked cardiac catheters and pacing leads. In: Proceedings of the Fourth Meeting of the World Federation for Ultrasound in Medicine and Biology, RW Gill, MJ Dadd, eds., Pergamon Press, Sydney, p. 399, 1985.

6. Breyer B, Cikes I, Ferek-Petric B: Ultrasonical marking of catheter. In: Recent Advances in Ultrasound Diagnosis 5, Kurjak A, Kossoff G, eds., Elsevier Science Publ, Amsterdam/New York, pp. 53–64, 1986.

7. Ferek B, Breyer B, Cikes I: Follow-up of ultrasonically marked lead. Clin Prog Electrophysiol and Pacing, abstr 4: 45, 1986.

8. Cikes I, Ferek B, Breyer B: Ultrasonically marker pacing system. Eur Heart J (abstr) 8: 31, 1987.

9. Breyer B, Cikes I, Ferek-Petric B: Ultrasonically marked lead, U.S. Patent No 4, 706.681, November 17, 1987.

10. Landzberg JS, Franklin JO, Langber JJ, Herre JM, Schiller NB: Echo guided transponder catheter placement in the right atrium. Circulation 76: IV-192, 1987.

11. Cikes I, Chandrasekaran K, Seward JB, Tajik AJ: Implantation and follow up of ultrasonically marked pacing system. JACC 11: 5A, 1988.

12. Ferek B, Cikes I: Echocardiography marker pacing system. Revue Europeenne de Technologie Biomedicale 6: 222, 1984.

13. Ferek-Petric B, Pasini M, Pustisek S et al.: Noninvasive detection of insulation break. PACE 7: 1063, 1984.

14. Levine PA: Clinical manifestations of lead insulation defects. J. Electrophys 1: 144, 1987.

15. Green GD, Forbes W, Bain WH et al.: Detection of faults in implantable cardiac pacemakers. Br Heart J 31: 707, 1969.

16. Smith D, McDonald R, Sloman G: Implanted cardiac pacemakers: experience with electronic testing. Cardiovasc Res 5: 236, 1971.

1.10. Transcatheter laser angioplasty and related techniques guided by echocardiography

WILLIAM J. BOMMER, GARRETT LEE, MING C. CHAN,
REGINALD I. LOW & DEAN T. MASON

Introduction

The feasibility of human laser radiation has opened up a variety of new areas of medical research. Within the cardiovascular field both directly aimed laser and catheter-directed laser firings have been used extensively in vitro and animal models [1–6]. Preliminary attempts have been reported in humans and ongoing investigations are being pursued for both catheter-directed and direct firing of lasers in both human coronary and peripheral vessels.

Although these studies have shown that laser energy is tremendously effective in ablating atherosclerotic plaque and thrombotic obstructions, a continuing concern has been the potential of vascular injury [7–9]. A number of techniques have been developed to reduce these problems; they include the use of a central guidewire, the focusing of laser free beams, the addition of cautery caps to prevent free beam penetration, and the use of additional imaging systems to align and monitor the laser firing [10–12]. It is in the search for additional imaging systems that echocardiography has developed as a potentially valuable adjunct for visualizing and monitoring intravascular and intracardiac laser procedures.

Laser therapy

The term *laser* is an acronym for Light Amplification by Stimulated Emission of Radiation. The laser light is achieved by inducing energy into a gas, liquid or solid crystal media. This energy is used to excite the light emitting electrons to a higher energy state or orbit. When the electron steps back to its lower energy level or orbit, it emits the excess energy in the form of a photon or light wave. When this photon approaches another excited electron, it causes that electron to step down to a lower energy level and emit and identical photon in synchrony with the initial photon. Further travel of these photons leads to multiple photon releases of gigantic proportions. The physical properties of the reaction dictate that all the photons will be travelling in the same direction with the same energy or light wavelength. In clas-

I. Cikes (ed.), *Echocardiography in Cardiac Interventions*, 99–115, 1989.
© 1989 *Kluwer Academic Publishers.*

sical wave theory, the wave phase of each of these photons will also be in synchrony leading to a coherent light source. This produces and even greater light energy since all of the light energy is additive rather that canceling as occurs in the more prevalent incoherent of phase variable light sources.

The lasers that have been used in medicine include argon (wavelength 488–514 nm), neodymium doped with yttrium-aluminium-garnet (YAG) (wavelength 1060 nm), CO_2 (wavelength 10,600 nm), and excimer (wavelength 193, 248, 308, 351 nm). Laser sources usually provide a total mirror at one end and a partial (95%) mirror at the other end. These mirrors confine the photons within the system and enhance the light multiplication process. However, the partial mirror allows some light to exit to be used for laser therapy. The exiting light can be aimed directly at the target (free beam directed) or focused into a laser conducting optical fiber. Currently, this laser fiber consists of quartz for the argon and neodymium – YAG laser although other conducting materials are being considered.

Laser radiation on vascular plaque or tissue delivers an intense energy to the molecules. The immediate solid and liquid matter become vaporized while more peripheral material shows charring, coagulation necrosis, and thermal effects further out from the central target. By varying the laser source, pulse duration, coolant media, and target absorption, specific types of damage may be achieved.

Ultrasound imaging

Ultrasonic imaging can be helpful in a number of applications. In the operating theater, direct visualization of coronary arteries and heart chambers is possible. The direct laser beam can be aimed or the catheter system can be positioned with visual imaging feedback. Further, intravascular and intracardiac optical systems have been developed to visualize lesions and the results of the laser techniques. However, they are not currently able to visualize vascular or cardiac anatomy in the presence of blood. It is in this area that ultrasound may prove useful. Ultrasound is unique in its ability to image structural anatomy as well as blood. The low intensity echoes returning from blood do not shadow or block out the larger intensity echoes from wall structures or vessels. Therefore in the operative room, the direct application of high frequency ultrasound transducers may allow visualization of the coronary arteries as well as the intravascular laser delivery system. In addition, transesophageal echocardiography may allow continuous monitoring of the cardiac chambers during an intraoperative procedure.

For non-operative procedures, direct visualization of the chambers or vessels is not possible. Since the laser technique evolved from the cardiac catheterization laboratory, fluoroscopy was the first imaging system used to visualize the laser procedure. Fluoroscopy does have certain advantages; the outer catheter guiding system can usually be visualized since it is often radio-opaque and the anatomy of the chambers or coronary arteries can be visualized with the injection of radio-opaque dye. Thus, the location of a guiding catheter within a coronary artery as well as the visualization of obstructions can be achieved with this system. However, limitations also exist; the quartz fiber used to conduct argon and neodymium-YAG laser sources is not presently radio-opaque. In addition, the relative position of the catheter and laser fiber tip within the vessel the relationship between the obstruction and the adjacent normal wall cannot be appreciated with these radiologic techniques. It is for these reasons that investigators have turned to other means of imaging to obtain more detailed information about laser delivery system position and results.

Ultrasound is fundamentally a different type of imaging procedure than fluoroscopy or angiography. Ultrasound consists of either single dimensional M-mode, two-dimensional (2-D) sector scanning or Doppler examinations. It has been the 2-D aspects of ultrasound that have been most appealing as an imaging technique. Since the standard 2-D sector scan provides a cross-sectional tomographic image, and the relationship of vessels, heart chambers, and indwelling catheter lines can be easily appreciated. In addition, quartz fibers which cannot be picked up on x-ray are easily defined with ultrasound. Lastly, laser firing creates a heat buildup and the creation of microbubbles which are easily displayed with the 2-D ultrasound technique. For these reasons ultrasound monitoring of laser positioning, firing and results has proved useful in the following vessels and chambers of the cardiovascular systems [13–15].

Venous system

Two-dimensional echo can easily visualize the major veins of the cardio-vascular system. Visualization of the veins in the thorax and abdomen can be routinely obtained. For peripheral studies a higher frequency transducer can provide images of veins down to several millimeters in diameter. Although intracerebral veins can be visualized in newborns, the overlying skull blocks imaging in older children. Veins are observed as relatively large echo free spaces and in general biphasic wall pulsations can be detected. Although laser applications for venous obstructions have not been well developed, there are several possibilities of applications. Venous systems can often develop blood clots, and although thrombolytic agents could be tried, the possibility of laser dissolution might be considered in a patient in whom thrombolytic therapy was contraindicated. Blood clots absorb light within the visible range and the argon laser spectrum appears to be particularly well suited for clot destruction [16,17]. Although a tumor mass frequently impinges upon the external wall, occasionally it can be found growing within the inferior vena cava. Selective use of laser might be effective in ablating this intravascular mass. More aggressive therapy might include the development or production of small communications between the portal and systemic venous system in patients with severe portal hypertension. The portal vein can be easily visualized with ultrasound and laser catheter might open up an intrahepatic portal venous anastomosis.

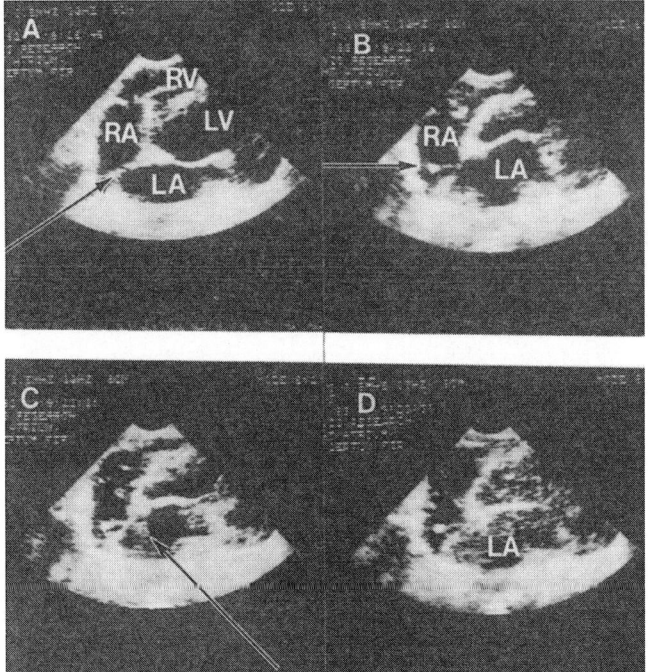

Fig. 1. Echocardiographic views obtained in the dog during laser septostomy. Figure A shows the 4 chamber view with an intact interatrial septum at the arrow. Figure B shows the introduction of the laser catheter as seen as the thicker echo in the right atrium. The thinner echo emerging from the thicker one represents the laser quartz fiber which has been advanced to impinge upon the interatrial septum. Figure C shows early firing of the laser fiber tip and the development of contrast echoes on the left atrial side of the interatrial septum appearing as bright microbubbles. In Fig. D, continued laser firing shows the bubbles filling the left atrium and passing into the left ventricle.
Abbreviations: RA – right atrium, RV – right ventricle, LA – left atrium, LV – left ventricle.
(Reprinted by permission of the American Heart Journal.)

Atrial chamber

Laser catheters can easily be visualized in the veins by 2-D echo and this can be used to direct the catheter system into the atria. Within the right atrium mechanical operations could be performed. Initial studies have shown that it is feasible to create an atrial septostomy using laser energy. In fact, the laser catheter is ideally suited for this since it can be advanced up the inferior vena cava and often assumes a position directly pointing at the intra-atrial septum (Figs. 1–3). This technique might prove useful in babies who require an intra-cardiac shunt for mixing but in whom a preformed Rashkin balloon cannot be passed because of a competent foramen ovale.

In addition to mechanical alterations, laser firing might be applied to influence electrical events. Both the sinus node and AV node lie in close approximation to atrial tissue. Apparent ablation of AV nodal function has been achieved with laser firing.

Ventricular chamber

Within the right ventricle the His bundle can be easily approached. Ablation of His bundle function has been performed with electrical discharges and laser energy firing may also prove useful since the His bundle lies so close to the surface (18). Although this may be feasible, certain problems will have to be overcome before this can be routinely performed. The detection of His

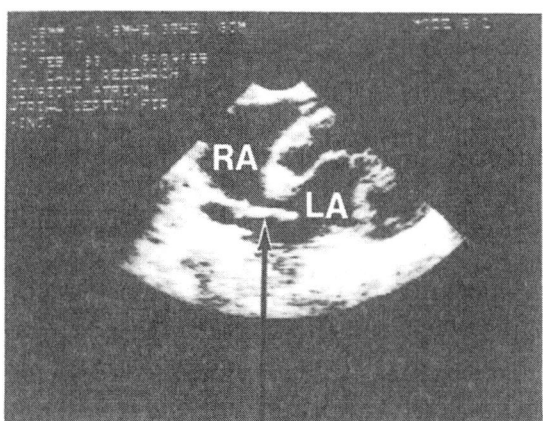

Fig. 2. Four chamber view of the right atrium and left atrium with the catheter position across the interatrial septum. The position of the catheter reveals that it is passed from the right atrium into the left atrium.
Abbreviations: RA – right atrium, LA – left atrium.
(Reprinted by permission of the American Heart Journal.)

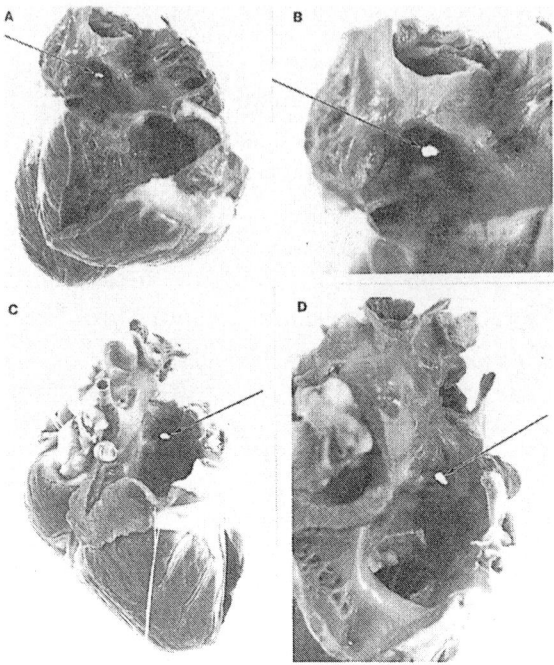

Fig. 3. Intraatrial septal defect. Figure A shows a view of the right atrium and right ventricle and the arrow points to the interatrial septum and its defect. Figure B is an expanded view and shows the roughened edges with dark carbonized border surrounding the atrial septal defect as delineated by the arrow. Figure C shows the same intraatrial defect from the left atrial side as indicated by the arrow. Figure D is an expanded view from the left atrial side showing the somewhat irregular intraatrial septal defect boundaries with slightly carbonized edges. This defect corresponds to the hole shown on the echocardiographic studies in figs. 1 and 2. (Reprinted by permission of the American Heart Journal.)

bundle location is usually obtained by placing a multipolar catheter alongside the tissue and recording His bundle spikes. Electrical depolarization through these electrodes is then easily achieved. However with laser, optimal firing is presently obtained with the distal tip of the catheter. Therefore, the tip would have to be aimed more perpendicular to the chamber wall or a deflection tip or cautery cap would have to be instituted. In addition, the laser tip would have to be movable along the outer wall of the monitoring electrodes to assure that it was lined up at the time of firing.

A second application in the right ventricle would be for elimination of arrhythmogenic foci [19]. This might be more feasible since the catheter tip could be directly aimed or pointed at the target. However, again this would require careful monitoring of the earliest site of electrical activation almost simultaneously with the positioning of the laser for firing. Although this would prove more complex than the electrical discharge systems, the laser shows the possibility of having a better demarcated zone of destruction than the electrical discharge.

Ventricles may often contain clot in the presence of low cardiac output or aneurysm from myocardial infarction. Again, anticoagulant or thrombolytic therapy may remain the therapy of choice. However, on occasional situations, the laser could be used to ablate left ventricular thrombi. This would have to be studied carefully to be certain that embolization does not become a problem during the procedure.

Cardiac valves

Another unique application would exist in performing valvuloplasties (Figs. 4, 5). Within the heart ultrasound is ideal at visualizing the valves as well as the chambers [20]. Ultrasound including Doppler can be applied to quantitate the level of valvular stenosis. Early studies have shown that it is possible for laser to open congential pulmonic stenosis [21]. It should be also feasible to open commissures and aortic valve stenosis as well as atrioventricular valve stenosis. During these procedures ultrasound is especially useful since it provides real time imaging of the valve leaflets, the laser catheter and guidance system, the effects of actual laser firing as well as the results of the valvuloplasty attempts. Both antegrade and retrograde laser passage during ultrasound monitoring have been used to effect valvuloplasties.

In addition to congenital or acquired stenosis, another possible area may be in the eradication of vegetations in infective endocarditis. The laser could be used to ablate the vegetative mass with presumably only the release of small innocuous amounts of gas products. The advantages of this technique

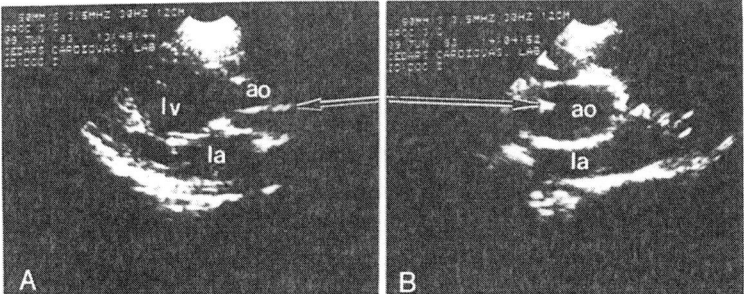

Fig. 4. Parasternal long axis view obtained in an animal. In fig. A, the catheter has been advanced until it impinges upon the aortic valve leaflets (arrow). The catheter position can also be seen in fig. B in this parasternal short axis view. Her it is shown to lie on the medial aspect of the aortic lumen. Both the direction as well as the relatively eccentric position of the catheter can be appreciated.
Abbreviations: AO – aorta, LV – left ventricle, LA – left atrium.

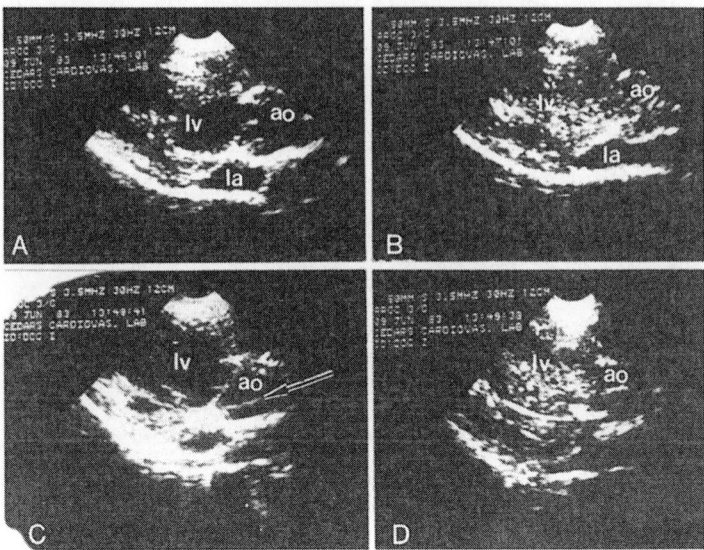

Fig. 5. Firing of the laser catheter in the aortic valve position. In fig. A the catheter tip has been advanced to the aortic valva and lies just below the visible aortic valve leaflet in the aorta. During laser firing in fig. B, contrast microbubbles fill the left ventricle and pass out into the aorta. Both the left ventricle and aorta are opacified. Following this, in fig. C, the catheter laser tip can again be seen in the aorta as it was along the border of the aortic valve leaflets. During a second firing, in fig. D, the left ventricle again appears to opacify prior to opacification of the aorta, which implies that the catheter tip has passed into the left ventricle and created a defect. This defect was confirmed at autopsy and pathologic examination.

would be the limited tissue destruction by the fairly selective laser energy with minimal destruction to adjacent tissue and apparently well tolerated effects of the laser firing.

Arterial system

The area that has received the greatest amount of investigation at this time has been the use of laser in the treatment of arterial disease [1–6, 10, 11, 22–29]. In congenital heart disease laser angioplasty has proved effective in enlarging in vitro coarctations in neonates [19]. In acquired heart disease two types of lesions predominate. The first is the fibrin clot which accumulates following embolization or thrombosis of a vessel and appears to be especially prominent in an acute myocardial infarction. Argon laser is ideally suited for clot dissolution, but whether laser will compete with traditional thrombolytic agents is unknown at this time. The second disease process involves the buildup of complex atherosclerotic plaques which impinge upon the vascular lumen. Within the heart, coronary artery obstructions are the most frequent source of problem. The laser has been shown to be effective in eliminating all types of plaques. Current studies suggest that recent or new accumulations which consist of more foam cells and fatty tissue are very easily ablated with laser. Organized plaques which contain more calcium can be more resistant but ultimately can be ablated with the laser.

The ultrasound has been applied in visualizing the main coronary arteries from transthoracic imaging windows. However, at this time, visualization of entire coronary arteries can only be accomplished during an intraoperative procedure. On the other hand, peripheral arteries can be easily visualized with ultrasound on a noninvasive basis. Thus, carotid and peripheral plaque obstructions can be detected. In addition, the placement of the catheter system within the lumen and its relationship to the obstruction can also be obtained. Lastly ultrasound allows a detailed examination of the plaque, and areas of calcium can be differentiated from areas of fatty infiltration. In the animals, visualization of anatomy, laser positioning, laser firing and angioplasty results have been shown in the cerebrovascular as well as peripheral circulations. High frequency ultrasound monitoring may prove especially valuable in ongoing human trials of peripheral vascular obstructions.

Laser catheter visualization

Although 2-D echo is useful at visualizing veins, chambers, valves, and arteries, it can also visualize guiding catheters and laser fibers. Initial work has shown that 2-D echo can visualize the outer guiding catheter with its lumen and can show the position of the fiber tip within the lumen (Fig. 6). In addition 2-D echo can identify the fiber tip particularly when it is fitted with a cautery cap [12]. Real-time visualization of this cap can be achieved and the

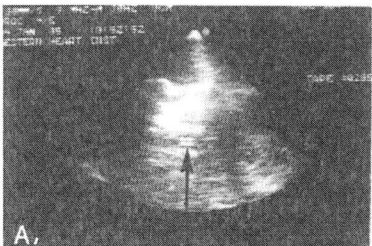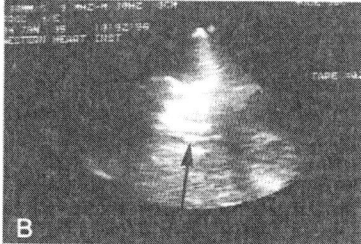

Fig. 6. Two-dimensional echocardiogrpahy of a catheter guiding system within the descending aorta. Figure A shows the catheter wall (arrow) and the luminal area is echo free secondary to being fluid filled at this time. In fig. B, the laser fiber has been advanced through the lumen and now occludes the lumen (the central echo free space disappears). Following this the laser fiber was advanced out of the catheter tip for aortic angioplasty in this canine study.

catheter can be moved back and forth to confirm its position prior to firing.

Perhaps the greatest advantage of any tomographic technique for laser firing is in its ability to predict the central position of the catheter within the vessel or chamber. Both long axis and short axis views can be used to project either the direction of the guiding catheter and laser tip or its position within the vessel. The long axis view allows visualization of the intravascular angle of the laser tip firing and its predicted impact site, which is helpful in preventing inadvertent penetration or perforation of normal vascular wall. The short axis position allows visualization of the catheter within the circular vessel, and is ideal for determining the coaxial position of the system. This permits firing directly along the central axis of the vessel and prevents tangential firing which may lead to vascular wall injury. Ultrasound is also useful for determining the precise distance between the laser tip and the catheter tip. This is useful in preventing ablation of the guiding catheter tip during laser therapy.

Laser firing

Ultrasound provides a somewhat unexpected confirmation of laser firing. Laser firing produces a tremendous amount of coherent light energy delivered to a small target. This results in excess heating and vaporization and perhaps photochemical dissociation of molecules. The resultant heated mass

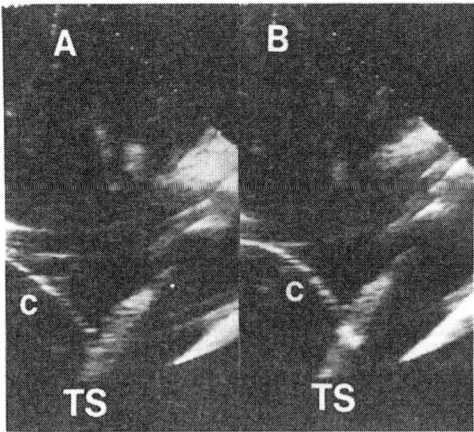

Fig. 7. The laser catheter has been advanced to superficially contact a tissue structure in fig. A. Firing of the laser produces a bright contrast effect within the tissue structure as represented by the bright echoes at the end of the catheter tip. Laser firing produces microbubbles within the tissue crater which persist in fig. B.
Abbreviations: C – catheter, TS – tissue structure.

vaporizes and appears as microbubbles on the ultrasound study [15] (Figs. 7, 8, 9]. Ultrasound is the most sensitive technique, far superior to angiography or other radiographic techniques, in picking up these microbubbles. It provides a unique opportunity to study the actual firing process.

The appearance of contrast can be used to confirm the exact time of the laser firing and show that the entire laser fiber optic system is intact. The disappearance rate of the contrast microbubble effect can be used as a guide to the blood flow velocity within the area following the firing. Both flow direction as well as relative velocity can be appreciated. Presumably much of the gas product may be water vapor. The water vapor should disappear rather rapidly once the bubbles cool. However, residual gases of nitrogen and light hydrocarbons may persist for a longer period of time. By observing and

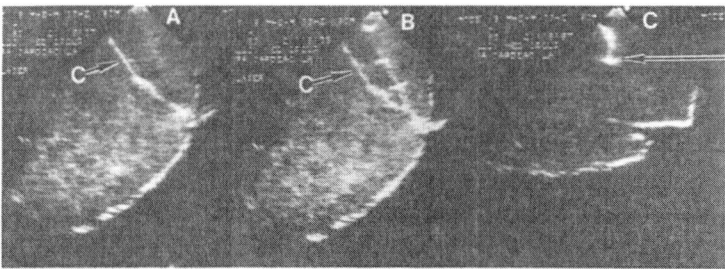

Fig. 8. A catheter which has been advanced into a blood suspension (fig. A). Laser firing produces microbubbles which can be seen rising from the catheter tip to the top of the echogram (fig. B). Following the firing an echo intense mass (arrow) is seen at the catheter tip (fig. C). Pathologic examination revealed this to be a thrombus.
Abbreviations: c – catheter.

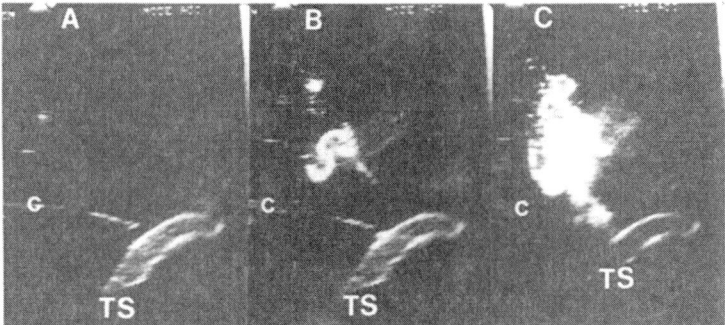

Fig. 9. A laser catheter tip has been advanced to lie adjacent to a tissue structure (fig. A). Following laser firing, in fig. B, a serpentine stream of echoes can be seen rising from the catheter tip and appearing in the middle of the echocardiogram. In fig. C, continued firing releases a barrage of microbubbles which rise from the surface of the tissue into a large cloud which eventually obscures visualization of the original catheter system.
Abbreviations: C – catheter, TS – tissue structure.

110

following the residual contrast effect, a better understanding of the gas process may by appreciated.

In addition to occasional residual contrast bubbles along the vessel wall and the catheter tip, a second less bright but larger and movable mass may develop at the vessel site or catheter tip. This is easily appreciated with ultrasound, and on pathologic examination, this echo mass has turned out to be thrombus (Figs. 10, 11). Again, the use of ultrasound to monitor the thrombus is unique for imaging systems. The visualization of this thrombus is obviously crucially important during the angioplasty procedure. The presence of a clot may interfere with further ablation attempts and may predispose the vessel to early occlusion following the procedure. In addition, the presence of the thrombus may lead to distal embolization. The thrombus on the fiber tip may be subject to embolization when the catheter is removed.

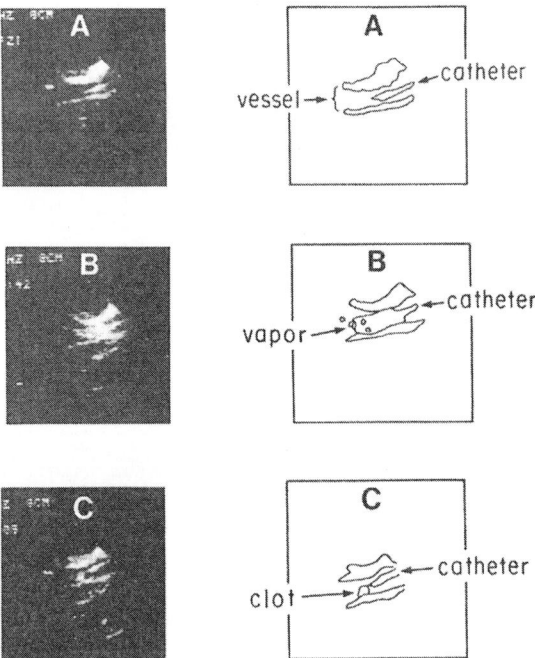

Fig. 10. Three echoes and corresponding schematic illustrations from a peripheral vascular study. Figure A shows the catheter within the lumen of the vessel. Figure B, taken during laser firing, shows an increased number of echoes on the catheter and numerous similar echoes which moved on real time examination. The moving echo targets were interpreted to represent microbubble vapor trails. Following disappearance of the microbubbles, fig. C shows a residual echo on the tip of the catheter. Pathologic examination revealed this to be a fibrin clot which is shown in fig. 11.

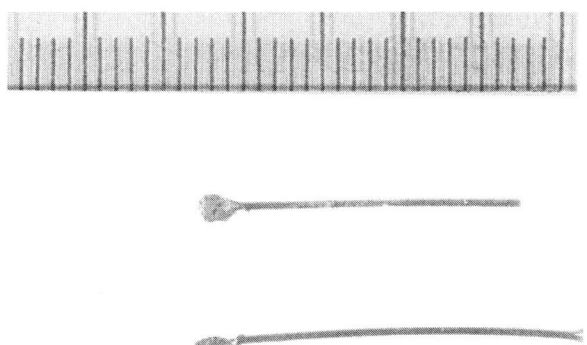

Fig. 11. Illustration of two catheters that were removed following laser ablation. The fibrin clot was found to be adherent to each catheter tip.

Complications

As important as the visualization of cardiac anatomy, catheter position, orientation, and laser firing, is the visualization of complications following laser angioplasty [8, 9]. As mentioned, gas embolization is a distinct possibility with laser firing. Ultrasound is perhaps the only imaging technique which can adequately visualize the bubble emboli as well as the presence of thrombus and its potential embolization role.

Additional complications seen by ultrasound include the indirect detection of coronary artery perforation leading to cardiac tamponade (Fig. 12).

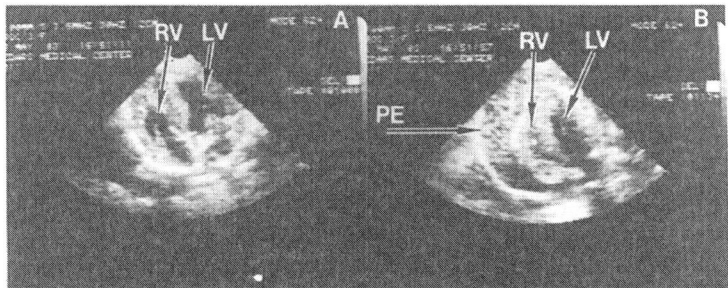

Fig. 12. Two four chamber views in a canine study. Figure B is obtained following laser firing and shows the development of a pericardial space which contains bright microbubble echoes following the laser firing. In addition the right ventricle and right atrium which were easily seen in fig. A, have been almost completely obliterated by the enlarging pericardial effusion representative of pericardial tamponade. The development of this sudden pericardial effusion with tamponade following coronary artery perforation could be rapidly detected using the real time two-dimensional sector scanning image. The pericardial effusion was not echo free because of the bright microbubble vapor trail left by the laser firing technique.
Abbreviations: RV – right ventricle, LV – left ventricle, PE – pericardial effusion.

112

The rather straight and somewhat inflexible quartz laser fibers have difficulty passing through torturous vessels. Both mechanical and thermal penetration of the coronary artery wall have been seen. Following coronary perforation, pericardial blood and early tamponade can be seen within seconds of laser firing. Two-dimensional echo provides an optimal way to evaluate this before hemodynamic changes can be appreciated. Instant recognition of this potentially lethal complication is needed during any angioplasty procedure. Two-dimensional echo may be unique in its ability to visualize both the pericardial blood as well as the results on cardiac function from this dramatic result.

An additional area of complication involves the obstruction or occlusion of a vessel following the angioplasty procedure. Again ultrasound is useful in detecting the development of a clot which will obstruct vascular flow. Visualization of both peripheral as well as coronary occlusions has been achieved. This will provide an early warning to the operator that additional procedures need to be performed. Vascular occlusion could also be monitored with ultrasound Doppler from an external position. The use of a pulse mode or continuous wave Doppler signal to detect blood flow both before and after the obstruction may prove useful in confirming the presence of a successful result.

Echocatheter system

Echocatheter systems using M-mode echo have shown the distance from the end of the catheter transducer to the vessel wall or obstruction. In addition to M-mode range information, small 2-D imaging systems can be assembled on catheters as small as several millimeters. Further miniaturization might allow coronary and peripheral vascular imaging from an even smaller intravascular catheter. These pictures would allow visualization of the entire circumferential wall of the vessel and provide detailed information about orientation and the coaxial nature of the laser catheter. Forward directing catheter tip information can also be obtained with ultrasound. Using either the previously described M-mode system or a Doppler transducer this information has been obtained in animal models [30]. The Doppler transducer has also been adapted to human use. The ability to obtain range gated blood flow velocities in front of the catheter tip before, during, and after laser firing has enabled confirmation of the effects and success of the laser angioplasty procedure.

Laser angioplasty is an especially exciting area of cardiovascular research. It perhaps offers us the very real chance of performing therapeutic maneuvers with a catheter based system. Combined with balloon angioplasty it may allow us to perform therapy on almost all patients with acquired heart disease and many patients with congenital heart disease without requiring surgery. Ultrasound offers a unique opportunity to position, aim, fire, and follow these procedures. The noninvasive nature of ultrasound, the ability to see through blood, the continuous monitoring available with ultrasound as well as its unique tomographic presentation offer distinct advantages over the other available imaging modalities. Perhaps ultrasound may be sufficient to provide the only imaging backup for laser angioplasty procedures. More likely, it will provide a very useful and complementary role to some of the other imaging modalities. Further developments in ultrasound should expand the horizons for its use, enabling safe and effective procedures and enhancing our understanding of laser therapy.

Summary

The transmission of laser through a fiberoptic catheter is a new experimental procedure to recanalize vessels obstructed by atherosclerotic disease or thrombus. However, limitations exist with present radiologic techniques in imaging the relative positions of the laser catheter, the obstruction, and the normal vessel wall so as to effectively ablate plaque without laser vascular injury. On the other hand, since two-dimensional ultrasound can provide a cross-sectional tomographic image, the relationship of vessels and indwelling catheters can be better appreciated. New development in ultrasound can enhance our understanding of laser therapy and enable its safe and effective clinical use in the cardiovascular system.

References

1. Lee G, Ikeda R, Kozina J, Mason DT: Laser dissolution of coronary atheromatous plaques. Am Heart J 102: 1074–1075, 1981.
2. Abela GS, Normann S, Cohen D, Flechman RL, Geiser EA, Conti CR: Effects of carbon dioxide, ND-YAG and argon laser radiation on coronary atheromatous plaques. Am J Cardiol 50: 1199–1205, 1982.
3. Choy DSL, Stertzer S, Rotterdam HZ, Bruno MS: Laser coronary angioplasty: experience with 9 cadaver hearts. Am J Cardiol 50: 1209–1211, 1982.
4. Lee G, Ikeda R, Herman I, Dwyer RM, Bass M, Hussein H, Kozina J, Mason DT: The qualitative effects of laser irradiation on human arteriosclerotic disease. Am Heart J 105: 885–889, 1983.
5. Lee G, Ikeda RM, Chan MC, Stobbe D, Kozina J, Jiang MC, Reis RL, Mason DT: Current and potential uses of lasers in the treatment of atherosclerotic disease. Chest 85: 429–434, 1984.
6. Selzer P, Murphy-Chutorian D, Ginsburg R, Wexler L: Optimizing strategies for laser angioplasty, Invest Radiol 20: 860–866, 1985.

114

7. Lee G, Ikeda RM, Theis JH, Chan MC, Stobbe D, Ogata C, Kumagai A, Mason DT: Acute and chronic complications of laser angioplasty. Vascular wall damage and formation of aneurysms in the atherosclerotic rabbit. Am J Cardiol 53: 290–293, 1984.

8. Lee G, Seckinger D, Chan MC, Embi A, Stobbe D, Thomson RV, Sanchez NA, Ikeda RM, Reis RL, Mason DT: Potential complications of coronary laser angioplasty. Am Heart J 106: 1577–1579, 1984.

9. Lee G, Ikeda RM, Chan MC, Lee MH, Rink JL, Reis RL, Theis JH, Low RI, Bommer WJ, Kung AH, Hanna ES, Mason DT: Limitations, risks, and complications of laser recanalization: A cautious approach warranted. Am J Cardiol 56: 181–185, 1985.

10. Lee G, Ikeda RM, Stobbe D, Ogata C, Theis J, Hussein H, Mason DT: Laser irradiation of human atherosclerotic obstructive disease: simultaneous visualization and vaporization achieved by a dual fiberoptic catheter. Am Heart J 105: 163–164, 1983.

11. Lee G, Ikeda RM, Stobbe D, Ogata C, Embi A, Chan MC, Reis RL, Mason DT: Intraoperative use of dual fiberoptic catheter for simultaneous in vivo visualization and laser vaporization of peripheral atherosclerotic obstructive disease. Cathet Cardiovasc Diagn 10: 11–16, 1984.

12. Lee G, Ikeda R, Chan M, Dukich J, Lee M, Theis J, Bommer W, Reis R, Hanna E, Mason D: Dissolution of human atherosclerotic disease by fiberoptic laser-heated metal cautery cap. Am Heart J 107, 777–778, 1984.

13. Perry LW, Galioto FM, Blair T, Shapiro SR, Ruckman RN, Scott LP: Two-dimensional echocardiography for catheter location and placement in infants and children. Pediatrics 67: 541, 1981.

14. Bommer WJ, Lee G, Riemenschneider T, Ikeda R, Stobbe D, Ogata C, Theis J, Reis R, Mason D: Laser atrial septostomy. Am Heart J 1152–1156, 1983.

15. Bommer WJ, Lee G, Rebeck K, Stobbe D, Ogata C, Ikeda R, Mendizabal R, Reist RL, Mason DT: Two-dimensional echocardiography of argon-laser vapor trails: monitoring of catheter position and prevention of potential complications (abstr). Circulation 68: 259, 1983.

16. Lee G, Ikeda RM, Stobbe D, et al.: Effect of laser radiation on human thrombus: demonstration of a linear dissolution dose relationship between clot length and energy density. Am J Cardiol 52: 876–877, 1983.

17. Lee G, Chan MC, Seckinger DL, et al.: Argon laser radiation of human clots: differential photoabsorption in red cell rich and red cell poor clots. Thromb Res 38: 561–565, 1985.

18. Narula O, Bharati S, Chan MC, Embi A, Lev M: Microtransection of the His bundle with laser radiation through a pervenous catheter: correlation of histologic and electrophysiologic data. Am J Cardiol 54: 186–192, 1984.

19. Lee G, Ikeda RM, Theis J, Stobbe D, Ogata C, Lui H, Reis RL, Mason DT: Effects of laser irradiation delivered by flexible fiberoptic system on left ventricular intend myocardium. Am Heart J 106: 587–90, 1983.

20. Lee G, Stobbe D, Chan MC, Bommer W, Riemenschneider TA, Ikeda RM, Mason DT: Effects of laser irradiation on cardiac valves: Transcatheter in vivo vaporization of aortic valve. Am Heart J 107: 394–395, 1984.

21. Riemenschneider T, Lee G, Ikeda R, Bommer W, Stobbe D, Ogata C, Rebeck K, Reis R, Mason D: Laser irradiation of congential heart disease: Potential for palliation and correction of intracardiac and intravascular defects. Am Heart J 106: 1389–1393, 1983.

22. Coelho JCU, Sigel B, Flanigan DP, Schuler JJ, Spigos DG, Nyhus LM: Detection of arterial defects by real-time ultrasound scanning during vascular surgery: an experimental study. J Surg Rev 30: 535, 1981.

23. Coelho JCU, Sigel B, Flanigan DP, Schuler JJ, Spigos DG, Tan WS, Justin J: An experi-

mental evaluation of arteriography and imaging ultrasonography in detecting arterial defects at operation. J Surg Res 32: 130, 1982.

24. Sahn DJ, Barratt-Boyes BG, Graham K, Kerr A, Roch A, Hill D, Brandt PWT, Copeland JG, Mammana R, Temkin LP, Glenn W: Ultrasonic imaging of the coronary arteries in open-chest humans: evaluation of coronary atherosclerotic lesions during cardiac surgery. Circulation 66: 1034, 1982.

25. Funai JT, Pandian NG, Isner JM, Clarke RH, Lojeski EW, Donaldson RF, Konstam MA, Salem DN: Utility of high-frequency two-dimensional echocardiography in the performance of laser coronary angioplasty-experimental studies. Clin Res 32: 672A, 1984.

26. Sahn DJ, Copeland JG, Temkin LP, Wirt DP, Mammana R, Glenn W: Anatomic ultrasound correlations for intra-operative open chest imaging of coronary artery atherosclerotic lesions in human beings. J Am Coll Cardiol 3: 169, 1984.

27. Ginsburg R, Kim D-S, Guthaner D, Toth J, Mitchell RS: Salvage of an ischemic limb by laser angioplasty: description of a new technique. Clin Cardiol 7: 54, 1984.

28. Choy DSJ, Stertzer SH, Myler RK, Marco J, Fournial G: Human coronary laser recanalization. Clin Cardiol 7: 377, 1984.

29. Lee G, Chan M, Ikeda R, Rink J, Dukich J, Peterson L, Lee K, Reis R, Mason D: Applicability of laser to assist coronary balloon angioplasty. Am Heart J 110: 1233, 1985.

30. Bommer W, Chan M, Lee G, Mason D, Rink J, Rink D, Chin M: Laser Doppler Angioplasty: A New Technique. Clin Res, in Press.

1.11. Echocardiographic assessment of coronary venous retroperfusion

SHEILA KAR & JOSEPH AREEDA

Numerous interventions have been improvised in the last decade, all aiming to decrease cardiac mortality and morbidity following myocardial infarction by reducing infarct size. Aggressive revascularization interventions such as thrombolysis, percutaneous angioplasty and coronary bypass surgery, have recently been performed during the acute phase, with remarkably favorable results. However, it has been established that the myocardium usually will remain alive for only 3–6 hours after an acute coronary occlusion and, therefore, the most favorable results for maintaining viability of the jeopardized myocardium will be dependent on the time elapsed from the onset of symptoms to the achievement of revascularization. It has also been noted that the first 2–3 hours is the most critical period affecting viability of myocardium [1]. Synchronized diastolic coronary venous retroperfusion using specially designed catheters and an electrocardiographically synchronized pump has been shown to immediately improve cardiac contractile and metabolic function and also reduce the infarct size after experimental coronary artery occlusion. This method has been proposed as a temporary clinical emergency treatment of acute myocardial ischemia, i.e., to provide support for periods of hours or days after an acute coronary occlusion, until other modes for permanent revascularization can be performed [2]. It is fortunate that computerized noninvasive imaging using artificial intelligence technology to enhance edge detection can provide more adequate echocardiographic diagnostic data. This now makes it possible to visualize the anatomic site, and quantify the extent of ischemia. It also enables further differentiation between potentially viable and irreversibly injured myocardium to provide an online evaluation of prognosis, and possibility of success or failure of targeted interventions.

Historical events

Experimental detection methods for regional localization and measurement of myocardial ischemia in the beating heart date back to 1935 when Tennant and Wiggins [3] demonstrated that altered ventricular contractile function

I. Cikes (ed.), *Echocardiography in Cardiac Interventions*, 117–130, 1989.
© 1989 *Kluwer Academic Publishers.*

118

resulting from acute ischemia could be observed by the use of mirrors attached to the walls of the moving left ventricle. Prinzmetal and Corday, in 1949, studied the simultaneous alterations in cardiac function against coronary flow by high speed direct cinematography [4–5], and later, nuclear and dye labeling methods were performed in the open chest canine model following thoracotomy. Subsequently, contrast roentgenographic angiographic and ventriculographic images provided much information about cardiac function in closed chest models, thus enabling comprehensive display of cardiac function without thoracotomy. Conventional contrast roentgenographic angiography or nuclear ventriculography were subsequently performed in canine species, and then the human, but these techniques were of limited use for repeat studies because they were considered potentially hazardous due to radiation exposure. In the search for simpler technologies that were considered safer, ultrasonic methods using M-mode echocardiography were attempted to study wall motion [7–9]. By 1980, 2-dimensional echocardiography (2DE) became the simplest, most acceptable noninvasive imaging method for repeated serial detection and study of the progressive alterations induced by myocardial ischemia [10–15]. The advantage of 2DE over other methods was the fact that serial tomographic views of the epicardial outline could be recorded and stop framed at comparable phases of end-systole and end-diastole. Computation of the endocardial and epicardial wall motion measurements was accomplished by several algorithms. These measurements were correlated with the visual interpretation during progressive alterations in wall movement of the left ventricle in both long and short-axis views under various experimental conditions. It also permitted subdivision of the endocardial and epicardial outlines around a geographic center in short-axis views which were subdivided into 8 pie shaped segments (Figs. 1, 2). Differences in area of change of each segment provided a quantitative index of regional anatomic contraction and ejection and physiological function. Thus, practical automatic computations were made of regional changes during each cardiac cycle over prolonged periods that permitted both regional and global measurements of comprehensive physiologic function. It also allowed us to integrate such changes in visual readings with quantitative displays which were validated by autopsy findings. These 2DE assessments provided comprehensive calculations and display of progressive alterations simultaneously with changes in regional and global cardiac function, thereby permitting serial, sequential, global and regional quantitative dysfunction to be accurately ascertained in vivo without thoracotomy [16–20].

Furthermore, phasic and comprehensive display of as many as 6 serial tomographic levels could be obtained corresponding to mitral, high, mid and low papillary and apical regions of the ventricle as well as a long-axis view

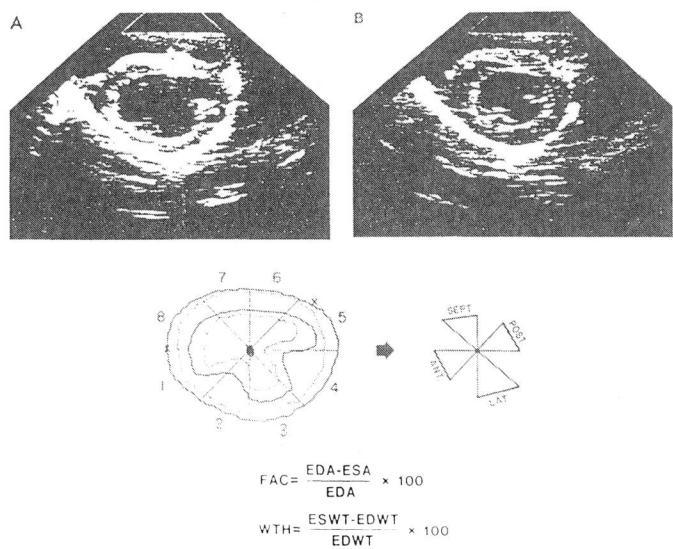

$$FAC = \frac{EDA\text{-}ESA}{EDA} \times 100$$

$$WTH = \frac{ESWT\text{-}EDWT}{EDWT} \times 100$$

Fig. 1. Two-dimensional echocardiography (2DE) short-axis cross section at the level of the papillary muscles at end-diastole (A) and end-systole (B) in a normal dog. The computer-assisted outlines of epicardium and endocardium during end-diastole (solid lines) and end-systole (dashed lines) are shown at the bottom. The cross sections are subdivided into 8 segments using a fixed-axis referencing system. The indexing line is derived connecting one of the junctions of the right and left ventricles (indicated by an X) to the endocardial diastolic geometric center of gravity. Systolic fractional area change (FAC) and wall thickening (WTH) are calculated for the entire section, as well as for each segment.

(Figs. 1–6). These could be assembled into a 3-dimensional model using a method described by Haendchen (Fig. 2). Based on this, innovative technology displaying 6 serial anatomic sections, each of which were subdivided into 8 sectors, was developed to both identify and quantitate measurements of normal and ischemic myocardium, and to provide comprehensive information to serially assess the beneficial-detrimental effects of reperfusion, pharmacologie interventions, and synchronized coronary venous retroperfusion on cardiac performance following acute coronary occlusion. These computerized techniques now permit us to quantify the dynamic changes in ischemic dysfunction that can instantly dictate the direction of interventional procedures.

120

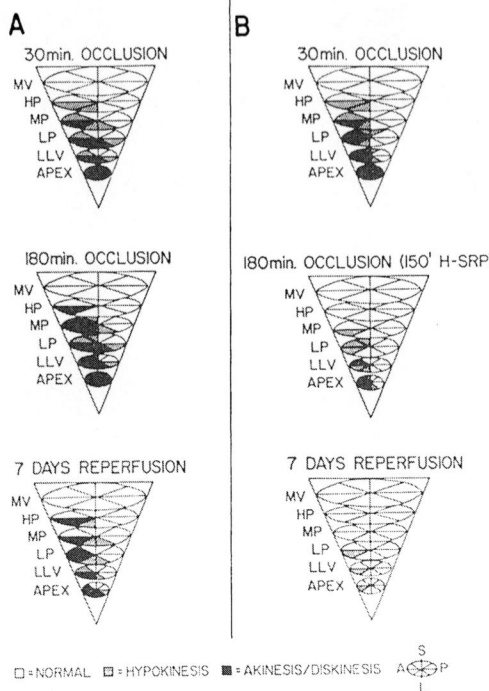

Fig. 2. Reconstruction of the ischemic zone derived from 2DE wall motion studies at several short-axis cross-sectional levels of the left ventricle in the same experiments illustrated in Figs. 5 and 6. The cross-sections are subdivided into 8 regions (as indicated in Fig. 2) and the wall motion is quantitatively discriminated in normal akinetic or dyskinetic, and hypokinetic (hypokinesis was defined as regional fractional area change below 2 standard deviations of mean values obtained in 50 normal dogs). MV = mitral valve level, HP = high papillary muscle level, LP = low papillary muscle level; LLV = low left ventricular level; apex = apical short-axis level. Note that 30 min occlusion of the LAD coronary artery caused more dysfunction in lower sections of the LV, while no wall motion abnormalities are seen at the MV level, which was above the site of the occlusion. Marked improvement in regional wall motion at all LV levels (but less at the lower LV levels) is observed in the dog in which the therapeutic intervention (hypothermic synchronized retroperfusion = HSRP) was applied from 30 minutes up to 3 hours of the occlusion period (panel B), as compared to no change or deterioration in regional function in the untreated dog (panel A). Myocardial reperfusion after 3 hours of LAD occlusion did not significantly improve segmental wall motion in the untreated dog (panel A, bottom). LAD = left anterior descending; S = septal; L = lateral; A = anterior and P = posterior wall.

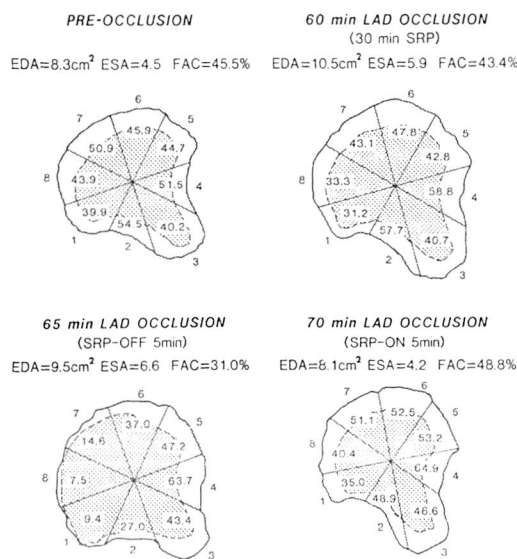

Fig. 3. Segmental wall motion analysis of short-axis endocardial outlines at the low left ventricular level, showing the rapid effect of synchronized retroperfusion (SRP). Continous lines and dashed lines indicate left ventricular endocardium at end-diastole and end-systole, respectively. Analysis was performed before (upper right) and after (lower left) a 5 minute interruption of retroperfusion and 5 minutes after resumption of retroperfusion (lower right). EDA = end-diastolic area; ESA = end-systolic area; FAC = systolic fractional area shange. (From Yamazaki S, Drury JK, Meerbaum S, et al. Synchronized coronary venous retroperfusion. Prompt improvement of left ventricular function in experimental myocardial ischemia. Reprinted with permission from the American College of Cardiology. JACC 5:655–63, 1985.)

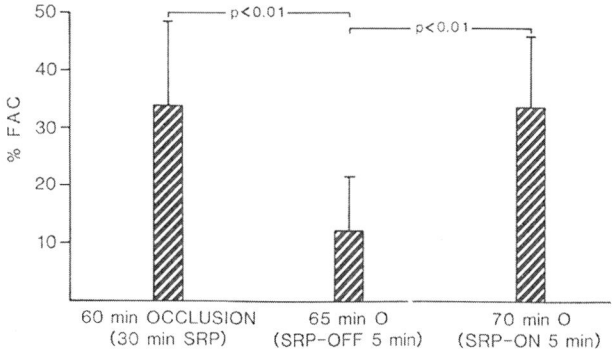

Fig. 4. Systolic fractional area change (FAC) in the ischemic segment of the left ventricle during synchronized retroperfusion (SRP) on-off-cycling (mean ± standard deviation). Note that at 1 hour coronary occlusion (O) with 30 minutes of retroperfusion, systolic fractional area change was increased by the treatment to near control levels (See Fig. 4). At 1 hour post-occlusion, synchronized retroperfusion was interrupted for 5 minutes. Two-dimensional echocardiographic measurements were obtained 5 minutes after interruption as well as 5 minutes after resumption of retroperfusion. It is seen that the retroperfusion induced improvement of segmental function was highly significant and rapid.

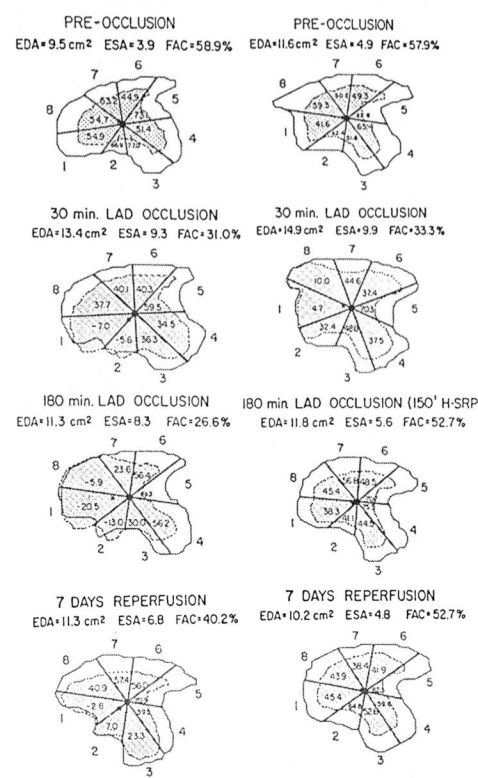

Fig. 5. Evaluation of the effectiveness of hypothermic synchronized retroperfusion (H-SRP) on left ventricular contraction abnormalities induced by coronary occlusion and reperfusion. Compared to untreated dogs (left panel), the dog pretreated with H-SRP exhibited a significant improvement in global and segmental wall motion at 180 minutes occlusion as well as on the seventh day of reperfusion. EDA = endocardial end-diastolic area; ESA = endocardial end-systolic area; LAD = left anterior descending. (From Haendchen RV, Corday E, Meerbaum S: Prevention of ischemic injury and early retroperfusion derangements by hypothermic reperfusion. Reprinted with permission from the American College of Cardiology. JACC 1: 1067–80, 1983.)

Clinical application

Signs of ischemia demonstrated by two-dimensional echocardiography:

– Dynamic alterations in regional-global endocardial wall motion kinetics
   akinesis
   dyskinesis
   diminished ejection fraction
   global $\left.\begin{array}{l} \\ \\ \end{array}\right\}$ fractional area of change.
   regional
– Conversion of normal systolic wall thickening to wall thinning.

123

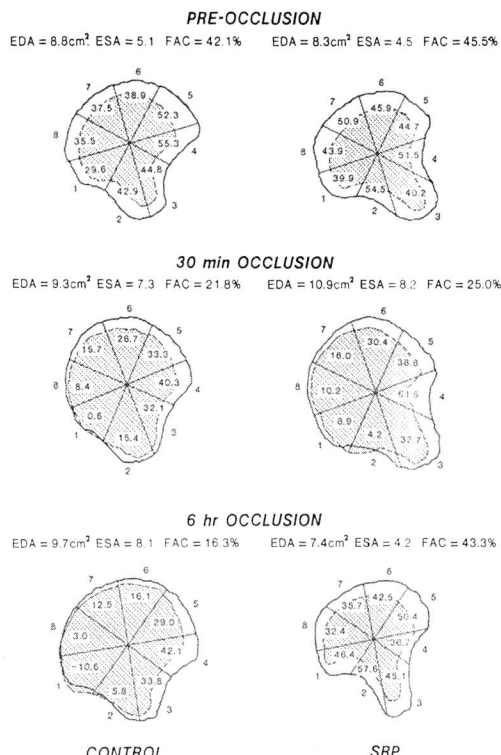

PRE-OCCLUSION
EDA = 8.8cm² ESA = 5.1 FAC = 42.1%   EDA = 8.3cm² ESA = 4.5 FAC = 45.5%

30 min OCCLUSION
EDA = 9.3cm² ESA = 7.3 FAC = 21.8%   EDA = 10.9cm² ESA = 8.2 FAC = 25.0%

6 hr OCCLUSION
EDA = 9.7cm² ESA = 8.1 FAC = 16.3%   EDA = 7.4cm² ESA = 4.2 FAC = 43.3%

CONTROL   SRP

Fig. 6. Two-dimensional echocardiographic computer-assisted segmental wall motion analysis of endocardial outlines in a low left ventricular level cross-section. Left ventricular endocardium is indicated with continuous lines at end-diastole and with dashed lines at end-systole (stippled area). Systolic fractional area change (FAC) was calculated for the entire cross-section as well as for individual segments (1 to 8) according to the formula: FAC = (EDA-ESA)/EDA × 100, where EDA = end-systolic area; ESA = end-systolic area. In this view, the interventricular septum is on the left and top and the anterior wall at the bottom. SRP = synchronized retroperfusion.

- Dilatation of the chamber cavity indicating cardiac decompensation.
- Reperfusion injury, viz, arrhythmia, diastolic thickening and the above physical alterations of dynamic function.

The crude quantitative wall motion indices of ischemia expressed as ballooning or contraction, were employed to define changes in cardiac function induced by ischemia and various interventions such as restoration of systemic blood pressure. These provided some real, but also some unreliable, information about physiologic function [21–22]. Fortunately, the recent developments previously cited now provide a simple, non-invasive, convenient and accurate method to validate the dynamic effects of an intervention with computer-assisted measurements (Figs. 1–6). This long sought advance in computer-assisted echocardiographic display and computation for diagnosis can now provide for more accurate treatment in the acute critical cardiac event.

Echocardiographic assessment of the efficacy of coronary venous synchronized retroperfusion

Gueret and Corday displayed innovative tomographic 3-dimensional display of progressive dynamic phasic wall motion by serial segmental analysis of 2DE short-axis sections following coronary artery occlusion, and then before and during the administration of nitroprusside. It quantified regional segmental and global alterations in the area of each tomographic level to produce an index of chamber volume ejection expressed as a fractional area of change [16, 23–25]. This 3-dimensional display portrayed dynamic changes in cardiac function at 6 tomographic levels. Thus, data could be immediately documented to control the online direction of an intervention. It also portrayed changing dynamics to indicate the reversibility of impaired cardiac dysfunction and efficacy of a pharmacologic intervention.

Assessment of global cardiac function

Our earliest left ventricular volume and ejection fraction were derived simultaneously by 2DE to define global function. Left ventricular volumes were calculated from 2DE sections using a Simpson's reconstruction model based upon several short-axis areas and length of the left ventricle [12, 16, 17]. But the application of this method for clinical studies is doubtful because of the limited number of short-axis cross-sections that may be obtained. However, several other models of volume reconstruction were reported, some of which applied measurements solely derived from apical views, which may be applicable clinically [25]. During acute myocardial ischemia [1], simple global ejection fraction does not represent a meaningful index of ventricular function because the non-ischemic contralateral side hypercontracts so that it minimizes actual effects of ischemic dysfunction. Thus, our new method of measurement of regional fractional area of change from tomographic slices at various levels was developed to provide more meaningful information regarding function in the beating heart (Figs. 5–6).

Quantitative measurement alterations of regional wall motion and thickness

Echocardiography provides several indices of regional myocardial performance such as systolic wall thickening, systolic fractional area change, radial shortening, and true circumferential shortening. In the experimental setting the following indices were developed for the analysis of two dimensional echocardiographic short-axis section contractility.

$$\% \text{ Fractional Area Change } = \frac{EDA - ESA}{ESA} \times 100$$

where EDA = endocardial end-diastolic area and ESA = endocardial end-systolic area

$$\% \text{ Wall thickening } = \frac{WTS - WTD}{WTED} \times 100$$

where WTES = wall thickness at end systole and WTED = wall thickness at end diastole.

Application of the ultrasonic test for viability

Fig. 1 illustrates the computer analysis of regional left ventricular function in two-dimensional echocardiography short-axis sections at the level of the papillary muscles. The previously mentioned indices are calculated for the overall section as well as for each segment. For regional wall motion analysis, computer programs subdivide this cross-section into 8 equal segments using either fixed or floating axis systems (with correction for intrathoracic cardiac motions). Using this method, a good correlation has been found between histochemical delineation of acutely ischemic myocardium [26] and phase of infarction without reperfusion which allowed us to consider echocardiographic quantification of wall motion as an ultrasonic test for myocardial viability.

Computation of intermittent regional dynamic ventricular wall function

Another advantage of computer-assisted 2DE is the possibility of calculating prompt sequential measurements of ischemic zone systolic fraction area change during the time of observation. For example, we could demonstrate prompt improvement of left ventricular function within minutes of synchronized retroperfusion [27]. Figures 3 and 4 illustrate the effects of temporary interruption of retroperfusion at 1 hour of coronary occlusion (30 minutes of retroperfusion). Interruption in treatment resulted in a rapid and major reduction in regional segmental fractional area change which was quickly restored with resumption of retroperfusion [25].

Significance of wall thickening changes

Previous studies have suggested that wall thickening and fiber shortening are closely correlated, and systolic thickening suddenly changing to thinning provides more information than endocardial motions. Several investigations, including our own [2, 29, 30], reported experimental studies on the relationship of wall thickening and thinning assessed by 2DE to the extent of myocardial infarction. Lieberman [20] reported an abrupt deterioration in systolic thickening in segments containing more than 20% transluminal extent of necrosis. He found wall motion abnormalities were less precise than thickening in discriminating between infarct and non-infarct size and could lead to infarct size overestimation. Pandian [31] found correlation between dyskinesis in echo and infarct size, but moderately overestimated the necrotic area and underestimated the risk area.

The benefits of a therapeutic intervention aimed at preventing permanent ischemic injury are demonstrated by the early occurrence of three cardinal signs:

1. Recovery of segmental wall motion,
2. Correction in diastolic wall thickening, and
3. Reduction in ventricular chamber volumes.

Figure 4 represents a wall motion study from experiments in which one group of animals was submitted to a period of three hours of untrated occlusion followed by 7 days of reperfusion. In a second group of dogs, hypothermic coronary venous retroperfusion was applied from 30 minutes up to 3 hours of the occlusion period, following which the myocardium was reperfused for 7 days. The figures clearly showed that in the first case the reperfusion was apparently instituted too late after the coronary occlusion, resulting in significant myocardial damage. In the second case, hypothermic synchronous coronary venous retroperfusion applied early after the coronary occlusion 'bought time' until the restoration of myocardial blood flow was instituted by means of reperfusion, resulting only in small focal areas of subendocardial necrosis. During the same experiment, hypothermic retroperfusion prevented the occurrence of an anticipated marked increase in diastolic wall thickness that characteristically persisted throughout a 7 day period in the suddenly reperfused control group without such retroperfusion support [1, 32].

Another example of the efficacy of coronary venous retroperfusion as demonstrated by echocardiography is shown in Figs. 5 and 6. The experiment was performed in an animal model. Sequential echocardiographic measurements of ischemic zone systolic fractional change and wall thickening are demonstrated in these figures. Both groups exhibited a markedly depressed fractional area change at 30 minutes postocclusion. This depressed regional dysfunction persisted throughout the 6 hour coronary occlusion period in the control dogs, but in the treated dogs, ischemic zone function was essentially restored after the start of the retroperfusion treatment. Systolic fractional area change and wall thickening in the nonischemic zone were not affected by either occlusion or retroperfusion. In the ischemic zone, end-diastolic wall thickness was first reduced by coronary occlusion, which also increased chamber volume. Systolic wall thickness tended to be restored with retroperfusion treatment, although differences between the groups were not significant, possibly because of large standard deviations in echocardiographic thickness measurements [2].

Current limitations of 2-D echocardiographic wall motion assessment of retroperfusion

In spite of the major advantages of ultrasound in the quantitation of regional wall motion abnormalities certain fundamental problems limit its usefulness. As with other imaging technologies such as contrast angiography or nuclear ventriculography that use segmental wall motion abnormalities to assess the size of an infarct, these techniques slightly overestimate the infarct size because segments adjacent to an infarction may also display hypokinesis, even in the absence of ischemia [32]. Tethering phenomena, marked spatial homogeneity of wall motion, thickening, and non-transmural infarction are some of the reasons put forth, however, it is possible to unmask the functional reserve or viability of the adjacent segments by increasing the diagnostic ability of echo images during a postextrasystolic potentiation of contractility [29]. The correlation can be further enhanced between the extent of abnormal wall motion and reduced blood flow, or myocardial necrosis. 2DE methods which integrate reconstruction of endocardial motion over the entire dynamic systolic contraction sequence have been reported to provide better definition of ischemic ventricular dysfunction than do methods that consider motion at solitary points of time, such as at end-diastole and end-systole.

Proposal for improvements

For improved analysis of regional contractility, recent advances in computerized quantification allow continuous display on a split video screen of two different heart cycles, one normal and another during ischemia [33–34]. For each ventricular region, immediate side by side comparison between these two frames increases the sensitivity of ventricular echocardiographic

128

detection of hypokinesis and facilitates the endocardial delineation. The present reconstruction of global quantitative measurements of function require multiple views which are manually drawn and digitized and thus tedious and time consuming, explaining perhaps the reason why echo quantification is not often used in the clinical setting. Recent improvements in computerized analysis of left ventricular wall motion have been published demonstrating better sensitivity and specificity in infarct area detection, as well as good reproducibility in 'hands off' computer tracing with automated endocardial edge detection [24, 35]. This technique is used in our institution in experimental and clinical studies to measure ischemic dysfunction during angioplasty, exercise stress testing and retroperfusion. These automated detection methods will allow simplified, objective online measurements for diagnosis and management of the critically ill patient, compared to the present pondorous, more subjective and questionable manual tracings. Problems do exist in employing these methods for clinical studies which have poor or marginal image quality. The introduction of innovative technology for enhanced echocardiographic imaging, for example, annular phased array transducer [36] will perhaps improve the resolution and penetration of the beam, and also provide better delineation of the endocardial borders which is mandatory for outline delineation from echocardiographic frames.

References

1. Berland J, Corday E: Echocardiography to demonstrate effects of interventions designed to reduce myocardial ischemia and infarct size. Echocardiography 3: 415–31, 1986.
2. Yamazaki S, Drury JK, Meerbaum S, et al.: Synchronized coronary venous retroperfusion. Prompt improvement of left ventricular function in experimental myocardial ischemia. J Am Coll Cardiol 5: 655–63, 1985.
3. Tennant R, Wiggers C: The effect of coronary occlusion on myocardial contraction. Am J Physiol 112: 351, 1935.
4. Corday E, Bergman HC, Schwartz LL, et al.. Studies on the coronary circulation. IV The Effect of shock on the heart and its treatment. Am Heart J 37: 560–81, 1949.
5. Prinzmetal M, Schwartz LL, Corday E, et al.: Studies on the coronary circulation. VI Loss of myocardial contractility after coronary artery occlusion. Ann Int Med 31: 429–49, 1948.
6. Prinzmetal M, Corday E, Spritzler R, et al.: Radiocardiography and its clinical application. JAMA 139: 617–22, 1949.
7. Jacobs JJ, Feigenbaum H, Corya BC, et al.: Detection of left ventricular assynergy by echocardiography. Circulation 48: 263–271, 1973.
8. Corya BC, Feigenbaum H, Rasmussen S, et al.: Anterior left ventricular wall echoes in coronary artery disease. Am J Cardiol 34: 652–57, 1974.
9. Corya BC, Rasmussen S, Knoebel SB, et al.: Echocardiography in acute myocardial infarction. Am J Cardiol 36: 1–10, 1975.
10. Heger JJ, Weyman AE, Wann LS, et al.: Cross-sectional echocardiography in acute myo-

cardial infarction. Detection and localization of regional left ventricular assynergy. Circulation 60: 531–538, 1979.

11. Horowitz RS, Morganroth J, Parrotto C, et al.: Immediate diagnosis of acute myocardial infarction by two-dimensional echocardiography. Circulation 65: 323–329, 1982.

12. Wyatt HL, Meerbaum S, Heng MK, et al.: Experimental evaluation of the extent of myocardial dyssynergy and infarct size by two-dimensional echocardiographic recognition of myocardial injury in man. Comparison with post-mortem studies. Circulation 63: 607–14, 1981.

13. Weiss JL, Bulkley BH, Hutchins GM, et al.: Two-dimensional echocardiographic recognition of myocardial injury in man. Comparison with post-mortem studies. Circulation 63: 401–408, 1981.

14. Nixon JV, Narahara KA, Smitherman TC: Estimation of myocardial involvement in patients with acute myocardial infarction by two-dimensional echocardiography. Circulation 62: 1248–55, 1980.

15. Gibson RS, Bishop HL, Stamm RB, et al.: Value of early two-dimensional echocardiography in patients with acute myocardial infarction. Am J Cardiol 49: 1110–19, 1982.

16. Gueret P, Meerbaum S, Wyatt HL, Corday E, et al.: Two-dimensional echocardiographic quantitation for left ventricular volumes and ejection fraction. Importance of accounting for dyssynergy in short-axis reconstruction models. Circulation 62: 1308–18, 1980.

17. Haendchen RV, Meerbaum S, Fishbein M, Corday, E, et al.: Extent of myocardial infarction delineated by two-dimensional echo analysis of left ventricular dysfunction (abstract). Clin Res 30: IIA, 1982.

18. Parisi AF, Moynihan PF, Folland ED, et al.: Quantitative detection of regional left ventricular contraction abnormalities by two-dimensional echocardiography. Circulation 63: 761–67, 1981.

19. Gillam LD, Hogan RD, Foale RA, et al.: A comparison of quantitative echocardiographic methods for delineating infarct-induced abnormal wall motion. Circulation 70: 113–22, 1984.

20. Lieberman AN, Weiss JL, Jugdutt BI, et al.: Two-dimensional echocardiography and infarct size. Relationship of regional wall motion and thickening to extent of myocardial infarction in the dog. Circulation 63: 739–46, 1981.

21. Anderson JL, Marshall HW, Bray BE, et al.: A randomized trial of intracoronary streptokinase in the treatment of acute myocardial infarction. New Engl J Med 308: 1312–18, 1982.

22. Charuzi Y, Beeder C, Marshall LA, et al.: Improvement in regional and global left ventricular function after intracoronary thrombolysis. Assessment with two-dimensional echocardiography (abstract). Am J Cardiol 52: 662, 1984.

23. Wyatt HL, Heng MK, Meerbaum S, Corday E, et al.: Cross-sectional echocardiography. II. Analysis of mathematical models for quantifying volume of the formalin-fixed left ventricle. Circulation 61: 1119–25, 1980.

24. Gueret P, Meerbaum S, Broffman J, Corday E, et al.: Differential effects of nitroprusside on ischemic and nonischemic myocardium demonstrated by two-dimensional echocardiography. Am J Cardiol 48: 59–68, 1982.

25. Shimoura K, Meerbaum S, Sakamaki T, Corday E, et al.: Relation between functional response to nitroglycerin and extent of myocardial necrosis in dogs. Mapping of the left ventricle by 2-dimensional echocardiography. Am J Cardiol 52: 177–83, 1983.

26. Wyatt HL, Meerbaum S, Heng MK, Corday E, et al.: Cross-sectional echocardiography. III. Analysis of mathematic models for quantifying volume of symmetric and asymmetric left ventricle. Am Heart J 100: 821–28, 1980.

27. Zwehl W, Levy R, Garcia E, Corday E, et al.: Validation of a computerized edge detection

algorithm for quantitative two-dimensional echocardiography. Circulation 68: 1127–35, 1983.

28. Meerbaum S, Fishbein M, Y-Rit J, Corday E, et al.: Two-dimensional echo measurement of regional cardiac function vs histochemical delineation of acutely ischemic myocardium (abstract). Clin Res 298: 222A, 1981.

29. Sakamaki T, Corday E, Meerbaum S, et al.: Relation between myocardial injury and post-extrasystolic potentiation of regional function measured by two-dimensional echocardiography. J Am Coll Cardiol 2: 52–61, 1983.

30. Heikkila J, Tabakin BS, Hugenholtz PG: Quantification of functional in normal and infarcted regions of the left ventricle. Cardiovasc RES 6: 516–31, 1972.

31. Pandian NG, Koyanagi S, Skorton DJ, et al.: Relations between 2-dimensional echocardiographic wall thickening abnormalities, myocardial infarct size and coronary risk area in normal and hypertrophied myocardium in dogs. Am J Cardiol 52: 1318–25, 1983.

32. Haendchen RV, Corday E, Meerbaum S, et al.: Prevention of ischemic injury and early reperfusion derangements by hypothermic retroperfusion. J Am Coll Cardiol 4: 1067–80, 1983.

33. Kerber RE, Marcus ML, Ehrhardt J, et al.: Correlation between echocardiographically demonstrated segmental dyskinesis and regional myocardial perfusion. Circulation 52: 1097–1104, 1975.

34. Force T, Bloomfield P, O'Boyle JE, et al.: Quantitative two-dimensional echocardiographic analysis of regional wall motion in patients with perioperative myocardial infarction. Circulation 70: 233–41, 1984.

35. Schnittger I, Fitzgerald PJ, Gordon EP, et al.: Computerized quantitative analysis of left ventricular wall motion by two-dimensional echocardiography. Circulation 70: 242–54, 1984.

36. Garcia E, Gueret P, Bennett M, et al.: Real time computerization of two-dimensional echocardiography. Am Heart J 101: 783–92, 1981.

37. Ryan T, Vasey CG, Armstrong WE, et al.: Application of annular phased array technology to two-dimensional echocardiography imaging (abstract). J Am Coll Cardiol 7: 146, 1986.

PART 2: Intrapericardial Interventions

2.1. Pericardiocentesis guided by ultrasound

I. CIKES, A. ERNST, J. A. CALLAHAN & M. E. GOLDMAN

Blind techniques of pericardiocentesis

The ancient beliefs of the harmful effects of pericardial effusion on cardiac function have inspired an idea about the possible treatment of the effusion by aspiration of pericardial fluid. The first recommendations of this method appeared in the 17th and 18th centuries, but no data on its accomplishment are available [1].

In 1798 Prince – Joseph Desault and in 1810 Dominique – Jean Larrey unsuccessfully attempted to drain pericardial fluid; both entered pleural space [2]. The first surgical aspiration of pericardial fluid through the trepanated sternum was done by F. Romero between 1801 and 1819 [3]. In 1840 Franz Schuh was the first who performed blind pericardiocentesis using a trocar inserted in the third and fourth parasternal interspace [4]. In 1911, A. B. Marfan introduced the subxiphoid approach which is still the most popular entry point for pericardiocentesis [5].

There have been several attempts to diminish the potential risk of pericardiocentesis.

Fluoroscopic guidance of the needle is not a reliable method, because it cannot differentiate pericardial effusion from cardiac mass.

In 1956 Bishop [6] introduced *ECG guided pericardiocentesis* using the needle for pericardiocentesis as an exploring electrode to detect the injury currents during the contact of the needle tip with the heart. When the needle tip is in contact with the visceral pericardium or when it punctures the ventricular wall, marked ST elevation can be seen, while the PR segment elevation is seen when needle punctures the atrial wall. This technique became unwarrantedly popular. However, it was shown that the heart can be punctured without provoking any current of injury [7]. This can occur when the area of puncture is electrically silent, as in cases of postinfarction fibrosis, tumor infiltration of the myocardium and infiltrative cardiomyopathies. Thus this technique can give a false sense of safety. By paying close attention to the ECG monitoring of pericardiocentesis, the operator can distract the attention from the techniques and may decrease the 'feel' and sensitivity of his hand for the needle [8]. Although the value of this technique has been

I. Cikes (ed.), *Echocardiography in Cardiac Interventions*, 133–145, 1989.
© 1989 *Kluwer Academic Publishers*.

questioned it is still recommended in recent textbooks of cardiology, surgery, anesthesiology and manuals for intensive and coronary care units.

The high incidence of severe complications and fatality using blind method (see Table 1) urged some authors to return to surgical pericardiostomy. Instead of percutaneous pericardiocentesis, they advocated 'open pericardiocentesis' as a safer and more efficient method. which, in addition, provides histological diagnosis [9]. However, the surgical pericardiocentesis is not free from significant complications either.

Table 1. Incidence of Complications of 'Blind' Pericardiocentesis (PC) 1956–1986.

First author	Year	Procedures No.	Complications	No.	%	Deaths No.	%
Bishop[6]	1956	40	Ventricular puncture	6	15	0	
Kilpatrick[4]	1965	20	Ventricular puncture	7	35	1	5
			Hypotension	3	15		
Frederiksen[21]	1971	21	Ventricular puncture	2	9.5	} 0	
			Atrial puncture	1	4.8		
Morin[22]	1976	6	Cardiac arrest	2	3.3	2	3.3
		86 (review)				16*	18.6
Pradham[23]	1976	5	RV perforation	1	20	0	
Silverberg[24]	1977	21	Cardiac arrest	1	4.8	0	
Krikorian[25]	1978	123	Hemopericardium	5	4	} 5	4
			Nonproductive PC	17	13.8		
Kwasnik[26]	1978	34	Ventricular puncture	2	5.8	} 0	
			Pneumothorax	1	2.9		
			Pneumoperithoneum	1	2.9		
Wong[27]	1979	52	Cardiac arrest	1	1.9	} 1	1.9
			Subdiaphragm. abscess	1	1.9		
			Ventricular puncture	5	9.6		
			Nonproductive PC	16	30.8		
Gubermann[28]	1981	46	RV laceration	3	6.5	} 2	4.3
			Nonproductive PC	3	6.5		
Fowler[29]	1986	44	RV laceration	3	6.8	} 2	4.5
			Nonproductive PC	3	6.8		
Total		498		81	16.2	29	5.8

* Died suddenly during or just after the procedure.

Echocardiographic guidance of pericardiocentesis

The most important advance in minimizing the hazards of pericardiocentesis was done when echocardiography was established as the procedure of choice for diagnosing of pericardial effusion. The false diagnosis of pericardial effusion was virtually eliminated, and selection of patients for pericardiocentesis has become reliable.

A- and M-mode. In 1970 Goldberg and Pollock [10] used a special transducer with a hole in the center to direct the needle during pericardiocentesis under A- and M-mode echocardiographic control. The needle tip was seen in A- and M-mode display as an echo arising at the needle tip – fluid interface. In one out of six patients in whom the procedure was performed the ventricle was punctured. There is no evidence that anyone followed this method in cardiology. The main disadvantage of pericardiocentesis guided under the control of A- and M-mode is the lack of spatial orientation.

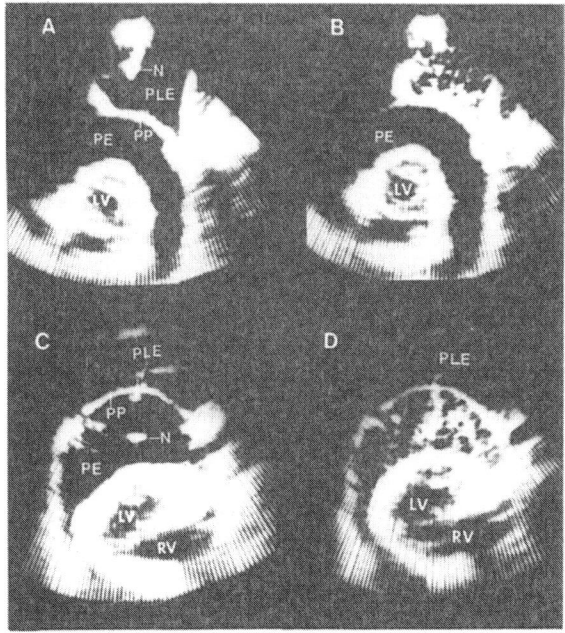

Fig. 1. Contrast echo pericardiocentesis to locate the needle tip in a patient with pericardial (PE) and pleural (PLE) effusion. Posterior thoracic route has been chosen because the largest accumulation of pericardial effusion occured behind left ventricle (LV). The needle was inserted first into pleural space (A), than through parietal pericardium (PP) into pericardial space (C). The position of the needle tip in pleural space (B) and pericardial sac (D) was confirmed by contrast method. Cardiac cavities are free of contrast.

Echo contrast method. By rapid injection of echo-producing contrast agents through the needle for pericardiocentesis, the cloud of bubbles will appear within the pericardial space. If the needle enters the cardiac cavity the bubbles will be noted within the relevant cavity (Figs. 1, 2).

Contrast echo pericardiocentesis has been reported in two separate studies: Chadraratna [11] with 16 patients and three inadvertant but asymptomatic myocardial perforations, and Goldman [12] with 13 patients and one asymptomatic right ventricular puncture. In 12 of the 13 patients in Goldman's series, the contrast was immediately visible in the pericardial cavity even when the needle itself was not seen.

Two-dimensional echocardiography can visualize some portions of the needle which are within the scanning plane, but the identification of the needle tip is difficult and uncertain. That can be facilitated by the contrast method: if, after injection of contrast, a jet appears at the presumed needle tip, it may be considered a true tip [13] (Fig. 2). However, the contrast method provides confirmation of needle location even if the needle tip is not visualized directly (Fig. 3). The next advantage of the contrast method is the immediate identification of the origin of blood-tinged evacuated fluid which could be pericardial, pleural or from cardiac cavities. The potential limitations of the contrast method are an inability to produce 'contrast effect' due to injection of unagitated fluid and a delay in visualizing contrast due to

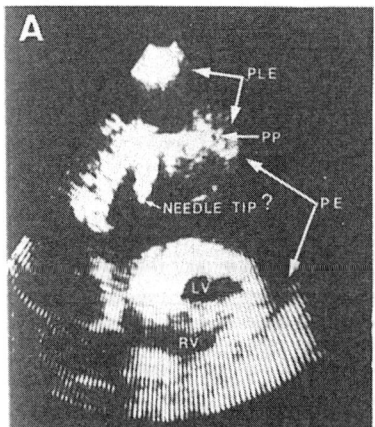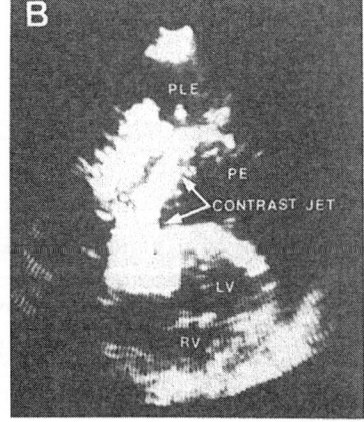

Fig. 2. The position of the needle tip during pericardiocentesis may be confirmed by contrast method. Panel A shows presumed needle tip in the pericardial effusion (PE). The patient had concomitant pleural effusion (PLE) and puncture was performed by posterior thoracic route through pleural effusion. If contrast jet appears at presumed needle tip it may be considered a true tip (panel B). Cardiac cavities are free of contrast. (From Cikes I, Ernst A: New aspects of echocardiography in the diagnosis and treatment of pericardial disease. In: The Practice of M-mode and Two-dimensional Echocardiography, J Roelandt, ed., Martinus Nijhoff Publishers, The Hague/Boston/London, 1983).

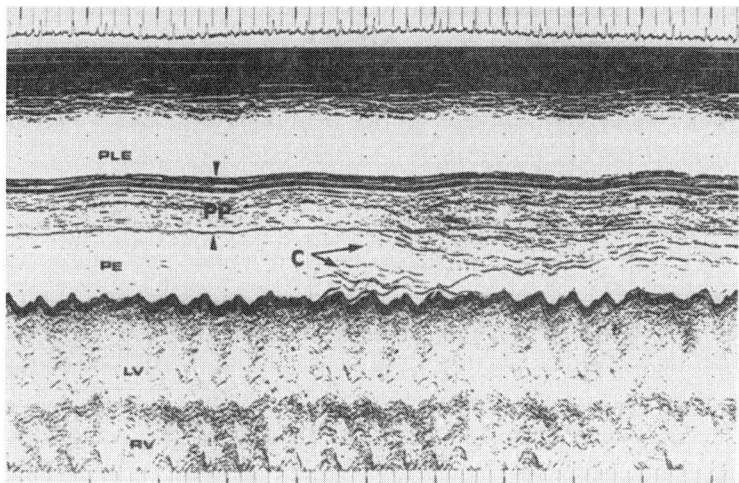

Fig. 3. M-mode contrast echocardiography to confirm the needle location. Although the needle tip is not visualized directly, contrast echoes (C) confirmed its location within the pericardial space. PP: parietal pericardium, PLE: pleural effusion, PE: pericardial effusion, LV: left ventricle, RV: right ventricle.

exudative or loculated pericardial effusion. The experience with the contrast method suggests that asymptomatic cardiac cavity punctures are not so infrequent as it is believed [12].

Two-dimensional echocardiography. Giving excellent spatial orientation, two-dimensional echocardiography is a most efficient tool for diagnosing, locating and quantifying pericardial effusion. By providing the exact relationship of the effusion to the thoracic and abdominal wall, easy selection of the optimal entry point and route for the pericardiocentesis needle is possible. It also confirms the location of the needle or catheter in the pericardial space with or without the use of the echo contrast method.

The procedure of pericardiocentesis can be monitored by two-dimensional echocardiography from *remote transducer* positions without continuous needle visualization, or by continuous needle visualization using a special *needle guide attachement*.

The procedure should start with complete echocardiographic examination, paying special attention to the quantity of pericardial fluid, its distribution within the pericardial sac and to its relationship to the thoracic and abdominal wall. It is important to check the width of the echo-free space from all possible entry points on the thoracic and abdominal walls [14,15]. It happens that patients are being referred by the echocardiographic laboratory to the physician who will perform the pericardiocentesis as having large pericardial effusion (often with estimated quantity) without details on distribu-

138

tion of the pericardial fluid within the pericardial sac. Thus, if the accumulation of the pericardial fluid occurs mainly around cardiac apex and behind the left ventricle, then the most common xiphocostal entry point will be inappropriate and hazardous due to the small echo-free space between the diaphragmatic parietal pericardium and right ventricular wall.

The most common approach for pericardiocentesis is left xiphocostal with the needle aimed to the left shoulder. It is generally considered the safest route [8]. Other possible approaches are right xiphocostal, apical, left and right parasternal, posterior thoracic and right-sided. Callahan [15] advocates as ideal an approach at which the pericardial fluid is closest to the transducer and from which the needle track avoids the heart or any underlying vital structure. In 132 reported procedures, subcostal entry was selected in 25% patients, whereas a chest approach was chosen in 64% (46% apical). If correctly carried out, the xiphocostal approach is extrapleural and extraperitoneal (Fig. 4). The apical approach is usually the shortest approach to the pericardial space, but it is transpleural, resulting in a greater possibility of pneumothorax and spreading of infection or malignant cells to the pleura and the lung. Potential advantages of the apical approach are in the smaller risk of bleeding if the thick apical wall is punctured and in the absence of larger coronary arteries in the apical region. This approach is specially preferrable in pulmonary hypertension to avoid the possibility of right ventricular puncture and serious bleeding complications [8].

After infiltration of local anesthetic a 16- to 18-gauge, thin-walled, Teflon-

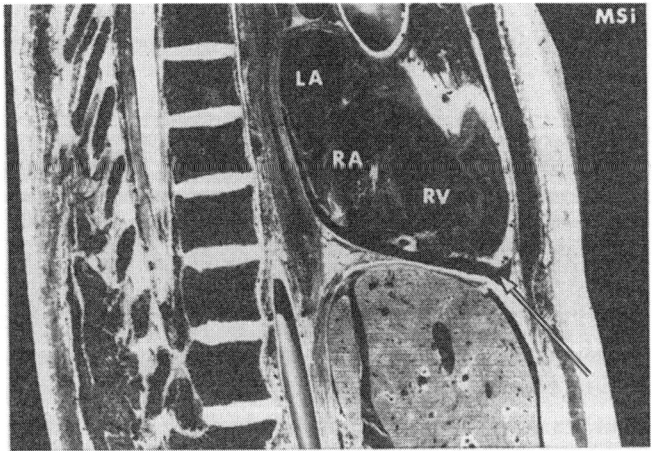

Fig. 4. Sagittal section of human heart and surrounding structures showing left xiphocostal approach for pericardiocentesis (arrow). This route is extrapleural and extraperitoneal. LA: left atrium, RA: right atrium, RV: right ventricle. (From Atlas of Sectional Human anatomy, JG Kortiké, H Sick (eds.), Urban & Schwarzenberg, Baltimore-Munich, 1983, with permission.)

sheathed, short-level needle is introduced toward the pericardial sac. From the xiphocostal approach, the needle should be introduced at a 30° to 40° angle to the frontal plane, and aimed toward the left shoulder or jugulum. The direction of the needle to the right shoulder carries a higher risk of injury of the right atrium and inferior vena cava, and should be reserved for the cases with a large accumulation of pericardial fluid in this direction [8,17]. The syringe is filled with anesthetic or saline. While advancing the needle, continuous aspiration and injection should be done. Gradual and deliberate needle advancement will significantly reduce the incidence of complications. The operator feels the pericardial entry as a distinct 'giving' or 'popping' sensation. The pericardial entering is confirmed by the free aspiration of pericardial fluid or by the appearance of echogenic microbubbles from the injected anesthetic or saline. Promptly after that the Teflon sheath is advanced and the needle is withdrawn.

The portion of plastic sheath can be visualized directly by two-dimensional echocardiographic scanning or by the contrast echocardiographic method (Fig. 5). The emptying of the pericardial sac is monitored by two-dimensional echocardiography with a remote transducer positioned outside of the sterile field. In the majority of patients this technique is sufficient [15]. If prolonged drainage of the pericardial sac is necessary, a flexible wire is introduced through the Teflon sheath followed by an introducer and side-hole catheter for continuous or intermittent drainage (Fig. 6).

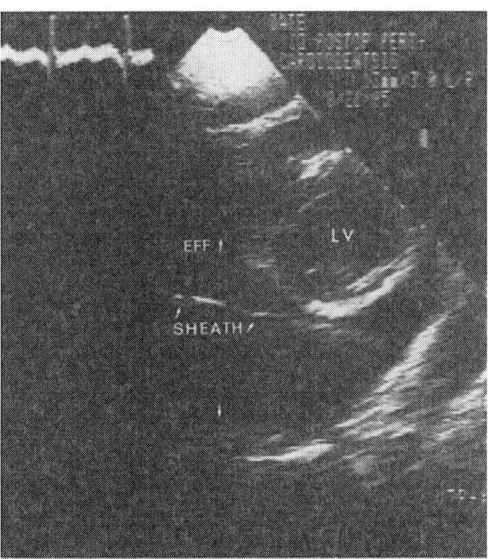

Fig. 5. Sheath inserted into pericardial space to allow complete drainage of effusion (EFF), LV: left ventricle.

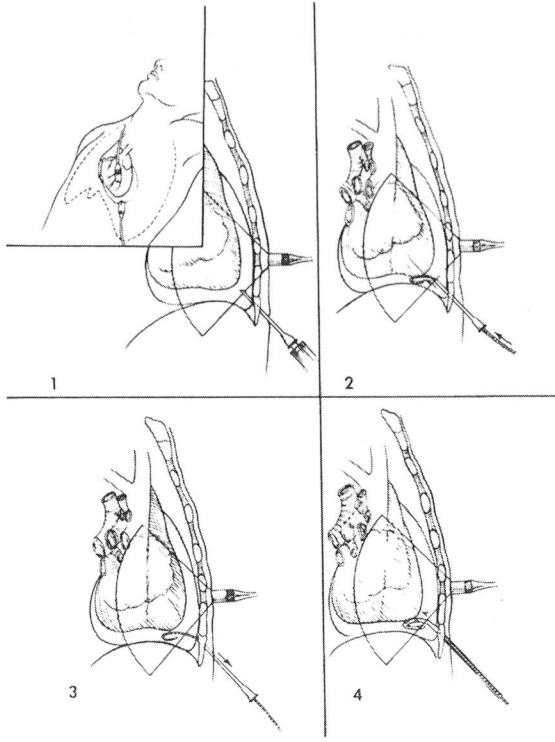

Fig. 6. Steps during pericardiocentesis guided by remote 2-D echocardiographic transducer: 1. Introduction of Teflon-sheathed needle into the pericardial sac. 2. Introduction of flexible guide-wire through the Teflon sheath. 3. Teflon sheath withdrawal. 4. Insertion of side-hole catheter, and guide-wire withdrawal.

Needle-guide attachment. Echocardiographic monitoring of the needle with a remote transducer during actual entry is time consuming and can give the spurious feeling of safety. If the needle is not in the scanning plane, it is not visible at all. Some portions of the needle can be seen in the scanning plane, but each point where the needle leaves or enters the scanning plane can be misinterpreted as a tip of the needle (Fig. 7). As previously described, the contrast study can help in identifying the true needle tip.

For safe echocardiographic guiding of the needle for pericardiocentesis, it is essential to keep the needle tip within the scanning plane. This can be achieved by having the needle guide attached to the transducer [13, 18, 19, 20]. This is now available as an optional part of many echoscopes, but in practice it is applied more in abdominal sonographic interventions. The needle can be positioned in the scanning plane at an adjustable angle by means of a flexible guide channel holder (Figs. 7, 8). Since the needle is angled relative to the ultrasound beam, the entire length of the needle in the plane is imaged. Thus, having visualized the needle tip and its target, the

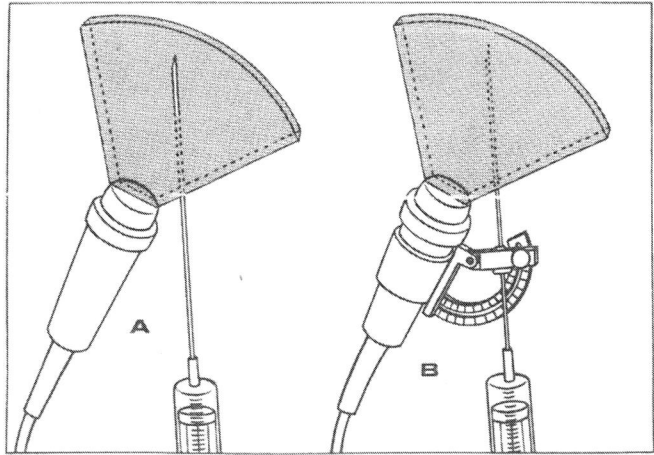

Fig. 7. Guiding the needle for pericardiocentesis with remote transducer position (A) with mis-identification of the tip at the point were the needle leaves the scanning plane. Needle guide attachment (B) assures the needle to be always in the scanning plane.

needle can be safely advanced to the pericardial sac under direct echocardiographic monitoring. It is easier to carry out this method when the thoracic approach is used in comparison to the xiphocostal approach, where the narrow field thwarts the optimal placement of the transducer and attached needle. The transducer and the needle guide should be chemically sterilized or a sterile glove can be used to cover the transducer.

In patients with concomitant pleural and pericardial effusion the pericardiocentesis can be performed through the posterior or lateral thoracic wall (Figs. 9, 10). Such a situation is more convenient, because the large pleural effusion assures an echo-free corridor toward the parietal pericar-

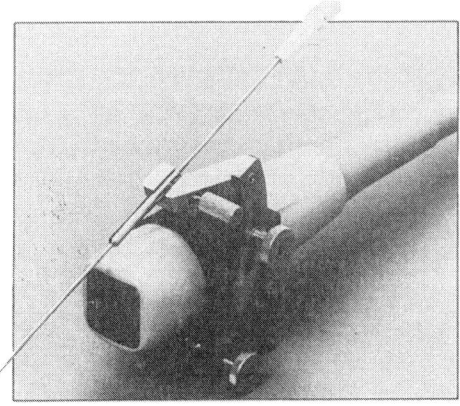

Fig. 8. Commercial needle guide attachment. Courtesy of Hewlett Packard Company.

142

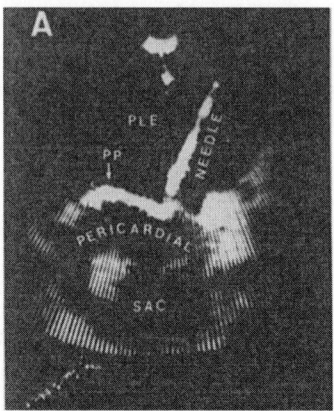 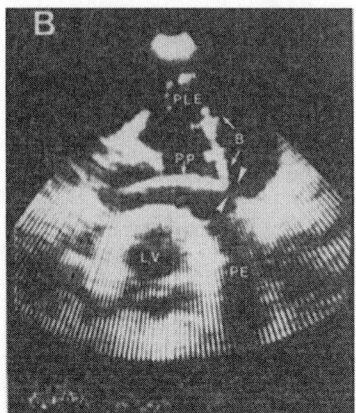

Fig. 9. Visualization of entire length of the needle for pericardiocentesis passing through the large pleural effusion (PLE) to the parietal pericardium (PP) and pericardial sac. Bioptom (B) and the window (arrows) in the parietal pericardium created during pericardial biopsy. PE: pericardial effusion, LV: left ventricle. (From Cikes I, Ernst A: New aspects of echocardiography in the diagnosis and treatment of pericardial disease. In: The Practice of M-mode and Two-dimensional Echocardiography, J Roelandt ed., Martinus Nijhoff Publishers, The Hague/ Boston/London, 1983.)

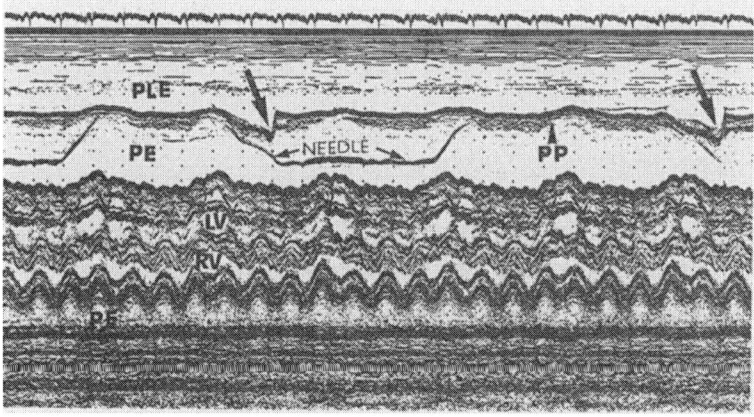

Fig. 10. M-mode tracing taken from left posterior thoracic wall during pericardiocentesis. The needle was inserted from pleural space (PLE) into the pericardial sac (PE). Fatt arrows show the invagination of parietal pericardium (PP) by needle tip. Due to lack of spatial orientation M-mode echocardiographic guidance of pericardiocentesis is not a safe procedure. LV: left ventricle, RV: right ventricle.

dium and the lung is pushed aside. In addition, the largest amount of pericardial fluid usually collects behind the left ventricular posterior wall [18–20]. In patients with such finding pericardial biopsy was performed using Trucut Travenol biopsy needle [19, 20]. A pericardial window created during biopsy for decompression can save repeted pericardiocentesis in recurent pericardial effusion with tamponade (Fig. 9B).

Complications

Although pericardiocentesis has been being performed since 1840, it is still a procedure with a high risk of morbidity and mortality. When using the 'blind' technique, it carries up to a 5% risk of fatal complications [4, 6, 21–29]; that exceeds the risk of some open heart surgical procedures. The most common major complications are hemopericardium from laceration of the coronary artery or cardiac cavity puncture and pneumothorax. Other complications include cardiac arrest, ventricular fibrillation, puncture of the peritoneal cavity or abdominal viscere, vasovagal reaction, acute pulmonary edema (too rapid empting of the pericardial sac) and nonproductive pericardiocentesis.

Eleven studies on 'blind' pericardiocentesis in the period from 1956 to 1986 are summarized in Table 1. In total of 498 reported procedures there were 29 (5,8%) deaths. Cardiac cavity punctures were reported in 35 (7%) procedures. On the contrary no fatal complications have been reported in six series [10–12, 15, 19, 30] where echocardiography was used for guidance (Table 2). Despite these reports, in practice, the echocardiographic guidance of pericardiocentesis has not been widely accepted and the role of echo-

Table 2. Incidence of Complications of Echo-guided Pericardiocentesis (PC) 1973–1988.

First author	Year	Echo-guidance	Proce-dures No.	Complications	No	%	Deaths No.
Goldberg[10]	1973	A- and M-mode	6	Ventricular puncture	1	16.7	0
Cikes[19]	1982	2D echo	17	LV puncture	1	5.9	0
Chandraratna[11]	1983	Contrast echo	16	LV puncture	2	12.5	0
				RV puncture	1	6.3	
Callahan[15]	1985	2D echo	132	RV puncture	2	1.5	0
				Pneumothorax	1	0.8	
Goldman[12]	1986	Contrast echo	13	RV puncture	1	7.7	0
Lengyel[30]	1988	2D echo	53	RV puncture	3	5.7	0
				Nonproductive PC	2	3.8	
Total			237		14	5.9	0

cardiography is usually restricted to diagnosing the pericardial effusion. To break off this habit, it seems necessary to have a larger series or cooperative studies showing the superiority of echo-guided pericardiocentesis. Such a multicentric cooperative study is now in progress in Europe [31].

Even with echo-guided pericardiocentesis cardiac cavity punctures still occur. In six studies with 237 procedures (Table 2) cardiac cavity punctures were reported in 11 (4,6%) cases. The absence of reported fatality is probably caused by its easy detection and rapid repositioning of the needle or surgical intervention. The difficulties in identifying the needle tip with a remote transducer and the inconvenience of using the needle guide attachment are the reason for punctures of the cardiac cavity. We believe that this complication could be avoided in the future by using a transducer specially designed for pericardiocentesis, or by ultrasonic marking of the needle tip (see Chapter 1.8).

References

1. Willius FA, Dry TJ: History of the Heart and the Circulation. WB Saunders Company, Philadelphia, p. 57, 1948.
2. Hochberg LA: Thoracic Surgery Before the 20th Century. 1st Ed. Vantage Press, New York, pp. 530–532, 1960.
3. Hochberg LA: Thoracic Surgery Before the 20th Century. 1st Ed. Vantage Press, New York, pp. 567–568, 1960.
4. Kilpatrick ZM, Chapman CB: On pericardiocentesis. Am J Cardiol 16: 722, 1965.
5. Marfan: Ponction du pericarde par l'epigastre. Ann de med et chir inf 15: 529, 1911.
6. Bishop LH Jr, Estes EH Jr, McIntosh HD: The electrocardiogram as a safeguard in pericardiocentesis. JAMA 162: 264, 1956.
7. Sobol SM, Thomas HM and Evans RW: Myocardial laceration not demonstrated by continuous electrocardiographic monitoring occurring during pericardiocentesis. N Engl J Med 292: 1222, 1979.
8. Tilkian AG, Daily EK: Cardiovascular Procedures. CV Mosby Company, St. Louis, pp. 233–256, 1986.
9. Alcan KE, Zabetakis PM, Marino ND, et al.: Management of acute cardiac tamponade by subxiphoid pericardiotomy. JAMA 247: 1143, 1982.
10. Goldberg BB, Pollack HM: Ultrasonically guided pericardiocentesis. Am J Cardiol 31: 490, 1973.
11. Chandraratna PAN, Reid CL, Nimalasuriya A, et al.: Application of 2-dimensional contrast studies during pericardiocentesis. Am J Cardiol 52: 1120, 1983.
12. Goldman M, Camunus J, Farhi J, Teichholz L, Mindich BP: Pericardiocentesis guided by two-dimensional contrast echocardiography: a new foolproof technique. JACC 7: 95A, 1986.
13. Cikes I: New echocardiographic possibilities in the etiological diagnosis and therapy of the pericardial diseases, Cardiovascular Diagnosis by Ultrasound: Transesophageal, Computerized, Contrast, Doppler Echocardiography, P Hanrath, W Bleifeld, J Souquet, eds., Boston, The Hague, pp. 188–201, 1982.

14. Callahan JA, Seward JB, Tajik AJ, et al.: Pericardiocentesis assisted by two-dimensional echocardiography. J Thorac Cardiovasc Surg 85: 877, 1983.
15. Callahan JA, Seward JB, Nishimura RA, et al.: Two-dimensional echocardiographically guided pericardiocentesis: experience in 117 consecutive patients. Am J Cardiol 55: 476, 1985.
16. Callahan JA, Seward JB: Diagnosis and treatment of pericardial effusion using ultrasonic guidance. In: Interventional Ultrasound Van Sonnenberg E., ed., Churchill Livingstone, New York, 1987.
17. Callaham M: Pericardiocentesis. In: Clinical Procedures in Emergency Medicine. Roberts JR, Hedges JR, eds., Saunders, Philadelphia, pp. 208–224, 1985.
18. Cikes I: Echocardiography in pericardial disease. In: Progress in Medical Ultrasound 3, Kurjak A, ed., Excerpta Medica, Amsterdam-Oxford-Princeton, pp. 227–240, 1982.
19. Cikes I, Ernst A: New aspects of echocardiography for the diagnosis and treatment of pericardial disease. In: The practice of M-mode and two-dimensional echocardiography, Roelandt J, ed., Martinus Nijhoff Pub, Hague/Boston/London, pp. 141–156, 1983.
20. Cikes I, Breyer B, Ernst A, Custovic F: Interventional Echocardiography. In: Interventional Ultrasound, Holm HH, Kristensen JK, eds., Munksgaard, Copenhagen, pp. 160–168, 1985.
21. Fredriksen RT, Cohen LS, Mullins CB: Pericardial windows or pericardiocentesis for pericardial effusion. Am Heart J, 82: 158, 1971.
22. Morin JE, Hollomby D, Gonda A, Long R, Dobell ARC: Menagement of uremic pericarditis: a report of 11 patients with cardiac tamponade and a review of the literature. Ann of Thorac Surg 22: 588, 1976.
23. Pradham DJ, Ikins PM: The role of pericardiectomy in the treatment of pericarditis with effusion. Am Surg 42: 257, 1976.
24. Silverberg S, Oreopoulos DG, Wife DG, et al.: Pericarditis in patients undergoing long term hemodialysis and peritoneal dialysis. Am J Med, 63: 874, 1977.
25. Krikorian JG, Hancock EW: Pericardiocentesis. Am J Med, 65: 808, 1978.
26. Kwasnik EM, Koster JK Jr, Lazarus JM, et al.: Conservative management of uremic pericardial effusions. J Thorac Cardiovasc Surg, 76: 629, 1978.
27. Wong B, Murphy J, Chang CJ, Hassenein K, Dunn M: The risk of pericardiocentesis, Am J Cardiol, 44: 1110, 1979.
28. Gubermann BA, Fowler NO, Engel PJ, Gueron M, Allen JM: Cardiac tamponade in medical patients. Circulation, 64: 633, 1981.
29. Fowler NO: Cardiac tamponade in medical patients: the rarity of Beck's triad. In: Progress in Cardiology 14, Yu PN, Goodwin JF, eds., Lea Febiger, Philadelphia, pp. 35–49, 1986.
30. Lengyel M: Data from questionnaire for Cikes I: European Cooperative Study on Pericardiocentesis. In preparation.
31. Cikes I: European Cooperative Study on Pericardiocentesis. In preparation.

PART 3: Contrast Echocardiography

3.1. Contrast echocardiography

J. ROELANDT, C. TIRTAMAN, W. B. VLETTER, F. J. TEN CATE,
D. ROMDONI, W. J. GUSSENHOVEN & H. RIJSTERBORGH

Echocardiography offers many advantages over other imaging techniques since it permits differentiation of cardiac structures from blood-filled cavities without using an exogenous contrast agent. This noninvasive and versatile method thus allows a quantitative assessment of cardiac structure and function. Information on blood flow can be obtained by the rapid injection of a biologically compatible solution containing microbubbles of gas which are dissolved in the solution and injected directly [1], or which may be produced by transient or stable cavitation during injection into the blood stream [2]. These microbubbles make the blood 'echogenic' and stream along with the blood enabling it to be imaged on its way through the cardiac chambers. The microbubbles of gas are completely removed from the blood by the 'sieve' action of the peripheral or pulmonary capillary bed [3]. Studies of blood flow dynamics were previously possible only with cine-angiocardiography.

The echocardiographic contrast effect was first described by Gramiak et al. in 1968 and they used it for identification of cardiac structures on M-mode echocardiograms [4]. Originally direct catheter injections of freshly prepared indocyanine green dye were employed as the contrast agent. It soon became apparent that the contrast effect could also be obtained after peripheral injection of commonly employed physiologic solutions. The method has been of enormous clinical potential and has been used for many years for the diagnosis (and exclusion) of intracardiac as well as extracardiac shunts and in the diagnosis of valvular insufficiency.

Color-coded Doppler flow imaging now provides an alternative method with many advantages to contrast echocardiography and most of these clinical uses will be displaced in the near future. Accordingly, research efforts have more intensely focused upon attempts to quantify cardiac function and myocardial blood flow. The development of experimental contrast agents with specific physiocochemical properties which have reproducible characteristics and/or are capable of pulmonary transmission [5–7] together with innovative videodensitometric techniques for quantitative analysis of two-dimensional contrast echocardiograms [8] have stimulated the interest in the field. The possibility of cardiac output [9], and ejection fraction measurement [10, 11] as well as the quantification of left-to-right shunts has been suggested

I. Cikes (ed.), *Echocardiography in Cardiac Interventions*, 149–177, 1989.
© 1989 *Kluwer Academic Publishers*.

150

[12]. Because of methodological and technical problems, however, these goals have not yet been achieved. Experimental studies have indicated the potential of studying myocardial regional perfusion [13–16] but a safe and reproducible contrast agent for human application is not yet available.

We will review the comparative clinical usefulness of contrast echocardiography and color Doppler flow imaging. The theoretical, technical and methodological problems relevant to the quantitative (videodensitometric) analysis of contrast echocardiograms will be discussed as this application represents an interesting current research goal.

General aspects of contrast echocardiography

Contrast agents[*]

Several mechanisms have been proposed to explain the echocardiographic contrast effect but it has been demonstrated that microbubbles of gas present in the injectate and/or the injecting apparatus are the predominant cause [1]. Hand agitated dextrose 5% in water and saline are currently the most commonly employed contrast agents for routine studies because they are inexpensive and lack toxicity. In most patients they yield adequate contrast intensity after both peripheral and central catheter injections. If this is not the case, hand agitated polygelin 3% colloid solution (Hemaccel[R]) can be used and may improve the contrast yield since its surfactant properties stabilize microbubbles of air in the solution [17]. If this is still insufficient, a 0.5 to 2 ml of 100% medical pure carbon dioxide followed by a 5 ml 'chaser' of saline or dextrose solution will always provide an adequate contrast effect [18,19]. Experimental studies with a large variety of substances such as perfluoro-carbon compounds (artificial blood) 10% liposyn, 75% dimethylsulfoxide, 0.5% paraldehyde and 8% propylene glucol, have been perfomed [20,21].

Recently, a whole area of potential new contrast agents has been developed by sonication of viscous sugar solutions [6]. A pharmacologically prepared contrast agent which holds great promise is SHU 454 (Echocon) [7]. It is a powder form of a biodegradable polysaccharide which when mixed with a diluent forms an echoreflective suspension of crystalloid (Fig. 1). Toxity studies with this new pharmacologically prepared contrast agents have confirmed that its use is associated with low risk.

It has further been demonstrated that the pulmonary transmission after peripheral venous injection is sufficient to delineate the boundary of the left ventricle. In addition, such contrast agents would allow regional myocardial perfusion studies although studies thus far have required intracoronary or

[*] State of the art 1986.

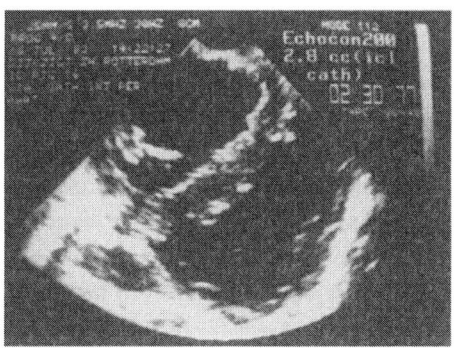

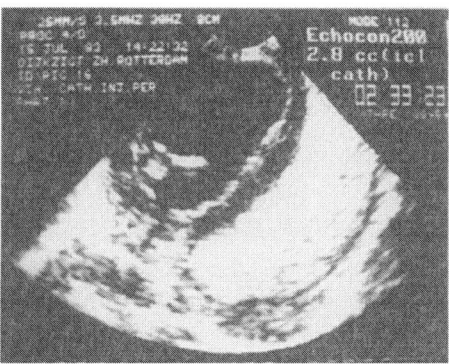

Fig. 1. Example of echocardiographic contrast effect of the right ventricle (RV) after peripheral venous injection of 2.8 ml Echocon (SSH-454) in an experimental animal. Note the homogeneous and dense contrast effect of the right ventricular cavity not causing overload as the thin RV wall structures behind the contrast filled cavity can still be identified. LV: left ventricular cavity.

intra-aortic injection of the contrast agent. The presently available contrast agents, however, do not permit measurement of physiologic microcirculatory transit time because their size is relatively large and not constant and cause blockage of the capillaries. It should also be realized that the physical characteristics of the carrier (diluent) must be considered as they may affect the imaging characteristics [22]. Carrier-induced toxic and hyperemic effects have been observed (see Chapter 3.2.).

Toxicity of contrast echocardiography

Problems of potential toxicity should especially be kept in mind during peripheral venous or right heart injections in patients with potential or known right-to-left shunting. The risk, however, has been estimated to be as low as 0.062% and the technique is certainly safer than currently available alternative diagnostic modalities [24]. With increasing interest in myocardial perfusion studies and left heart studies following peripheral venous injection, blockage of regional microcirculation due to a significant amount of large microbubbles should be considered as a potential cause of side effects. Both animal [25] and human studies [26] have not demonstrated gross toxicity but adverse effects on myocardial performance have been reported, which may have consequences in patients with marginal function [27, 28]. Cardiac depression may result from the properties of the vehicle of the contrast material or transient mechanical obstruction of the capillaries by the micro-bubbles. Displacement of O_2 carrying seems negligable. Safety must remain a prime concern of all clinicians involved in contrast echocardiography.

Qualitative contrast echocardiography

M-mode and two-dimensional contrast echocardiography each have their own specific advantages and disadvantages for clinical problem solving. In general, two dimensional echocardiography is superior when abnormal anatomy or patterns of blood flow need to be studied. Because of its better time resolution M-mode echocardiography has advantages when time relations are to be examined. When performing routine echocardiographic contrast studies using peripheral venous injection, there is large variability in contrast effect even when the procedure is carefully standardized. This is most likely due to the variability of microbubbles of air present in the injectate, connection of the syringe to the injecting apparatus, individual variations of venous circulation and differences of respiration and arm/head position between injections. Adequate transmission from the injection site to the central circulation may further be limited by a sluggish injection and/or slow venous blood flow. Because of their low weight, microbubbles of air tend to move against the vascular wall where blood flow is slower. All these factors increase the chance that a variable amount of microbubbles of air dissolve before they reach the heart.

Quantitative contrast echocardiography

M-mode echocardiography

Different types of measurements can be made from M-mode contrast echo-cardiograms which are pertinent for studying both physiologic and patho-physiologic events of intracardiac blood flow [29] (Table 1).

Timing of contrast appearance yields important physiologic and diagnos-

Table 1. Analysis of M-mode contrast echocardiograms.

- Timing of appearance
- Pattern of opacification
- Clearance time
- Cyclical opacification
- Relative intensity
- Slope of trajectories

---

tic information. Left heart contrast appearing a few cycles after right heart opacification implies an intracardiac shunt, whereas a consistent delay of 6-8 cardiac cycles suggests intrapulmonary right-to-left shunting [30]. In total anomalous pulmonary venous drainage contrast appears in early diastole in the mitral valve orifice, whereas it arrives in mid-diastole in transposition of the great arteries with right-to-left shunting at atrial level. The timing of echo contrast appearance in the left heart after peripheral contrast injection in patients with a ventricular septal defect may help in the assessment of right ventricular hemodynamics [31]. The pattern of opacification often provides clues to the diagnosis of complex congenital heart disease [32]. Atrial and ventricular clearance time of echo contrast is prolonged in patients with a low output state or valvular insufficiency [33]. Relative clearance time of both right and left ventricle or the great vessels can also be examined and yields information on shunt size [12].

Cyclical opacification of a great artery proves its ventriculo-arterial connection [34]. In the presence of an intracardiac shunt, the relative intensities of contrast in both the right and left heart cavities and great vessels contain information on the shunt size [12, 34]. The slopes of contrast trajectories on M-mode echocardiographic tracings represent the velocity component of the blood moving in the direction of, or away from, the transducer, thus providing information similar to that obtained using pulsed Doppler techniques [35]. A correlation between invasive measured pulmonary blood velocities and the velocity of contrast trajectories on M-mode recordings has been demonstrated by Japanese investigators [36].

Two-dimensional echocardiography

A quantitative videodensitometric analysis of contrast echocardiograms would be possible if indicator dilution theory and techniques could be applied to contrast two-dimensional echocardiography. This requires a constant relationship between the concentrations of a contrast agent and the contrast intensity. However, several problems exist and are related to the contrast agents, ultrasound physics and the instrumentation.

A. Problems related to contrast agents (Table 2)

Quantitative contrast echocardiography requires predetermined acoustical properties of the contrast agent used. Although gas containing microbubbles have optimal echogenic qualities they are less optimal from a physical point of view. Microbubbles of gas are unstable resulting in an unpredictable contrast effect. Acoustic theory further indicates that the size of the microbubbles should be smaller than half of the wavelength of the incident sound beam in order to make them omnidirectional scatterers rather than reflectors. In addition, the relative backscattering ratio is strongly related to the size of the microbubble. In practice, they should be smaller than 100 microns in diameter. However, such small microbubbles are highly unstable in solution and will only persist for a few seconds in the circulation. Thus, the key to the application of microbubbles of gas for echo contrast imaging lies in making them stable so that they survive long enough in the blood stream.

Table 2. Assumptions for videodensitometric analysis of contrast echocardiograms.

- Known and reproducible properties of ultrasound scatterers
- Volume concentration of ultrasound scatterers must be known
- Known and constant intensity of the sound field
- Video level proportional to the number of ultrasound scatterers
- Lifetime of ultrasound scatterers must be longer than measurement time

The backscattering properties of a microbubble of gas must remain constant during echocardiographic measurement. As a consequence its size should remain constant. The density and size of microbubbles of gas in solution is influenced by numerous physical factors including temperature, surface tension, viscosity and partial pressure of the gas in the circulation. Furthermore, all microbubbles must have identical characteristics and therefore they all must have the same dimension. Encapsulation materials such as gelatin (soft-shelled microbubbles) and polysaccharides (hard-shelled microbubbles) can be used. Such encapsulated microbubbles can be made precise to a diameter of approximately 75 microns with a standard deviation of ± 0.7 microns [37]. Current attempts to manufacture smaller microbubbles are underway. The 'microballoons' may contain air, nitrogen or carbon dioxide and are suspended in a viscous liquid or gelatin matrix which dissolves from the bubbles when injected in the blood stream. Clearly, the encapsulating and suspending materials must be biologically compatible, nontoxic and should not interfere with the reflective characteristics of the microbubbles of gas. Recently, a new methodology applying sonication to cavitate and agitate high viscous solutions with air has been developed [6]. These microbubbles are fairly uniform and small (microbubble size approx. 10 microns) and most of them pass the microcapillary circulation without obstructing it. They also persist so long that they may appear in the left ventricular cavity and myocardium after a right-sided injection [38]. Until now, these agents were used in experimental studies but their toxicity needs further evaluation before they can be used clinically. Also pharmacologically prepared substances able to pass a capillary bed and derived from SHU-445 are now being tested in animal studies.

In addition to the need to know the quantity of backscattered energy per microbubble, the amount of microbubbles or scatterers injected must also be known in order to have an indication of their concentration in the heart or myocardium during echocardiographic measurement. Bolus dynamics and blood flow characteristics are further unknown factors influencing the concentration of scatterers in a cardiac cavity after a peripheral injection.

B. Problems related to ultrasound physics and instrumentation

An important prerequisite for quantitative contrast echocardiography is that the sound field intensity must be known and remain constant in the volume sampled for contrast intensity. This will be difficult to achieve in practice as there are different structures with different acoustic properties interfering with the sampling sound beam during the cardiac cycle.

A high concentration of scatterers may give rise to secondary scatterers (reverberations) which may result in an unknown quantity of ultrasound energy reflected on the transducer. This effect can theoretically be avoided by the use of microbubbles with a dimension of at most 1/10 of the wave length of the interrogating sound beam.

Uniform scatterers are necessary for an accurate display of intracardiac cavities not affected by side lobe artifacts. Indeed, the accuracy of display of a contrast filled medium is determined by the ratio between main and side lobe sensitivity, and thus depends on uniformity of contrast material.

Commercially available video systems cannot represent the full dynamic range of the echo amplitudes. This introduces measurement errors. These errors are further influenced by the signal processing and time-gain compensation of the echographic system resulting in nonlinear and unevenly compensated image distribution of echo amplitudes [23]. Therefore it appears that physical characteristics of imaging (beam profiles, attenuation of sound), processing of and presentation of the echo data presently limit the quantitative analysis of echo intensities. All the above considerations make clear that at present accurate quantitative videodensitometric analysis of contrast echocardiograms is not yet possible. Many studies published so far have demonstrated that computer-based videodensitometric analysis is possible [8] but the results should be considered qualitative or semi-quantitative at best. The subject, however, is an exciting and valid research goal.

Clinical application of contrast echocardiography

Echocardiographic structure identification

Contrast echocardiography was originally used for identifying cardiac structures on M-mode echocardiograms [4] and later for validation of two-dimensional echocardiography [39]. Abnormal venous connections, such as a persistent left superior vena cava entering the right atrium through a dilated coronary sinus, or the rare form entering directly into the left atrium, are readily diagnosed using left antecubital vein contrast injections [40]. Other structures that peripheral contrast injections can aid in correctly identifying include the Eustachian valve, at the level of the inferior vena cava – right atrial junction, the inter-atrial patch and its function after Mustard's operation for transposition of the great arteries, aneurysm of the interatrial septum, and space occupying lesions in the right atrium and ventricle. Direct catheter injections of echo contrast were used to identify the common pulmonary venous chamber in patients with total anamolous pulmonary venous return.

With the availability of high resolution two-dimensional echocardiographic systems providing excellent structure definition the use of contrast echocardiography for structure identification has decreased dramatically.

Demonstration (or exclusion) of shunts

Since echocardiographic contrast is entirely removed from the circulation by the pulmonary capillary bed [3], the appearance of contrast in the left heart after a peripheral venous injection is diagnostic for a right-to-left shunt. The pattern and appearance time of the echo contrast in the left heart are determined by the level of the shunt and the relative pressures in the cardiac chambers. Shunts as small as 5% can detected by contrast echocardiography [41]. Recently, it has been shown that pulmonary wedge injections can yield left heart contrast. This may be used to demonstrate and often localize left-to-right shunts without requiring left heart catheterization [42, 43]. Agents capable of crossing the pulmonary circulation after intravenous injection may provide direct echo contrast imaging of left-to-right shunts. Videodensitometric analysis of both positive (and negative) contrast effects may further allow to quantify the magnitude of intracardiac shunts [21].

Peripheral contrast echocardiography can be used to diagnose a shunt at the atrial level by taking advantage of the small right-to-left shunt present in early systole in an uncomplicated atrial septal defect [44, 45]. The specificity is 100% and the sensitivity 88% which is better than either oxymetry or nuclear medicine techniques. 'Negative contrast effect' [46] in our experience is not a sensitive sign to diagnose atrial septal defects (Fig. 2). In right-to-left

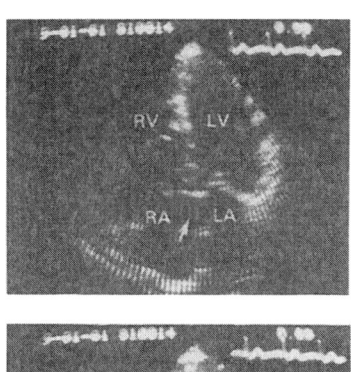

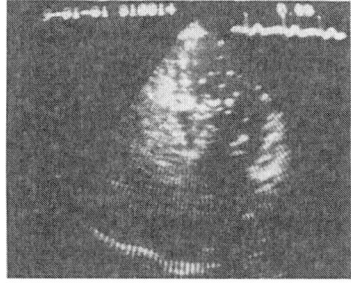

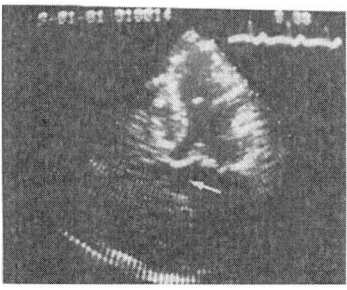

Fig. 2. Apical four chamber views obtained from a patient with an atrial septal defect of the primum type. The defect is indicated by the arrow on the upper panel. The middle panel shows opacification of the right-sided heart after peripheral venous injection of 5 ml of dextrose 5% in water. Echocontrast appears in the left ventricle (LV) indicating right-to-left shunting. The negative contrast effect proving the atrial septal defect is seen on the lower panel (arrow) when noncontrast blood flows from the left atrium (LA) into the right atrium (RA). RV = right ventricle.

158

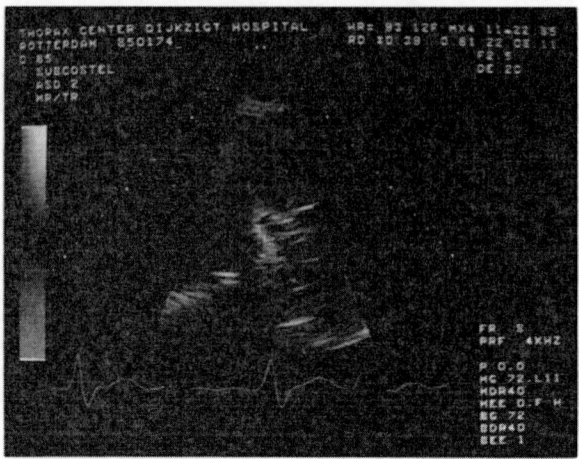

Fig. 3. Subcostal view of a patient with an atrial septal defect of the secundum type. Left-to-right shunting blood flow towards the transducer is visualized during diastole and encoded in red.

shunting at atrial level, the peripherally injected contrast should appear in the left ventricle only one or two heartbeats after appearance in the right ventricle. If there is a delay of more than two cardiac cycles, the diagnosis of intrapulmonary shunting should be considered. Of course, patients with an atrial septal defect with significant left-to-right shunting will always have signs of right ventricular volume overload on their baseline echocardiograms [47]. Color Doppler flow imaging greatly improves our capabilities to diagnose the various types of atrial septal defects. It facilitates imaging of the localization of the defect (Fig. 3).

Positive contrast studies may be obtained in patients with only a patent foramen ovale and this has consequences for the diagnosis of an atrial septal defect. On the other hand, the detection of a patent foramen ovale may sometimes have important clinical consequences in individual patients. Unexplained cyanosis in patients with patent foramen ovale may occur after right ventricular myocardial infarction. These patients will have a strongly positive contrast study. In patients suspected of having had a paradoxical systemic embolism the diagnosis is supported by a positive contrast study.

Although there is some bidirectional flow across a ventricular septal defect, peripheral venous contrast studies often fail to show the right-to-left shunting in the absence of pulmonary hypertension. Right-to-left shunting of contrast material occurs when the right ventricular systolic pressure approaches 50% of the systolic systemic pressure [48]. The shunting occurs in protodiastole during isovolumic relaxation of the left ventricle. With increasing pressure, specific patterns of right-to-left shunting blood-flow can be

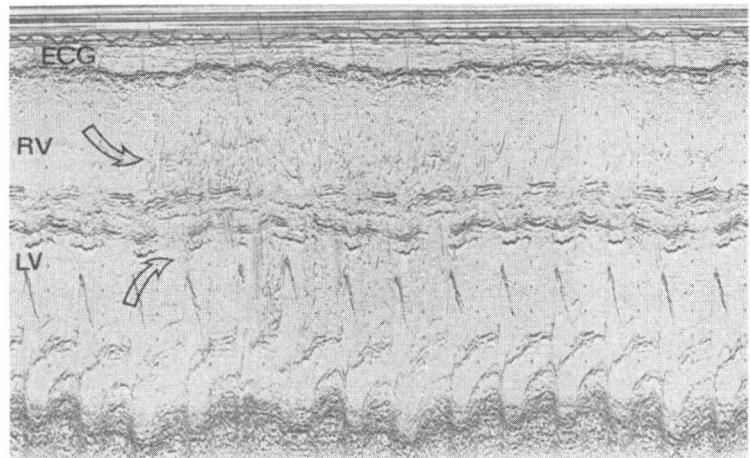

Fig. 4. M-mode echocardiogram of a patient with a ventricular septal defect and moderately severe pulmonary hypertension. After peripheral venous injection of echo-contrast, it appears first in the right ventricle (RV) in early diastole (see arrow) and one cardiac cycle later in the left ventricle (LV) during the early diastolic (isovolumic) phase (see arrow). The echo-contrast does not appear in the mitral valve funnel. This pattern is compatible with a ventricular septal defect and right-to-left shunt. Note the increased shunting after the ventricular premature beat. ECG: electrocardiogram.

observed [31]. In uncomplicated ventricular septal defects, right-to-left shunting may occasionally be observed during Valsalva maneuver or ventricular premature beats and in patients with post-infarction ventricular septal defect, contrast echoes may be seen passing from the right to the left ventricle, possibly as a result of inequalities in compliance and relaxation between both ventricles (Fig. 4). Negative contrast effect can also be used for detecting uncomplicated and post-infarct ventricular septal defects [49]. Direct left ventricular echo contrast injections are now increasingly used in the catheterization laboratory (Fig. 5). The method is certainly a better technique than angiography for the detailed assessment of the interventricular septum and blood flow patterns in the presence of atrioventricular canal defects [50] and for the demonstration of small (additional) muscular septal defects [51] (Fig. 6). Left ventricle to right atrium shunts have been demonstrated with left ventricular contrast injections.

Color-coded Doppler flow imaging has great promise for detecting the presence, localization, direction and timing of ventricular septal defects. Unsuspected additional and multiple defects are readily recognized with this new technique and it is quite obvious that it will replace contrast echocardiography for the diagnosis of most conditions with intracardiac shunts in the routine echo laboratory (Figs. 7 and 8).

160

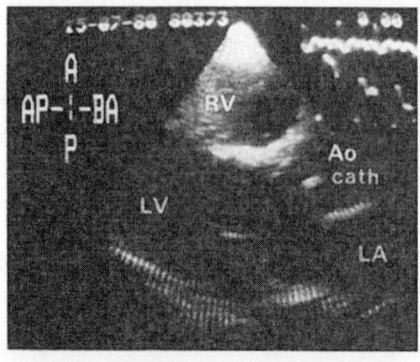

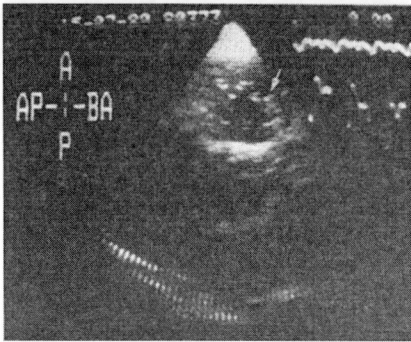

Fig. 5. Parasternal long axis views of a patient with a high ventricular septal defect before (upper panel) and after (lower panel) catheter injection of echo contrast in the left ventricular outflow tract. Echoes appear in the right ventricular outflow tract (arrow) proving a small left-to-right shunt.

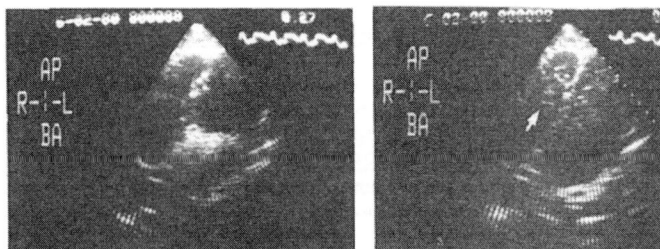

Fig. 6. Apical four chamber view of a patient with a small ventricular septal defect. A bolus of echo constrast is injected into the left ventricle (LV) via a catheter (left panel). During the next systole, a small amount of echo contrast passes via the muscular ventricular septal defect into the right ventricle (RV) indicated by the arrow on the right panel. This ventricular septal defect was not demonstrated by oximetry.

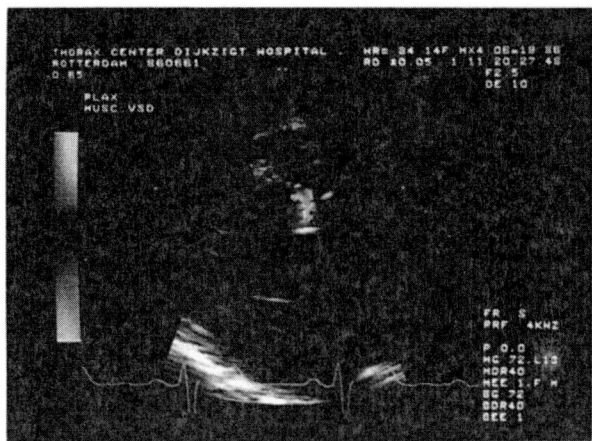

Fig. 7. Parasternal long axis view (PLAX) visualizing the apical area of the left ventricle with color-coded Doppler flow imaging. A small jet through the midventricular septum was unexpectedly visualized during systole proving a muscular septal defect.

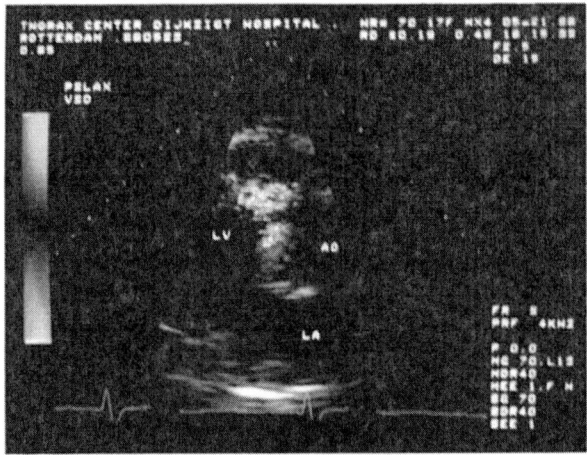

Fig. 8. Long axis view and a left-to-right shunt through a high ventricular septal defect which was unexpectedly visualized in a patient with a systolic murmur. Note similarity of information with contrast echocardiography after left ventricular catheter injection shown in Fig. 5. Ao = aorta; LA = left atrium; LV = left ventricle.

Analysis of complex congenital heart disease

Using information obtained by peripheral contrast injections from both the parasternal and suprasternal transducer positions it is possible to determine the position of the great vessels and their ventriculo-arterial connections [34]. Together with the ability to detect and localize shunts, contrast echocardiography offers important advantages to the pediatric cardiologist who needs to analyze complex congenital heart disease, particularly in neonates. Characteristic contrast echocardiographic patterns may be seen in univentricular hearts with either one of two atrioventricular valves, tricuspid atresia, overriding tricuspid valve, 'double-inlet' left ventricle, and atrioventricular canal defects [52]. In general, the more complex the congenital defect, the more likely is the existence of lesion specific echocardiography and blood flow patterns. Here too, color-coded Doppler flow imaging may replace contrast echo to a large extent in the near future.

Diagnosis of valvular insufficiency

Direct visualization of the regurgitant jet is only exceptionally possible by contrast echocardiography (Fig. 9). Color Doppler flow imaging allows direct visualization of the regurgitant jet in virtually all patients (Fig. 10). Analysis of the timing – more specifically the moment of appearance of the contrast bolus in the inferior vena cava after an upper extremity vein injection allows the examiner to diagnose or exclude tricuspid insufficiency with a high degree of certainty. The inferior vena cava can be imaged in nearly all patients studied, since there are no 'window problems' due to overlying bones or lung. If contrast appears in the inferior vena cava synchronous with the v-wave of the atrial pressure curve, the diagnosis of tricuspid insufficiency can be made [53, 54] (Figs. 11 and 12). Contrast is frequently seen to appear synchronous with the a-wave (presystolic) or in no definite relation to the cardiac cycle: this does not suggest tricuspid insufficiency, and is frequently seen in normals during deep respiration and in conditions affecting right

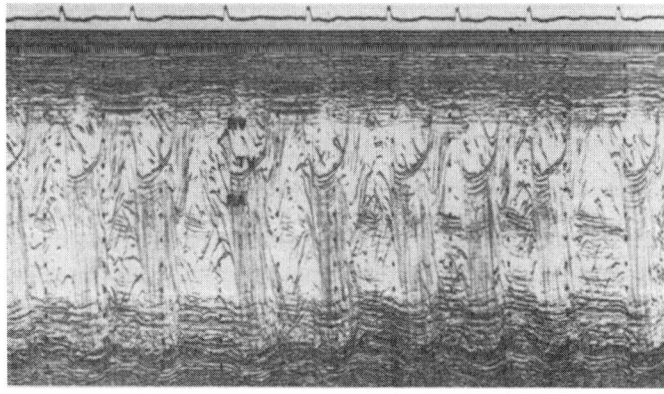

Fig. 9. Contrast echocardiogram of the tricuspid valve showing regurgitation of echo contrast during systole into the right atrium (RA). RV = right ventricle; TV = tricuspid valve.

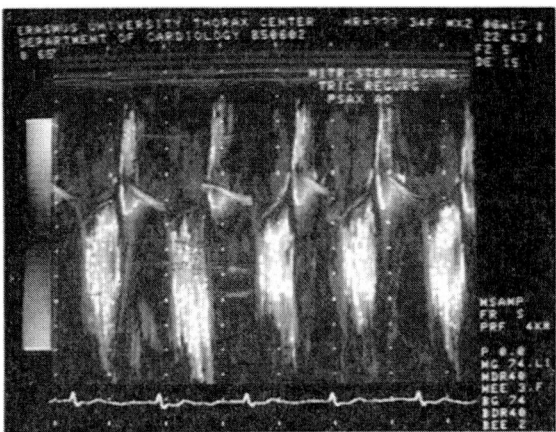

Fig. 10. Regurgitant blood flow velocity is sampled along a single Doppler line aimed through the regurgitant jet in a patient with tricuspid regurgitation. The blood flow velocity and its dispersion at each point along this interrogating Doppler beam axis is displayed in color and superimposed on the M-mode echocardiogram. This V-mode Doppler echocardiogram allows an accurate analysis of timing and direction of blood flow. Note similarity with the data obtained by contrast echocardiography shown in fig. 9.

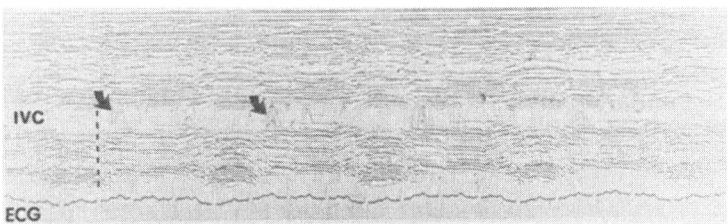

Fig. 11. M-mode echocardiogram showing the inferior vena cava (IVC) and a 'V-wave synchronous' appearance of echo contrast (see arrows) in a patient with atrial fibrillation and a fast ventricular rate. The pattern is diagnostic for tricuspid regurgitation.

ventricular filling (pulmonary stenosis, constrictive pericarditis, tricuspid stenosis, pulmonary hypertension, and rhythm disturbances). Specific echo contrast patterns have been seen in pulmonary insufficiency (a steep positive slope in early diastole across the pulmonary valve), but their sensitivity and specificity remains a subject for further study. The use of contrast echocardiography for the detection of right-sided valve lesions is now being replaced by Doppler echocardiography which offers greater sensitivity and allows semi-quantitative assessment of the severity in most patients. In addition, right ventricular and pulmonary arterial systolic pressure can be estimated from the peak systolic velocity across the valve (Fig. 13).

Demonstration of left-sided valvular insufficiency requires catheter injection and thus cardiac catheterization [55]. However, it is a sensitive

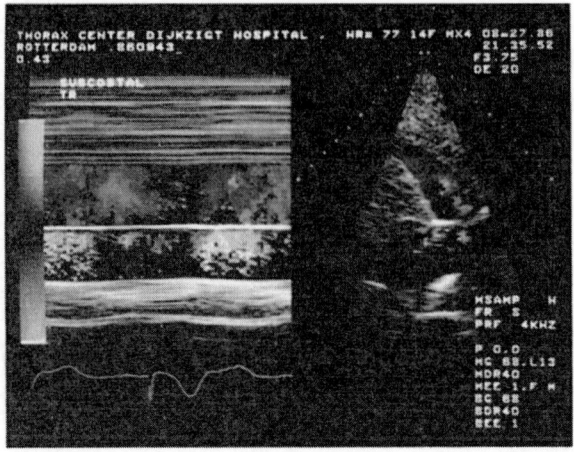

Fig. 12. A systolic subcostal view of the inferior vena cava and hepatic vein of a patient with tricuspid regurgitation. Note flow reversal (towards transducer and encoded in red) in the hepatic vein, which is diagnostic when occuring in systole. For a better timing analysis a single Doppler line is selected and indicated on the flow map. The blood flow velocity and its dispersion are superimposed on the M-mode echocardiogram of the IVC (at left). Reversal of flow occurs during systole and is diagnostic for tricuspid regurgitation.

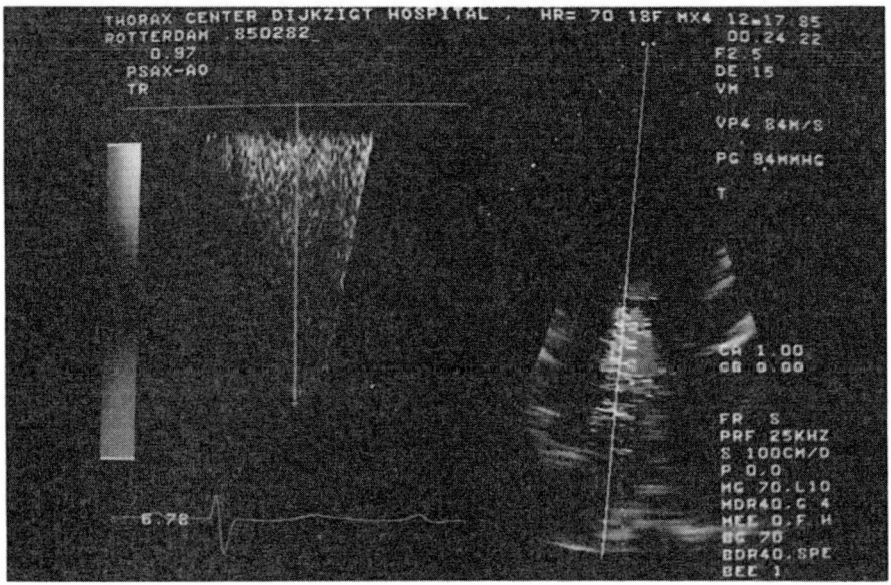

Fig. 13. Continuous-wave Doppler interrogation of the tricuspid regurgitant jet is performed along the sound beam axis shown on the color Doppler flow map at right. Peak systolic velocity (VP) is 4.84 m.s.$^{-1}$ corresponding to a peak systolic pressure difference (PG) of 94 mmHg between the right ventricle and right atrium. Adding clinically estimated central venous pressure provides an estimated right ventricular systolic pressure of approximately 105 mmHg, indicating severe pulmonary hypertension.

method for the detection (or exclusion) of valvular insufficiency since as little as 10% of the forward stroke volume is detected [56].

Echo-ventriculography can be considered in situations with poor hemo-dynamics or when contraindications to radiographic contrast agents (allergy, renal insufficiency) or ionizing radiation (pregnancy) exist [57] (Figs. 14–17). Further advantages are that multiple injections can be performed and many different cardiac views can be obtained for analysis since entirely nontoxic contrast agents are used, and that hand injections of small amounts of fluid

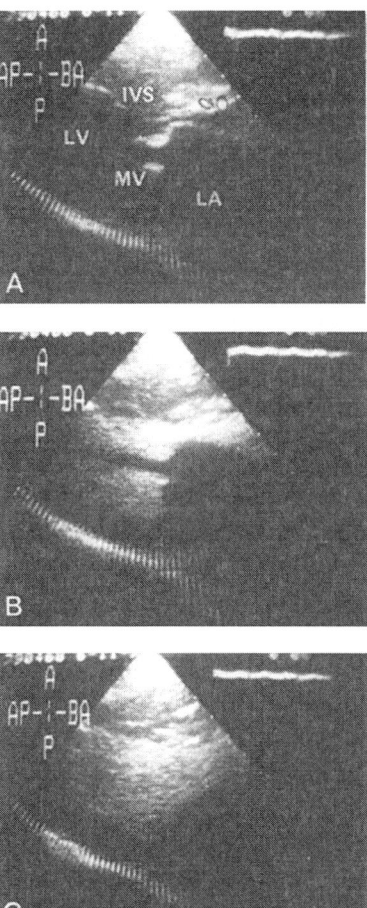

Fig. 14. Parasternal long axis views of a patient with mitral valve stenosis before (upper panel) and after injection of echo contrast via a catheter in the left ventricle. The middle panel shows a frame recorded during diastole. The negative shadow caused by the non-contrast blood flowing from the left atrium into the left ventricle visualises the transmitral blood flow pattern. During systole (lower panel) the contrast does not pass into the left atrium excluding mitral in-competence. IVS = interventricular septum; LA = left atrium; LV = left ventricle, MV = mitral valve.

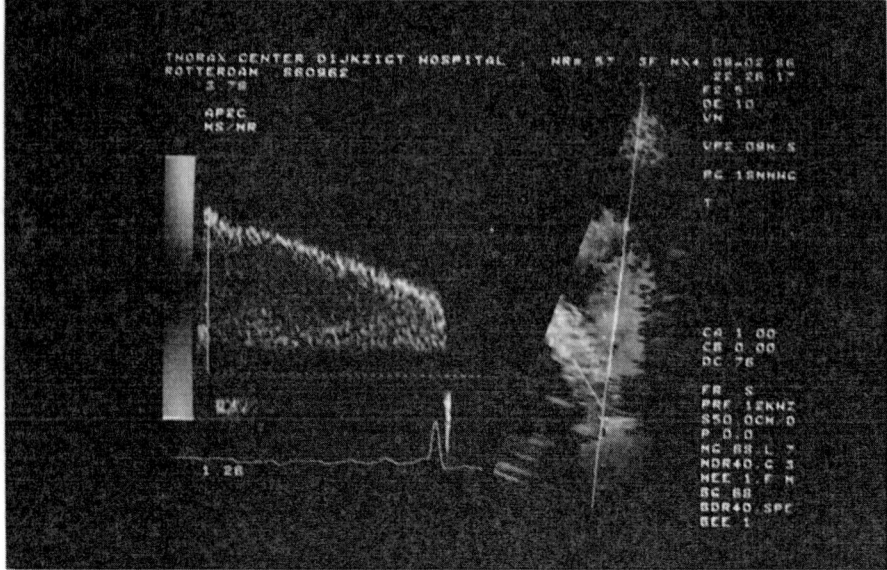

Fig. 15. A diastolic apical long axis view of a patient with mitral stenosis is shown to the right. The stenotic jet is visualized and bends off towards the apex as it hits the left ventricular wall. Continuous wave Doppler sampling is performed along a sound beam indicated on the flow map and the spectral velocity output is shown to the left. The angle between the jet flow and sound beam can be adjusted on the flow map allowing an accurate calculation of blood flow velocity. As an example the velocity has been measured in early diastole (indicated by the cursor on the spectral velocity output) and automatically calculated by machine software. The peak velocity (VP) in this beat is 2.09 m.s.$^{-1}$ representing a pressure difference of 18 mmHg at that particular moment in diastole. Transmitral blood flow is readily visualized not requiring the injection of echo contrast.

do not cause the premature beats frequently seen during standard cardiac angiography (Table 3).

Other uses in the catheterization laboratory are guiding the needle and verification of catheter tip position after transseptal puncture [58] and pericardiocentesis with pericardial biopsy and fenestration [59, 60].

Table 3. Advantages of contrast echoventriculography.

- Multiple injections and cardiac views for analysis.
- High sensitivity for detection of shunts and valvular insufficiency.
- No adverse effects:
  no toxic contrast (allergy, renal failure)
  no ionizing energy (pregnancy)
- Avoidance of arrhythmias
- Decrease of cost

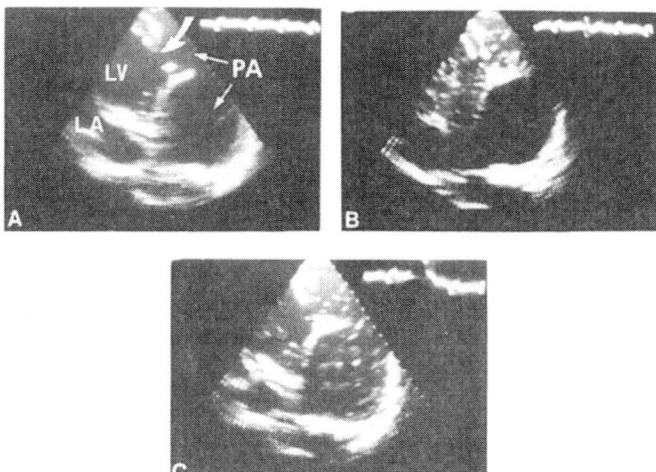

Fig. 16. Apical views of the left ventricle (LV) and left atrium (LA) aforeshortened to the left in the four chamber plane. The patient had a large post-myocardial infarction pseudo-aneurysm (PA). The defect in the lateral LV wall is indicated by the arrow in panel A. Echo contrast injected into the left ventricle passes via the defect into the anterior part of the PA (panel B) and subsequently opacifies it completely (panel C). The echo contrast remains circulating in the PA during many cardiac cycles.

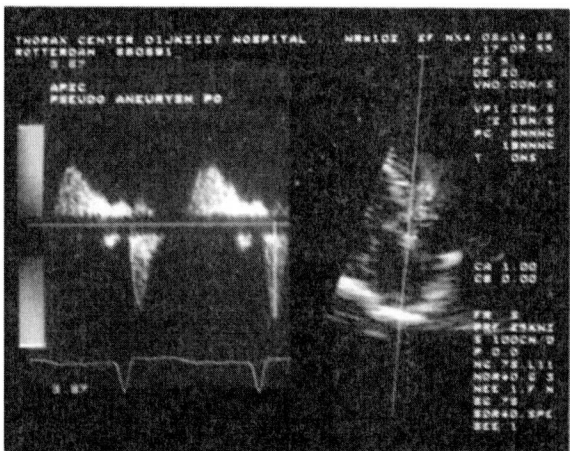

Fig. 17. Diastolic apical long axis view with color Doppler flow map of a patient with a postero-basal pseudo-aneurysm of the left ventricle. The mosaic of colors indicates inflow of blood from within the pseudo-aneurysm into the ventricle. Continuous wave Doppler sampling is performed along a sound beam indicated on the flow map and a spectral velocity output is shown to the left. Note the systolic flow away from the transducer into the pseudo-aneurysm and the diastolic outflow in the direction of the transducer into the left ventricle. Unlike with contrast echocardiography a direct and comprehensive diagnosis is possible with the color Doppler mapping technique.

Intraoperative contrast echocardiography

Some investigators have used contrast echocardiography before chest closure to evaluate mitral valve operations [61, 62]. Residual valvular regurgitation after commissurotomy and reconstructive surgery of the mitral and tricuspid valve as well as residual shunting after repair of intracardiac defects are readily demonstrated (Fig. 18). In some instances this information made us to decide to put the patient again on extracorporeal circulation and reoperate (see Chapter 5.1.). Obviously, more data are necessary before this approach will find a more widespread application. Although in an early stage it is anticipated that intraoperative echocardiography has the potential to become an important clinical method [63] but here too color Doppler flow imaging may ultimately become the superior method.

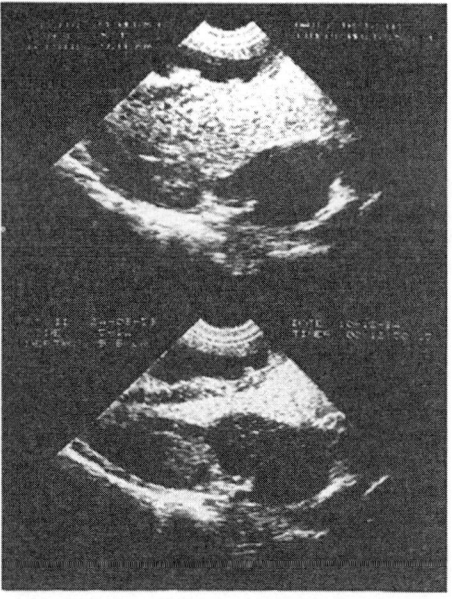

Fig. 18. Intraoperative echocardiographic contrast study after mitral valve repair. The transducer is placed on the right ventricular outflow tract and a left ventricular long axis cross-section is imaged. The LV cavity is opacified after injection of saline and some echo contrast has passed into the left atrium during systole (upper panel) indicating a small degree of mitral incompetence. During diastole (lower panel) the opening of the mitral valve is seen. The inflow pattern is visualized as a negative shadow caused by the low contrast containing blood flowing from the LA into the LV.

Experimental applications

Videodensitometry of contrast echocardiograms. Contrast agents which opacify the left ventricle after peripheral venous injection would have great potential clinical utility since left ventricular ejection fraction assessment is possible from contrast agent dilution analysis. Bommer et al. [64] described in 1978 a method of obtaining dilution curves of echocardiographic contrast by videodensitometry. They focused an analogue photometer on the video screen over the middle of the right ventricular cavity during two-dimensional echocardiographic contrast studies. The dilution curves were reproducible on multiple echocardiographic contrast injections to an accuracy of 15%. Time course of decay allowed separation of patients with normal cardiac output and/or tricuspid regurgitation. Subsequently, a good correlation with cardiac output measurements was found [9, 65]. We have used an image processing computer to analyse video recordings of contrast injections in order to follow the decay of density after left ventricular and pulmonary wedge injections [10] (Figs. 19 and 20). The decay phase was found to be mono-

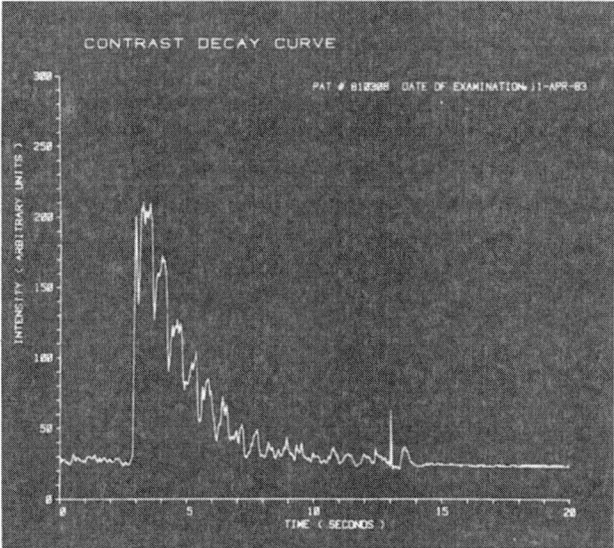

Fig. 19. Videodensity (expressed in arbitrary units) decay curve representing 'washout' of echo contrast from within the left ventricle in a normal subject. The insert shows the apical four chamber view with a rectangular sample area designated within the left ventricular cavity for measuring the videodensity. The steep decay of the curve indicates a rapid 'washout' of the contrast material and corresponds to a normal cardiac output. Note the similarity of this videodensity curve to the indicator-dilution type of curve. The stepwise decrease of videodensity represents the difference in videodensity between complete mixing and inflow of noncontrast containing blood and reflects ejection fraction.

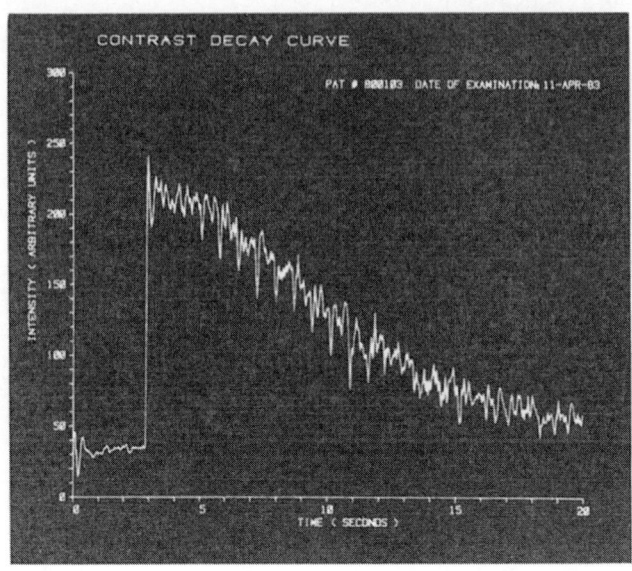

Fig. 20. Videodensity decay curve of a patient with congestive heart failure. Note the slower 'washout' of echo contrast indicating a low cardiac output. Valvular insufficiency would result in a similar videodensity curve.

exponential and had some characteristics of indicator-dilution curves as predicted theoretically. A meaningful calculation of the area under the curve, however, could not be made mainly because of variability of contrast intensity from injection to injection and limitations due to video 'overload' immediately after each injection. Thus, contrary to the studies of others. It seems that at present ejection fraction and cardiac output measurements cannot be made reliably using routine contrast dilution techniques. Further research in this area is attractive and the advantages are obvious. Indeed, ejection fraction determination does not require definition of the endocardial border of the left ventricle, nor does it require assumptions regarding the geometry.

Other investigators used computer-based video-densitometric techniques to analyse video recordings of left ventricular contrast echocardiograms for quantitating left-to-right shunts [12, 21]. Time-density histograms were generated from right and left ventricular outflow tracts after injection of echo contrast in the left ventricle in patients with left-to-right ventricular shunts. The percentage of left-to-right shunts was calculated and compared with standard Fick and dye dilution techniques. A good correlation between the three methods was reported.

Myocardial contrast echocardiography

Myocardial contrast echocardiography is a technique whereby a solution of microbubbles of air is injected into the circulation resulting in an echocardiographically detected myocardial contrast effect (see Chapter 3.3.). DeMaria et al. [66] demonstrated in dogs that the intracoronary injection of a suspension of 30 micron microbubbles (polysaccharide encapsulated microbubbles) increased the echo reflectivity of the myocardium. Subsequently, Bommer et al. [67] showed that the contrast effect was diminished, and the wash-out time of the echo-contrast was altered in areas of the myocardium made ischemic by coronary artery occlusion. Armstong et al. [68] injected gelatin-encapsulated microbubbles into the aortic root as a marker for the detection of regions of abnormally perfused myocardium and compared the findings with simultaneous distribution of radioactive microspheres in the coronary arteries of these dogs. Contrast intensity was measured from the videoscreen with a lightmeter. There was no linear correlation between echo-contrast intensity and the absolute level of myocardial blood flow. Ischemic areas of the left ventricle induced by coronary artery occlusion were accurately identified and the technique was more accurate than echocardiographic wall motion analysis for detecting the ischemic areas. An example of myocardial opacification after aortic root injecton of SSH-454 is shown in Fig. 21.

These earlier observations have subsequently been confirmed in several studies [69, 70] and the data have been extended to quantitation of fixed coronary artery stenosis [15, 16] and dynamic coronary artery flow [14]. Sakamaki et al. [70] correlated areas of acutely ischemic myocardium delineated by myocardial contrast two-dimensional echocardiology with pathologic specimen and found a good correlation (r = 0.88). The perfusion deficiency, however, slightly overestimated the extent of myocardial necrosis but was more accurate than wall motion. Tei et al. [15] and Maurer et al. [16] measured dynamic myocardial appearance and disappearance of echocardiographic contrast. They found that after significant coronary artery stenosis (70%) myocardial contrast disappearance rate was prolonged. Subsequently Ten Cate et al. [14] demonstrated that dynamic coronary flow during control, hyperemia and severe ischemia can be estimated from the myocardial contrast disappearance rate. A moderate correlation was found between the epicardial coronary flow and the myocardial contrast disappearance rate, however. At present, contrast echocardiography provides a reproducible accurate and quantitative visualization of myocardial perfusion defects which correlates with postmortem staining and tracer microsphere technique in animal experiments. It is too early to predict whether contrast echocardiography will become a practical and reproducible method for

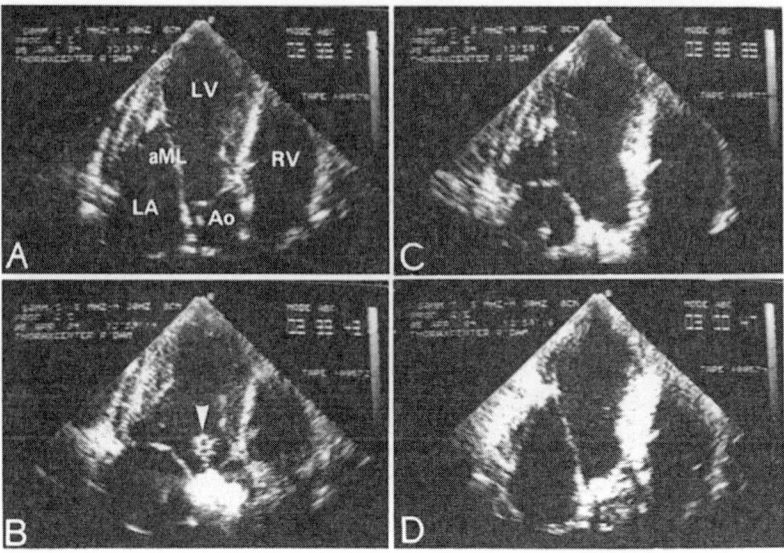

Fig. 21. Myocardial opacification after injection of Echocon (SSH-454) in the aortic root. Panel A shows the initial phase of injection in diastole and some echo contrast is visible above the aortic valve. In panel B the aortic root is opacified and some echo contrast is also seen regurgitating into the left ventricular outflow tract during isovolumic relaxation (arrow). Immediately thereafter the interventricular septum becomes opacified (panel C) followed by the left ventricular free wall and apical area (panel D).

assessment of the actual level and distribution of regional myocardial perfusion in normal and ischemic conditions. As was discussed in previous sections the safety and the adequate and reproducible echogenicity of the echo contrast agents remain major problems to be solved. We recently demonstrated the feasibility and safety of intracoronary injection of polygelin colloid solution [70]. This and other contrast agents contain small microbubbles of air which have to pass the coronary capillary bed. A rapid 'washout' of these microbubbles of air consistent with capillary transit time is necessary and they should not cause alterations in blood flow by e.g. hyperemic effects. Preliminary results reported by Feinstein et al. [71, 72] and Armstrong et al. [73] indicate that serial changes in contrast intensity can be detected in patients following percutaneous transluminal angioplasty when pre- and postdilatation contrast injections are compared. Other problems which must be considered for quantitative analysis are related to the echo amplitude measurements from the videodata (Table 2).

Nonetheless, the potential of the method is enormous if quantifiable contrast agents would become available that can pass the microcirculation of the lung (peripheral venous injection) obviating the need for direct coronary or aortic root injection. The method is relatively inexpensive, is minimally invasive and would be readily applied in the cardiologist's office, stress laboratory and for continuous surveillance in the coronary care unit. New developments in the field of radionuclide imaging and digital angiography are greatly competitive for such applications, however. In a symposium on this subject in the Journal of the American College of Cardiology (1984) the present state of the field of videodensitometric analysis has been reviewed extensively. From the data presented it appears that despite many methodological and technological problems a method using two-dimensional echocardiography which allows the simultaneous quantitation of myocardial function and perfusion may become available.

References

1. Meltzer RS, Tickner EG, Sahines T, Popp R: The source of ultrasound contrast effect. J Clin Ultrasound 8: 121–7, 1980.
2. Kremkau FW, Gramiak R, Carstensen E, Shah P, Kramer H: Ultrasonic detection of cavitation at catheter tips. Am J Roentgenol 110: 177–83, 1970.
3. Meltzer RS, Tickner EG, Popp RL: Why do the lungs clear ultrasonic contrast? Ultrasound in Med & Biol 6: 263, 1980.
4. Gramiak R, Shah RM: Echocardiography of the aortic root. Invest Radiol 3: 356–366, 1968.
5. Schartl M, Fritzsch TH, Friedman W, Lange L: Quantitative myocardial perfusion studies with a new safe contrast agent. J Am Coll Cardiol 3: 469, 1984.
6. Feinstein SB, Ten Cate FJ, Zwehl W, Ong K, Maurer G, Tei C, Shah PM, Meerbaum S, Corday E: Two-dimensional contrast echocardiography 1. In vitro development and quantitative analysis of echo contrast agents. J Am Coll Cardiol 3: 14–20, 1984.
7. Smith MD, Ling Kwam OI, Reiser HJ, DeMaria AN: Superior intensity and reproducibility of SHU-454, a new right heart contrast agent. J Am Coll Cardiol 3 (4): 992–998, 1984.
8. Ong K, Maurer G, Feinstein S, Zwehl W, Meerbaum S, Corday E: Computer methods for myocardial contrast two-dimensional echocardiography. J Am Coll Cardiol 3: 1212–1218, 1984.
9. DeMaria AN, Bommer W, Kwam OIL, Riggs K, Smith M, Waters J: In vivo correlation of thermodilution curves obtained from contrast two-dimensional echocardiograms. J Am Coll Cardiol 3: 999–1004, 1984.
10. Meltzer RS, Bastiaans OL, Lancée CT, Pièrard L, Serruys PW, Roelandt J: Videodensitometric processing of contrast two-dimensional echocardiographic data. Ultrasound in Med & Biol 8: 509–514, 1982.
11. Wann LS, Stickels KR, Mabrah VS, Gross CM: Digital processing of contrast echocardiograms: a newer technique for measuring right ventricular ejection fraction. Am J Cardiol 53: 1164–1168, 1984.
12. Hagler DJ, Tajik AJ, Seward JB, Ritman EL: Future prospects – videodensitometric quantitation of left-to-right shunts with contrast echocardiography. In: Contrast Echocardiography, Meltzer RS, Roelandt J (ed.), Martinus Nijhoff, The Hague: p. 298–303, 1982.
13. Kemper AJ, O'Boyle JE, Sharma S, Cohen CA, Kloner RA, Khuri SF, Parisi AF: Hydrogen peroxide contrast-enhanced two-dimensional echocardiography: real time in vivo delineation of regional myocardial perfusion. Circulation 68: 603–611, 1983.

174

14. Ten Cate FJ, Drury JK, Meerbaum S, Noordsy J, Feinstein S, Shah PM, Corday E: Myocardial contrast two-dimensional echocardiography: experimental examination at different coronary flow levels. J Am Coll Cardiol 3: 1219–1226, 1984.

15. Tei C, Kondo S, Meerbaum S, Ong K, Maurer G, Wood F, Sakamaki T, Shimoura K, Corday E, Shah PM: Correlation of myocardial echo contrast disappearance rate ('washout') and severity of experimental coronary stenosis. J Am Coll Cardiol 3: 39–46, 1984.

16. Maurer G, Ong K, Haendchen R, Torres M, Tei C, Word F, Meerbaum S, Shah P, Corday E: Myocardial contrast two-dimensional echocardiography: comparison of contrast disappearance rates in normal and underperfused myocardium. Circulation 69: 418–430, 1984.

17. Ernst A, Cikes I: Polygelin colloid solution as a new echocardiographic agent. J Cardiovasc Ultrasonography 2: 143–145, 1984.

18. Meltzer RS, Serruys PW, Hugenholtz PG, Roelandt J: Intravenous carbon dioxide as an echocardiographic contrast agent. J Clin Ultrasound 9: 127–131, 1981.

19. Gaffney FA, Jui-Chin L, Peshock RM, Bush L, Buja M: Hydrogen peroxide contrast echocardiography. Am J Cardiol 52: 607–609, 1983.

20. Mattrey RF, Andre MP: Ultrasonic enhancement of myocardial infarction with perfluorocarbon compounds in dogs. Am J Cardiol 54: 206–210, 1984.

21. Valdes-Cruz LM, Sahn DJ: Ultrasonic contrast studies for the detection of cardiac shunts. J Am Coll Cardiol 3: 978–985, 1984.

22. Zwehl W, Areeda J, Schwartz G, Feinstein S, Ong K, Meerbaum S: Physical factors influencing quantitation of two-dimensional contrast echo amplitudes. J Am Coll Cardiol 4: 157–164, 1984.

23. Kondo S, Tei C, Meerbaum S, Corday E, Shah PM: Hyperemic response of intracoronary contrast agents during two-dimensional echocardiographic delineation of regional myocardium. J Am Coll Cardiol 4: 149–156, 1984.

24. Bommer WJ, Shah PM, Allen H, Meltzer R, Kisslo J: The safety of contrast echocardiography. Report of the Committee on contrast echocardiography for the American Society of Echocardiography. J Am Coll Cardiol 3: 6–13, 1984.

25. Gillam MD, Kaul S, Fallon JT, Hedley-White ET, Slater CE, Weyman AE: Sequelar of echocardiographic contrast: studies of myocardium, brain and kidney. Circulation 70: (suppl. II) II-6, 1984.

26. Santoso T, Roelandt J, Mansjoer H, Abdurahman M, Meltzer RS, Hugenholtz PG: Use of polygelin colloid solution for contrast myocardial perfusion imaging in humans. J Am Coll Cardiol 8: 1985.

27. Holt G, Reeves W, Rieder M, Daley L, Murthy V, Christensen C: Negative inotropic effects of intracoronary echo-contrast agents. J Am Coll Cardiol 5: (abstract) 474, 1985.

28. Levine RA, Gillam LD, Guerrero JL, Weyman AE: Wall motion abnormalities following myocardial echo contrast injection are caused by microbubbles. J Am Coll Cardiol 5 (abstract): 474, 1985.

29. Meltzer RS, Vered Z, Roelandt J, Neufeld HN: Systemic analysis of contrast echocardiograms. Am J Cardiol 52: 375–380, 1983.

30. Hernandez A, Strauss AW, McKnight R, Hartman AF Jr.: Diagnosis of pulmonary arteriovenous fistula by contrast echocardiography. J Pediatrics 93: 258–261, 1978.

31. Serwer GA, Armstong BE, Anderson PAW, Sherman D, Benson W, Edwards SB: Use of contrast echocardiography for evaluation of right ventricular hemodynamics in the presence of ventricular septal defects. Circulation 58: 327–336, 1978.

32. Seward JB, Tajik AJ, Hagler DJ, Ritter DG: Peripheral venous contrast echocardiography. Am J Cardiol 39: 202–212, 1977.

33. Tsuyuguchi N, Nohara R, Suwo M, Yoshimatsu S, Tamagawa M, Shigeta H, Hashimoto

M, Kaneko R: Evaluation of cardiac function by contrast echo disappearance time. J Cardiography 11: 467–475, 1981.

34. Mortera C, Hunter S, Tynan M: Contrast echocardiography and the suprasternal approach in infants and children. Eur J Cardiol 9: 437–454, 1979.

35. Levine RA, Teichholtz LE, Goldman ME, Steinmetz MY, Baker M, Meltzer RA: Microbubbles have intracardiac velocities similar to those of red blood cells. J Am Coll Cardiol 3: 28–33, 1984.

36. Shiina A, Kondo K, Nakasone Y, Tsuchiya M, Yaginuma T, Hosoda S: Contrast echocardiographic evaluation of changes in flow velocity in the right side of the heart. Circulation 63: 1408–1416, 1981.

37. Tickner EG: Precision microbubbles for right side intracardiac and flow measurements. In Contrast Echocardiography. Meltzer RS, Roelandt J (ed.), Martinus Nijhoff, The Hague: p. 313–324, 1982.

39. Tajik AJ, Seward JB, Hagler DJ, Mair DD, Lie JT: Two-dimensional real time ultrasonic imaging of the heart and great vessels. Technique, image orientation, structure identification and validation. Mayo Clin Proc 53: 271–303, 1978.

40. Stewart JA, Fraker TD, Slosky DA et al.: Detection of persistent left superior vena cava by two-dimensional contrast echocardiography. J Clin Ultrasound 7: 357–360, 1979.

41. Pieroni DR, Varghese PJ, Freedom RM, Row RD: The sensitivity of contrast echocardiography in detecting intracardiac shunts. Cathet Cardiovasc Diagn 5: 19-29, 1979.

42. Meltzer RS, Serruys PW, McGhie J, Verbaan N, Roelandt J: Pulmonary wedge injection yielding left-sided echocardiographic contrast. Brit Heart J 44: 390–394, 1980.

43. Reale A, Pizzuto F, Gioffre A, Nigri A, Romeo F, Martuscelli E, Mangieri E, Scibilia G: Contrast echocardiography transmission of echoes to the left heart across the pulmonary vascular bed. Eur Heart J: 1 101–106, 1980.

44. Valdes-Cruz LM, Pieroni DR, Roland JM, Varghese PH: Echocardiographic detection of intracardiac right-to-left shunts following peripheral vein injections. Circulation: 54 558–562, 1976.

45. Serruys PW, van den Brand M, Hugenholtz PG, Roelandt J: Intracardiac right-to-left shunts demonstrated by two-dimensional echocardiography after peripheral vein injection. Brit Heart J 42: 429–437, 1979.

46. Weyman AE, Wann LS, Caldwell RL, Hutwitz RA, Dillon JC, Feigenbaum H: Negative contrast echocardiography a new method for detecting left-to-right shunts. Circulation 59: 498–505, 1979.

47. Roelandt J, Serruys PW: Real-time cross-sectional contrast echocardiography. In W. Bleifeld, Effert S, Hanrath H, Mathey D (eds.) Evaluation of cardiac function by echocardiography. Berlin, Springer Verlag: p. 152, 1980.

47. Kronik G: Contrast echocardiography in patent formane ovale. In Contrast Echocardiography, Meltzer RS, Roeland J (ed.), Martinus Nijhoff, The Hague: p. 137–152, 1982.

48. Serruys PW, van den Brand M, Hugenholtz PG, Roelandt J: Intracardiac right-to-left shunts demonstrated by two-dimensional echocardiography after peripheral vein injection. Brit Heart J 42: 429, 1979.

49. Farcot JC, Boisante L, Rigand M, Bardet J, Bourdarias JP: Two-dimensional echocardiographic visualization of ventricular septal rupture after acute myocardial infarction. Am J Cardiol 45: 370, 1980.

50. Hagler DJ, Tajik AJ, Seward JB, Mair DD, Ritter DAG: Real-time wide-angle sector echocardiography atrioventricular canal defects. Circulation 59: 140–150, 1979.

51. Seward JB, Tajik AJ, Hagler DJ: Two-dimensional contrast echocardiography. In Pediatric echocardiography – cross-sectional, M-mode and Doppler, N.R. Lündstrom (ed.), Elsevier/North Holland Biomedical, Amsterdam: p. 239, 1980.

176

52. Seward JB, Tajik AJ, Hagler DJ: Contrast echocardiography in the assessment of cyanotic and complex congenital heart disease peripheral venous, invasive and unique applications. In Contrast Echocardiography. Meltzer RS, Roelandt J (ed.), Martinus Nijhoff, The Hague: p. 235–277, 1982.

53. Lieppe W, Behar VS, Scallion R, Kisslo JA: Detection of tricuspid regurgitation with two-dimensional echocardiography and peripheral vein injections. Circulation 57: 128–132, 1978.

54. Meltzer RS, van Hoogenhuyze DCA, Serruys PW, Haalebos MMP, Roelandt J, McGhie J, Vletter WB, Gorissen W: The diagnosis of tricuspid regurgitation by contrast echocardiography. Circulation 63: 1093–1099, 1981.

55. Reid CL, Kawanishi DT, McKay CR, Eilkayam U, Rahimtoola SH, Chandraratna PAN: Accuracy of evaluation of the presence and severity of aortic and mitral regurgitation by contrast two-dimensional echocardiography. Am J Cardiol 52: 519–524, 1983.

56. Kerber RE, Kioschos JM, Lauer RM: Use of an ultrasonic contrast method in the diagnosis of valvular regurgitation and intracardiac shunts. Am J Cardiol 34: 722–727, 1974.

57. Meltzer RS, Serruys PW, McGhie J, Hugenholtz PG, Roelandt J: Cardiac catheterization under echocardiographic control in a pregnant woman. Am J Med 71: 481–484, 1981.

59. Kronzon I, Glassman E, Cohen M, Winer H: The use of two-dimensional echocardiography during transseptal cardiac catheterization. J Am Coll Cardiol 4: 425–428, 1984.

60. Cikes I, Ernst A: New aspects of echocardiography for the diagnosis and treatment of pericardial disease. In: The practice of M-mode and two-dimensional echocardiography, Roelandt J (ed.), Martinus Nijhoff, The Hague: p. 141–156, 1983.

61. Goldman ME, Mindich BP, Teichholtz LE, Burgess N, Staville K, Fuster V: Intraoperative contrast echocardiography to evaluate mitral valve operations. J Am Coll Cardiol 4: 1035–1040, 1984.

62. Gussenhoven EJ, van Herwerden LA, Ligtvoet KM, Bos E, Roelandt J, Witsenburg M: Intraoperative two-dimensional echocardiography in congenital heart disease. J Am Coll Cardiol 9: 565–572, 1987.

63. Goldman ME, Mindich BP: Intraoperative cardioplegic contrast echocardiography for assessing myocardial perfusion during open heart surgery. J Am Coll Cardiol 4: 1029–1034, 1984.

64. Bommer W, Neef J, Neumann A, Weinert L, Lee G, Mason DT, DeMaria AN: Indicator-dilution curves obtained by photometric analysis of two-dimension echo-contrast studies. Am J Cardiol 41: 370, 1978.

65. DeMaria AN, Bommer W, Rasor J, Tickner G, Mason DT: Determination of cardiac output by two-dimensional echocardiography. In: Echocardiology, Rijsterborgh H (ed.), Martinus Nijhoff, The Hague. p. 245, 1981.

66. DeMaria AN, Bommer WJ, Riggs K, Dejee A, Keown M, Ling Kwam O, Mason DT: Echocardiographic visualization of myocardial perfusion by left heart and itnracoronary injections of echo contrast agents. Circulation 60 (suppl. II): II-143, 1980.

67. Bommer WJ, Rasor J, Tickner G, Tadeka P, Miller L, Lee G, Mason DT, DeMaria AN: Quantitative regional myocardial perfusion scanning with contrast echocardiography. Am J Cardiol 47: 403, 1981.

68. Armstrong WF, Mueller TM, Kinney EL, Tickner EG, Dillon JC, Feigenbaum H. Assessment of myocardial perfusion abnormalities with contrast-enhanced two-dimensional echocardiography. Circulation 66: 166–173, 1982.

69. Tei C, Sakamaki T, Shah PM, Meerbaum S, Shimoura K, Kondo S, Corday E: Myocardial contrast echocardiography. A reproducible technique of myocardial opacification for identifying regional perfusion deficits. Circulation 67: 585–593, 1983.

70. Santoso T, Roelandt J, Mansyoer H, Abdurahman N, Meltzer RS, Hugenholtz PG:

Myocardial perfusion imaging in humans by contrast echocardiography using polygelin colloid solution. J Am Coll Cardiol 6: 612–20, 1985.

71. Feinstein SB, Lang R, Neumann A, Al-Sadir J, Carroll JD, Keller MW, Powsner SM, Borow KM: Intracoronary contrast echocardiography in humans: perfusion and anatomic correlates. Circulation 72: III-57 (abstr), 1985.

72. Lang RM, Feinstein SB, Feldman T, Neumann A, Chua KG, Borow KM: Contrast echo-cardiography for evaluation of myocardial perfusion: effects of coronary angioplasty. J Am Coll Cardiol 8: 232–5, 1986.

3.2. New echocardiographic contrast agents

RICHARD S. MELTZER, XIE FENG, MICHELE NANNA &
RAYMOND GRAMIAK

1. Introduction

Echocardiographic contrast was first described at the University of Rochester by Gramiak and Shah in 1968 [1, 2]. This was important in the rapid growth of M-mode echocardiography starting about then, since it allowed accurate structure identification by correlation with contrast injections made in the cardiac catheterization laboratory in known chambers and vessels.

The contrast targets in 'standard' contrast agents are merely the microbubbles present in any biocompatible solution which is injected (e.g., 5% dextrose or saline solutions or even the patient's own blood) [3]. By 'standard' contrast agents we mean those in routine use in echocardiography laboratories throughout the world – dextrose, saline, indocyanin green, and the patient's own blood. This chapter will discuss other agents.

Virtually any solution gives contrast, though trouble in obtaining adequate contrast occasionally occurs, especially with injections through small bore needles and catheters distant from the heart – such as in a small gauge butterfly needle inserted into a small hand vein. This is caused by slow flow to the central circulation and the opportunity for 'margination' and even dissolution, as well as simple dilution due to a less concentrated delivery to the heart than a direct bolus. Though there is some mystique and even a sort of folklore around the best technique for obtaining adequate and good quality contrast (3-way stopcocks, double syringe or agitation and air exclusion techniques, rapid injection, large bore catheters in proximal veins, etc.), the basic common-sense rule of thumb is that 'the more gas, the more contrast.' Further tips on the optimal technique for obtaining contrast have been published by Schiller & Goldstein [4]. Unfortunately, since increasing the amount of injected gas, though microscopic, increases the chance of gas embolus, a direct corolary of the above rule is 'the more contrast, the more the risk of gas embolus.' It would certainly be better to have inadequate contrast than toxicity due to gas embolus, especially since the clinical setting for contrast injection is usually the suspicion of an intracardiac shunt. With adequate precautions, however, standard contrast has been found extremely safe – no permanent sequelae in over 50,000 contrast echocardiographic

I. Cikes (ed.), *Echocardiography in Cardiac Interventions*, 179–189, 1989.
© 1989 *Kluwer Academic Publishers.*

studies surveyed [5] and only 1 reported stroke in the literature [6].

The stimulus for the search for new contrast agents is largely the desire to create an agent that can pass the pulmonary capillaries and yield contrast on the left side of the heart [7–11]. This would allow better imaging of the left heart, detection of left-to-right shunts, myocardial perfusion imaging, improved systemic ultrasound arteriography (carotid, etc.), and should yield important information about organ (e.g., renal) perfusion. The following discussion, organized by agents, relates to the 'non-standard' agents that have been proposed in the literature but are not in routine clinical use.

2. Specific agents

2.1. Carbon dioxide

Since carbon dioxide is absorbed very rapidly into the blood, it is safer than intravascular air, oxygen, or nitrogen, in that bubbles are less likely to permanently occlude a vessel and cause ischemia. There was therefore a large experience with intravascular carbon dioxide in radiology, especially for intravenous injection in the diagnosis of pericardial effusion in the pre-echocardiographic era [12–14]. Rather large volumes of carbon dioxide (up to 200 cc) were injected without reported toxicity, so there seems to be a large margin of safety. It should be noted that the patients were in the left lateral decubitus position with the right side up to enhance safety during these injections of larger amounts of carbon dioxide: the carbon dioxide stays trapped in the right atrium until dissolved into the blood, and never travels further in the cardiovascular system. Further, experimental animals tolerate 7.5 cc/kg of carbon dioxide rapidly injected into the left ventricle or carotid artery with minimal cardiorespiratory effects [12]. Carbon dioxide has even been injected intra-coronary in humans without reported adverse effect [15], though the current authors would not recommend this practice!

Ziskin reported the use of carbon dioxide as an ultrasound contrast agent in 1972 in an *in vitro* experiment [43].

Because of the large reported use and proven safety margin of intravenous carbon dioxide, we tried using small amounts [1–3 cc of medically pure carbon dioxide) as an echocardiographic contrast agent and found it safe and efficacious in human subjects [16]. Others have confirmed this independently using pulmonary wedge injections [17], and subsequently using intravenous injections [18]. Though carbon dioxide does cause better contrast, it does not go through the lungs for the same reason that other gas injected intravenously does not pass the pulmonary capillaries [8]. Therefore, it has only restricted

181

applicability in the few patients where contrast is needed but cannot be obtained by standard intravenous injections.

2.2. Sodium bicarbonate – ascorbic acid mixture to generate CO2

Jiang et al. from China have reported in a preliminary study the use of a mixture consisting of 4 ml of 5% sodium bicarbonate and 2 ml of 5% ascorbic acid injected into the left ventricle [19]. They reasoned that this mixture generates carbon dioxide and therefore should be safer than injecting air, as per the discussion above in section 2.1. The mixture is mixed and directly injected, and it generates carbon dioxide immediately. They reported that injections yielded contrast in all 9 patients studied and that there were no adverse symptomatic or hemodynamic effects. The full study was published in China [20].

We see little advantage in using sodium bicarbonate/ascorbic acid as a contrast agent since it does not pass the lungs and offers little advantage over 'standard' contrast agents.

2.3. Hydrogen peroxide

In 1970, Merin, Neal, and Gramiak used 0.3% hydrogen peroxide to obtain ultrasound contrast in an experimental model, but this observation was not published until 1974, and was reviewed in 1982 [21].

Want et al. reported on animal [22] and human [23] studies with intravenous hydrogen peroxide in 1979, noting good right heart contrast effects, no left heart contrast, and no significant toxicity.

Independently of these studies, in 1980 we began using hydrogen peroxide as an echocardiographic contrast agent in experimental animals [9]. The rationale for this is that when injected into blood and combined with the peroxidase in leukocytes, oxygen results. Further, there was a prior experience with human use of intravascular and epicardial hydrogen peroxide suggesting that low doses might be non-toxic, though higher doses clearly can cause air embolism [24–26]. In our animal studies we used high doses intravenously and noted transmission of echocardiographic contrast to the left heart, as well as hemodynamic toxicity [9].

Hydrogen peroxide contrast echocardiography was again independently discovered in 1983 by Gaffney et al. [27]. These authors used 0.3% hydrogen peroxide passed through a millipore filter and diluted with heparinized saline solution and mixed with a drop of blood in the syringe before injection.

182

Studies in dogs, normal adults, and 36 patients with various cardiac disorders produced dense, sustained contrast with no complications.

Kemper et al. in Parisi's laboratory in Boston have been using hydrogen peroxide as a contrast agent for myocardial perfusion imaging in experimental animals for several years. They mix 1 ml of blood with 1 to 2 ml of 0.3% hydrogen peroxide and inject in the aortic root or coronary arteries [28]. Myocardial perfusion is imaged in this manner by contrast echocardiography.

We see little likelihood that hydrogen peroxide will become a contrast agent in widespread use in humans, since at concentrations that yield contrast its toxic potential is significant.

2.4. Gelatin

Gelatin is a substance which for many years was available for intravenous use as a plasma expander, but has been removed from the market in the US by the FDA due to occasional allergic reactions. It is a surfactant and stabilizes microbubbles to the point that they can be densely packed together and centrifuged (when bubbles in gelatin are centrifuged they rise since they are lighter than the gelatin) without causing coalescence, under certain conditions. This was originally developed by Rasor Associates, a small company in Sunnyvale, California, which is now defunct [29]. These bubbles were partially investigated *in vitro* by us [3] and *in vivo* by Carroll et al. [30], both at Stanford. Though these microbubbles seemed promising, due to commercial and proprietary considerations they were withdrawn and this promising direction of investigation could no longer be followed.

Using commercial gelatin from Grayslake, Inc. (Grayslake, Ill.) we succeeded in generating precision microbubbles and employing them in an *in vitro* flow system as a contrast echocardiographic agent for quantitative studies [31]. Further studies with precision microbubbles in gelatin are currently underway in our laboratory in a canine model.

It is possible that gelatin might be the base or part of newer contrast agents in the future, but currently no sterile preparation is available for human use except polygelin colloid solution (see section 2.5 below), which is not available in the U.S.A.

2.5. Polygelin colloid solution

Polygelin colloid solution is a gelatin-based solution available commercially in Europe and most of the developing countries as a 3.5% solution from

Hoechst under the trade name Haemaccel (R). As with gelatin, it is a surfactant and stabilizes small microbubbles, thus it can be used as a contrast agent. It is not available in the US. It is used as a plasma expander largely. It was investigated in Zagreb, Yugoslavia by Ernst and Cikes for use as an echo-cardiographic contrast agent in humans [32]. Of 100 patients, the Hoechst Haemaccel (R) brand of polygelin colloid solution was a more effective contrast agent than 5% dextrose in 79, equally good in 21, and less effective in 0. No side effects were noted.

Further, Santoso et al. from Jakarta, Indonesia, report the use of direct intra-coronary injections of Hemaccel (R) in 25 patients at cardiac catheterization [33]. Six patients had nonagitated and a subsequent 19 patients had hand-agitated solution injected. Myocardial contrast was seen on two-dimensional echocardiography in 3/6 of the initial patients and 19/19 of the subsequent patients. The contrast effect lasted from 15 to 60 seconds. One patient had transient second-degree atrioventricular block after a right coronary wedge injection, one had a QRS axis shift and 2 others had transient T wave changes. There were no aortic blood pressure changes and no significant changes in total CK, CK-MB, or SGOT, or left ventricular contractility assessed by 2D echocardiography.

Though polygelin colloid solution may become a significant contrast agent in Europe and outside the U.S., the F.D.A.'s opposition effectively precludes its use within the United States.

2.6. Saccharide particles

A proprietary microbubble technoloy that Rasor Associates originally termed Suger Encapsulated Microbubbles (SEM) was acquired by the German firm of Schering, Inc. (Berlin) and for the past several years they have been developing a contrast agent or a series of such agents for commercial introduction. Though several American investigators have requested to use this substance both in experimental animals and human subjects, Berlex (the American subsidiary of Schering) has not been forthcoming and in the U.S. investigation of SHU-454 has largely been limited to the laboratory of Anthony DeMaria [34]. In this instance injections in 9 dogs were reported to show superior intensity and reproducibility.

Other reports using the same or a similar polysaccharide contrast agent called Echoson (R) also provided by Schering, Berlin, have appeared [35, 36]. These have been very difficult to evaluate due to the effort to preserve the proprietary and commercial nature of the ultrasound agent. The mechanism of contrast seems to be formation of bubbles rather than acoustic imaging of the polysaccharide itself. However, the mechanism by which this agent causes bubbles to form is currently not in the public domain. Further disclosure of the chemical and physical contents of the agent and the nature of its interaction with its diluent and the mechanism of bubble formation would be desirable before introduction into human use.

2.7. Fluorochemicals

Matsuda et al. reported the use of a perfluorochemical emulsion (Fluosol (R)) in 18 open-chested dogs [37]. They noted appearance of contrast in the right heart after the injection of Fluosol (R) into the inferior vena cava. Left heart contrast followed and were 'clear' in 16 of the dogs and 'weak' in the other 2. The solution of surfactants which were added to Fluosol (R) were also used as a contrast agent in 6 of the dogs and the left heart was opacified after intravenous injection in all 6. However, opacification was less intense than when Fluosol (R) was used. When 95% oxygen was mixed with the Fluosol (R), left heart contrast intensity was reported to be subjectively greater. The myocardial wall echoes were also reported enhanced by the intravenous Fluosol (R) injections.

Valdes-Cruz and Sahn also reported on left heart opacification after intravenous injection of 20% Oxypherol, a synthetic oxygen carrying fluorocarbon, gasified separately with oxygen and carbon dioxide [11]. They found left heart contrast after both, with similar intensities of right and left heart contrast which were both fairly weak compared to other agents tested.

Mattrey reported on ultrasonic enhancement of myocardial infarction with perfluorocarbon compounds in 9 dogs [38]. The enhancement was either diffuse or localized to the rim of the infarction. Initial studies suggested to the authors that the mechanism of the enhancement was related to perfluorocarbon accumulation in macrophages within the infarction zone.

The mechanism of contrast with fluorocarbons may be different from that with most other agents. it is possible that the acoustic properties of these very heavy liquids are such that the acoustic impedance mismatch with blood allows direct imaging of the fluorocarbon in the fluid state as contrast, without the necessity to be associated with gas. This is perhaps why concentration in the reticuloendothelial system can lead to contrast.

Although these effects are interesting, the current authors consider perfluorocarbons to be low intensity contrast targets and in need of significant improvement before adequate intensity for most clinical applications is reached.

2.8. Fat emulsions

Several authors have noted that fat emulsions (e.g., Intralipid (R) and others) can yield contrast when infused intravenously, and there are some claims that this contrast can pass through the lungs and yield contrast on the left side of the heart [11]. This raises the question of whether the fat microparticles are passing through the pulmonary capillaries in a liquid phase and yielding contrast by acoustic impedance mismatch with the surrounding blood on the left side of the heart, as might be the case in the preceding section about fluorocarbons. However, once again this effect is fairly weak and the current authors do not feel that it is of sufficient intensity to be clinically useful in most settings.

2.9. Microbubbles formed by high-intensity sonication

The group headed by Dr. Steven Feinstein, formerly in Dr. Eliot Corday's laboratory at Cedars-Sinai Hospital and currently in Chicago, has created great excitement by their careful work over the past several years on new ultrasound agents [39–42]. They have progressed in an elegant manner from *in vitro* work through animal work to human studies [42] using their sonicated agents for myocardial perfusion imaging and occasionally trans-pulmonary transmission or renal perfusion imaging, etc. This exciting work will largely be reviewed in the following Chapter 3.3. by Dr. Corday.

2.10. Other contrast agents

Many other agents have been reported as potential ultrasound contrast agents *in vitro*, in experimental animals or in humans. Some of them include isopropyl alcohol [43], milk [43], Decholin [43], Renografin 60 and 76 [43, and in many recent studies of myocardial perfusion imaging reviewed in Chapter 3.3.), carbonated water [43], ether [9, 43], 0.5% paraldehyde in experimental animals [11] and human subjects [23], 8% propylene glycol [11], salt-poor albumin gasified with carbon dioxide [11], a supersaturated solution of saccharides [11], 75% dimethylsulfoxide (DMSO) [11], 2 degree centigrade normal saline solution gasified with carbion dioxide [11], gelatin and collagen microspheres, sonicated human plasma, ether [9], etc.

3. General considerations about microbubbles, viscosity, surface tension and directions for future research

In the late 1970's we realized that one of the reasons that indocyanin green dye was in widespread use was that it was a surfactant and stabilized small bubbles. We measured the surface tension associated with it and with gelatin solutions then being used to produce experimental contrast echo agents [3]. For microbubbles to go through the lungs after intravenous injection they have to pass the capillary microcirculation [8, 39, 40, 44]. In order for this to occur, they have to be protected from 'implosion' due to surface tension effects by either a surfactant decreasing the driving force for implosion or a mechanical 'prop' preventing it, in the form of a solid coat or a liquid of high viscosity. Both approaches have been found efficacious *in vitro* in stabilizing microbubbles [41, 45, 46]. A combination of both approaches may be additive. Currently, much of the technology involved with solid coats, especially saccharides, is proprietary (see section 2.6 above).

Some further interesting avenues for investigation include the development of a liquid contrast agent, and the development of a technique to make microbubbles grow rather than implode by physical chemical techniques at the pulmonary capillary/alveolar level (altering inhaled gas composition or by hyperbaric techniques).

4. Conclusion

A multiplicity of potential agents has been reported for contrast echocardiography. Though there have been many reports of transpulmonary transmission, no agent currently in clinical use routinely attains left heart contrast after intravenous injection. One of the major problems in development of new agents is the lack of characterization of the microbubble spectrum (size and concentration) of the agent once it is injected, and how this changes in the heart and great vessels and quantitatively how it is affected by passage through a capillary bed. Advances in this area, in surfactant and liquid physical chemistry relating to viscosity, etc., are likely to allow the creation of safe and effective contrast agents within the next few years that can transit capillary beds. This will allow myocardial perfusion imaging, better peripheral ultrasound arteriography, and ultrasound quantification of organ perfusion (such as renal blood flow), etc. This goal is attainable and will be a major breakthrough in medical diagnosis.

References

1. Gramiak R, Shah PM: Echocardiography of the aortic root. Investigative Radiology 3: 356–66, 1968.
2. Gramiak R, Shah PM, Kramer DH: Ultrasound cardiography: contrast studies in anatomy and function. Radiology 92: 939–48, 1969.
3. Meltzer RS, Tichner EG, Sahines TP, Popp RL: The source of ultrasonic contrast effect. J Clin Ultrasound 8: 121–7, 1980.
4. Schiller NB, Goldstein JA: Methodology in contrast echocardiography. In: Meltzer RS, Roelandt J (eds.), *Contrast Echocardiography*. The Hague: Martinus Nijhoff, 1982: 47–50.
5. Bommer WJ, Shah PM, Allen H, Meltzer R, Kisslo J: The safety of contrast echocardiography: report of the committee on contrast echocardiography for the American Society of Echocardiography. J Am Coll Cardiol 3: 6–13, 1984.
6. Lee F, Ginzton L: A central nervous system complication of contrast echocardiography. J Clin Ultrasound 11: 292–4, 1983.
7. Bommer WJ, Mason DT, DeMaria AN: Studies in contrast echocardiography: Development of new agents with superior reproducibility and transmission through the lungs. Circulation 59–60 (Suppl. II): II-17, 1979.
8. Meltzer RS, Tickner EG, Popp RL: Why do the lungs clear ultrasonic contrast? Ultrasound in Med & Biol 6: 263–9, 1980.
9. Meltzer RS, Sartorius OEH, Lancee CT, Serruys PW, Verdouw PD, Essed C, Roelandt J: Transmission of ultrasonic contrast through the lungs. Ultrasound in Med & Biol 7: 377–84, 1981.
10. Meltzer RS, Vermeulen HWJ, Valk NK, Verdouw PD, Lancee CT, Roelandt J: New echocardiographic contrast agents: transmission through the lungs and myocardial perfusion imaging. J Cardiovasc Ultrasonography 1: 277–82, 1982.
11. Valdes-Cruz LM, Sahn DJ, Ultrasonic contrast studies for the detection of cardiac shunts: J Am Coll Cardiol 3: 978–85, 1984.
12. Oppenheimer MJ, Durant TM, Stauffer HM, Stewart GH, Lynch PR, Barrera F: In vivo visualization of intracardiac structures with gaseous carbon dioxide. Am J Physiol 186: 325–334, 1956.
13. Turner AF, Meyers HL, Jacobson G, Lo W: Carbon dioxide cineangiography in the diagnosis of pericardial disease. Am J Roent Rad Ther 97: 342–349, 1966.
14. Phillips JH, Burch GE, Hellinger R: The use of intracardiac carbon dioxide in the diagnosis of pericardial disease. Am Heart J 61: 784–55, 1961.
15. Tambe A, McLaughlin WR, Zimmerman HA: Double contrast medium technic for coronary blood flow studies. Am J Cardiol 21: 117 (abstract), 1968.
16. Meltzer RS, Serruys PW, Hugenholtz PG, Roelandt J: Intravenous carbon dioxide as an echocardiographic contrast agent. J Clin Ultrasound 9: 127–31, 1981.
17. Reale A, Pizzuto F, Gioffre PA, Nigri A, Romeo F, Martuscelli E, Mangieri E, Scibilia G: Contrast echocardiography: transmission of echoes to the left heart across the pulmonary vascular bed. Eur Heart J 1: 101–6, 1980.
18. Munoz S, Berti C, Pulido C, Bolanco P: Two-dimensional contrast echocardiography with carbon dioxide in the detection of congenital cardiac shunts. Am J Cardiol 53: 206–10, 1984.
19. Jiang L, Pu SY, Yang MZ, Lu YZ, Chen HZ: Left heart contrast echocardiography using a carbon dioxide producing agent. Circulation 70 (Suppl. II): II-5 (abstract), 1984.
20. Jiang L, Pu SY, Yang MZ, Lu YZ, Chen HZ: Left heart catheterization – 2D echo contrast imaging in the diagnosis of aortic and mitral regurgitation. J Cardiovasc Dis China 12: 36–7, 1984.

188

21. Gramiak R: Contrast agents for diagnostic ultrasound. In: Meltzer RS, Roelandt J (eds.), *Contrast Echocardiography*. The Hague: Martinus Nijhoff, 1982.
22. Wang X, Wang J, Huang Y, Cai C: Contrast echocardiography with hydrogen peroxide. I. Experimental study. Chinese Med J 92: 595–99, 1979.
23. Wang X, Wang J, Hanrong C, Lu C: Contrast echocardiography with hydrogen peroxide. II. Clinical application. Chinese Med J 92: 693–702, 1979.
24. Finney JW, Jay BE, Race GJ, Urschel HC, Mallams JT, Balla GA: Removal of cholesterol and other lipids from experimentalanimal and human atheromatous arteries by dilute hydrogen peroxide. Angiology 17: 223–8, 1966.
25. Urschel HC, Morales AR, Finney JW, Balla GA, Race GJ, Mallams JT: Cardiac resuscitation with hydrogen peroxide. Ann Thor Surg 2: 655–82, 1966.
26. Takahashi M, Horiguchi Y, Murakami K: Effects of epicardial perfusion with hydrogen peroxide for ischemic myocardium. Jap Heart J 10: 53–58, 1969.
27. Gaffney FA, Lin JC, Peshock RM, Bush L, Buja LM: Hydrogen peroxide contrast echocardiography. Am J Cardiol 52: 607–9, 1983.
28. Kemper AJ, O'Boyle JE, Sharma S, Cohen CA, Kloner RA, Khuri SF, Parisi AF: Hydrogen peroxide contrast-enhanced two-dimensional echocardiography: real-time in vivo delineation of regional myocardial perfusion. Circulation 68: 603–11, 1983.
29. Tickner EG, Rason NS: Noninvasive assessment of pulmonary hypertension using the bubble ultrasonic resonance pressure (BURP) method. Report HR-62917-1A to National Heart, Lung, and Blood Institute, Bethesda, MD. April, 1977.
30. Carroll BA, Turner RJ, Tickner EG, Boyle DB, Young SW: Gelatin encapsulated nitrogen microbubbles as ultrasonic contrast agents. Invest Radiol 15: 260–66, 1980.
31. Meltzer RS, Klig V, Teichholz LE: Generating precision microbubbles for use as an echocardiographic contrast agent. J Am Coll Cardiol 5: 978–82, 1985.
32. Ernst A, Cikes I, Custovic F: Polygelin colloid solution as an echocardiographic contrast agent. J Cardiovascular Ultrasonography 3: 143–5, 1984.
33. Santoso T, Roelandt J, Mansyoer H, Abdurahman N, Meltzer RS, Hugenholtz PG: Myocardial perfusion imaging in humans by contrast echocardiography using polygelin colloid solution. J Am Coll Cardiol 6: 612–20, 1985.
34. Smith MD, Kwan OL, Reiser HJ, DeMaria AN: Superior intensity and reproducibility of SHU-454, a new right heart contrast agent. J Am Coll Cardiol 3: 992–8, 1984.
35. Schartl M, Fritzsch T, Friedmann W, Lange L: Quantitative myocardial perfusion studies with a new safe echo contrast agent. J Am Coll Cardiol 3: 563 (abstract), 1984.
36. Miszalok V, Fritzsch T, Schartl M: Myocardial perfusion defects in contrast echocardiography: spatial and temporal localisation: Ultrasound in Med & Biol 12: 581–6, 1986.
37. Matsuda M, Kuwako K, Sugishita Y, Ito I, Akatsuka T: Contrast echocardiography of the left heart by intravenous injection of perfluorochemical emulsion. J Cardiography 13: 1021–28, 1983.
38. Mattrey RF, Andre MP: Ultrasonic enhancement of myocardial infarction with perfluorocarbon compounds in dogs. Am J Cardiol 54: 206–10, 1984.
39. Feinstein SB, ten Cate FJ, Zwehl W, Ong K, Maurer G, Tei C, Shah PM, Meerbaum S, Corday E: Two-dimensional contrast echocardiography. I. In vitro development and quantitative analysis of echo contrast agents. J Am Coll Cardiol 3: 14–20, 1984.
40. Feinstein SB, Shah PM, Bing RJ, Meerbaum S, Corday E, Chang BL, Santillan G, Fujibayashi Y: Microbubble dynamics visualized in the intact capillary circulation. J Am Coll Cardiol 4: 595–600, 1984.
41. Keller MW, Feinstein SB, Briller RA, Powsner SM: Automated production and analysis of echo contrast agents. J Ultrasound in Med 5: 493–8, 1986.
42. Lang RM, Feinstein SB, Feldman T, Neumann A, Kok GC, Borow KM: Contrast echo-

cardiography for evaluation of myocardial perfusion: effects of coronary angioplasty. J Am Coll Cardiol 8: 232–5, 1986.

43. Ziskin MC, Bonakdarpour A, Weinstein DP, Lynch PR: Contrast agents for diagnostic ultrasound. Investigative Radiol 7: 500–05, 1972.

44. Kort A, Kronzon I: Microbubble formation: in vitro and in vivo observation. J Clin Ultrasound 10: 117–20, 1982.

45. Bommer WJ, Miller L, Takeda P, Mason DT, DeMaria AN: Contrast echocardiography: pulmonary transmission and myocardial perfusion imaging using surfactant stabilized microbubbles. Circulation 64 (Suppl. IV): IV-203 (abstract), 1981).

46. Koenig K, Meltzer RS: Effect of viscosity on the size of microbubbles generated for use as echocardiographic contrast agents. J Cardiovasc Ultrasonography 5: 3–4, 1986.

3.3. Myocardial perfusion study by contrast echocardiography

ELIOT CORDAY & ISTVAN HAJDUCZKI

Two-dimensional echocardiography which can visualize wall motion abnormalities and changes in systolic wall thickening and thinning induced by transient or permanent ischemia has been widely studied and applied in the diagnosis of coronary artery disease [1]. The experimental principles of ischemic blood flow and myocardial kinetics have been well understood [2–3], but the imaging of the underlying myocardial perfusion defect and perfusion flow rates could not be quantitated by practical noninvasive method. Only widely used and invasive coronary angiography using contrast fluoroscopy could outline the coronary vascular anatomy, and ventriculography visualize chamber volumes and systolic contraction defects. It has been demonstrated in animal experiments that contrast-enhanced two-dimensional echocardiography can be used to identify and quantitate regional myocardial perfusion defects, infarct areas and perfusion flow rates. The recent introduction of the method in the experimental animal and human studies now provides the potential to evaluate not only myocardial perfusion but simultaneous myocardial function as well [4–11].

The myocardial echo-contrast effect is presumed to be due to the microbubbles introduced into the capillaries which increases the reflectance of the myocardium by their presence in the arteriolar or capillary bed.

A wide variety of echo-contrast agents has been recently applied for myocardial contrast echocardiography as carrier solutions for microbubbles, such as gelatin-encapsulated microbubbles, Renografin-76, Renografin-saline mixture, indocyanin-green, dextrose, sorbitol, dextran in different concentrations. Early ultrasound contrast-agents consisted of microbubbles generated by hand agitation [4–8, 12–14], but recently a new method has been introduced by using sonication [15–17]. This method was proposed to provide microbubbles in a higher concentration and in more uniform and smaller size. Attempts were also made to inject a substance into the blood stream which generates gas bubbles in vivo. Substances such as sodium bicarbonate and ascorbic acid were used to produce carbon dioxide, or diluted hydrogen peroxide to release oxygen bubbles. Recently, several new commercially prepared polysacharid suspensions have also been tried [9–10,18].

To achieve a more satisfactory magnitude of echographic opacification of

I. Cikes (ed.), *Echocardiography in Cardiac Interventions*, 191–206, 1989.
© 1989 *Kluwer Academic Publishers.*

the myocardium, echo-contrast agents were applied either into the aortic root [10–11], or directly via intracoronary injections [4–8, 13–14, 16). Attempts were also made to achieve myocardial opacification of the left ventricle by injecting the contrast agent retrogradely, via the coronary venous circulation [12], or through a catheter in a right sided, pulmonary wedge position [17].

Delineation and quantitation of myocardial ischemic and infarcted zones

Several studies have demonstrated that myocardial contrast echocardiography can accurately define not only the endocardial outline of the cardiac chambers and structural elements such as papillary muscles and cardiac valves, but also regional and global myocardial areas, by introducing microbubbles containing echo-contrast solutions into the coronary circulation.

When the coronary arteries are normal, aortic root or selective injections into the left main, left anterior descending or circumflex coronary arteries will opacify regional myocardial areas of the left ventricle and the positive, echo-contrast filled area will distinctly delineate the myocardial region normally supplied by the individual arteries (Fig. 1).

Intracoronary injection of a contrast agent can detect and sharply outline the underperfused 'area at risk' during acute coronary occlusion in the dog (Fig. 2). If the echocontrast agent is injected into the left main coronary artery proximal to the coronary occlusion, the region supplied by that occluded artery will be visualized as a negative, echo-contrast free area.

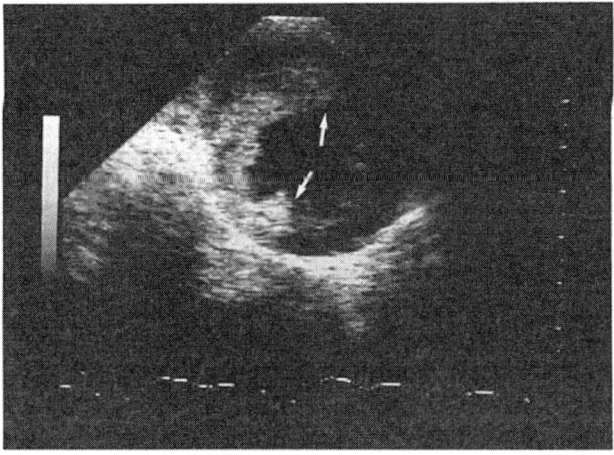

Fig. 1. Opacification of the myocardium in the short axis view at mid-papillary level after selective injection of contrast material into the left anterior descending coronary artery. The myocardial region supplied by the artery is sharply outlined by a positive echo contrast area (arrows).

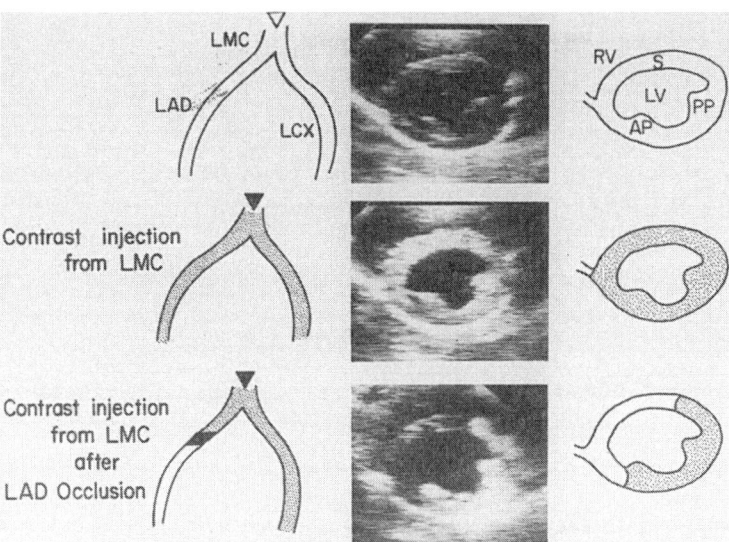

Fig. 2. This illustration indicates the quality of myocardial contrast echocardiographic opacification in two-dimensional echocardiographic cross sections after left main coronary artery injection of saline-Renografin echo contrast agent. The *top panel* shows a midpapillary level short axis view of the left ventricle before coronary artery occlusion and before contrast injection. Note the epicardial and endocardial outlines, with relatively echolucent intervening myocardium. The same cross section appears in the *midpanel* after contrast agent injection from the left main coronary artery in the preocclusion state. The entire circumference of the left ventricular myocardium is opacified. The *lower panel* shows the effect of a left main coronary artery contrast agent injection after left anterior descending coronary artery occlusion. Note that a substantial portion of the interventricular septum and a part of the left ventricular anterior wall are devoid of contrast echo. This negative echo contrast area represents the underperfused myocardium during the coronary artery occlusion. (From Sakamaki T, Meerbaum S, Corday E. Verification of myocardial contrast two-dimensional echocardiographic assessment of perfusion defects in ischemic myocardium. Reprinted with permission from the American College of Cardiology. JACC 3: 34–39, 1984.)

Comparison of the location and extent of contrast opacified myocardium, and the location and extent of left ventricular segmental assynergy after coronary occlusion on the same site, demonstrates a significant concordance [4] (Fig. 3). The percent fractional area change in the segments supplied by the occluded coronary artery is significantly depressed compared to pre-occlusion. The segments that exhibit reduced contraction in the under-perfused zones were also visualized by the contrast echocardiogram obtained from the same site before coronary occlusion. There is a sharp correlation between the contrast-perfused area and the segments with reduced con-tractility.

Myocardial contrast echocardiographic technique was validated against monastral blue dye delineation of underperfused ischemic regions and also

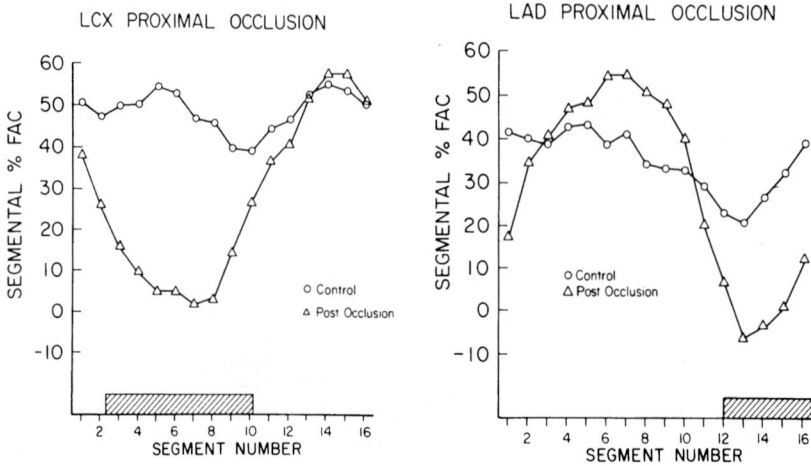

Fig. 3. Left panel: The relationship between contrast-outlined area after the proximal left circumflex artery (LCX) injection of echo-contrast material and asynergic segments after its subsequent occlusion. The left ventricular short axis section at the high papillary level was divided into 16 subsegments; the anti clockwise division starting at the line connecting the center of gravity and the junction of the septum and anterior papillary muscle. Segmental fractional area change (% FAC) was defined for each subsegment. The hatched area (segments 3–10) indicates the myocardial segments filled with the contrast agent. The segments in which % FAC was reduced after occlusion (open triangles) as opposed to the control (open circles) correspond to the area opacified with the contrast. Right panel: The relationship between the myocardial segments outlined by contrast echoes after the proximal left anterior descending artery (LAD) injection and asynergy of the segments after its subsequent occlusion. The segmental % FAC was measured at the midpapillary muscle level of short axis cross section. The hatched area (segments 12–16) indicates the contrast outlined area after the proximal LAD injection. The segmental asynergy after LAD occlusion (open triangles) corresponds to the contrast-filled areas (open circles = segmental % FAC before occlusion). (From Tei C, Sakamaki T, Shah PM, Meerbaum S, Shimoura K, Kondo S, Corday E: Myocardial contrast echocardiography: A reproducible technique of myocardial opacification for identifying regional perfusion deficits. Circulation 67: 585–591, 1983. Reprinted by permission of the American Heart Association, Inc.)

to the extent of myocardial infarction outlined with triphenyl-tetrazolium chloride [5]. An agitated Renografin-saline (3:2) mixture was injected into the left main coronary artery in the control state and than after left anterior descencing coronary artery occlusion. The underperfused regions distal to the left anterior descending coronary artery occlusion appeared as 'negative' or contrast free areas. These negative areas were determined by planimetry and expressed as percent of left ventricular muscle area visualized in short-axis sections. Perfusion defects assessed by contrast two-dimensional echo-cardiography correlated well with those delineated by monastral blue dye ($r = 0.91$) after 45 minute of coronary occlusion. There was also a close relationship ($r = 0.88$) between the extent of contrast echo free area and the

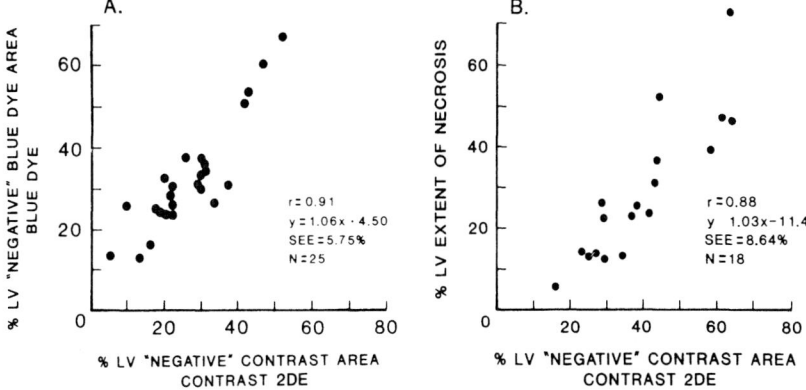

Fig. 4. Left panel: This graph shows a comparison between contrast echocardiography and blue dye staining, using linear regression analysis. Right panel: comparison between contrast echocardiographic measurement and extent of necrosis determined postmortem, using linear regression analysis. (From Sakamaki T, Tei C, Meerbaum S, Shimoura K, Kondo S, Fishbein MC, Y-Rit J, Shah PM, Corday E. Verification of myocardial contrast two-dimensional echocardiographic assessment of perfusion defects in ischemic myocardium. Reprinted with permission from the American College of Cardiology. JACC 3: 34–38, 1984.)

extent of necrosis determined by tripehnyl tetrazolium chloride staining after 5 hour occlusion of the left anterior descending coronary artery (Fig. 4).

Determination of myocardial blood flow

Despite the remarkable advances in coronary angiography which have contributed much for the practical delineation of coronary anatomy, it has provided little information about the all important degree of myocardial perfusion [19]. Therefore, all the attempts which are aimed to quantitate the extent of myocardial perfusion deficiencies and myocardial blood flow have specific importance. As a relatively noninvasive state of the art procedure, two-dimensional contrast echocardiographic imaging has been proposed to provide practical clinical methodology to actually measure not only regional myocardial perfusion defects but also myocardial blood flow rates.

The basic assumption is that the rate of ultrasonic contrast decay reflects the rate of washout of microbubbles by myocardial blood flow. Computerized measurement of contrast-induced echo intensities as indicators of myocardial blood flow in experimental studies provide the potential for an essentially noninvasive, economical and convenient method for the evaluation of regional myocardial perfusion.

One of the preliminary observations was that the time required for the echo contrast disappearence from ischemic myocardium is significantly

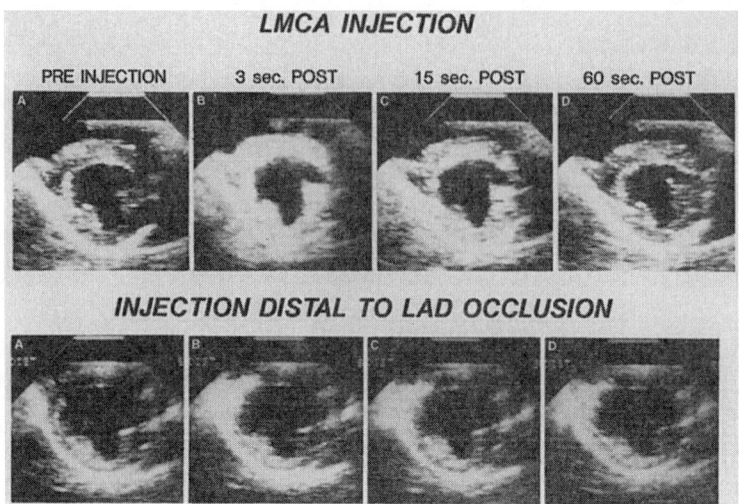

Fig. 5. The figure illustrates the visual observation of echo-contrast disappearence from normal and ischemic myocardium. Upper panel: contrast injection into the left main coronary artery during control state results in global opacification at the myocardial cross-section, followed by brightness decrease to preinjection level within 60 sec. Lower panel: contrast injection distal to intracoronary balloon occlusion of the LAD results in regional myocardial opacification (8–11 o'clock). Contrast disappearance is significantly slower than during control state, with myocardial opacification persisting for several minutes. (From Maurer G, Ong K, Haendchen R, Torres M, Tei C, Wood F, Meerbaum S, Shah PM, Corday E: Myocardial contrast two-dimensional echocardiography: comparison of contrast disappearence rates in normal and underperfused myocardium. Circulation 69: 418–29, 1984. Reprinted by permission of the American Heart Association, Inc.)

prolonged, compared to normally perfused regions (Fig. 5). An agitated 1:1 mixture of Renografin-76 and saline was injected into the left main coronary artery of dogs which resulted in global opacification of the left ventricular myocardium in the two-dimensional echocardiographic short axis sections. Following the contrast agent injections, echo opacification increased to a peak brightness that successively decreased to the control level. The visual appreciation of two-dimensional echocardiographic images showed that the return to preinjection brightness occurred generally within 1 minute. On the other hand, when the contrast agent was injected distal to the balloon occlusion of the left anterior descending coronary artery through the central lumen of the balloon catheter, the contrast disappearence from the underperfused myocardial region was significantly slower, and contrast opacification on two-dimensional echocardiographic images persisted well beyond 1 minute.

To quantify the visual observation of different time courses of contrast echocardiographic opacification in the myocardium, a computerized video-

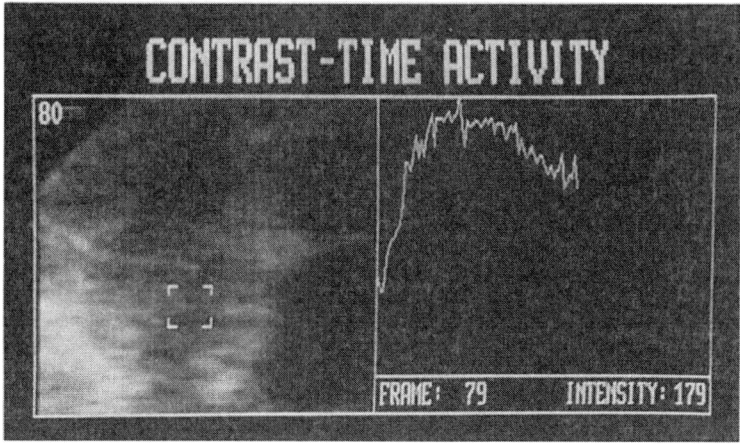

Fig. 6. Computerized videodensitometric analysis of contrast disappearence from the myocardium following echo-contrast injection into the left anterior descending coronary artery. A rectangular region of interest is placed between the epicardial and endocardial border in each frame and the gray level within the region of interest defined. The figure shows the generation of the time-activity curve.

densitometric procedure was developed [20] (Fig. 6). Contrast echo intensities were determined throughout the contrast opacification of the myocardium and time intensity curves were generated. By defining the peak and baseline intensities a monoexponential function was fitted between the two points. Decay rate constants were computed and then converted to biological half lives (Fig. 7).

Other potential indexes characterizing myocardial perfusion peak echo contrast intensity, upstroke half-time, time from echo contrast appearance to peak intensity, total duration of contrast appearence-disappearence, can also be defined by this technique [4]. Using this videodensitometric method, studies were performed to define echo-contrast disappearence half lives producing different coronary flow levels experimentally [13–14, 16].

Serial contrast agent injections were performed into the left anterior descending coronary artery during control state, then after occlusion of the same artery. The echocontrast agent was injected distal to the site of the stenotic plug which resulted in localized myocardial opacification of the underperfused area. The mean contrast disappearance half-life values of the area supplied by the left anterior descending coronary artery increased significantly following contrast injections after insertion of the stenotic plug, compared to the baseline level (Fig. 7). It was demonstrated that the echo contrast washout half-life is inversely proportional to the level of coronary blood flow.

Attempts were made to derive echo contrast disappearence half-life values

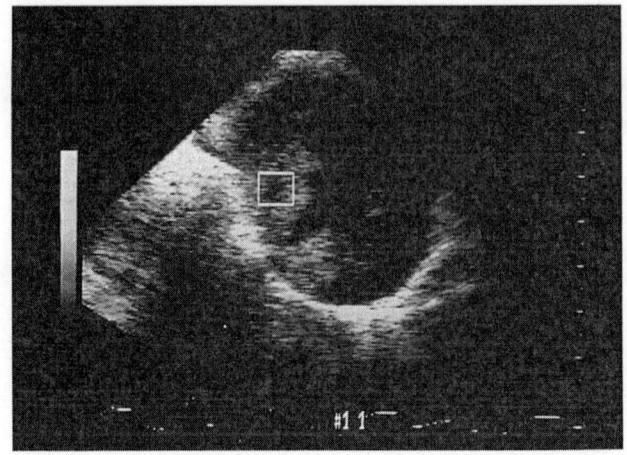

A

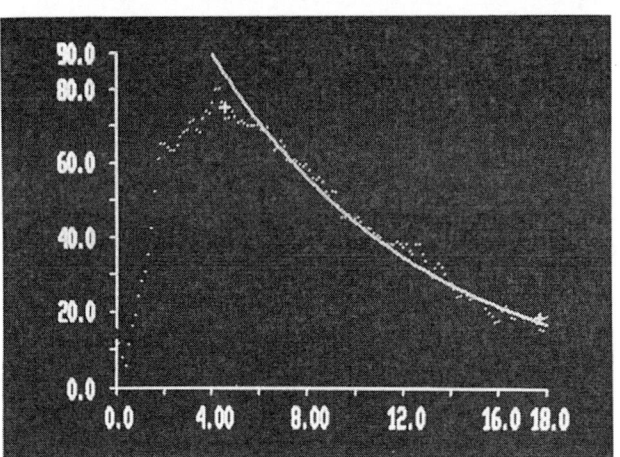

on different severity of experimentally induced coronary stenosis by inserting intracoronary plugs into the coronary artery, reducing the flow by 50%, 70% and 100% [14]. A small but statistically significant increase in mean half-life values was noted with 50% stenosis, and the difference from the mean of control half-lifes increased with successively more severe degrees of coronary stenosis (Fig. 8).

Echo contrast characteristics were studied, not only at decreased, but also at increased myocardial blood flow [16]. Echo contrast injections were performed into the left anterior descending, or left circumflex coronary artery in dog experiments after decreasing the flow in the corresponding artery by a hydraulic occluder or increasing it by a dipyridamol injection. Echo contrast indexes provided a significant differentiation between control

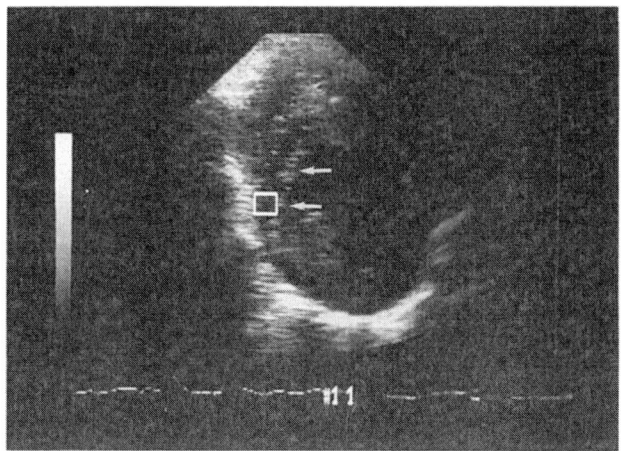

B

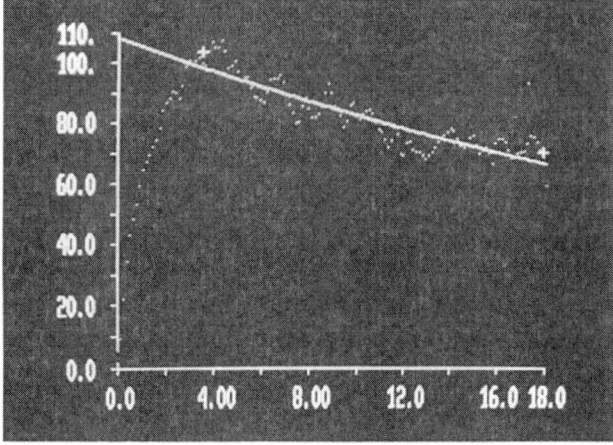

Fig. 7. Echo-contrast disappearence from normal (A) and ischemic myocardium (B). The generated time-activity curves disclose a rapid washout of contrast material from the normal myocardium and a prolonged disappearance from the ischemic myocardium. The analysis of the time-activity curves resulted in a contrast disappearence half life 6.5 sec from the normal and 13.0 sec from the ischemic myocardium. Both left ventricular short axis sections are shown at end-systole. Note the differences in end-systolic wall thickness in the region of the left anterior descending coronary artery (arrows). The lack of systolic thickening on the short axis sections of panel B is the result of the occlusion of the left anterior descending coronary artery. Contrast agent was injected distal to the intracoronary balloon occlusion.

coronry flow and flow reduction greater than 50%, or hyperemia induced by dipyridamol. Contrast disappearance half-life measured in the ischemic myocardium during coronary flow reduction increased significantly from a control level of 5.2 ± 0.3 sec to 9 ± 2 sec and decreased during dipyridamol induced hyperemia to 2 ± 2 sec (Fig. 9). From preliminary information in this

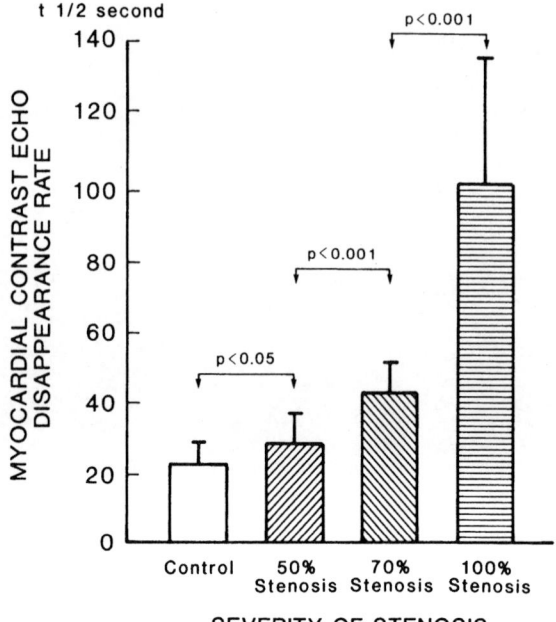

Fig. 8. Myocardial contrast echo disappearance rate index (t 1/2) for varying degrees of coronary stenosis, derived by computerized analysis of myocardial images during intra-coronary injections (From Tei C, Kondo S, Meerbaum S, Ong K, Maurer G, Wood F, Sakamaki T, Shimoura K, Corday E, Shah PM: Correlation of myocardial contrast disappearance rate ('washout') and severity of experimental coronary stenosis. Reprinted with permission from the American College of Cardiology. JACC 3: 39–46, 1984.)

study, it appears that a 30 percent resting flow reduction will be detected by the analysis of washout parameters. Evaluation of the other portions of the time-activity curves showed that parameters like upstroke half-time, time to peak intensity also correlated well with different levels of myocardial blood flow.

Peak echo contrast intensities were also correlated with myocardial blood flow determined by radioactive microspheres or electromagnetic flow probe [18], and a statistically significant correlation was found [21] between the two parameters over a wide range of flows.

Limitations

Although the potentials of myocardial contrast echocardiography are promising, there are significant limitations to be overcome. Fundamental to all quantitative echocardiographic contrast methods is the need to use uniform contrast agents with sufficiently small (3–5 micron) microbubbles which, while producing a satisfactory opacification, can readily pass in the myo-

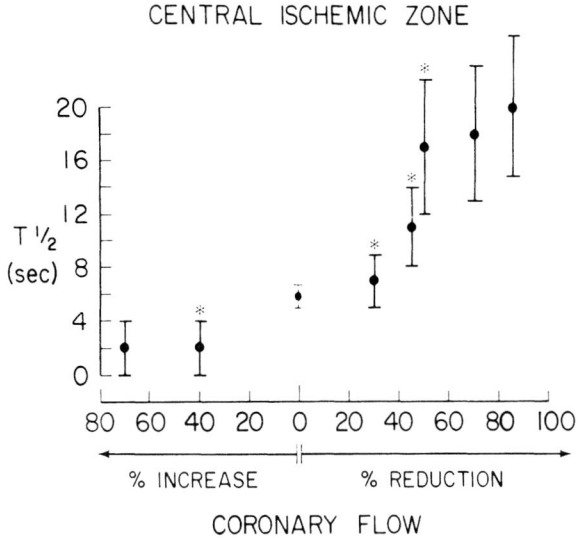

CENTRAL ISCHEMIC ZONE

Fig. 9. Relation between percent of coronary artery flow reduction or increase from the control level and the myocardial contrast decay-phase half-life (T 1/2) for the center of the ischemic zone. Coronary artery flow reduction results in a distinct increase in T 1/2, although T 1/2 decrease during dipiridamol-induced hyperemia. Values are mean ± standard deviation.* $p < 0.05$ compared with control. From Ten Cate F, Drury K, Meerbaum S, Noordsy J, Feinstein SB, Shah PM, Corday E: Myocardial contrast two-dimensional echocardiography: experimental examination at different coronary flow levels. Reprinted with permission from the American College of Cardiology. JACC 3: 1219–26, 1984.)

cardial microcirculation, and to use carrier solutions without significant adverse effects. The size of the microbubbles plays a crucial role in myocardial contrast echo studies since large bubbels can become entrapped in the microcirculation affecting measurements of myocardial perfusion rate, and because of the entrapment can produce temporary ischema as well [22]. The half-life of the two-dimensional echocardiographic contrast opacification observed in the different myocardial perfusion studies has a wide variety ranging from 22–23 sec using hand agitated Renografin-saline mixture [18] with mean bubble size of 16 ± 7 micron to $5.2. \pm 0.3$ sec, using sonicated 50% Dextrose [20] with a mean bubble size of 12 ± 6 micron. These half-life values are larger than a physiologically measured tissue transit time of 2.0 ± 3.2 sec [23], suggesting that temporary entrapment of larger microbubbles in the capillaries results in a prolonged contrast disappearence. The microcirculatory blockade and subsequent ischemia are probably the underlying causes of the reported transient decrease of wall motion in the region of contrast echo opacification [24, 25]. We realize that our presently available echo contrast agents provide an echo contrast decay which probably reflects both the rate of washout by coronary blood flow, as well as the rate at which microbubbles collapse and then dissolve in the capillary circulation. The simple squeezing effect of myocardial contraction should also be considered.

The size of the microbubbles published in the different studies ranges from 6 ± 2 micron generated by sonication in 70% Sorbitol [15] to 75 ± 1 micron of the gelatin-encapsulated gas-bubbles [11]. In an attempt to standardize the measurement technique of sonicated microbubbles we used a KONTRON 2000 Cardio Image Analyzer [26]. A drop of sonicated solution was placed on a hemocytometer and the microscopic image viewed through a TV-camera. Recordings were made within 30–60 seconds after completion of the sonication and the recorded images were analyzed by the computer, measurements previously calibrated by microspheres of known sizes. The sizes and concentrations of microbubbles generated by 30 second sonication in the most frequently used carrier agents are summarized in Table 1. The size of the bubbles ranges from 10.9 ± 8.4 to 16.5 ± 14.9 with a wide range of concentrations and more than 50 percent of the generated bubbles are larger than 10 micron.

Table 1. Size, concentration and percent of microbubbles less than 10 micron in diameter. Mean + SD of 10 measurements of microbubble characteristics generated by 30 second soni-cation in different microbubble-carrying solutions (Iopamidol is a low-osmolality, non-ionic angiographic contrast agent).

Carrier solution	Microbubble			
	Size (micron)	Range (micron)	Conc. $\times 10^4$/ml	< 10 %
70% Sorbitol	10.9 ± 8.4	4–13	311 ± 59	43
70% Dextrose	12.1 ± 9.5	3–26	166 ± 38	23
Renografin-76	16.5 ± 14.9	7–32	229 ± 37	19
Renografin-saline	14.3 ± 12.6	3–32	33 ± 4	26
Iopamidol	15.1 ± 125	3–26	19 ± 8	19

Using this automated measurement technique we could establish that certain factors such as the use of surfactants in the carrier solutions, or the duration of sonication, may influence the size and concentration of the generated microbubbles (Table 2).

The site of echo contrast agent injections also varies in different studies which apply them intracoronary or into the aortic root because the ideal right heart or intravenous application of the agents currently appears far from practical. It has, however, been reported that newly developed contrast agents such as biodegradable sacharid pass in satisfactory amounts into the

Table 2. Size, concentration and percent of microbubbles with less than 10 micron diameter generated in 70% Sorbitol. Sonication was performed for 30 seconds, 10 seconds and using different surfactants (NLS = N-Lauryl-Sarcosine, LPC = L-Phosphatyldicholine). * p < 0.001 against surfactants and 10 second of sonication.

Microbubble	70% Sorbitol			
	30 Sec sonication	+ NLS	+ LPC	10 Sec sonication
Size (microns)	10.9 ± 8.4*	8.6 ± 5.2	8.7 ± 4.2	7.9 ± 6.4
Concentration ($\times 10^4$/ml)	311 ± 59*	940 ± 190	663 ± 218	125 ± 36
< 10 micron (%)	43*	81	76	84
Mean $\pm$ SD)				

pulmonary circulation after intravenous injection, producing left heart opacification [27].

We must realize as we review modern microbubble research that unless microbubbles are of small and uniform size, any research study claiming the ability to provide sound scientific myocardial perfusion rates are misleading. Therefore, it appears that failed attempts to assess the extent of regional perfusion deficiencies or to study the effects of success or failure of an intervention during myocardial perfusion, or in physiologic conditions such as reperfusion or retroinfusion, or treatment with pharmacologic agents, the conclusion might lack true capability as a scientific instrument.

Clinical implications

In spite of recent reports on transient adverse affects due to the presence of microbubbles partly due to the physiochemical properties of carrier solutions of intracoronary administered echo contrast agents, current evidence suggests that gaseous microbubble containing solutions can be delivered into the myocardial circulation with safety, especially when the microbubbles are extremely small [28–29].

Contrast echocardiography appears to offer several advantages over the current techniques such as thallium scintigraphy in the study of regional blood flow. The lower cost, the higher resolution of echocardiography, the ability to make frequent and serial studies, and to obtain information immediately and in real time, makes the method attractive.

Potential already exists for clinical use of this contrast technique to determine myocardial infarction size and to assess the amount of myocardium in jeoppardy from partial coronary occlusion. Because of the above mentioned adventages contrast enhanced myocardial two-dimensional echocardiographic imaging could be the ideal technique to evaluate the results of interventions such as intracoronary thrombolysis with streptokinase or coronary balloon angioplasty.

Preliminary reports have been published recently on clinical studies using myocardial contrast echocardiography to evaluate changes in regional myocardial perfusion during percutaneous transluminal coronary angioplasty [30–31], cardiac surgery [32], and during routine aortic root hypothermia to identify the myocardial segments with the poorest cardioplegic perfusion and, therefore, probably at greatest jeopardy for intraoperative ischemia [33].

The attempts to correlate myocardial perfusion blood flow with myocardial ultrasound contrast are promising, however, due to the present lack of satisfactory echo contrast agents such clinical application of the methodology should be considered in light of the potential problems.

In spite of the existing limitations which need to be overcome, myocardial contrast echocardiography remains a highly desirable and apparently achievable technique [34]. It is hoped that uniform and small bubble sizes can soon be provided so that computerized measurements of echo induced intensities in experiments and clinical studies can provide a strong, practical potential to study myocardial perfusion. Present myocardial two-dimensional echocardiographic achievements designed to provide adequate, reproducible images which can be individually validated are expected to be applied as a relatively inexpensive but valuable technique suitable for the practitioner's office, the stress laboratory, and for continuous and improved surveillance in the coronary care facility [34].

References

1. Wyatt HL, Meerbaum S, Hong MK et al.: Experimental evaluation of the extent of myo cardial dyssynergy and infarct size by two-dimensional echocardiography. Circulation 63: 607–14, 1981.
2. Tennant R, Wiggers C: The effect of coronary occlusion on myocardial contraction. Am J Physiol 112: 351, 1935.
3. Prinzmetal M, Schwartz LL, Corday E, et al.: Studies on the coronary circulation. VI. Loss of myocardial contractility after coronary artery occlusion. Ann Int Med 31: 429, 1948.
4. Tei C, Sakamaki T, Shah PM et al.: Myocardial contrast echocardiography: A reproducible technique of myocardial opacification for identifying regional perfusion deficits. Circulation 67: 585, 1983.
5. Sakamaki T, Tei C, Meerbaum S et al.: Verification of myocardial contrast two-dimensional echocardiographic assessment of perfusion defects in ischemic myocardium. J Am Coll Cardiol 3: 34, 1984.

6. Kaul S, Panfian NG, Okada RD et al.: Contrast echocardiography in acute myocardial ischemia: I. In vivo determination of total left ventricular 'area at risk'. J Amer Coll Cardiol 4: 272, 1984.

7. Santoso T, Roelandt J, Mansyoer H et al.: Myocardial perfusion imaging in humans by contrast echocardiography using polygelin colloid solution. J Am Coll Cardiol 6: 612, 1985.

8. DeMaria AN, Bommer WJ, Riggs K et al.: Echocardiographic visualization of myocardial perfusion by left heart and intracoronary injections of echo contrast agents (abstr). Circulation 60 (suppl III): 143, 1980.

9. Kemper AJ, O'Boyle JE, Cohen CA et al.: Hydrogen peroxide contrast echocardiography: Quantification in vivo of myocardial risk area during coronary occlusion and of the necrotic area remaining after myocardial reperfusion. Circulation 70: 309, 1984.

10. Armstong WF, West SR, Mueller TM et al.: Assessment of location and size of myocardial infarction with contrast enhanced echocardiography. J Am Coll Cardiol 2: 63, 1983.

11. Armstong WF, Mueller TM, Kinney EL, Tickner EG, Dillon JC, Feigenbaum H: Assessment of myocardial perfusion abnormalities with contrast-enhanced two-dimensional echocardiography. Circulation 66: 166–172m 1982.

12. Maurer G, Punzengruber C, Haendchen RV et al.: Retrograde coronary venous contrast echocardiography: Assessment of shunting and delineation of regional myocardium in the normal and ischemic canine heart. J Amer Coll Cardiol 4: 577, 1984.

13. Maurer G, Ong K, Haendchen R et al.: Myocardial contrast two-dimensional echocardiography: comparison of contrast disappearence rates in normal and underperfused myocardium. Circulation 69: 418, 1984.

14. Tei C, Kondo S, Meerbaum S et al.: Correlation of myocardial echo-contrast disapperence rate ('washout') and severity of experimental coronary stenosis. J Amer Coll Cardiol 3: 39, 1984.

15. Feinstein SB, Ten Cate F, Zwehl W et al.: Two dimensional contrast echocardiography. I. In vitro development and quantitative analysis of echo contrast agents. J Am Coll Cardiol 3: 14–20, 1984.

16. Ten Cate FJ, Drury JK, Meerbaum S et al.: Myocardial contrast two-dimensional echocardiography: Experimental examination at different coronary flow levels. J Amer Coll Cardiol 3: 1219, 1984.

17. Ten Cate FJ, Feinstein S, Zwehl W, Meerbaum S, Fishbein M, Shah PM, Corday E: Two-dimensional contrast echocardiography. II. Transpulmonary studies. J Amer Coll Cardiol 3: 21–17, 1984.

18. Armstrong WF: Assessment of myocardial perfusion with contrast enhanced echocardiography. Echocardiography 3: 355–70, 1986.

19. White CW, Creighton WB, Doty DB et al.: Does visual interpretation of the coronary angiogram predict the physiologic importance of a coronary stenosis? N Engl J Med 310: 819–24, 1984.

20. Ong K, Maurer G, Feinstein S et al.: Computer methods for myocardial contrast two-dimensional echocardiography. J Am Coll Cardiol 3: 1212–9, 1984.

21. Kemper AJ, Force T, Kloner R, et al.: Contrast echocardiographic estimation of regional myocardial blood flow after acute coronary occlusion. Circulation 72: 1115, 1985.

22. Feinstein SB, Shah PM, Bing RJ et al.: Microbubble dynamics visualized in the intact capillary circulation. J Am Coll Cardiol 3: 595, 1984.

23. Sarelius I, Duling B: Direct measurement of microvessel hematocrit, red cell flux, velocity a Am J Physiol 243: H1018–27, 1982.

24. Gillam LD, Kaul S, Fallon JT et al.: Functional and pathologic effects of multiple echocardiographic contrast injections on the myocardium, brain and kidney. J Amer Coll Cardiol 5: 474, 1985.

25. Levine RA, Gillam LD, Guerrero JL et al.: Wall motion abnormalities following myo-cardial echo contrast injection are caused by microbubbles (Abstr). J Amer Coll Cardiol 5: 474, 1985.

26. Pincu M, Rajagopalan R, Drury K et al.: Factors influencing the physical characteristics of sonicated myocardial echo contrast agents. J Amer Coll Cardiol 7: 189A, 1986.

27. Smith M, Kwuan L, Nissem S et al.: Left heart opacification after peripheral venous injection: pulmonary transmission of ZK44012, a new echo contrast agent (Abstr). Circulation 73 (suppl III): 228, 1986.

28. Bommer WJ, Shah PM, Allen H et al.: The safety of contrast echocardiography. Report of the committee on contrast echocardiography for the American Society of Echocardiography. J Amer Coll Cardiol 3: 6–12, 1984.

29. Lang R, Borow KM, Neumann A et al.: Effect of intracoronary injections of sonicated microbubbles on left ventricular contractility in humans (Abstr). J Amer Coll Cardiol 7: 189A, 1986.

30. Lang R, Feinstein SB, Feldman T et al.: Contrast echocardiography for evaluation of myo-cardial perfusion: effects of coronary angioplasty (Abstr). Circulation 74 (supl II): 474, 1980.

31. Griffin B, Timmis AD, Sowtin E: Contrast perfusion echocardiography in humans: Experience with PTCA (Abstr). Circulation 74 (suppl II): 474, 1981.

32. Smith J, Feinstein JB, Kapelanski DP et al.: Transesophageal echocardiographic determination of myocardial perfusion during cardiac surgery (Abstr). Circulation 74 (suppl II): 475, 1986.

33. Goldman ME, Mindich BP: Intraoperative cardiolegic contrast echocardiography for assessing myocardial perfusion during open heart surgery. J Amer Coll Cardiol 4: 1029–34, 1984.

34. Meerbaum S: Promise and status of myocardial contrast-enhanced two-dimensional echocardiography: delineation of ischemic risk zone and quantitation of myocardial perfusion defects. J Amer Coll Cardiol 7: 395–6, 1986.

35. Corday E, Shah PM, Meerbaum S: Seminar on contrast two-dimensional echocardiography: applications and new developments. Part I. Introduction. J Amer Coll Cardiol 3: 1–5, 1984.

PART 4: Transesophageal Echocardiography

4.1. Transesophageal echocardiography — technique and standard views

MICHAEL SCHLÜTER, BURKHART A. LANGENSTEIN &
PETER HANRATH with the technical assistance of Volker Siglow

In 1971, Side and Gosling from Guy's Hospital Medical School in London, England, reported that 'the close proximity of the mediastinal vessels, especially the aortic arch, to the esophagus has stimulated the development of an ultrasonic Doppler shift esophageal probe as a nonsurgical technique for estimating aortic arch blood velocity in the conscious patient' [1]. This brief report, dealing with continuous-wave Doppler recordings from the descending thoracic aorta in humans, was the first to make use of esophageal ultrasonography. Two experimental studies using this approach with prototype transducer systems to assess blood flow dynamics and wall motion of the thoracic aorta in dogs followed in 1972 and 1975 [2, 3].

M-mode echocardiography

At the time of these initial reports, M-mode echocardiography had gained considerable clinical importance due to the immediate and noninvasive availability of essential information on cardiac morphology and dynamics that it provided. However, it was also realized that ultrasonic access to the heart from the chest wall was severely compromised or not even possible in a certain population (patients with obesity, narrow intercostal spaces, emphysema, or barrel-chested diseases). To circumvent these restrictions, and 'because of the proximity of the esophageal transducer to cardiac structures, and lack of bony structures and lung interfaces', Frazin and co-workers, in 1976, advocated the technique of esophageal or 'posterior' M-mode echocardiography [4]. By means of a prototype device consisting of a 3.5 MHz nonfocused transducer attached to a 3 mm coaxial cable, transesophageal recordings of aortic root and valve, left atrium, mitral valve, and right ventricle (identified by green dye injection) could be obtained.

Another motivation for the development of transesophageal M-mode echocardiography was provided by Matsumoto et al. [5] who, in 1979, used the technique to monitor left ventricular performance during cardiothoracic surgery. These investigators reported that the technique 'provides a readily accessible location for continuous cardiac examination; the location is stable,

I. Cikes (ed.), *Echocardiography in Cardiac Interventions*, 209–225, 1989.
© 1989 *Kluwer Academic Publishers*.

and monitoring not only does not interfere with the operation, but also can be performed before the chest is open and while it is being closed'. The esophageal probe used in these investigations was simply a commercially available ultrasound transducer, the cable of which was reinforced with copper wire and tygon tubing, thereby restricting the flexibility of the assembly.

In Frazin's as well as Matsumoto's approach, the examiner's control of transducer orientation and, thus, reproducibility of the esophageal echocardiograms was limited because of the rather primitive instrumentation. Controlled manipulation of sound beam orientation became possible only when the transducer head was attached to the tip of a standard gastroscope from which the fiber optics system had been removed to make way for the transducer cable [6].

Initial studies with transesophageal M-mode echocardiography using a gastroscope were aimed at assessing left ventricular functional reserve during exercise in normal volunteer subjects [7] as well as in patients with aortic regurgitation [8] or hypertrophic cardiomyopathy [9]. Results obtained during supine bicycle ergometry proved transesophageal imaging to be superior to the transthoracic approach in exercise studies. Esophageal transducer position remained stable throughout the examination, and respiration and chest wall excursions did not degrade left ventricular imaging. High-quality transesophageal echocardiograms were obtained, and changes in left ventricular cavity dimension could be recorded with good reproducibility, to derive functional parameters such as fractional shortening and peak fiber shortening rate. Transesophageal M-mode echocardiography has also been employed to assess left ventricular anterolateral wall motion in normals and patients with coronary artery disease [10], to measure left and right atrial sizes [11], and to determine the mechanism of the decrease in cardiac output during positive end-expiratory pressure [12].

Continuing the work begun by Matsumoto et al. [5], several authors have used the technique in recent years to detect intracardiac air bubbles during neuro-surgical procedures and after cardiopulmonary bypass [13–16]. It has been claimed that 'transesophageal echocardiography is a very sensitive and convenient method for detecting air embolism in its early stages, being at least as sensitive as the (conventionally used) Doppler device' [13].

Two-dimensional echocardiography

The well recognized lack of lateral image information inherent in M-mode echocardiography led to the development of a rotational multi-crystal device suited for cross-sectional cardiac imaging from the esophagus as early as

1973 [17]. In 1980, a single-crystal high-speed rotational scanner for horizontal cross-sectional images of the heart, displayed within a 240° sector, was introduced by Hisanaga et al. [18]. Concurrently, DiMagno et al. [19] obtained sagittal cardiac images in animal experiments with a linear array. The most promising approach to transesophageal cross-sectional imaging, however, appeared to be the incorporation of a miniature phased array transducer into a gastroscope [20]. This instrument had a 3.5 MHz transducer head which obtained horizontal sections of the heart within an 84° sector. Depth of focus was 2 to 10 cm in front of the array and axial resolution was about 1 mm. Overall dimensions of the transducer head were 35 mm (length) × 15 mm × 16 mm, and gastroscope diameter was 9 mm. The transducer was interfaced to a commercial phased array sector scanner.

A transesophageal investigation is usually performed with the patient lying supine or in a left lateral decubitus position, after he has fasted for about eight hours. Premedication consists of a light sedation of 5 to 10 mg diazepam. Local anesthesia of the pharyngeal region is usually not necessary. In patients in whom an esophageal disease is suspected, a barium swallow x-ray is performed prior to the examination. Failure to swallow the gas-

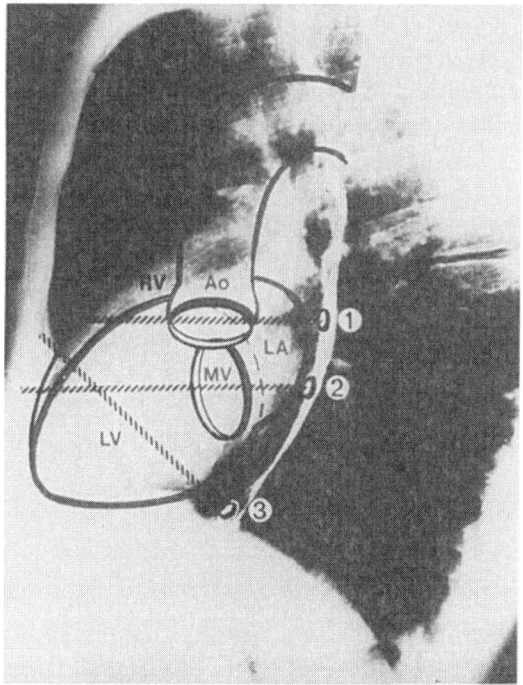

Fig. 1. Lateral view barium passage chest x-ray with superimposed sketch of cardiac structures and contours. Esophageal transducer positions are labeled 1, 2 and 3. Ao = aorta; LA = left atrium; LV = left ventricle; MV = mitral valve; RV = right ventricle.

troscope occurs rarely, although mild but transient gagging is encountered during introduction of the gastroscope. In cases of hypersalivation, excessive fluid accumulation is removed with a suction pump.

Although two-dimensional imaging greatly enhances spatial orientation and structure identification [21, 22], transesophageal cross-sectional images are still unfamiliar to most echocardiographers. The various tomographic planes through the heart are achieved by translating and rotating the gastroscope within the esophagus (Fig. 1). Several 'standard' transesophageal cross-sectional views have been proposed to be the most useful [23].

Aortic valve view. The gastroscope is always inserted into the esophagus with the transducer facing anteriorly. It is advanced to a depth of 35 to 40 cm from the patient's teeth when, as an orientational landmark, the typical tricuspid echo appearance of the aortic valve is seen within the ultrasonic sector during diastole (Fig. 2). The transducer is then situated behind the roof of the left atrium (Fig. 1: position 1), and the ultrasonic beams traverse the heart from dorsal to ventral, resulting in an image of part of the left atrial cavity, aortic root, and right ventricular outflow tract. Calcific or inflammatory lesions of the aortic valve (Fig. 3), as well as malformations such as a bicuspid valve (Fig. 4) may be recognized in this view. A recent case report on a patient with aortic valve endocarditis [24] has stressed the importance of transesophageal echocardiography as an 'adjunct to precordial echocardiography for demonstrating detailed morphologic information about the aortic root relevant to surgical decision making.'

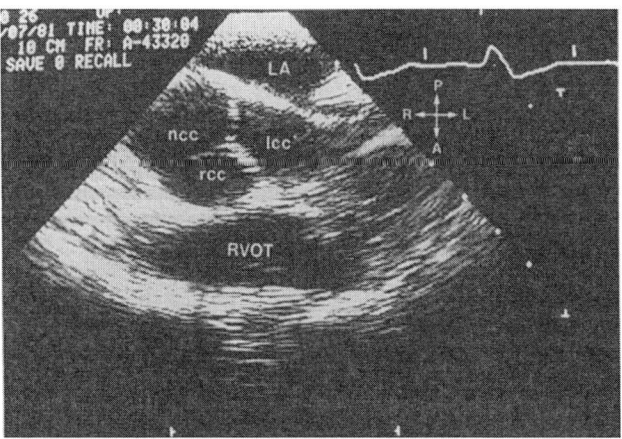

Fig. 2. Transesophageal cross-sectional view of the normal aortic root in diastole. Top of figure is dorsal, bottom of figure is ventral. Esophageal transducer faces anteriorly. A = anterior; L = left; LA = left atrium; lcc = left coronary cusp; ncc = noncoronary cusp; P = posterior; R = right; rcc = right coronary cusp; RVOT = right ventricular outflow tract.

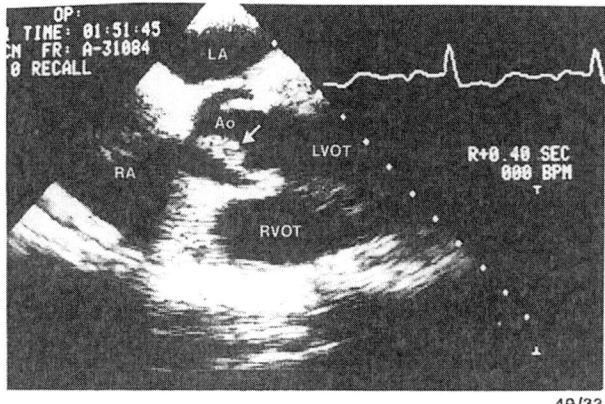

49/33

Fig. 3. Transesophageal view of thickened aortic cusp. With respect to Fig. 2, esophageal transducer is slightly rotated medially. LVOT = left ventricular outflow tract; RA = right atrium; other abbreviations as before.

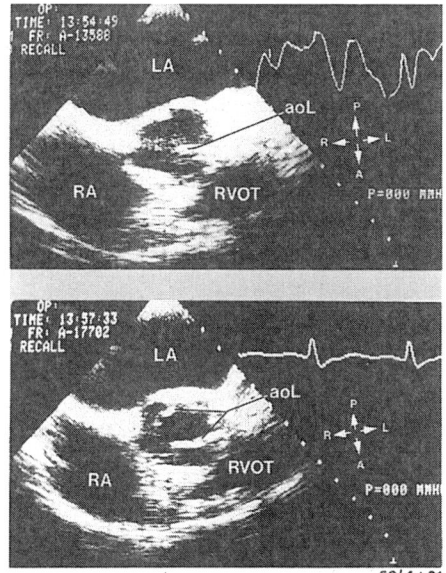

59/4+21

Fig. 4. Transesophageal visualization of a bicuspid aortic valve. Top panel: diastole; bottom panel: systole. Left atrium is dilated. Image orientation as in Fig. 3. aoL = aortic leaflets; other abbreviations as before.

Mitral valve view. After slight advancement of the gastroscope by 1 to 2 cm and counterclockwise rotation by about 20°, the transducer is still at atrial level (Fig. 1: position 2), yet faces left laterally to transverse the inferior left atrium, mitral valve, and left ventricular cavity (Fig. 5). The ultrasonic plane

214

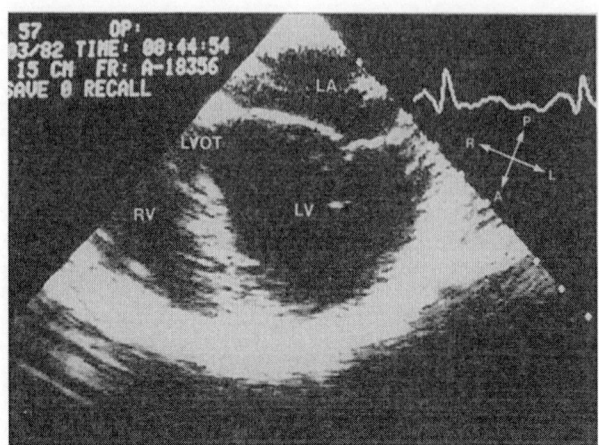

Fig. 5. Normal transesophageal view of the mitral valve. Esophageal transducer faces left laterally. The anterior (septal) mitral leaflet is to the left, the posterior mitral leaflet to the right of the ultrasonic sector. True long axis of the heart is not contained in this view; the distal border of the left ventricular cavity represents the anterolateral wall, not the cardiac apex. Abbreviations as before.

is horizontal but, because of the tilted situs of the heart within the chest, this is an oblique cardiac section. It does not contain the long axis of the heart, and the distal left ventricular wall (near the bottom of the ultrasonic sector) is not the cardiac apex but the anterolateral wall.

This view is one of the most frequently used in transesophageal investigations. It is particularly valuable for direct inspection of morphological dis-

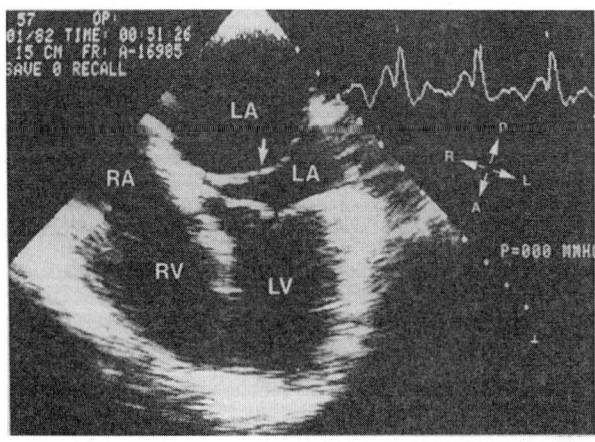

Fig. 6. Transesophageal recording from a patient with cor triatriatum. Image orientation as in Fig. 5. The membrane (arrow) subdividing the left atrium is clearly outlined. Abbreviations as before.

orders of the left atrium and mitral valve [25–28]. Figure 6 shows a transesophageal echocardiogram from an adult patient with cor triatriatum. The intraatrial membrane, which is rarely identified from precordial transducer positions, is clearly visualized. Ambiguous external echo information is also often encountered in chordal rupture of the mitral leaflets or in mitral valve prolapse. Transesophageal echocardiography readily distinguishes between these two entities. Figures 7 and 8 show ruptured chordae tendineae of the posterior mitral leaflet being pushed back into the left atrium with ventricular systole [29], and prolapse of the posterior mitral valve leaflet, respectively.

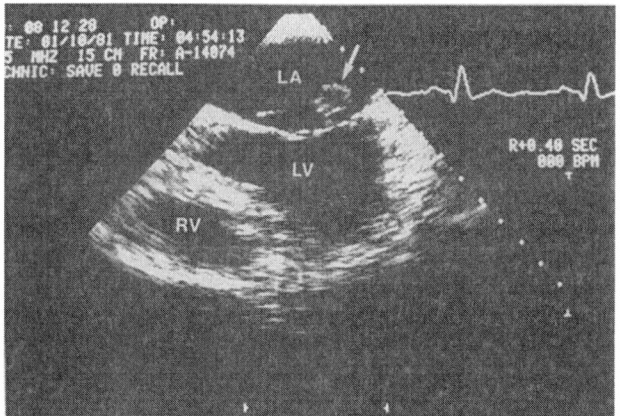

Fig. 7. Systolic transesophageal view from a patient with ruptured chordae tendineae (arrow) of the posterior mitral leaflet, representing as a coiled echo structure in the left atrium. Image orientation as in Fig. 5. Abbreviations as before.

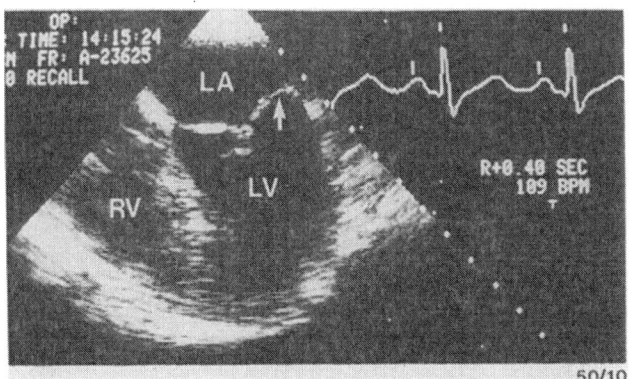

Fig. 8. Transesophageal view of a posterior mitral valve prolapse (arrow). Image orientation as in Fig. 5. Abbreviations as before.

Left ventricular short axis view. As the gastroscope is advanced further, it curves ventrally with the esophagus, and the ultrasonic plane will no longer be horizontal but tilted slightly upwards (Fig. 1: position 3). Thereby, a true short axis view of the left ventricle at the level of the papillary muscles can be obtained (Fig. 9). This view may be useful in the assessment of regional wall motion abnormalities or distribution of myocardial hypertrophy when these phenomena affect this particular cardiac region. At present, the view is primarily used for intraoperative monitoring of left ventricular performance [30].

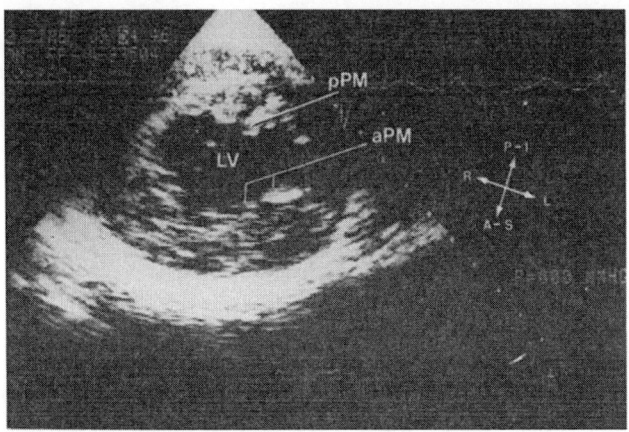

Fig. 9. Transesophageal left ventricular short axis view at the level of the papillary muscles. Image plane is no longer horizontal, but tilted upwards. aPM = anterolateral papillary muscle; A-S = anterosuperior; P-I = posteroinferior; pPM = posteromedial papillary muscle; other abbreviations as before.

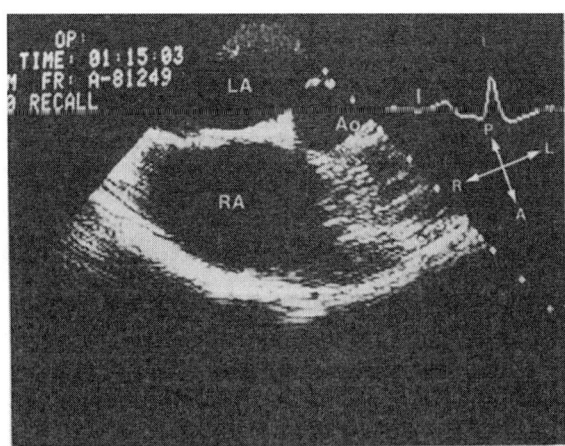

Fig. 10. Transesophageal view of both atria at a level slightly above the aortic valve. Abbreviations as before.

Biatrial view. If the gastroscope is rotated clockwise from position 3 (Fig. 1) by about 40°, so that the transducer faces right medially, and is withdrawn to the left atrial esophageal level, both atria can be viewed. The left atrial cavity is imaged in the upper half and the right atrial cavity in the lower middle part of the ultrasonic sector, separated by the roughly horizontal echo of the inter-atrial septum (Fig. 10). Next to the mitral valve view, this is the second most useful view in two-dimensional transesophageal echocardiography for mor-phologic studies. In conjunction with the former view, it will aid in the investi-gation of anomalous left atrial masses and structures [25, 27, 28, 31]; it is also particularly valuable for the detection of pathologic right atrial structures such as the right atrial membrane shown on Fig. 11.

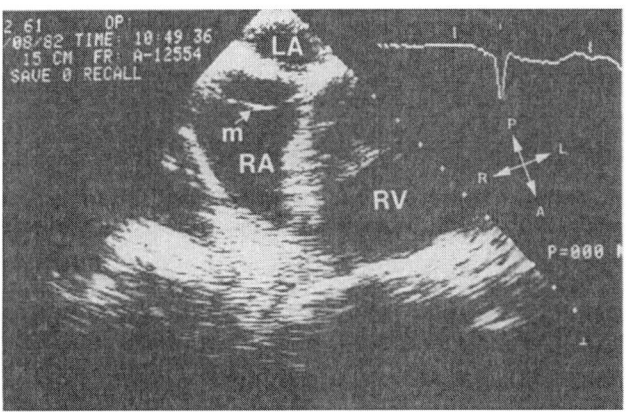

Fig. 11. Right atrial membrane (m) visualized in transesophageal biatrial view. Image orienta-tion as in Fig. 10. Abbreviations as before.

Because the interatrial septum is close to the esophageal transducer and runs almost perpendicular to the ultrasonic beam, the detection of atrial septal defects is greatly facilitated in this view [32, 33]. Figure 12 is an example from a patient with an ostium secundum defect. The biatrial view has also been employed to detect aneurysms of the interatrial septum [34] and spontaneous echo contrast within the left atrium [35].

Pulmonary artery view. The last of the standard transesophageal cross-sectional views is obtained when the gastroscope is rotated counterclockwise by 20° to face anteriorly again, and is withdrawn by another 2 cm. The great cardiac vessels are imaged, with the ascending aorta in a horizontal orienta-tion and the main and right pulmonary arteries in a longitudinal cross-section (Fig. 13).

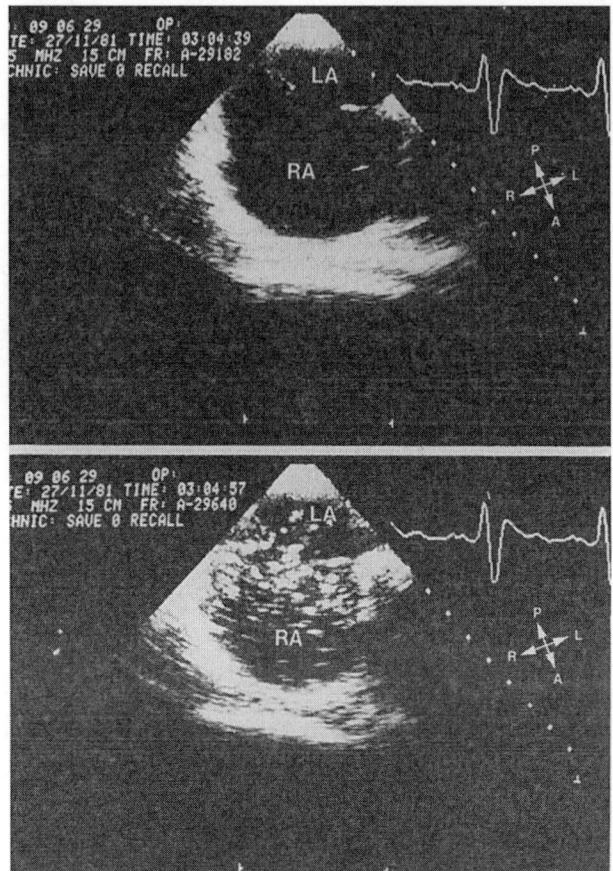

Fig. 12. Transesophageal visualization of an ostium secundum atrial septal defect. Image orientation as in Fig. 10. Top panel: direct visualization as discontinuity in interatrial septum. Bottom panel: contrast opacification of right atrium with passage across the defect into left atrium after intravenous injection of saline. Abbreviations as before.

Non-standardized views. Two of the several non-standardized views in transesophageal cross-sectional echocardiography are shown in Fig. 14. The esophageal level of both views is slightly above the aortic root, and they differ somewhat in their rotational degree for imaging the origins of the left main and right coronary artery. The more distal parts of the coronary arteries cannot be imaged. At roughly this elevational plane, yet with a left lateral rotation corresponding to the mitral valve view, the left atrial appendage can be inspected [36]. Figure 15 shows this view, with a thrombus filling most of the appendage. Transesophageal echocardiography for investigation of the descending thoracic aorta at various levels has also been reported [33, 37–40].

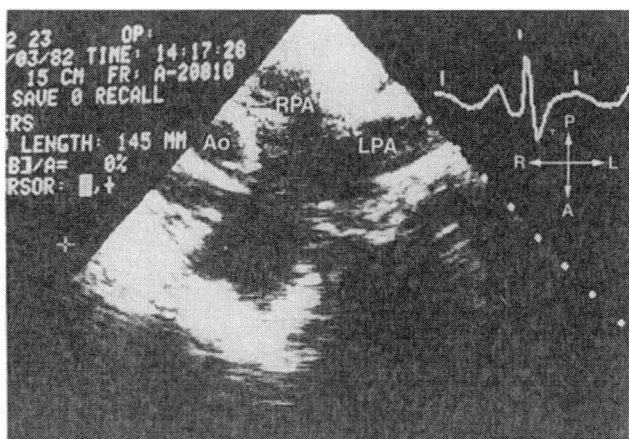

Fig. 13. Transesophageal image of main pulmonary artery and pulmonary bifurcation in a longitudinal cross-section. Ascending aorta is transected perpendicularly. Transducer faces anteriorly. LPA = left pulmonary artery; RPA = right pulmonary artery.

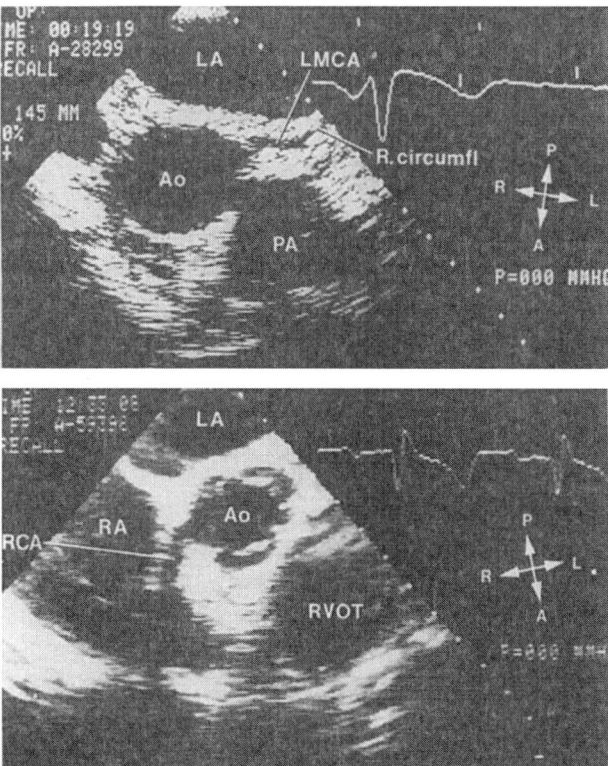

Fig. 14. Transesophageal views of origins of left (top panel) and right (bottom panel) coronary artery. LMCA = left main coronary artery; PA = pulmonary artery; RCA = right coronary artery; R. circumfl = right circumflex coronary artery.

220

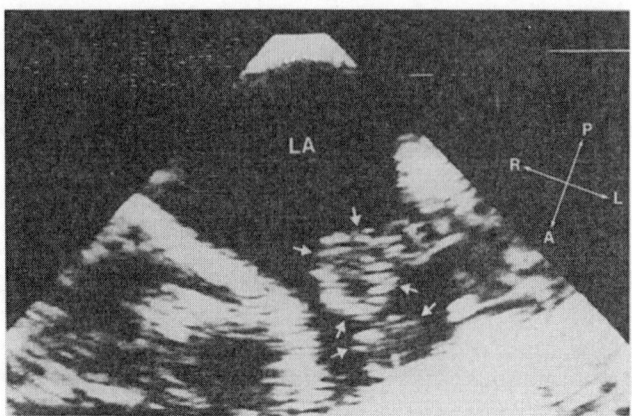

Fig. 15. Transesophageal view of a thrombus (arrows) within the left atrial appendage.

Applications. The main field of application for two-dimensional transesophageal echocardiography today is intraoperative monitoring [30, 41, 42]. The technique is highly suited, and superior to electrocardiography, for an immediate detection of intraoperative myocardial ischemia and infarction [43–45], as well as for an assessment of the immediate effects of coronary artery bypass grafting on regional myocardial function [46]. Other authors have reported its use for the detection of systemic or venous embolisms (due to air or matter) during various surgical procedures [47–53] and as a guide to surgical tumor excision [54]. It may also be employed to study patients in the coronary care unit [55] or investigate cardiac function in patients undergoing cardiopulmonary resuscitation [56].

Doppler echocardiography

As has been mentioned at the beginning of this article, the first probes to be used for transesophageal ultrasonography were continuous-wave Doppler probes. A pulsed Doppler system operating at a frequency of 7.5 MHz, in combination with 4.0 MHz 'echo track' instrumentation, was employed by Wells et al. [57] in 1979 to measure blood velocity and vessel diameter in the pulmonary artery and descending aorta in six healthy, conscious humans.

Transesophageal Doppler echocardiography has been used to study patients with left-sided valvular regurgitation by the M-mode [58] as well as by the cross-sectional technique [59]. The rationale for this approach, especially for assessing mitral regurgitation, was that: 1. the directions of blood flow through the mitral orifice and ultrasound emerging from an esophageal transducer are nearly parallel; thus, the angle-dependent sensitivity for velocity detection is highest; and 2. scanning of the left atrium for eccentric regurgitant jets is easily accomplished. The recognition of abnormal flow within the cardiac chambers fhas been greatly facilitated with the recent advent of Doppler color flow mapping [60], and initial experience with the transesophageal application of this modality has been reported [61].

Discussion

Transesophageal echocardiography, particularly for cross-sectional and Doppler imaging is a valuable adjunct to conventional precordial echocardiography in the aforementioned group of patients with obesity, obstructive pulmonary disease, or deformities of the thorax. Even in patients without any of these abnormalities, transesophageal echocardiography may yield improved diagnostic information because of the anatomically unrestricted ultrasonic access to the heart from the esophagus, the ability of freely scan cardiac structures such as atria and mitral valve, and the availability of new imaging planes that cannot be achieved from transthoracic transducer positions.

It is imperative, however, that the examiner has had basic training in endoscopy. Furthermore, a certain learning period for becoming accustomed to the unfamiliar looking transesophageal echocardiograms will be necessary. As in the early stages of M-mode echocardiography, contrast injections may be helpful in this respect. One must also be aware of the fact that, unlike transthoracic echocardiography, the transesophageal technique is associated with some degree of patient discomfort, and the decision to perform a transesophageal study should be carefully weighed. It is contraindicated in patients with a diverticulum or obstructive esophageal disease, and in patients with previous esophageal surgery or radiation therapy.

In unconscious patients, the diagnostic potential of transesophageal echocardiography will come to full advantage. Most promising is the intraoperative application of the technique for continuous monitoring of mechanical cardiac function as well as for detection of intracardiac air. Future perioperative transesophageal studies may include the Doppler determination of cardiac output in the main pulmonary artery, and the immediate evaluation of prosthetic valve competence before sternal closure by either contrast or Doppler echocardiography. The use of 5 MHz phased array transducers and the application of Doppler color flow mapping may further increase the clinical importance of transesophageal echocardiography as a diagnostic tool in selected patients and as an intraoperative monitoring device.

222

References

1. Side CD, Gosling RG: Non-surgical assessment of cardiac function. Nature 232: 335–6, 1971.
2. Olson RM, Shelton DK: A nondestructive technique to measure wall displacement in the thoracic aorta. J Appl Physiol 32: 147–151, 1972.
3. Daigle RE, Miller CW, Histand MB, McLeod FD, Hokanson DE: Non-traumatic aortic blood flow sensing by use of an ultrasonic esophageal probe. J Appl Physiol 38: 1153–1160, 1975.
4. Frazin L, Talano JV, Stephanides L, Loeb HS, Kopel L, Gunnar RM: Esophageal echocardiography. Circulation 54: 102–108, 1976.
5. Matsumoto M, Oka Y, Strom J, Frishman W, Kadish A, Becker RM, Frater RWM, Sonnenblick EH: Application of transesophageal echocardiography to continous monitoring of left ventricular performance. Am J Cardiol 46: 95–105, 1980.
6. Hanrath P, Kremer P, Langenstein BA, Matsumoto M, Bleifeld W: Transösophageale Echokardiographie. Ein neues Verfahren zur dynamischen Ventrikelfunktionsanalyse. Dtsch med Wochenschr 106: 523–525, 1981.
7. Matsumoto M, Hanrath P, Kremer P, Tams C, Langenstein BA, Schlüter M, Weiter R, Bleifeld W: Evaluation of left ventricular performance during supine bicycle exercise by transesophageal M-mode echocardiography in normal subjects. Br Heart J 48: 61–66, 1982.
8. Kremer P, Hanrath P, Langenstein B, Matsumoto M, Tams C, Bleifeld W: The evaluation of left ventricular function at rest and during exercise by transesophageal echocardiography in aortic insufficiency. Am J Cardiol 47: 412 (Abstract), 1981.
9. Hanrath P, Schlüter M, Kremer P, Thier W, Meenen S, Weiter R: The assessment of left ventricular function in hypertrophic cardiomyopathy by echocardiography. Eur Heart J 4 (Suppl F): 39–46, 1983.
10. Matsuzaki M, Masuda Y, Ikee Y, Takahashi Y, Sasaki T, Toma Y, Ishida K, Yorozu T, Kumada T, Kusukawa R: Esophageal echocardiographic left ventricular anterolateral wall motion in normal subjects and patients with coronary artery disease. Circulation 63: 1085–1092, 1981.
11. Toma Y, Masuda Y, Matsuzaki M, Annò Y, Uchida T, Hiroyama N, Tamitani M, Murata T, Yonezawa F, Moritani K, Katayama K, Ogawa H, Kusukawa R: Determination of atrial size by esophageal echocardiography. Am J Cardiol 52: 878–880, 1983.
12. Terai C, Uenishi M, Sugimoto H, Shimazu T, Yoshioka T, Sugimoto T: Transesophageal echocardiographic dimensional analysis of four cardiac chambers during positive end-expiratory pressure. Anesthesiology 63: 640–646, 1985.
13. Furuya H, Suzuki T, Okumura F, Kishi Y, Uefuji T: Detection of air embolism by transesophageal echocardiography. Anesthesiology 58: 124–129, 1983.
14. Furuya H, Okumura F: Detection of paradoxical air embolism by transesophageal echocardiography. Anesthesiology 60: 374–377, 1984.
15. Oka Y, Moriwaki KM, Hong Y, Chuculate C, Strom J, Andrews IC, Frater RWM: Detection of air emboli in the left heart by M-mode transesophageal echocardiography following cardiopulmonary bypass. Anesthesiology 63: 109–113, 1985.
16. Oka Y, Inoue T, Hong Y, Sisto DA, Strom JA, Frater RWM: Retained intracardiac air. Transesophageal echocardiography for definition of incidence and monitoring removal by improved techniques. J Thorac Cardiovasc Surg 91: 329–338, 1986.
17. Eggleton RC: Ultrasonic visualization of the dynamic geometry of the heart. Proceedings 2nd World Congress on Ultrasonics in Medicine, Exerpta Medica, International Congress Series 277: 10 (Abstract), 1973.

18. Hisanaga K, Hisanaga A, Hibi N, Nishimura K, Kambe T: High speed rotation scanner for transesophageal cross-sectional echocardiography. Am J Cardiol 46: 837–842, 1980.

19. DiMagno EP, Buxton JL, Regan PT, Hattery RR, Wilson DA, Suarez JR, Green PS: Ultrasonic endoscope. Lancet 1: 629–631, 1980.

20. Souquet J, Hanrath P, Zitelli L, Kremer P, Langenstein BA, Schlüter M: Transesophageal phased array for imaging the heart. IEEE Trans Biomed Eng BME-29: 707–712, 1982.

21. Schlüter M, Langenstein BA, Polster J, Kremer P, Souquet J, Engel S, Hanrath P: Transesophageal cross-sectional echocardiography with a phased array transducer system. Technique and initial clinical results. Br Heart J 48: 67–72, 1982.

22. Hanrath P, Schlüter M, Langenstein BA, Polster J, Engel S: Transesophageal horizontal and sagittal imaging of the heart with a phased array system. Initial clinical results. In: Hanrath P, Bleifeld W, Souquet J (eds.): Cardiovascular Diagnosis by Ultrasound. Boston, Martinus Nijhoff Publishers, p 280–288, 1982.

23. Schlüter M, Hinrichs A, Thier W, Kremer P, Schröder S, Cahalan MK, Hanrath P: Transesophageal 2-dimensional echocardiography. Comparison of ultrasonic and anatomic sections. Am J Cardiol 53: 1173–1178, 1984.

24. Gussenhoven EJ, van Herwerden LA, Roelandt J, Bos E, de Jong N: Detailed analysis of aortic valve endocarditis: comparison of precordial, esophageal and epicardial two-dimensional echocardiography with clinical findings. J Clin Ultrasound 14: 209–211, 1986.

25. Thier W, Schlüter M, Krebber HJ, Polonius MJ, Klöppel G, Becker K, Hanrath P: Cysts in left atrial myxoma identified by transesophageal cross-sectional echocardiography. Am J Cardiol 51: 1793–1795, 1983.

26. Ezekowitz MD, Smith EO, Rankin R, Harrison LH, Krous HF: Left atrial mass: diagnostic value of transesophageal 2-dimensional echocardiography and indium-111 platelet scintigraphy. Am J Cardiol 51: 1563–1564, 1983.

27. Schlüter M, Langenstein BA, Thier W, Schmiegel WH, Krebber HJ, Kalmar P, Hanrath P: Transesophageal two-dimensional echocardiography in the diagnosis of cor triatriatum in the adult. J Am Coll Cardiol 2: 1011–1015, 1983.

28. Nellessen U, Daniel WG, Lichtlen RP: Bedeutung der transösophagealen Echokardiographie in der Diagnostik kardialer und parakardialer raumfordernder Prozesse. Z Kardiol 75: 91–98, 1986.

29. Schlüter M, Kremer P, Hanrath P: Transesophageal 2-D echocardiographic feature of flail mitral leaflet due to ruptured chordae tendineae. Am Heart J 108: 609–610, 1984.

30. Schiller NB: Evaluation of cardiac function during surgery by transesophageal 2-dimensional echocardiography. In: Hanrath P, Bleifeld W, Souquet J (eds.): Cardiovascular Diagnosis by Ultrasound. Boston, Martinus Nijhoff Publishers, p 289–293, 1982.

31. Nellessen U, Daniel WG, Matheis G, Oelert H, Depping K, Lichtlen PR: Impending paradoxical embolism from atrial thrombus: correct diagnosis by transesophageal echocardiography and prevention by surgery. J Am Coll Cardiol 5: 1002–1004, 1985.

32. Hanrath P, Schlüter M, Langenstein BA, Polster J, Engel S, Kremer P, Krebber HJ: Detection of ostium secundum atrial septal defects by transesophageal cross-sectional echocardiography. Br Heart J 49: 350–358, 1983.

33. Erbel R, Mohr-Kahaly S, Drexler M, Schreiner G, Börner N, Schuster S, Henkel B, Pfeiffer C, Meyer J: Erweiterung der kardialen Diagnostik mittels transösophagealer Echokardiographie. Med Klin 81: 251–257, 1986.

34. Schreiner G, Erbel R, Mohr-Kahaly S, Krämer G, Henkel B, Meyer J: Nachweis von Aneurysmen des Vorhofseptums mit Hilfe der transösophagealen Echokardiographie. Z Kardiol 74: 440–444, 1985.

224

35. Erbel R, Stern H, Ehrenthal W, Schreiner G, Treese N, Krämer G, Thelen M, Schweizer P, Meyer J: Detection of spontaneous echocardiographic contrast within the left atrium by transesophageal echocardiography. Clin Cardiol 9: 245–252, 1986.
36. Aschenberg W, Schlüter M, Kremer P, Schröder E, Siglow V, Bleifeld W: Transesophageal two-dimensional echocardiography for the detection of left atrial appendage thrombus. J Am Coll Cardiol 7: 163–166, 1986.
37. Börner N, Erbel R, Braun B, Henkel B, Meyer J, Rumpelt J: Diagnosis of aortic dissection by transesophageal echocardiography. Am J Cardiol 54: 1157–1158, 1984.
38. Stern H, Erbel R, Börner N, Schreiner G, Meyer J: Spontaner Echokontrast, registriert mittels transösophagealer Echokardiographie bei Aortendissektion Typ III. Z Kardiol 74: 480–481, 1985.
39. Engberding R, Bender F, Grosse-Heitmeyer W, Müller US, Schneider D: Diagnose thorakaler Aortenaneurysmen durch kombinierte transthorakale und transösophageale 2D-Echokardiographie. Z Kardiol 75: 225–230, 1986.
40. Engberding R, Bender F, Müller US, Grosse-Heitmeyer W: Aneurysms and dissections of the descending thoracic aorta – identification by transesophageal two dimensional echocardiography. J Am Coll Cardiol 7: 138A (Abstract), 1986.
41. Goldman ME, Mindich BP: Intraoperative two-dimensional echocardiography: new application of an old technique. J Am Coll Cardiol 7: 374–382, 1986.
42. Roizen MF, Beaupre PN, Alpert RA, Kremer P, Cahalan MK, Schiller N, Sohn YJ, Cronnelly R, Lurz FW, Ehrenfeld WK, Stoney RJ: Monitoring with two-dimensional transesophageal echocardiography. Comparison of myocardial function in patients undergoing supraceliac, suprarenal-infraceliac, or infrarenal aortic occlusion. J Vasc Surg 1: 300–305, 1984.
43. Beaupre PN, Kremer PF, Cahalan MK, Lurz FW, Schiller NB, Hamilton WK: Intraoperative detection of changes in left ventricular segmental wall motion by transesophageal two-dimensional echocardiography. Am Heart J 107: 1021–1023, 1984.
44. Smith JS, Cahalan MK, Benefiel DJ, Byrd BF, Lurz FW, Shapiro WA, Roizen MF, Bouchard A, Schiller NB: Intraoperative detection of myocardial ischemia in high-risk patients: electrocardiography versus two-dimensional transesophageal echocardiography. Circulation 72: 1015–1021, 1985.
45. Shively BK, Schiller NB: Transesophageal echocardiography in the intraoperative detection of myocardial ischemia and infarction. Echocardiography 3: 433–443, 1986.
46. Topol EJ, Weiss JL, Guzman PA, Dorsey-Lima S, Blanck TJJ, Humphrey LS, Baumgartner WA, Flaherty JT, Reitz BA: Immediate improvement of dysfunctional myocardial segments after coronary revascularization: detection by intraoperative transesophageal echocardiography. J Am Coll Cardiol 4: 1123–1134, 1984.
47. Cucchiari RF, Nugent M, Seward JB, Messick JM: Air embolism in neurosurgical patients: Detection and localization by two-dimensional transesophageal echocardiography. Anesthesiology 60: 353–355, 1984.
48. Cucchiara RF, Seward JB, Nishimura RA, Nugent M, Faust RJ: Identification of patent foramen ovale during sitting position craniotomy by transesophageal echocardiography with positive airway pressure. Anesthesiology 63: 107–109, 1985.
49. Glenski JA, Cucchiara RF, Michenfelder JD: Transesophageal echocardiography and transcutaneous O_2 and CO_2 monitoring for detection of venous air embolism. Anesthesiology 64: 541–545, 1986.
50. Roewer N, Beck H, Kochs E, Kremer P, Schröder E, Schöntag H, Jungbluth KH, Schulte am Esch J: Nachweis venöser Embolien während intraoperativer Überwachung mittels transösophagealer zweidimensionaler Echokardiographie. Anästh Intensivther Notfallmed 20: 200–205, 1985.

51. Roewer N, Beck H, Kochs E, Kremer P, Schröder E, Schulte am Esch J: Detection of venous embolism during intraoperative monitoring by two-dimensional transesophageal echocardiography. Anesthesiology 63: A169 (Abstract), 1985.

52. Heinrich H, Kremer P, Winter H, Wörsdorfer O, Ahnefeld FW: Transösophageale zwei-dimensionale Echokardiographie bei Hüftendoprothesen. Anaesthesist 34: 118-123, 1985.

53. Topol EJ, Humphrey LS, Borkon M, Baumgartner WA, Dorsey DL, Reitz BA, Weiss JL: Value of intraoperative left ventricular microbubbles detected by transesophageal two-dimensional echocardiography in predicting neurologic outcome after cardiac operations. Am J Cardiol 56: 773–775, 1985.

54. Topol EJ, Biern RO, Reitz BA: Cardiac papillary fibroelastoma and stroke. Echocardiographic diagnosis and guide to excision. Am J Med 80: 129–132, 1986.

55. Hinrichs A, Schlüter M, Roewer N, Schmiegel W, Kremer P, Hanrath P: Clinical value of transesophageal two-dimensional echocardiography in mechanically ventilated coronary care unit patients. Circulation 68 (Suppl III): III-95 (Abstract), 1983.

56. Clements FM, de Bruijn NP, Kisslo JA: Transesophageal echocardiographic observations in a patient undergoing closed-chest massage. Anesthesiology 64: 826–828, 1986.

57. Wells MK, Histand MB, Reeves JT, Sodal IE, Adamson HP: Ultrasonic transesophageal measurement of hemodynamic parameters in humans. ISA Transactions 18: 57–61, 1979.

58. Schlüter M, Langenstein BA, Hanrath P, Kremer P, Bleifeld W: Assessment of transesophageal pulsed Doppler echocardiography in the detection of mitral regurgitation. Circulation 66:784–789, 1982.

59. Shively B, Cahalan M, Benefiel D, Schiller N: Intraoperative assessment of mitral valve regurgitation by transesophageal Doppler echocardiography. J Am Coll Cardiol 7:228A (Abstract), 1986.

60. Miyatake K, Okamoto M, Kinoshita N, Izumi S, Owa M, Takao S, Sakakibara H, Nimura Y: Clinical applications of a new type of real-time two-dimensional Doppler flow imaging system. Am J Cardiol 54:857–868, 1984.

61. Goldman ME, Thys D, Ritter S, Hillel Z, Kaplan J: Trans-esophageal real time Doppler flow imaging: a new method for intraoperative cardiac evaluation. J Am Coll Cardiol 7:1A (Abstract), 1986.

4.2. Transesophageal echocardiography – an overview of applications

BRUCE SHIVELY & NELSON B. SCHILLER

Introduction

Among newer ultrasound imaging modalities, transesophageal echocardiography (TEE) is one of the most promising and rapidly evolving. Although the concept has been around for the past decade its proliferation into a wide variety of clinical applications has occured mainly in the past years. Early M-mode studies demonstrated the accuracy of anatomic presentation by TEE and more recent two-dimensional (2D) investigations have assessed intraoperative changes in left ventricular (LV) size and contractility in response to altered loading conditions and changes in anesthesia dosage. Clinically, TEE is being used as an intraoperative monitoring tool with which the anesthesiologist is able to detect ischemia or infarction by observing regional changes in wall motion. Although most widely used in intubated anesthetized patients, applications in awake resting or exercising patients have been described. For example, dynamic exercise (upright bicycle) was performed in groups of patients with aortic insufficiency or coronary disease while a TEE probe maintained a stable image of the left ventricle. Other intraoperative applications of TEE have included detection of intracardiac air in neurologic and cardiac procedures. It is routine practice in our institution to preoperatively assess patients undergoing upright craniotomy for patent foramen ovale with contrast echocardiography. Those having right to left intra-atrial shunts routinely have TEE during the procedure. Most recently, Doppler has been added to our TEE capabilities. Using pulse wave and color Doppler we routinely assess the success of mitral valve repair procedures in aleviating mitral regurgitation.

Early studies using TEE

TEE was introduced by Frazin et al. [1], who in 1975, afixed a single crystal M-mode transducer to a catheter. Their device, likened to a lozenge on a string, allowed them to study the feasibility of obtaining accurate M-mode measurements of the aortic root and left atrium and mitral filling slope in

I. Cikes (ed.), *Echocardiography in Cardiac Interventions*, 227–248, 1989.
© 1989 *Kluwer Academic Publishers*.

conscious patients who were able to swallow the probe. Based on their excellent results, they recommended that TEE be used to study patients who presented technical barriers to conventional precordial imaging. Frasin's method, however, had a major flaw in that they could not reproducibly image the left ventricle. This one deficiency inhibited the growth of this technique until 1980 when Matsumoto [2] and associates successfully recorded LV dimensions, wall thickness and derived LV functional indices on a transducer afixed to a stiffer assembly. Their initial experience was limited to use in intubated anesthestized patients and they thus became the first group to perform TEE. In their experiments they were able to make observations about the effects on the heart of changes in LV loading conditions as well on the influence of sternal and pericardial opening and closure.

Matsumoto et al. [3] studied a total of 21 cardiac surgery patients with serial observations at six predetermined points during surgery. In six patients undergoing coronary bypass grafting and six having aortic or mitral valve replacement for regurgitation, LV volumes, ejection fraction (EF) and velocity of circumferential fiber shortening (Vcf) were measured and indices of end-diastolic wall stress and stiffness were calculated from the TEE generated M-mode tracings and pulmonary capillary wedge pressures. Immediately after the correction of regurgitant lesions, the expected large decreases in preload indices (LV end-diastolic volume and wall stress) were found to be associated with decreases in EF and Vcf. Decreases in Vcf and EF were not found in those having coronary bypass surgery, probably due to the minimal preload decreases in this group. Possible changes in contractility were not addressed in this study, in part due to limited data on loading conditions. No effect of cardiopulmonary bypass or the surgical procedure on the calculated stiffness constant of compliance ($-dp/dv$) of the LV was shown in either patient group. A good correlation (after valve replacement) between calculated TEE and dye dilution stroke volumes was observed, pointing to the potential substitution of TEE for more conventional hemodynamic monitoring. The influence of pericardial and sternal closure on diastolic filling and apparent septal motion were also examined. Following both pericardial and sternal closure, decreases in preload indices were accompanied by decreases in cardiac output, compliance and increases in the LV stiffness constant. These findings have theoretical importance regarding the role of these 'containing' structures in determining cardiac performance as well as practical implications for intraoperative patient monitoring.

Finally, Matsumoto and his group noted effects of the opening and closure of the mediastinum on septal motion. Prior to their study, controversy had developed in the echocardiographic literature [4] concerning whether or not the apparent changes in septal motion observed after open heart surgery were due to increased anteromedial translational motion of the whole heart, paradoxical septal motion due to uncertain causes, or actual contractile dysfunction of the septal myocardium due to surgical injury. The intraoperative observations of this study established that septal thickening is preserved but that increased translation of the heart is not the only factor affecting apparent septal motion after surgery. They observed a delay of inward motion of the septal endocardium (relative to posterior wall motion) appearing with pericardiotomy and at least partially reversed after sternal closure. Unfortunately, in the absence of right and left ventricular pressure data the authors were unable to definitely explain this apparent role of the pericardium in maintaining synchronous LV contraction.

The next technical advance was the use of a gastroscope housing with tilt and azimuth controls (Fig. 1). An M-mode transducer was mounted at the end of this device (Fig. 5) and allowed almost complete control over the position of the transducer footprint against the esophageal mucosa. With improved control came improved image quality and the ability to standardize cardiac views. In Japan, Matasuzaki's group [5] and Fukagawa [6] used this device to study anterior and septal wall motion in patients with coronary disease. Matsuzaki's group successfully imaged almost all 21 of their study patients and noted that, in the classification of anterior wall motion into five categories ranging from hyperdynamic to dyskinetic, TEE agreed more closely with angiography than precordial echocardiography. The authors felt that this difference was due to the heart's anteromedial systolic motion minimizing apparent wall excursion when viewed precordially. In a similar study, Fukagawa found that abnormalities of both septal and anterior wall motion by TEE were associated with proximal left anterior descending artery lesions, while isolated anterior wall motion abnormalities accompanied distal lesions.

A modified gastroscope M-mode tipped probe was also used in studies by Kremer [7] and Matsumoto [8], who reported on the influence of exercise on M-mode indices of LV size (end-diastolic dimension) and function (fraction shortening). Employing premedication with atropine and oropharyngeal

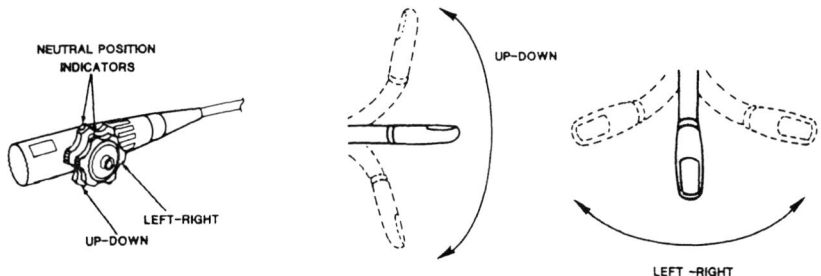

Fig. 1. Illustration of tilt (center) and azimuth (right) controls of Diasonics Echoscope. (Drawing courtesy of Diasonics, Inc., Milpitas, CA.)

anesthesia, these authors were able to maintain esophageal intubation with a 9 mm probe in awake patients during supine bicycle exercise. Among their findings was that the response to exercise of patients with symptomatic aortic insufficiency (AI) was distinct from that found in normals/asymptomatic AI patients. In the symptomatic patients, LV size increased and fractional shortening decreased at peak exercise compared to rest while in the normal/asymptomatic AI group opposite changes were seen. Despite the considerable advantages of exercise TEE (stable probe position and superior resolution) no further reports of this methodology have appeared, possibly because of poor patient acceptance and inconvenience of the technique.

Technical advances in TEE

Between 1980 and 1986 both phased-array and mechanical 2D TEE probes have been developed. Hisanaga et al. [9] has developed a number of innovative devices. One of these is a mechanical scanner encased in an oil-filled bag and capable of scanning over a wide (180° to 260°) scan angle. Owing to the proximity of the TEE transducer to the posterior heart and great vessels, a wide scan angle is advantageous because it can simultaneously interrogate all nearby structures. High frequency transducer crystals (e.g. 7–10 MHz) can also be easily incorporated into mechanical systems to take full advantage of the proximity of the heart and the airless pathway from the transducer. Both Hisanaga [11] and Reifert and Strohm [12] have claimed that structures difficult to define with precordial imaging are easily appreciated through the esophagus. Another noteworthy device reported by Hisanaga [10] is the combination of a horizontally oriented rotating scanner and vertically oriented linear scanner on the same probe. With this device it is possible to simultaneously display images from each of these orthogonal scan planes.

Although mechanical scanners have advantages, the prevailing state-of-the-art during the early 1980's has led to the predominance of phased array transducers for TEE. Lacking noise and vibration of the mechanical systems, phased arrays offer a higher line density and frame rate and can be more readily miniturized. M-mode, 2D and Doppler are also more easily interfaced within the same crystal assembly. Nevertheless, the limited scan angle, relatively high expense of phased array electronics, the inherently higher resolution of mechanically driven crystals and rapid progress in microelectronics make a reappearance of mechanical scanners for TEE applications likely.

Among the various phased array devices that have been developed, that reported by Souquet et al. [13, 14] was incorporated into TEE probe, the

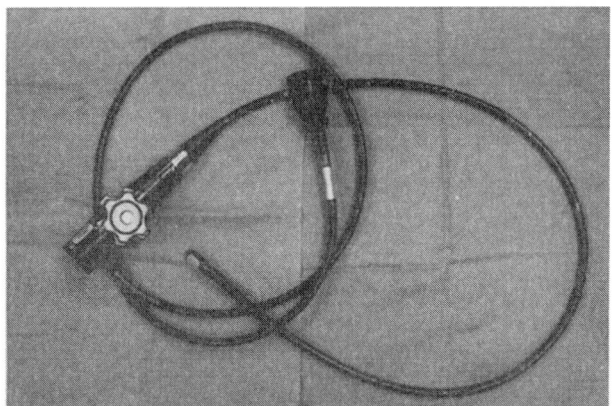

Fig. 2. Diasonics Echoscope transesophageal echocardiographic probe.

Diasonics Echoscope (Fig. 2). With this instrument the vast majority of the work described in the rest of this review was performed.

Case reports involving TEE imaging

Many case reports have appeared describing the application of TEE to a variety of clinical problems. Ezekowitz et al. [15] and Thier et al. [16] reported the detection of left atrial myxomas by TEE, previously only suspected due to inadequate precordial imaging. In Thier's paper, the detection of echo-free spaces or cysts within the tumor and their surgical documentation was described. Schlüter et al. [17] illustrated the value of TEE in two cases of cor triatriatum in which the diagnosis was made by this technique after precordial echocardiography had failed to image the obstructing membrane. Nissensen and his group [18] reported an unusual case in which masses in both atria were found by precordial echocardiography in a patient who had sustained a number of pulmonary emboli. By TEE the masses were seen to represent the two ends of a 12 cm long thrombus lodged across a secundum atrial septal defect. Another instance of pulmonary embolism in progress detected by TEE, with a clot observed traversing the right arium, also appears in the literature [19].

The localization of the entrance tear of a type III aortic dissection was reported by Borner's group [20] and Engbending et al. [21] found TEE superior to precordial echocardiography in the detection of descending aortic aneurysms. Venishi et al. [22] performed M-mode TEE in several severly injured patients during the chest compression phase of cardiopulmonary resuscitation (CPR). These observations lend support to the thoracic pump theory of the mechanism of CPR in the production of systemic blood flow. They refute the role of direct cardiac compression by showing that the mitral valve remains open during chest compression. Thus, the heart merely serves as a conduit during CPR.

Detection of intracardiac air embolism by TEE

Air entering the central circulation, even in amounts as little as 5 ml/kg, may be attended by circulatory collapse and death. Imaging and Doppler TEE has been found to be sensitive in detecting small amounts of intracardiac air in two surgical situations where the risk of this complication is substantial: neurologic and open heart surgery.

The practice of conducting neurologic surgical procedures in the upright position allows air to enter the central circulation because of low or negative superior vena caval pressure and fixation of the intracranial veins to their attachments to the skull. An air bolus entering the right atrium from central access may cause obstruction and shock. Lesser degrees of air embolization may induce a rise in pulmonary artery and right atrial pressure favoring paradoxical air embolization across a patent foramen ovale (PFO). Furuya and et al. [23] conducted a canine experiment to test the sensitivity of TEE to intracardiac air of various ammounts; TEE detected only 0.01 ml/kg given as a bolus. Since this quantity is a small fraction of the dose capable of impeding pulmonary gas exchange or raising pulmonary pressures, TEE was judge more sensitive than any other monitoring device available. In their clinical setting, the authors responded to the immediate detection of air in the right heart by initiating preventative maneuvers such as aspiration of air from PA catheters. These authors also observed that TEE could also simultaneously monitor the left heart and aorta for the appearance of paradoxical embolism. In a later communication [24] they documented the value of TEE in a case report. The high sensitivity of TEE to the detection of air was also studied by Cucciara and associates [25] in a series of 15 patients. In another report, these authors [26] employed a brief interval of 15 cm of positive end expiratory pressure (PEEP) accompanied by intravenous saline contast injection to test for PFO prior to upright neurologic surgery. They recommended that this valsalva maneuver analog was appropriate just prior to neurosurgery to identify those patients in whom a PFO placed them at risk for paradoxical embolization. In our own institution we test for PFO in the echocardiography laboratory by performing a valsalva maneuver simultaneously with administration of saline contrast and precordial imaging. In those neurosurgical patients in whom PFO is detected by appeance of left sided bubbles, TEE monitoring is conducted throughout the operation.

At the University of California San Fransisco, we have monitored over 3,000 patients with TEE and have found it common to encounter mobile intracardiac targets (bubbles) during open heart surgery. These targets are small air bubbles and their common occurance suggests that air readily gains access to the central circulation during the course of this type of surgery. However, possibly because the surgeon routinely conducts air removal maneuvers, these targets have not been associated with neurological events. A study seeking an association between left heart air by TEE and neurologic complications was reported by Oka's group [27]. In 15 patients, TEE detected air in 11 and in these, one patient sustained a stroke and two had prolonged episodes of post operative disorientation. In this extremely limited series, only four patients without detected intracardiac air were available as a control group, precluding the conclusion that TEE detection of air predicts neurological events. Topol et al. [28] in reporting a larger series of 82 patients, detected air after cardiopulmonary bypass in 41% and found it to be more frequent after cardiotomy (75%) than after routine coronary artery grafting (10%). Neurologic events were neither associated with the presence of intracardiac air nor with its apparent quantity.

From these data, we conclude that TEE is indicated in monitoring for air embolism (venous and paradoxical) during upright neurosurgical procedures because immediate intervention can prevent complications. In open heart surgery where it is routine to perform air maneuvers, TEE commonly shows microbubbles that probably represent small quantities of air and are not associated with neurological consequences. For this reason, monitoring for air embolism is not a major reason for utilizing intraoperative TEE.

Left ventricular function during anesthesia

TEE has been used to study the effects of anesthesia and loading conditions (i.e. preload and afterload) on segmental and global LV function. Quantitation of myocardial depression related to Halothane and similar agents has been achieved by observing changes in area ejection fraction (diastolic area-systolic area/diastolic area) measured from the short axis LV view papillary muscle level. One of the studies addressing the issue of the characteristic effects on LV performance among anesthetic agents was that of Smith et al. [29] who evaluated the influence of two anesthetic regimes in a population determined angiographically to have depressed ejection fractions (< 40%). They showed that the outcome of surgery as guaged by patient survival and morbid events was the same in a regimen of a high dose narcotic (Fentanyl alone) compared to a lower dose of Fentanyl plus intermittent doses of the inhalational anesthetic Isoflurane. The regimen that included Isoflurane might be expected to be associated with a more negative hemodynamic impact and poorer outcome than the Fentanyl only regimen in this population. However, the study demonstrated that the lowered systemic vascular resistance of the second regimen offset its greater contractility depression. This study also demonstrates that it is difficult to predict the impact of a change in an anesthetic regimen without a method that provides an accurate, direct measure of LV preload and contractility. Clearly more studies of this type are needed and TEE is an ideal method with which to implement them.

Matsumoto [14] was able to track changes in hemodynamic status during surgery by estimating cardiac output from changes in the LV M-mode minor axis dimension. Another study by Oka et al. [30] used the opening of the aortic leaflets (systolic time intervals) and aortic root motion to follow changes in circulatory performance. Intraoperative LV preload has been monitored using the LV end diastolic area or dimension from the short axis view. This direct measure of LV filling has been compared to the standard indirect measure, the pulmonary capillary wedge pressure (PCW). The PCW may not reliably reflect LV preload if the LV compliance changes throughout the period of observation. The interoperative setting is one where several major dynamic circulatory mediators can be expected to strongly influence LV compliance. For example, anesthetic concentration, hypothermia and ischemia may all appear, persist, intensify or resolve during an operation. However, because the end diastolic area is a direct analog of preload, it should continue to represent LV filling independent of compliance. Beaupre et al. [31] in studying how closely PCW represented LV size, found that during surgery PCW and LV end diastolic areas often changed in different directions. Since PCW monitoring requires a pulmonary artery catheter and TEE does not, the relative safety and more informative nature of TEE suggest that TEE should assume a greater role in surgical monitoring.

Decreased preload due to hypovolemia or depression of ventricular contractility can cause hypotension. The value of TEE in readily separating these diverse mechanisms of shock at the termination of cardiopulmonary bypass was studied by Topol et al. [32]. At the University of California San Fransisco, the usefulness of this application of TEE has been apparent to us from very early in our experience. The appearance of a hyperdynamic LV with a small cavity is an indication for fluid replacement, in spite of input and output records which may suggest that fluid balance has been maintained. On the other hand, a globally or segmentally depressed ventricle with normal or increased end diastolic volume may require inotropic support not fluid replacement to ameliorate hypotension.

TEE in the intensive care unit

Patients in the intensive care unit (ICU) often have severe hemodynamic embarrasment and are very difficult to study with conventional precordial echocardiography. Thus TEE is ideally suited for the study of these patients and the benefits of obtaining these highly resolved TEE images far outweighs the relatively minimal discomfort and very small risk it imparts to the patient. In these hemodynamically unstable subjects, the use of postive end expiratory pressure (PEEP) is often inhibited by its known detrimental effects on cardiac output. In order to ascertain the mechanisms by which PEEP exerts this noxious influence it is desirable to determine its effect on cardiac chamber size and contractile function. Terai and co-workers [33] used TEE to evaluate 16 intubated patients at PEEP settings of zero, ten and 15 cm water while also recording thermodilution cardiac output, heart rate and intra-arterial pressure. As PEEP was initiated, the size of the LV, left atrium and right atrium decreased and the ejection fraction increased. The authors inferred from these data that LV filling and not contractility is impeded by PEEP. contractility is impeded by PEEP.

Because RV failure had attended the use of an LV assist device in one patient, Hershon and associates [34] studied the effects of LV assist pumps on right ventricular function. TEE was performed in patients having LV assist during cardiopulmonary bypass and revealed that RV volume fell and RV EF rose in direct relation to pulmonary artery pressure but not in relation to changes in interventricular septal position. Their speculation prior to the study had been that the RV failure might have been due to a Bernheim effect (interference by an encroaching septum with RV function) but the TEE data did not support it.

Transesophageal echocardiography/Doppler

TEE provides highly resolved ultrasound images obtained under conditions that are optimal for the ultrasound examination. Some of these same conditions (i.e. target proximity and airless pathway) are also optimal for the Doppler flow velocity examination. Because imaging and Doppler can be performed from the same reflected sonic radiation and with the same ultrasonic crystals, the use of Doppler with TEE to assess intracardiac blood flow velocity and to detect and localize the jets characteristic of valve stenosis or regurgitation is a natural extension of this important area of cardiac ultrasound. Some recent work in this area has centered on the incorporation of continuous wave ultrasound crystals into a TEE probe for assessment of cardiac output [35–38]. Lacking imaging capabilities, the Doppler signal is obtained 'blindly' in these studies by manipulating the TEE probe so as to maximize the audible flow signal. The usual target in these studies is flow in the descending aorta and the recorded time velocity curves are analysed in order to calculate the mean systolic blood flow velocity. The product of this mean flow velocity and the time of flow (duration of systole) is an expression of the distance blood is propelled during the period of systolic flow. This calculation of the distance blood travels is multiplied by the cross sectional area through which blood flow is occuring (in this case the descending aorta) to provide a close approximation of the stroke volume. The distance the blood is propelled can conveniently be referred to as the stroke distance and if only directional changes are sought this value by itself can be followed without the need for factoring in the relatively static aortic diameter. A number of studies show that [35–38] changes in thermodilution cardiac output may be reliably predicted by stroke distance fluctuations. The results obtained in these studies provide a further rationale for limiting the intra-operative use of flow directed pulmonary artery catheters when TEE is available.

As with precordially performed Doppler echocardiography, TEE is an ideal method of detecting valvular insufficiency. The use of TEE guided Doppler intraoperatively has been a subject of interest by both anesthesiologist and cardiologist investigators. The first reported observation valvular regurgitation by Doppler TEE was reported by Schlüter and coworkers [39] who intraoperatively studied patients with mitral regurgitation (MR). In 12 surgical patients, angiographically documented to have MR, all also had the regurgitant flow identified by Doppler. Although in a number of patients, precordial pulsed Doppler failed to detect MR, it should be noted that Doppler instrumentation in the early 1980's was insensitive when compared to the current generation of color flow instruments; presently even 'physiologic' degrees of mitral regurgitation are detected. Schlüter's investigation made no effort to quantitate MR by Doppler.

At the University of California at San Fransisco (Moffitt/Long Hospitals), our anesthesiology researchers, directed by Dr. Michael Cahalan, have studied MR with intraoperative TEE Doppler and have found it possible to estimate the severity of the lesion with resonable accuracy [40]. Among those submitting to mitral valve surgery (replacement or valvuloplasty) our data suggest that angiographically significant levels of MR can be identified by pulsed Doppler mapping of the distance the systolic jet penetrates towards the superior wall of the left atrium and more readily by color flow mapping. Moreover, the postoperative precordial Doppler findings were correlated with TEE Doppler intraoperative estimation of MR severity. The availability of an accurate intraoperative method of assessing MR severity should be valuable in making intraoperative decisions about valve replacement, repair or nonintervention.

We have been able to accumulate the most experience with intraoperative Doppler evaluation of the mitral valve because the plane and direction of the echo beam is the same as the vector of transmitral inflow and regurgitation; these circumstances are conductive to obtaining a high quality Doppler flow signals. The planes of forward and retrograde flow across the other valves are not as favorable for Doppler study, a situation which limits their suitability for TEE Doppler evaluation. Color flow mapping Doppler techniques appear to lend themselves well to the evaluation and detection of regurgitant lesions of these other valves and have proved to be the method of choice for their study [41].

Ischemia and infarction in coronary artery disease studied by TEE

As a method of intraoperatively monitoring segmental contractile function, TEE is both sensitive and specific. Its potency in this application is probably the major reasons for its growing clinical importance. Owing to the seminal work of Tennant and Wiggers [42] the intimate linkage between local myocardial blood supply and contractile performance became an accepted fact. Later investigators [43] expanded upon these original observations by showing that segmental ischemic contractile hypokinesis was not an all or none phenomenon by establishing that small reductions in coronary blood flow can decrease segmental shortening. Subsequently, diastolic function was also been shown to be highly vulnerable to minor decreases in blood supply [44]. It has also been established that echocardiography is far more sensitive than ECG for identification of ischemia or infarction, particularly when the subendocardium is ischemic [45]. When studied in coronary care unit patients with acute myocardial infarction, precordial echocardiography also proves to be more sensitive than ECG in detecting, sizing and localizing proven acute myocardial infarction [46]. In view of echocardiography's sensitivity in detecting ischemia and since ECG is typically the exclusive intraoperative monitor for ischemia, anesthesiologists charged with the care high risk surgical patients have demonstrated intense interest in intraoperative TEE.

In discussing wall motion abnormalities and ischemia detection, it must be emphasized that not all wall motion abnormalities are the result of decreased segmental blood supply. Cardiopulmonary bypass is associated with several nonischemic factors capable of altering local or global contractility. For example, thoracotomy by itself has been identified as a cause of septal wall motion abnormalities [3]. The mechanism in this case is probably a change in cardiac motion resulting from a change in thoracic anatomy rather than local myocardial dysfunction. Another nonischemic wall motion abnormality arising during coronary bypass grafting, is a reversible decrease in septal systolic thickening [4]. In this instance, changes in the sequence of myocardial activation have been shown to change the timing, velocity and systolic excursion of the endocardium [47, 48].

In ranking nonischemic influences on segmental LV function, the most important appear to be contractility and loading conditions. However, in hearts with normal coronary flow, changes in contractility and loading to the degree likely to occur in a clinical setting are not expected to stimulate changes in segmental contraction. Data supporting this expectation was presented by Roizen et al. [49] who studied the impact of alterations in both loading and contractility induced by large elevations in plasma catecholamine levels arising during the tumor manipulations of pheochromocytoma excision. The relatively young age of the patients in this study placed them in a group at low risk for having heart disease. As expected, surgical manipulation produced marked elevations in end-diastolic and end systolic area and in calculated area ejection fraction. At the times of marked elevations in aortic pressure, heart rate, wall stress and oxygen demand, segmental wall motion abnormalities did not appear. Surgery they experienced marked swings in end-diastolic and end systolic areas and in ejection fraction. During periods of markedly elevated aortic pressure, heart rate and myocardial oxygen demand, regional wall motion abnormalities were not deteted.

Vascular surgical techniques require occlusion of the proximal arterial supply to insure a bloodless field and to minimize blood loss. Such occlusions are attended by a number of risks to the patient. Abdominal aortic aneurysm repair requires that the aorta be cross clamped above the repair site. The higher clamp is applied (i.e. the closer to the diaphragm) the greater the rise in peripheral vascular resistence it will provoke. This feature of abdominal aortic aneurysm surgery provides an opportunity to employ TEE to study the influence of abrupt rises in afterload on segmental and global LV performance. Roizen and associates took advantage of this opportunity to observe the hemodynamic and cardiac consequences of abrupt, cross clamp related changes in afterload [50]. Among a group of patients having TEE monitoring during surgery, 12 had cross clamp aortic occlusion above the level of the celiac axis. In these patients aortic pressure rose 58% and PCW 38% while end-diastolic and end-systolic area rose markedly and area ejection fraction fell sharply. With lower levels of aortic occlusion (supra and infra renal) only minimal changes in these variables occured. Coronary disease was highly prevalent in this study group and was manifest by a history of anginal symptoms in 90% as well as a large percentage with either myocardial infarction within two months prior to surgery or a depressed ejection fraction. In 11/12 patients with supraceliac cross clamping, new systolic wall motion abnormalities appeared just after application of the clamp. Conversely, there were no cross clamp related wall motion abnormalities in those with cross clamping below the renal arteries. Thus, increased afterload was clearly demonstrated to exert a powerful influence on LV performance if there is preexisting disease.

Segmental wall motion abnormalities do not always arise because of ischemia and not all motion abnormalities of previously infarcted segments arise because of acute ischemia. For example, dilated cardiomyopathy develops areas of myocardium that are more intensely scarred than others and Chagas' disease causes apical scarring. These fibrosed regions exhibit contraction abnormalities that are either manifest under all conditions or are latent, becoming accentuated or unmasked in the face of altered loading conditions or contractility. It is important to realize that in the late stages of ischemic cardiomyopathy, 'normal' (at least in the sense of not being infarcted) regions may experience acute changes in wall motion related to local fluctuations in wall stress or tethering forces. Without any drop in coronary perfusion (i.e. without the development of ischemia) a change in loading or contractility might provoke a wall motion change in areas that are partially scarred. Erroneous interpretation of such wall motion changes might lead to the diagnosis of ischemia or infarction. Finally, a ventricle appearing to be completely normal at rest may harbor a region of prior subendocardial infarction. In the absence of ischemia, such a previously damaged region might become unmasked by changing loading conditions that under normal circumstances would alter wall motion in a more uniform fashion. There is experimental data regarding the potential importance of these interactions and effects [51–54].

Early studies on the use of TEE to identify and detect intraoperative ischemia were not always optimally designed or reported. For example, when Roizen et al. [50] studied patients undergoing aortic cross clamping he detected numerous transient wall motion abnormalities at the time of cross clamping in a population of patinets in whom angina and/or previous myocardial infarction was highly prevalent. These results support the hypothesis that wall motion changes arising in this manner are due to increased oxygen demand in the face of greatly increased afterload. By failing to report on simultaneous ECG monitor changes or on the rate of post operatively detected infarction among these patients, the study leaves open the possibility that the large increases in wall stress caused by the superceliac occlusion of the aorta might have unmasked or increased areas of abnormal wall motion from previous subendocardial infarction.

Intraoperative improvements in the motion of previously abnormal myocardial segments have been found by studies using TEE monitoring. However, the reports documenting these changes may also suffer from the same design problems as those reporting the appearance of new abnormalities. For example, a report by Topol et al. [55] is worthy of consideration because it raises some concern about study protocol design issues in TEE intraoperative studies. In this project, 20 patients going to coronary artery bypass grafting were monitored for wall motion changes. A manual, off-line computerized method, developed by the authors, was used to quantitate segmental wall motion changes. Specifically, this computer measured both segmental thickening, as well as the usually measured endocardial inward motion, because experimental evidence has shown that thickening changes are far more indiciative of myocardial ischemia than endocardial motion. The most striking finding of this study was that there was immediate improvement in the systolic thickening of many myocardial segments following grafting of a stenosed coronary artery supplying that segment. While the authors suggest that the changes resulted from amelioration of chronic ischemia in the revascularized segments, questions regarding the role of profound alterations in loading conditions as another responsible (or at least partially responsible) factor in the observed changes are not satisfactorily answered. While the study did address this problem by matching pulmonary wedge pressures and arterial pressures before and after grafting, the actual degree of match was never specified. Furthermore, the authors did not use the preferred measures of preload and afterload, end-diastolic area and end systolic wall stress to express loading conditions, in a setting where ventricular volumes and filling pressures change dramatically. This study and its important findings highlight the critical nature of controlling the multiple variables in addition to ischemia that may influence TEE measures of regional wall motion.

The influence of the level of the short axis slice from which the LV is monitored during the period of observation is another major area of concern when one attempts to assess the mechanisms responsible for changes in regional wall motion. Most studies attempt to maintain stable probe position during the monitoring period so that a change in a segment is not the result of moving in or out of a neighboring abnormality. In spite of rigorous attempts to avoid this error, slight but significant shifting or tilting of the scan plane can result from manipulating of the probe's controls during attempts to maintain image quality. We employ painstaking attempts to maintain consistency in the morphology and position of LV landmarks such as the papillary muscle tips but are, at times, frustrated by large volume shifts which compress the anatomy and appear to bring neighboring segments into view. In an effort to more effectively deal with this problem we begin the examination by conducting multiple short axis interrogations so that all identifiable preexisting abnormalities can be located. As a further refinement, we have recently added a digitizing frame-grabber to our video recording system so that we can store one cycle reference beats on floppy disc (Microsonics Crop., Indianapolis, IN). During surgery we can constantly refer to these reference cycles without rolling the tape back. Our intial experience suggests that this device will greatly improve our efforts to control translocational artifacts.

The first documented myocardial infarction occuring during intraoperative TEE monitoring was reported by our group at the University of California, San Francisco [56]. The patient was a young woman with severe mitral stenosis and normal coronary arteries undergoing mitral valve replacement. Just after achieving hemodynamic stability post cardiopulmonary bypass, a large area of anterior akinesis was seen. When compared to her prebypass hemodynamic data, there had been no changes in arterial pressure, PCW or heart rate nor had any change occured in her single lead (V5) ECG monitor. Postoperatively, a large anterior wall myocardial infarction was documented by both ECG and enzyme pattern. The cause of the event was judged to be due to either coronary embolization or an accident of surgical technique.

The sensitivity and specificity of TEE in the detection of myocardial infarction and/or ischemia has been addressed in three studies. Kremer et al. [57] studied 43 high risk patients having either aortic reconstruction, coronary artery bypass grafting or valve replacement. The studies were read blindly at a time remote from the operation and, therefore, did not address the question of the accuracy of an 'on the spot' determination. The studies were classified according to three groups: those showing no new wall motion abnormalities, those with transient wall motion abnormalities which resolved by the end of surgery and those with persistent abnormalities. Postoperative MI was sought by serial postoperative ECG's and CKMB determination. Among the 8 patients with no intraoperative wall motion changes or with transient changes there were no infarctions detected. However, five of seven patients with persistent abnormalities had evidence of MI in the region implicated by TEE (Fig. 3a). Finding that TEE detects intraoperative infarction with high sensitivity and specificity is of considerable importance and has been borne out by subsequent studies.

An extention of this work was conducted at our institution by Smith [58] who prospectively studied 50 'high risk' patients (21 having coronary artery surgery and 29 having vascular procedures). Intraoperative monitoring was performed with seven lead ECG's (limb leads plus V5) and with TEE. Postoperatively, all had serial ECG's, CKMB determinations and 18 had scinti-

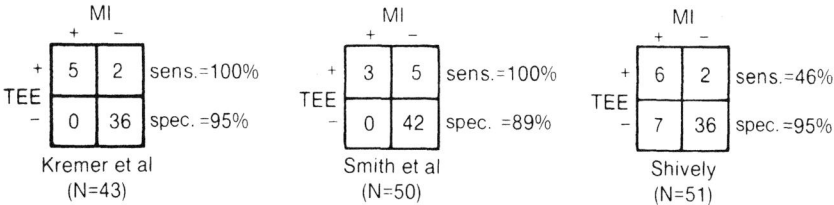

Fig. 3a–c. Summarized data on the detection of MI by TEE. 6a (left), 6b (center), 6c (right).

242

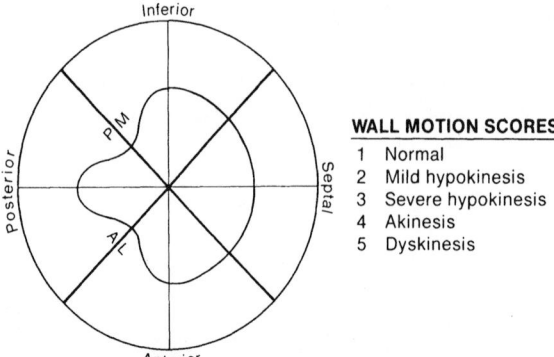

Fig. 4. Qualitative wall motion scoring system used by Smith et al. [58] and Shively et al. [59].

graphic infarct-avid imaging scans. Echocardiographers blinded to other clinical data read the TEE's, scoring them according to a scheme that divides the LV in quandrants and scores wall function (thickening) according to one of five categories (Fig. 4). Of the eight patients with persistent wall motion abnormalities at the conclusion surgery, three had evidence of MI (Fig. 3b). The sensitivity and specificity values for TEE were high (as in the Kremer study) but, owing to the low incidence of myocardial infarction in the group, the positive predictive value was a modest (though useful) 38%. Sixteen of the fifty patients in this group had evidence of transient wall motion abnormalities. Only three of these had accompanying ECG changes and none had evidence of a rise in pulmonary capillary wedge pressure. While it is entirely possible that these results demonstrate that ischemia can occur frequently without ECG evidence there is no way of knowing this with certainty. One observation supporting the identity of these transient abnormalities as ischemic events is the observation that they did not tend to occur in regions served by patent coronary arteries.

In third study from the University of California, San Fransisco, Shively et al. [59] retrospectively evaluated our experience with intraoperative myocardial infarction and persistent, TEE detected wall motion abnormalities. Between June 1982 and July 1985, 178 patients underwent TEE and coronary bypass grafting. Of these, 57 patients also had postoperative studies adequate for the diagnosis or exclusion of myocardial infarction. In this study, among our inclusionary requirements were serial ECG's, serial CKMB's, and a technetium infarct-avid imaging scan; the diagnosis of myocardial infarction was made if any two of these three were positive. Of the 57, six had myocardial infarctions that were proven to have occured more than 24 hours after surgery; these were not considered intraoperative myocardial infarctions. Of the remaining 51, 13 (26%) had intraoperative infarctions (12/13 with positive scans). The high incidence of MI in this retrospective study reflects selection bias towards patients with a stronger clinical likelihood of having had intraoperative infarction in that more postoperative tests were ordered in these individuals than in the other 121 undergoing TEE monitoring but not studied. TEE studies were read by three readers according to the method of Smith et al. described above. Of 13 patients with MI, only six were detected by new persistent wall motion changes. Of 38 without MI, only 2 had persistent wall motion changes (Fig. 3c). The high specificity for MI seen in the other studies was confirmed but the sensitivity was unexpectedly lower. A likely explanation for the discrepency is that all three studies are small samples and, as such, are prone to sampling error. Because of the small numbers of myocardial infarctions in all three studies, the 95% confidence limits around the values obtained for sensitivity are very wide. For example, in the Shively study, 46%–27% and in the other two, even wider. Thus, the sensitivity of TEE for intraoperative infarction detection remains undefined but the high specificity has been firmly established in all three studies.

There is a number of mitigating factors that might explain why Shively et al. found an apparent lowered sensitivity of TEE for intraoperative infarction. An important factor might be that some infarctions occur in the early, unmonitored postoperative period rather than being truely 'intraoperative'. Since the TEE probe is removed before the patient leaves the operating room and since this period is marked by wide swings in loading conditions and myocardial oxygen demand a high occurance rate of undetected infarction during this period is plausible. Another contributing factor may be the relatively limited area of myocardium monitored by TEE. While it has been reasoned that the mid papillary muscle area is a watershed region and thus likely to manifest ischemia in the distribution of either coronary artery it is also possible that the omission of the apex by this imaging techniquel imparts insensitivity to the technique. Support for this interpretation comes from the observation that scintigraphy showed most of these intraoperative infarctions to involve at least some of the apex. Another major factor in this insensitivity is that a high proportion of the false negative TEE studies occured in patients with severe diffuse hypokinesis. In these patients, incoordinate contraction patterns make identification of changes in wall motion very difficult. Finally, canine [38] and clinical [39] studies suggest that small infarctions involving up to 6% of the total LV mass may occur in the absence of echocardiographically detectible wall motion abnormality.

Future directions of TEE

Some of the technical considerations associated with TEE include the necessity for the passage of with a stiff, bulky (9 mm diameter) gastroscope discourages the frequent use of TEE in the ambulatory or conscious in-patient. Even if patient discomfort were not a factor, TEE provides only a limited number of imaging planes. On the other hand, standard transcutaneous echo-cardiography provides a plethora of planes and imaging windows. With the use of TEE there is also a risk os esophageal laceration; this risk is, of course, nonexistent with precordial echocardiography.

The ascendency and wide dissemination of standard echocardiography has been the product of heavy commercial investment (often unprofitable) and intense competition (often unsuccessful). Conversely, the comparatively languid development of TEE can be attributed to highly restrained entre-preneurial interest. Diasonics (Milpitas, Ca., as Varian Associates, Palo Alto) fabricated the first TEE probe. These instruments, while of excellent quality, have evolved very little from their original configuration and remain coupled to imaging systems which are, in terms of circa 1980 image quality and technology, obsolete. As a result of this situation, the only way to acquire TEE for clinical applications is to invest in nearly antiquated technology that has no prospects of being improved. This situation resulted in large reservoir of pent up interest that exploded when the Hewlet Packard Corp. offered a 5 MHz high resolution color flow probe. Five other manufacturers have fol-lowed them and there are at least 400 centers in the U.S. performing this exam-ination. The dissemination of this technology might be even further facili-tated, if echocardiographic instruments were designed specifically for the operating room. Many of the features of instruments designed for clinical use are of no value in the operating room and merely add to the expense. In a busy hospital surgical suite, there is need for three or more instruments operating simultaneously. For a state of the art instrument configured for routine clinical use and equipped with a TEE probe and color flow mapping capability, the cost is around $170,000. Equiping an operating suite with three of these instruments would easily cost in excess of $500,000. A solu-tion to this problem might include construction of 'strip-down' operating room instrument. This device would not require strip chart recorder or M-mode capability but should be equiped with a digital image acquisition, storage device and color flow Doppler. Since monitoring is conducted inter-mittently in each patient, it might be possible to attach two or more probes to a single central phased array unit much in the same way computer terminals are networked to a CPU. A second central unit could also be located in the postoperative intense care unit, enabling continuation of monitoring until hemodynamic stability is established.

In conclusion, the unique high resolution images and highly reliable nature of TEE data ensures that this technique will eventually be found in most operating rooms and intensive care installations.

Addendum

Since the preparation of this manuscript the use of TEE in the outpatient setting has grown. The major ambulatory applications of TEE include assessment of prosthetic valve function, mitral regurgitation, left atrial mass evaluation, detection of aortic ring abscess, assessment of aortic dissection and congenital heart disease evaluation.

References

1. Frazin L, Talano JV, Stephanides L, et al.: Esophageal echocardiography. Circulation 54: 102–108, 1976.
2. Matsumoto M, Oka Y, Lin YT, et al.: Transesophageal echocardiography for assessing ventricular performance. NY State J of Med, 1979, January, 19–21.
3. Matsumoto M, Oka Y, Strom J, et al.: Application of transesophageal echocardiography to continuous intraoperative monitoring of left ventricular performance. Am J Cardiol 46: 95–105, 1980.
4. Righetti A, Crawford MH, O'Rourke RA, et al.: Interventricular septal motion and left ventricular function after coronary bypass surgery. Am J Cardiol 39: 372–377, 1977.
5. Matsuzaki M, Matsuda Y, Ikee Y, et al.: Esophageal echocardiographic left ventricular anterolateral wall motion in normal subjects and patients with coronary artery disease. Circulation 63: 1085–1092, 1981.
6. Fukagawa K: Prediction of left anterior descending coronary artery disease by esophageal echocardiography. Jpn Heart J 173–183, 1981.
7. Kremer P, Hanrath P, Langenstein B, et al.: The evaluation of left ventricular function at rest and during exercise by transesophageal echocardiography in aortic insufficiency.
8. Matsumoto M, Hanrath P, Kremer P, et al.: The evaluation of left ventricular function by transesophageal M-mode exercise echocardiography. In Cardiovascular Diagnosis by Ultrasound; Hanrath P, Bleifeld W, Souquet J, eds. Martinus Nijhoff, pub, pp. 227–236, 1981.
9. Hisanaga K, Hisanaga A, Hibi N, et al.: High speed rotating scanner for transesophageal cross-sectional echocardiography. Am J Cardiol 46: 837–842, 1980.
10. Hisanaga K, Hisanaga A, Nagata K, et al.: Transesophageal cross-sectional echocardiography. Am Heart J 100: 605–609, 1980.
11. Hisanaga K, Hisanaga A: Transesophageal cross-sectional echocardiography with a mechanical scanning system. In Cardiovascular Diagnosis by Ultrasound; Hanrath, Bleifeld, Souquet, eds. Martinus Nijhoff, pub, pp. 239–245, 1982.
12. Reifart N, Strohm WD: Detection of atrial septum defects by transesophageal two-dimensional echocardiography with a mechanical sector scanner. In Cardiovascular Diagnosis by Ultrasound; Hanrath P, Bleifeld W, Souquet J, eds. Martinus Nijhoff, pub. pp. 247–250, 1982.
13. Souquet J, Hanrath P, Zitelli L, Kremer P, Langenstein BA, Schlüter M: Transesophageal phased array for imaging the heart. IEEE Trans Biomed Eng BME-29: 707–712, 1982.
14. Souquet J: Phased array transducer technology for transesophageal imaging of the heart: current status and future aspects. In Cardiovascular Diagnosis by Ultrasound; Hanrath, Bleifeld, Souquet, eds. Martinus Nijhoff pub., pp. 251–259, 1982.
15. Ezekowitz MD, Smith EO, Rankin R, et al.: Left atrial mass: diagnostic value of trans-

esophageal 2-dimensional echocardiography and Indium-111 platelet scintigraphy. Am J Cardiol 51: 1563–1564, 1983.

16. Thier W, Schlüter M, Krebber HJ, et al.: Cysts in left atrial myxomas identified by transesophageal cross-sectional echocardiography. Am J Cardiol 51: 1793–1795, 1983.

17. Schlüter M, Langenstein BA, Thier W, et al.: Transesophageal two-dimensional echocardiography in the diagnosis of cor triatriatum in the adult. J Am Coll Cardiol 2: 1011–1015, 1983.

18. Nellessen U, Daniel WG, Matheis G, et al.: Impending paradoxical embolism from atrial thrombus: correct diagnosis by transesophageal echocardiography and prevention by surgery. J Am Coll Cardiol 5: 1002–1004, 1985.

19. Roewer N, Beck H, Kochs E, et al.: Detection of venous embolism during intraoperative monitoring by two-dimensional transesophageal echocardiography. Anesthesiology 63: A169, 1985.

20. Borner N, Erbel R, Braun B, et al.: Diagnosis of aortic dissection by transesophageal echocardiography. Am J Cardiol 54: 1157–1158, 1984.

21. Engberding R, Bender F, Muller US, et al.: Aneurysms and dissections of the descending thoracic aorta - identification by transesophageal two-dimensional echocardiography. J Am Coll Cardiol 7: 138A, 1986.

22. Uenishi M, Sugimoto H, Sawada Y, et al.: Transesophageal echocardiography. during external chest compression in humans. Anesthesiology 60: 618, 1984.

23. Furuya H, Suzuki T, Okumura O, et al.: Detection of air embolism by transesophageal echocardiography. Anesthesiology 58: 125–124, 1983.

24. Furuya H, Okumura F: Detection of paradoxical air embolism by transesophageal echocardiography. Anesthesiology 60: 374–377, 1984.

25. Cucchiara RF, Seward JB, Nishimura RA, et al.: Identification of patent foramen ovale during sitting position craniotomy by transesophageal echocardiography with positive airway pressure. Anesthesiology 63: 107–109, 1985.

26. Cucchiara RF, Nugent M, Seward JB, et al.: Air embolism in upright neurosurgical patients: detection and localization by two-dimensional transesophageal echocardiography. Anesthesiology 60: 353–355, 1985.

27. Oka Y, Moriwaki KM, Hong Y, et al.: Detection of air emboli in the left heart by M-mode transesophageal echocardiography following cardiopulmonary bypass. Anesthesiology 63: 109–113, 1985.

28. Topol EJ, Humphrey LS, Borkon AM, et al.: Value of intraoperative left ventricular microbubbles detected by transesophageal two-dimensional echocardiography in predicting neurologic outcome after cardiac operations. Am J Cardiol 56: 773–775, 1985.

29. Smith JS, Cahalan MK, Benefiel DJ, et al.: Fentanyl versus fentanyl and isoflurane in patients with impaired left ventricular function. 1986, in press.

30. Oka Y, Moriwaki K, Hong Y, et al.: Left ventricular stroke volume and systolic time interval determined by transesophageal aortic valve echogram. Anesthesiology 59: A162, 1983.

31. Beaupre PN, Cahalan MK, Kremer PF, et al.: Does pulmonary artery occlusion pressure adequately reflect left ventricular filling during anesthesia and surgery? Anesthesiology 59: A3, 1983.

32. Topol EJ, Humphrey LS, Blanck TJJ, et al.: Characterization of post-cardiopulmonary bypass hypotension with intraoperative transesophageal echocardiography. Anesthesiology 59: A2, 1983.

33. Terai C, Uenishi M, Sugimoto H, et al.: Transesophageal echocardiographic dimensional

analysis of four cardiac chambers during positive end-expiratory pressure. Anesthesiology 63: 640-646, 1985.

34. Hershon JJ, Farrar DJ, Compton PG, et al.: Right ventricular dimensions with transesophageal echocardiography during an operating room model of left heart assist. Trans Am Soc Artif Intern Organs 30: 129–132, 1984.

35. Freund PR, Padavich CA: A comparison of cardiac output techniques: transesophageal Doppler versus thermodilution cardiac output during general anesthesia in man. Anesthesiology 63: A191, 1985.

36. Kumar A, Minagoe S, Thangathurai D, et al.: Non-invasive measurement of cardiac output during general anesthesia by continuous wave Doppler esophageal probe: comparison with simultaneous thermodilution cardiac output. Anesthesiology 63: A68, 1985.

37. Colley PS, Barnes SR: Feasibility of transesophageal measurement of cardiac output during surgery using Doppler ultrasound. Anesthesiology 63: A170, 1985.

38. Kumar A, Minagoe S, Thangathurai D, et al.: The continuous wave Doppler esophageal probe: a new method for measurement of cardiac output during surgery. J Am Coll Cardiol 7: 2A, 1986.

39. Schlüter M, Langenstein BA, Hanrath P, et al.: Assessment of transesophageal pulsed Doppler echocardiography in the detection of mitral regurgitation. Circulation 66: 784–789, 1982.

40. Shively B, Cahalan M, Benefiel D, et al.: Intraoperative assessment of mitral valve regurgitation by transesophageal Doppler echocardiography. J Am Coll Cardiol 7: 228A, 1986.

41. Goldman ME, Thys D, Ritter S, et al.: Transesophageal real time Doppler flow imaging: a new method for intraoperative cardiac evaluation. J Am Coll Cardiol 7: 1A, 1986.

42. Tennant R, Wiggers CJ: The effect of coronary occlusion on myocardial contraction. Am J Physiol 112: 351–361, 1935.

43. Vatner SF: Correlation between acute reductions in myocardial blood flow and function in conscious dogs. Circ Res 47: 201–297, 1981.

44. Hess OM, Osakada G, Lavelle JF, et al.: Diastolic myocardial wall stiffness and ventricular relaxation during partial and complete coronary occlusions in the conscious dog. Circ Res 52: 387–400, 1983.

45. Battler A, Froelicher VF, Gallagher KP, et al.: Dissociation between regional myocardial dysfunction and ECG changes during ischemia in the conscious dog. Circulation 62: 735–744, 1980.

46. Gibson RS, Bishop HL, Stamm RB, et al.: Value of early two dimensional echocardiography in patients with acute myocardial infarction. Am J Cardiol 49: 1110–1119, 1982.

47. Abbasi AS, Eber LM, MacAlpin RN, et al.: Paradoxical motion of interventricular septum in left bundle branch block. Circulation 49: 423–427, 1983.

48. Feigenbaum H: Echocardiography 4th ed. Philadelphia, Lea & Febiger, p. 231, 1986.

49. Roizen MF, Hunt TK, Beaupre PN, et al.: The effect of alpha-adrenergic blockade on cardiac performance and tissue oxygen delivery during excision of pheochromocytoma. Surgery 94: 941–945, 1983.

50. Roizen MF, Beaupre PN, Alpert RA, et al.: Monitoring with two-dimensional transesophageal echocardiography. Comparison of myocardial function in patients undergoing supraceliac, suprarenal-infraceliac, or infrarenal aortic occlusion. J Vasc Surg 1: 300–305, 1984.

51. Kerber RE, Abboud FM: Effect of alterations of arterial blood pressure and heart rate on segmental dyskinesis during acute myocardial ischemia and following coronary reperfusion. Circ Res 36: 145–155, 1975.

52. Kerber RE, Abboud FM, Marcus ML, et al.: Effect of inotropic agents on the localized dyskinesis of acutely ischemic myocardium. Circulation 49: 1038–1046, 1974.
53. Kerber RE, Marcus ML, Ehrhardt J, et al.: Effect of intra-aortic balloon counterpulsation on the motion and perfusion of acutely ischemic myocardium. Circulation 53: 853–859, 1976.
54. Lima JAC, Becker LC, Melin JA, et al.: Impaired thickening of nonischemic myocardium during acute regional ischemia in the dog. Circulation 71: 1048–1059, 1985.
55. Topol EJ, Weiss JL, Guzman PA, et al.: Immediate improvement of dysfunctional myocardial segments after coronary revascularization: Detection by intraoperative transesophageal echocardiography. J Am Coll Cardiol 5: 1123–1134, 1984.
56. Beaupre PN, Kremer PF, Cahalan MK, et al.: Intraoperative detection of changes in left ventricular segmental wall motion by transesophageal two-dimensional echocardiography. Am Heart J 107: 1021–1023, 1984.
57. Kremer P, Cahalan MK, Beaupre P, et al.: Intraoperative myocardial ischemia detected by transesophageal two-dimensional echocardiography. Circulation 68 (Supp. III): 332, 1983.
58. Smith JS, Cahalan MK, Benefiel DJ, et al.: Intraoperative detection of myocardial ischemia in high-risk patients: electrocardiography versus two-dimensional transesophageal echocardiography. Circulation 72: 1015–1021, 1985.
59. Shively B, Watters T, Benefiel D, et al.: The intraoperative detection of myocardial infarction by transesophageal echocardiography. J Am Coll Cardiol 7: 2A, 1986.

4.3. Transesophageal echocardiographic imaging of the thoracic aorta in aortic dissection

R. ERBEL, S. MOHR-KAHALY, M. DREXLER, N. WITTLICH,
N. BÖRNER & J. MEYER

Introduction

Only the combination of rapid medical and surgical therapy can improve prognosis of aortic dissection [1]. Therefore it is necessary that the diagnosis is established with high accuracy. In type A dissection (dissection of the ascending aorta) operative therapy and in type B dissection (dissection of the descending aorta) medical therapy is recommended [1, 2].

Clinic

In patients with aortic dissection, acute chest pain is a leading symptom. Quite often a pulse difference between the left and right arm can be detected. In about 10% of the patients neurological symptoms are most prominent. Aortic insufficiency is present in 70% of the patients with type A and 10% of patients with type B. Pericardial effusion can be found in 10%, hypotension in 20%, pleural effusion in 10% of cases [1].

Chest X-ray examination

In up to 18% of the patients a negative chest X-ray examination is found [2]. Specific signs of aortic dissection are a disparity in size between the ascending and descending aorta, a double aortic shadow, different radiolusancy, irregular contour, loss of sharpness, displaced intimal calcification as well as cardiac dilatation and signs of pericardial effusion.

Computed tomography

After the first report of the detection of aortic dissection by computed tomography, published by Harris et al. [3], other authors could confirm their results [4–7]. The most important sign is the detection of an intimal flap.

I. Cikes (ed.), *Echocardiography in Cardiac Interventions*, 249–260, 1989.

Contrast agent injections are necessary to differentiate between true and false lumen, because of differential density between the two lumina and compression deformity of the true lumen by the false lumen, and delayed flow in the false lumen by dynamic scanning [6–11]. A differentiation is possible in 50%, and in 50% a displaced intimal calcification can be detected [6, 9]. In most cases an aortic dilatation is present. By computed tomography pericardial effusion as well as pleural effusion can be detected. Aortic insufficiency cannot be identified. Only rarely can the rupture location be imaged.

Echocardiography

Already in 1973 Nanda et al. described the diagnosis of aortic dissection by M-mode echocardiography [12]. In 6 patients a dilatation of the aortic root and a double contour of the posterior wall of the aorta was visualized. Very soon false positive cases were published according to an ectasia of the sinus of Valsalva [13, 14]. Suprasternal imaging became particularly important to evaluate the aortic arch [15]. Two-dimensional echocardiography has improved the sensitivity and specificity of the method. In order to image the whole thoracic aorta not only parasternal and apical, but also right parasternal and subcostal views are necessary [17–23]. Specific signs of aortic dis-

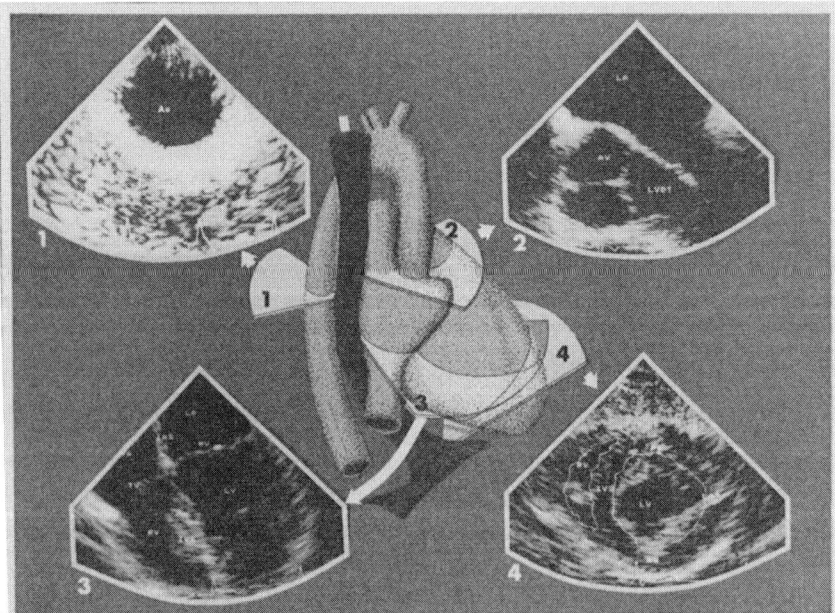

Fig. 1. Schematic drawing with the standard scannings of the arch and the descending aorta by transesophageal and transgastric echocardiography.

section are aortic dilatation and imaging of an intimal flap [21–23]. The limitation of transthoracic echocardiography is related to reduced image quality in patients with pulmonary emphysema, obesity and thorax deformation as well as mechanical ventilation. Only in 17% of the patients can the whole thoracic aorta be visualized [17,19].

The limitations of transthoracic echocardiography were overcome by transesophageal echocardiography [24, 25] (Fig. 1). After local anesthesia a flexible echoscope is introduced in the left lateral supine position. To avoid severe adverse gastric reactions, sedation with 10 mg diazepam or even better analgesia with 0.5 mg Bumorphin is necessary. Of course in all patients with suspected aortic dissection and hypertension, antihypertensive therapy has to be started immediately. The best control can be achieved by intravenous application of natrium nitroprusside or nifedipine.

Echotomographically the whole thoracic aorta, particularly in the descending part, can be visualized (Fig. 2) similar to computed tomographic images (Fig. 3). But also the aortic root can be imaged. Limitations are related to interposition of the trachea in visualization of the aortic arch.

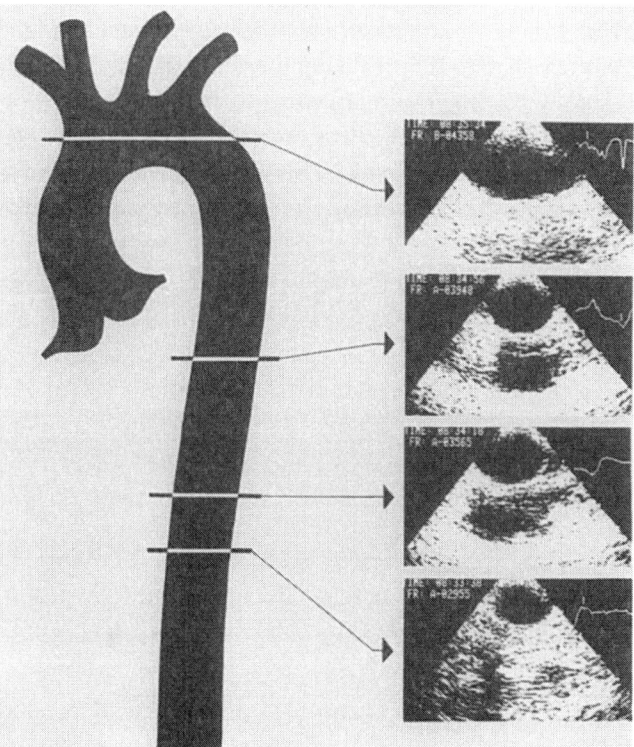

Fig. 2. Echotomographic imaging of the thoracic aorta by transesophageal echocardiography in multiple planes.

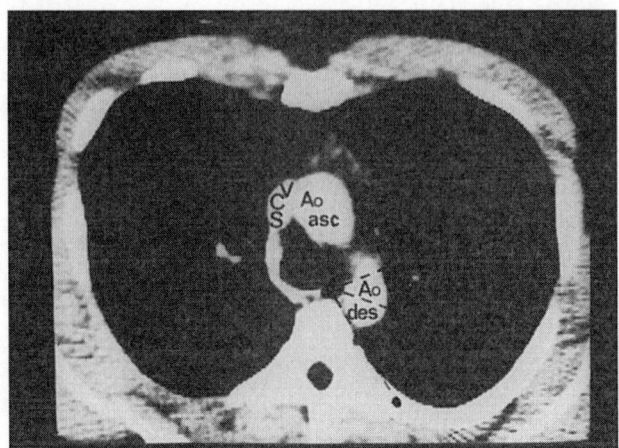

Fig. 3. Computed tomographic image of the thorax with the scanning of the descending aorta from the oesophagus. Illustrated is also the trachea, the aorta ascendens and the vena cava superior [25].

The intimal flap is separating the true and false lumen (Fig. 4). In most cases the true lumen is compressed by the false lumen. The differentiation can be done by M-mode [1] with demonstration of a systolic enlargement of the true lumen, [2] by the detection of spontaneous echocardiographic contrast in the false lumen (Fig. 4) with thrombus formation related to the reduced blood flow [26], [3] by pulsed Doppler echocardiography with demonstration of a systolic forward flow in the true lumen and a delayed flow or no flow in the false lumen (Fig. 5).

The type of aortic dissection should be described: Type A including the ascending aorta (Fig. 6) and type B including the descending aorta (Fig. 7).

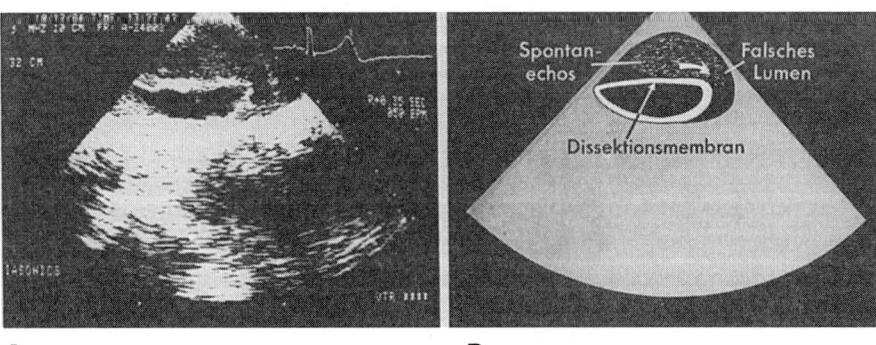

A **B**

Fig. 4. Type III aortic dissection demonstrating the intimal flap only in the descending part of the thoracic aorta with spontaneous echocardiographic contrast in the false lumen [26].

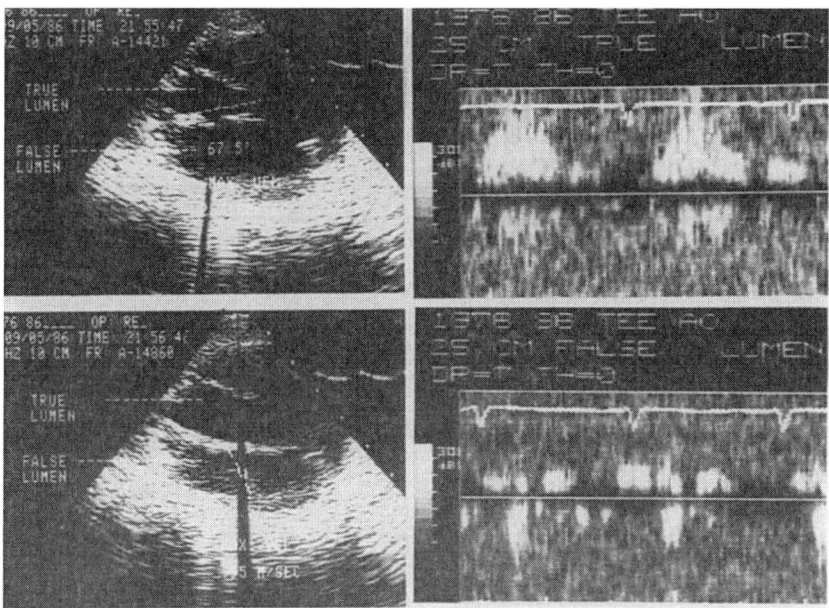

Fig. 5. Pulse Dopplerechocardiography of the true lumen (upper part) and the false lumen (lower part) demonstrating normal systolic blood flow in the true lumen and delayed and only reduced flow velocities in the false lumen.

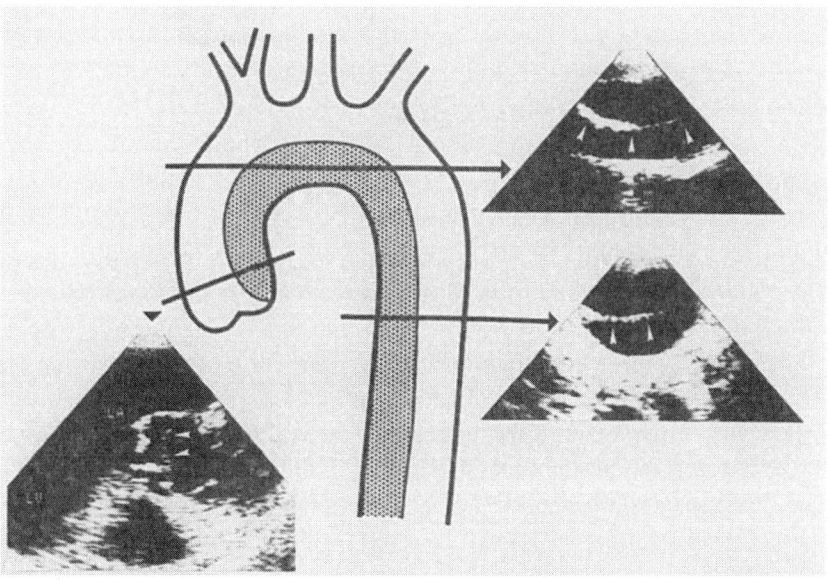

Fig. 6. Type I aortic dissection with 3 scan planes in the aortic root, aortic arch and aorta descendens demonstrating the intimal flap [25].

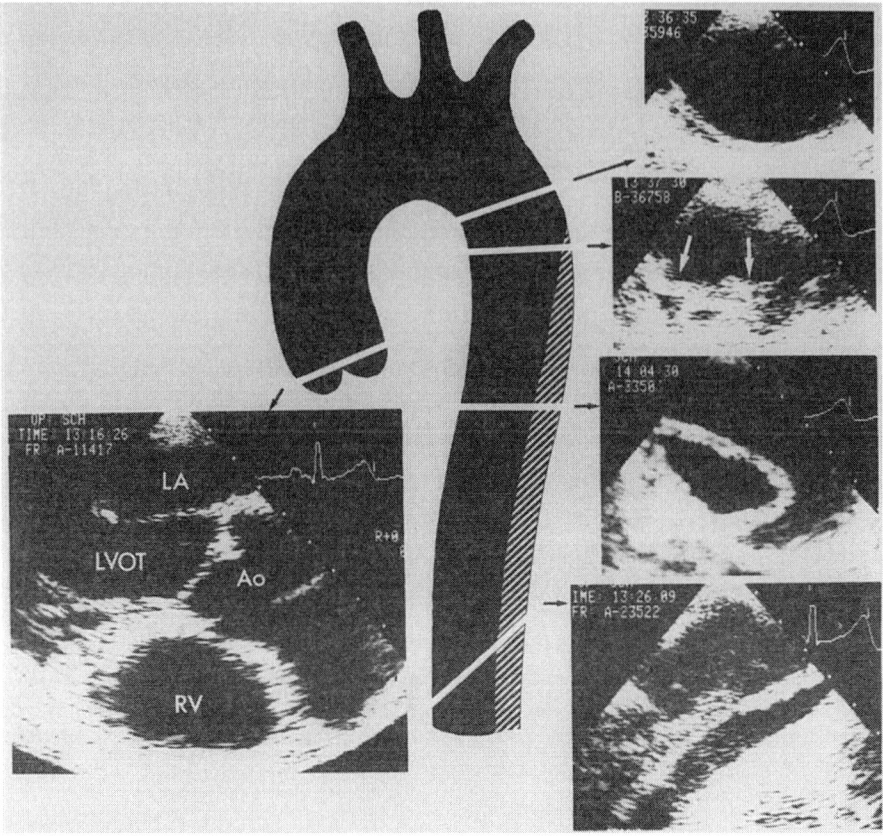

Fig. 7. Compression of the true lumen by the false lumen filled with dense spontaneous echo-cardiographic contrast [25].

The detection of the entry tear has to be found (Fig. 8).

Aortic dissection has to be differentiated to ectasia of the aorta with or without mural thrombus formation (Figs. 9/10). As for computed tomography, central displacement of intimal calcification is helpful to differentiate between the two clinical entities.

It is necessary to differentiate artefacts in the aorta ascending from true aortic dissection (Fig. 11), in order to avoid a false positive diagnosis. In 5 patients where an aortic replacement has been done, it could be demonstrated that artefacts as demonstrated in Fig. 11 are not related to true intimal flaps. They are possibly related to slice thickness artefacts on reverberation.

Another differential diagnosis is aortic rupture leading to mediastinal hematoma with compression of the left atrium, as shown in Fig. 12.

The diagnostic possibilities of echocardiography were improved by color-coded Doppler [27]. Transthoracically, the true and false lumen can be dif-

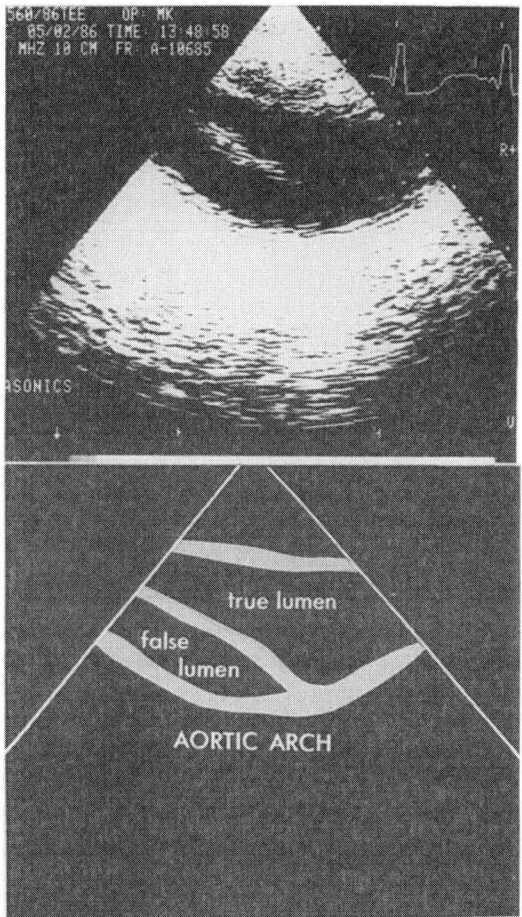

Fig. 8. Start of aortic dissection in the aortic arch in type III dissection imaged by transesophageal echocardiography.

ferentiated by blood flow imaging. Furthermore, using transesophageal echocardiography now, not only functional and morphological information but also blood flow information can be provided for cardiac surgery [28, 29].

Sensitivity and specificity

In 164 consecutive patients with suspected aortic dissection, sensitivity and specificity of transesophageal echocardiography, angiography and computed tomography were compared. The results are given in Table 1 [29]. It is important to underline, that in no patient computed tomography or angio-

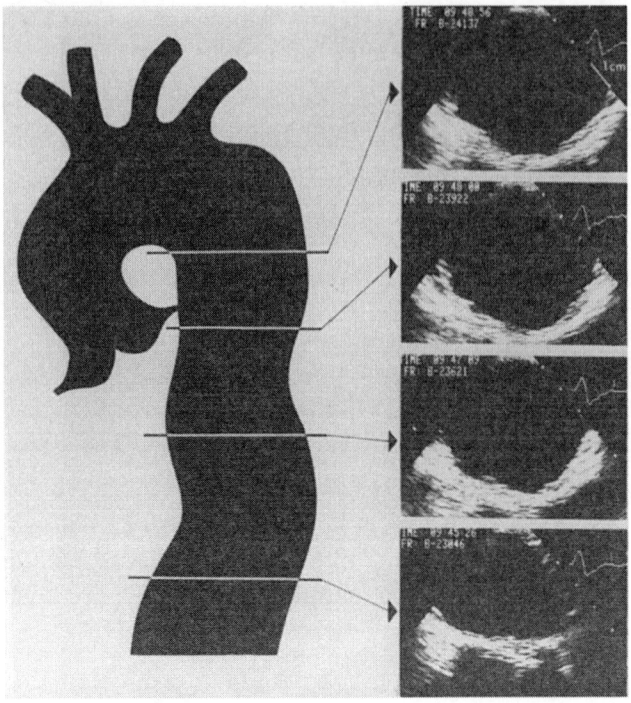

Fig. 9. Ectasia of the aorta without aortic dissection demonstrated by transesophageal echocardiography. Even plaque formations at the aortic wall are visualized.

Table 1. Sensitivity and specificity of transesophageal echocardiography (TEE), computed tomography (CT) and aniography (n = 164) [30].

	TEE	CT	Angio
Sensitivity (%)	99	83	88
Specificity	98	100	94
(+) pred. accuracy	98	100	96
(−) pred. accuracy	99	86	84

No case with negative TEE but positive CT or Angio.

graphy could detect aortic dissection where echocardiography was negative. One false negative result is related to a localized dissection in the aortic root which was found by cardiac surgery in a patient with aortic ectasia and severe aortic insufficiency. Clinically, the dissection had no relevance.

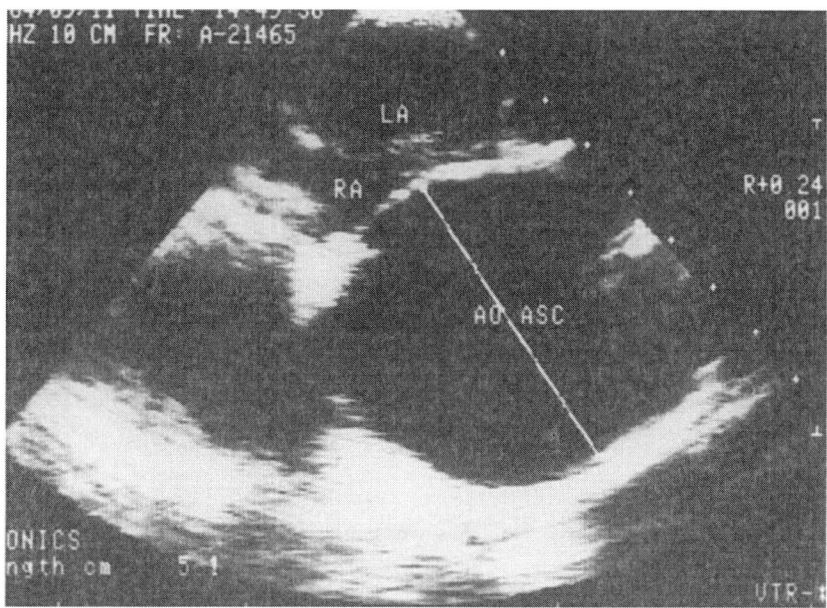

Fig. 10. Ectasia of the aorta ascendens analyzed by transesophageal echocardiography. Aortic dissection was excluded. The diameter of the ascending aorta was 5.1 cm.

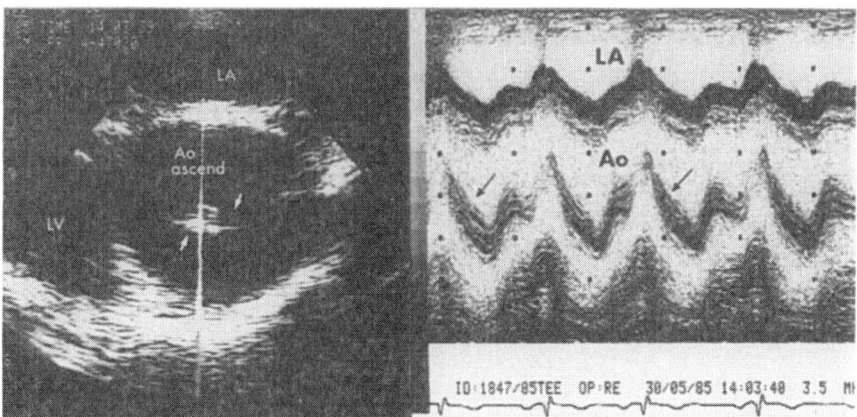

Fig. 11. Transesophageal echocardiographic imaging of the aorta ascendens demonstrating in the lumen of the aorta an artefact suggesting an intimal flap. It is only a reverberation of the aortic wall and demonstrates an artefact and has not to be mixed with a true aortic dissection.

258

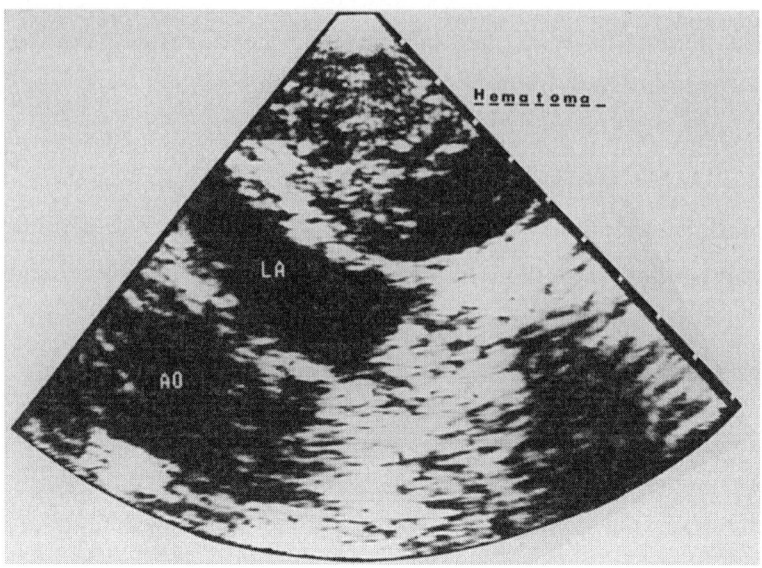

Fig. 12. Transesophageal echocardiographic image in a patient with suspected aortic dissection. In this patient aortic rupture with mediastinal hematoma developed a compressing of the left atrium.

Summary

Ultrasound examination of the aorta from different positions allows a clear differentiation between aortic dissection type A (aorta ascendens and aortic arch) and type B (aorta descendens). Immediately after taking into account the diagnosis of aortic dissection medical therapy with lower blood pressure has to be started independently on further diagnostic procedures. In type A dissection, cardiac surgery with replacement of the ascending aorta and possibly aortic valve replacement has to be performed. In type B dissection, medical therapy is recommended. Surgery is only performed in cases with complications and persistent chest discomfort.

The accuracy of echocardiography supplemented by transesophageal echocardiography has reached such a level that now surgery can be performed based only on this method [30, 31]. In all cases where the diagnosis is not established and in patients where coronary artery disease is suspected, angiography and coronary angiography should be performed.

References

1. Doroghazi RM, Slater EE: Aortic dissection. McGraw-Hill, New York 1983.
2. Earnest F, Muhm JR, Sheedy PF: Roentgenographic findings in thoracic aortic dissection. Mayo Clin Proc 54: 43–50, 1979.
3. Harris RD, Usselman JA, Vint VC, Warmath MA: Computerized tomographic diagnosis of aneurysms of the thoracic aorta. J Comp Ass Tomogr 3: 81–91, 1979.
4. Sanders JH, Malave S, Niemann HL, Moran JM, Roberts AJ, Michaelis LL: Thoracic aortic imaging without angiography. Arch Surg 114: 1326–9, 1979.
5. Suchato C, Pekanan P, Singjaroen T, Sereerat P: Indication of dissecting aortic aneurysm on noncontrast computed tomography. J Comp As Tomogr 4: 115–6, 1980.
6. Heiberg E, Wolverson M, Sundaram M, Conners J, Susman N: CT findings in thoracic aortic dissection. Am J Roentgenol 136: 13–7, 1981.
7. Lardé D, Bellor C, Vasile N, Frija J, Ferrané J: Computed tomography in dissection of the thoracic aorta. Radiology 136: 147–51, 1980.
8. Godwin JD, Herfkens RL, Skiöldebrand CG, Ferderle MP, Lipton MJ: Evaluation of dissections and aneurysms of the thoracic aorta by conventional and dynamic CT scanning. Radiology 136: 125–33, 1980.
9. Gross SC, Barr I, Eyler WR, Khaja F, Goldstein S: Computed tomography in dissection of the thoracic aorta. Radiology 136: 135–41, 1980.
10. Moncada R, Churchill R, Reynes C, Gunnar RM, Salines M, Love L, Demos TC, Pifarre R: Diagnosis of dissecting aortic aneurysm by computed tomography. Lancet 1: 238–41, 1981.
11. Egan TJ, Niemann H, Hermann RJ, Malve SR, Sanders JH: Computed tomography in the diagnosis of aortic aneurysm, dissection or traumatic injury. Radiology 136: 141–6, 1980.
12. Nanda NC, Gramiak R, Sha Ph: Diagnosis of aortic root dissection by echocardiography. Circulation 48: 506–13, 1973.
13. Krueger SK, Starke H, Forker AD, Eliot RS: Echocardiographic mimics of aortic root dissection. Chest 67: 441–4, 1975.
14. Hirschfeld DS, Rodriguez HJ, Schiller NB: Duplication of aortic wall seen by echocardiography. Br Heart J 38: 949–50, 1976.
15. Kasper W, Meinertz T, Kersting F, Lang K, Just H: Diagnosis of dissecting aortic aneurysm with suprasternal echocardiography. Am J Cardiol 42: 291–4, 1978.
16. Schweizer P, Erbel R, Lambertz H, Effert S: Two-dimensional suprasternal echocardiography in dissection of the thoracic aorta. In: Echocardiology, H. Rijsterburgh, eds., M. Nijhoff, The Hague, 55–60, 1981.
17. Iliceto S, Ettorre G, Francioso G, Antonelli G, Biaco G, Rizzon P: Diagnosis of aneurysm of the thoracic aorta. Comparison between two noninvasive techniques: two-dimensional echocardiography and computed tomography. Eur Heart J, 5: 545–55, 1984.
18. Mintz GS, Kotler MN, Segal BL, Parry WR: Two-dimensional echocardiographic recognition of the descending thoracic aorta. Am J Cardiol 44: 232–8, 1979.
19. Bubenheimer P, Schmuzier M, Roskamm: Ein- und zweidimensionale Echokardiographie bei Aneurysmen und Dissektionen der Aorta. Herz 5: 226–40, 1980.
20. Victor MF, Mintz GS, Kotler MN, Wilson AR, Segal BL. Two-dimensional echocardiographic diagnosis of aortic dissection. Am J Cardiol 48: 1155–9, 1981.
21. Roudat R, Billes MA, Gateau P, Besse P, Dallocchio M: Two-dimensional echocardiography in the diagnosis of aortic dissection in 41 patients (Abstr.). Circulation 64. Suppl. IV: 314, 1981.
22. Nakamura K, Suzuki S, Satomi G, Adachi F, Hirosawa K, Takao A, Hashimoto A, Toluyasu Y, Kusakabe K, Yamazaki T, Shigeta A: Two-dimensional echocardiographic

and angiographic features of aneurysm of the ascending aorta in patients with annulo-aortic ectasia. J Cardiogr 11: 239–52, 1981.

23. Bubenheimer P: Fortschritte in der Diagnose der Aortendissektion durch TM- und 2D-Echographie. Cardiology 68: (Suppl. 1): 66–74, 1981.

24. Börner N, Erbel R, Braun B, Henkel B, Meyer J, Rumpelt J: Diagnosis of aortic dissection by transesophageal echocardiography. Am J Cardiol 54: 1157–8, 1984.

25. Erbel R, Börner N, Steller D, Brunier J, Thelen M, Pfeiffer C, Mohr-Kahaly S, Meyer J: Detection of aortic dissection by transesophageal echocardiography. Br Heart J 58: 45–51, 1987.

26. Stern H, Erbel R, Börner N, Schreiner G, Meyer J: Spontaner Echokontrast, registriert mittels transösophagealer Echokardiographie bei Aortendissektion Typ III. Z. Kardiol 74: 480–81, 1985.

27. Mohr-Kahaly S, Erbel R, Börner N, Drexler M, Wittlich N, Iversen S, Oelert H, Meyer J: Kombination von Farb-Doppler und transösophagealer Echokardiographie in der Notfalldiagnostik bei Aortendissektionen vom Typ I. Z. Kardiol 75: 616–20, 1986.

28. Takamoto S, Kyo S, Matsumura M, Hojo H, Yokote Y, Omoto R: Total visualization of thoracic dissecting aortic aneurysm by transesophageal Doppler Color Flew mapping. Circulation 74: Suppl. II–132, 1986.

29. Mohr-Kahaly S, Erbel R, Rennollet H, Wittlich N, Drexler M, Oelert H, Meyer J: Ambulatory follow-up of aortic dissection by transesophageal two-dimensional and color-coded Doppler echocardiography. Circulation (in press).

30. Erbel R, Ergberding R, Daniel W, Roelandt J, Visser L, Rennollet H: Echocardiography in diagnosis of aortic dissection. Lancet 1: 457–461, 1989.

31. Lass J, Schlüter G, Haverist A, Daniel W, Hendricks Ph, Borst HG: Präoperative Diagnostik bei akuter Aortendissektion Typ A. Thorac. Cardiovasc. Surg. 35: Suppl. I–22, 1987.

4.4. Detection of cardiac and extracardiac masses by transesophageal echocardiography

WERNER G. DANIEL, ULRICH NELLESSEN, ANDREAS MÜGGE,
EBERHARD SCHRÖDER & PAUL R. LICHTLEN

The diagnosis of cardiac tumors and thrombi was almost completely restricted to necropsy until echocardiography became available. Actually, the non-invasive identification of left atrial myxomas during lifetime was one of the earliest diagnostic applications of M-mode echocardiography at all [1]. Due to the rapid development in cardiac ultrasound techniques during the last 15 years, today, this method can be considered as the diagnostic approach of choice for the assessment of abnormal masses localized in and around the heart [2–7]. This is in particular true for the two-dimensional technique which allows a clear imaging of most cardiac regions. A further improvement of the imaging quality and the insight in anatomical structures which are usually not demonstrable by the transthoracic approach (as the left atrial appendage and the vena cava superior) could recently be obtained by the introduction of transesophageal echocardiography.

Intracardiac masses

Except a recent study from our laboratory [8] to our knowledge there is no systematic comparison between transthoracic and transesophageal echocardiography concerning the detection rate of intracardiac tumors and thrombi. In this paper it could be shown that in all six patients with a left or right atrial myxoma, tumors could be detected equally accurate with both techniques. Of nine patients with a thrombus in the left or right heart, a correct diagnosis was established by the transesophageal as well as by the transthoracic approach in eight cases; in one patient, an isolated thrombus within the left atrial appendage could be visualized by transesophageal imaging alone.

Although conventional transthoracic echocardiography seems to be of comparable accuracy in the detection of intracardiac tumors and thrombi, the transesophageal image provides additional information regarding the acoustic properties of a mass, its mobility and wall adherence [8–10] (Fig. 1–6). Thus, by the transesophageal technique, Thier et al. [11] could clearly show zones of echolucency within atrial myxomas representing cysts which were missed on the transthoracic view (Fig. 5). Furthermore, masses within

I. Cikes (ed.), *Echocardiography in Cardiac Interventions*, 261–271, 1989.
© 1989 *Kluwer Academic Publishers.*

262

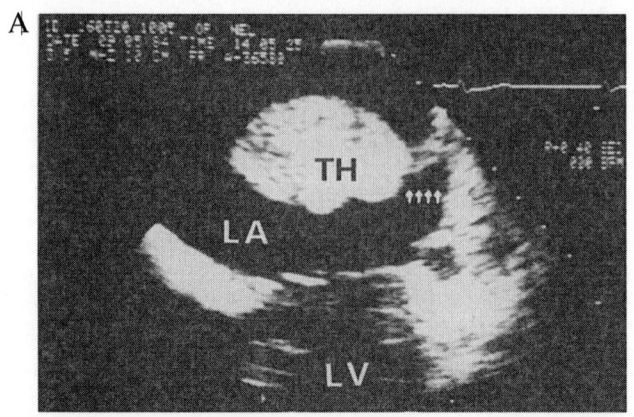

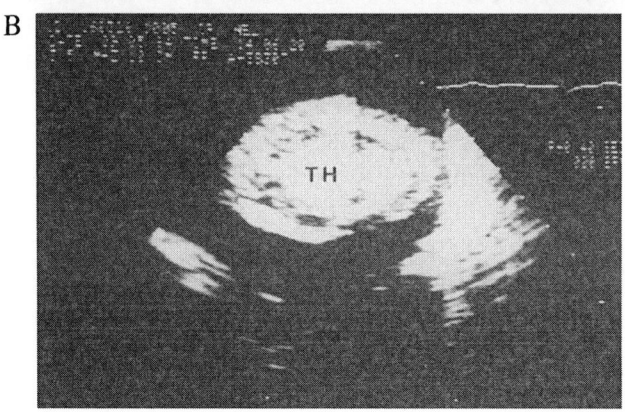

Fig. 1. Transesophageal echocardiogram of a patient with mitral stenosis and a large thrombus (TH) within the left atrium (LA) fixed to the lateral atrial wall by a small pedicle (arrows) (A); a slightly different view (B) shows various circular layers of different densities within the thrombus. LV = left ventricle.

the vena cava superior (Fig. 7, 8) and the left atrial appendage are usually not or only difficult detectable from ultrasound windows of the anterior chest wall.

Left atrial appendage thrombi

Only recently, Herzog et al. [12] reported the first three cases in which they successfully could image a thrombus within the left atrial appendage by transthoracic echocardiography. These authors used a modified short axis parasternal cross-sectional view at the aortic valve level and a sufficient visualization of the atrial appendage was possible only during maximal dis-

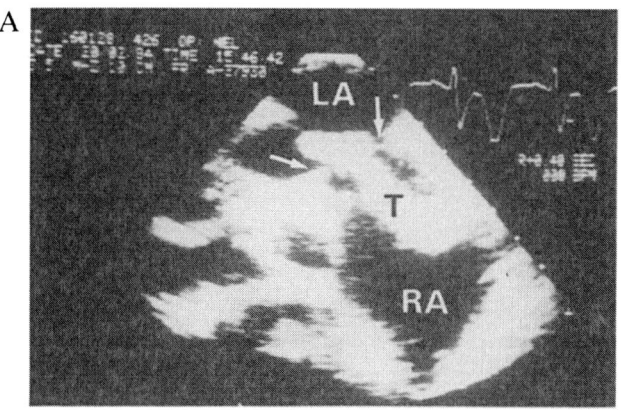

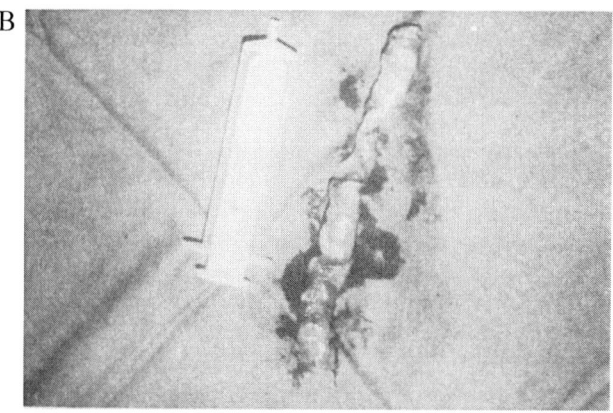

Fig. 2. Transesophageal echocardiogram (A) of a patient with a thrombus (T) in the left (LA) and right (RA) atria overriding the interatrial septum (arrows) and surgical specimen of the thrombus (B).

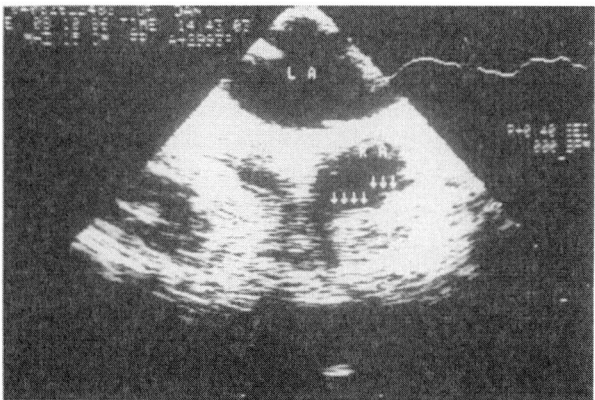

Fig. 3. Transesophageal echocardiogram of a thrombus (arrows) in the right atrium (RA) following mitral valve replacement. LA = left atrium.

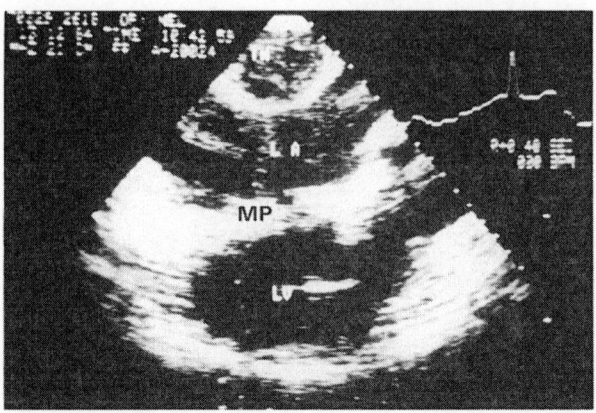

Fig. 4. Transesophageal echocardiogram of a patient with a thrombus (TH) in the left atrium (LA) following mitral valve replacement. The interior of the thrombus shows a very low echodensity; at surgery, the thrombus was found to be filled with semiliquid clots of blood. MP = mitral prosthesis; LV = left ventricle.

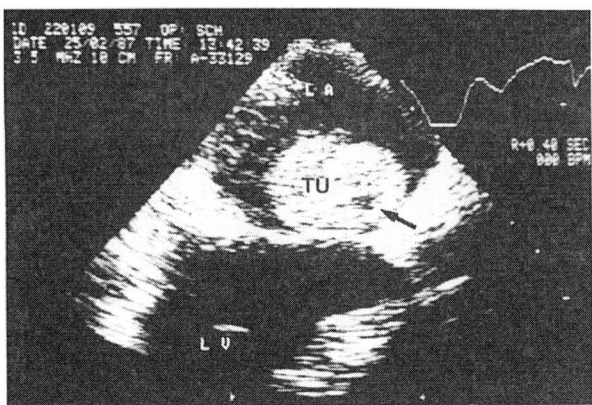

Fig. 5. Transesophageal echocardiogram of a patient with a left atrial myxoma (TU) showing an area of echolucency (arrow) representing a large cyst subsequently proven by surgery. LV = left ventricle.

tension of the left atrium in late ventricular systole. Usually, however, the atrial appendage is considered as 'blind' [13] and 'inaccessible to current techniques of echocardiographic study' [14].

In contrast, the left atrial cavity can clearly be visualized in various horizontal sections from an esophageal transducer position and the atrial appendage is demonstrable in virtually all patients (Fig. 9). Accordingly, Aschenberg et al. [15] detected thrombi in the atrial appendage in six of 21 consecutive patients with mitral stenosis using this technique. Sensivity and specificity of transesophageal echocardiography for detection of atrial appendage thrombi was 100% in this report. All thrombi were subsequently

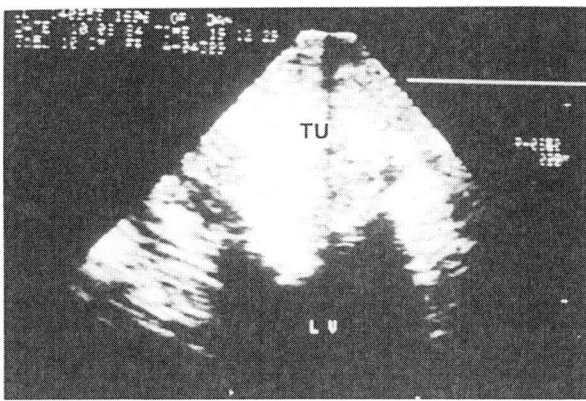

Fig. 6. Transesophageal echocardiogram of a patient with left atrial myxoma (TU) filling almost completely the left atrium and prolapsing into the left ventricle (LV).

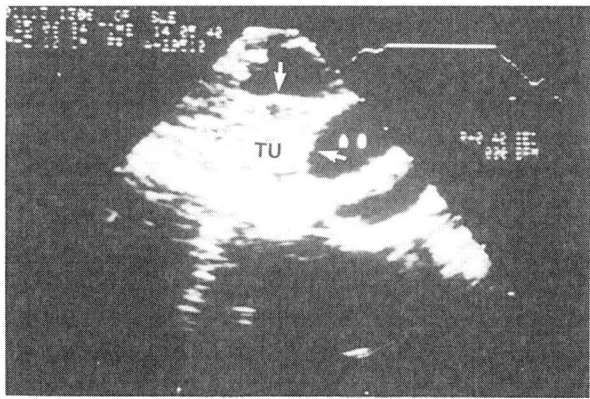

Fig. 7. Transesophageal echocardiogram of a patient with a tumor (TU) almost completely obstructing the vena cava superior (arrows). AO = aorta.

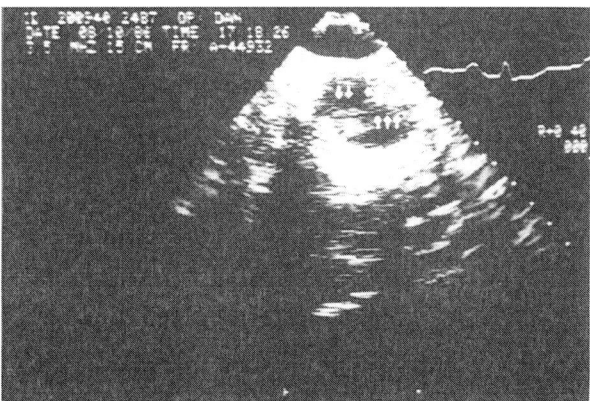

Fig. 8. Transesophageal echocardiogram of a patient with phlebographically proven thrombi (arrows) in the vena cava superior.

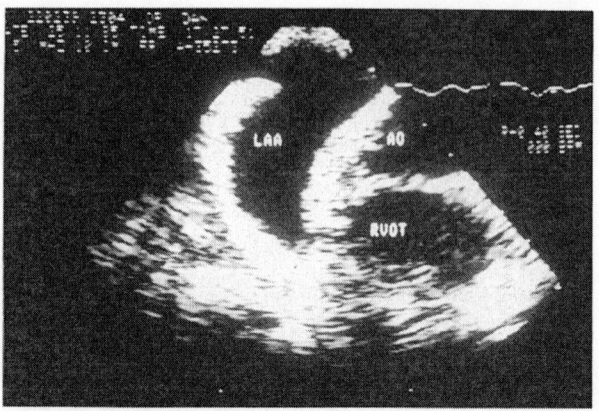

Fig. 9. Transesophageal echocardiogram showing a normal left atrial appendage (LAA). AO = aorta, RVOT = right ventricular outlow tract.

confirmed by surgery and all had been missed on the transthoracic echocardiogram. These findings are in good agreement with our observations in 29 consecutive patients with otherwise unexplained arterial embolism where isolated left atrial appendage thrombi could be documented in 14 cases (48.3%) by the transesophageal approach (Fig. 10, 11); the transthoracic echo had failed in all cases [16]. Interestingly, left atrial appendage thrombi were also found in patients without mitral stenosis and even in sinus rhythm (at least at the time of the study).

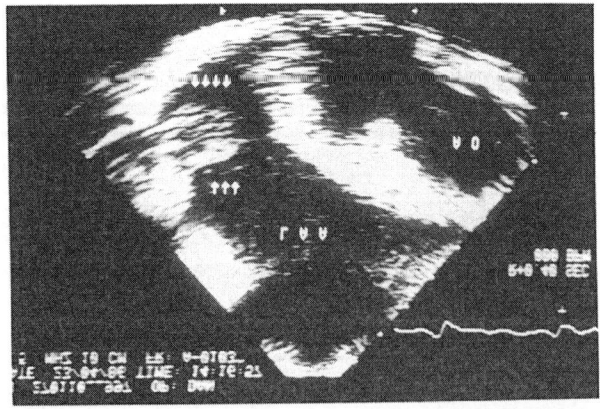

Fig. 10. Transesophageal echocardiogram showing a thrombus (arrows) in the left atrial appendage (LAA). AO = aorta.

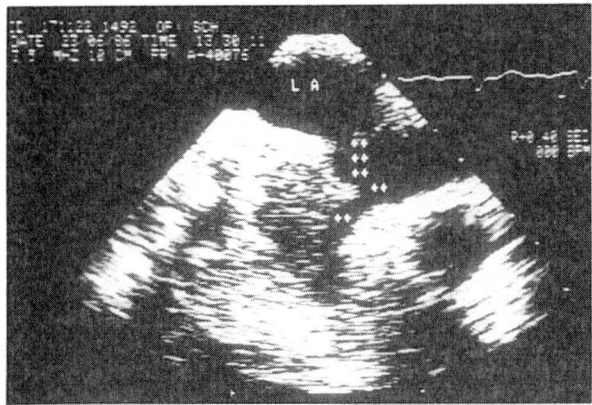

Fig. 11. Transesophageal echocardiogram with a thrombus (arrows) almost completely filling the left atrial appendage. LA = left atrium.

Left atrial spontaneous echo contrast

A phenomenon which has to be carefully differentiated from thrombotic and tumorous intracardiac masses is the appearance of spontaneous echo contrast. Dynamic clouds of spontaneous echos curling up slowly in a circular or spiral shape have been described in the left ventricle in patients with large aneurysms or dilative cardiomyopathy [16], they were found in the dilated left atrium in mitral stenosis [17–20] and could be occasionally observed in patients with aortic dissection within the false lumen of the aorta [21]. Common to all these conditions is a slow blood flow situation.

Transesophageal echocardiography seems to improve the detection rate

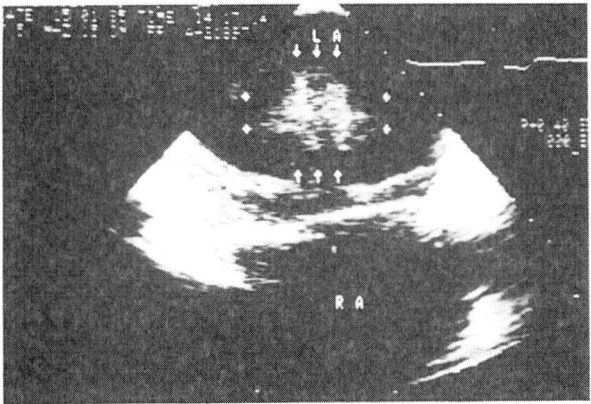

Fig. 12. Transesophageal echocardiogram of a patient with mitral stenosis and discrete spontaneous echo contrast (arrows) in the left atrium (LA). RA = right atrium.

268

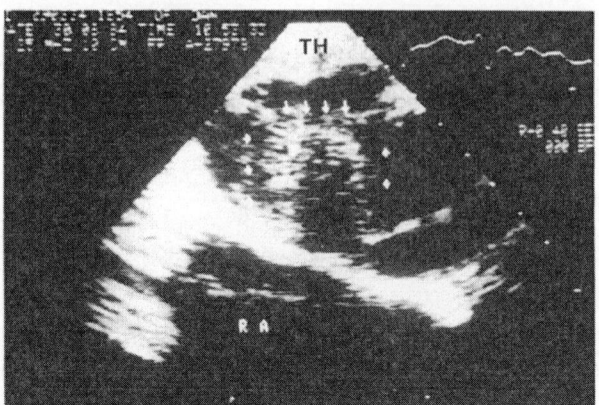

Fig. 13. Transesophageal echocardiogram showing a thrombus (TH) and marked spontaneous echo contrast (arrows) in the left atrium. RA = right atrium.

of spontaneous echo contrast in the left atrium markedly [19, 20] (Fig. 12, 13). Sixty-one of 122 (50%) consecutive patients with mitral stenosis or after mitral valve replacement studied in our laboratory during the last years showed atrial spontaneous echo contrast when investigated from the esophageal window. Patients with spontaneous echo contrast had significantly larger left atrial diameters and significantly more often left atrial thrombi and/or a history of arterial embolism than those without. Thus, left atrial spontaneous echo contrast in patients with mitral stenosis or mitral prosthesis seems to be an indicator of an increased thrombembolic risk and can easily be assessed by transesophageal echocardiography.

Extracardiac masses

Whereas the echocardiographic features of intracardiac masses have been described extensively, only few reports are published on the value of this technique for diagnosing extracardiac tumors and cysts [23–28]. As long as a tumor shows a cystic structure, its identification by ultrasound is usually easy (Fig. 14). Solid tumors may demonstrate a more highly reflective echo pattern than the surrounding tissue; a clear separation from adjacent structures, however, remains usually difficult or even impossible. In addition, some regions around the heart are almost inaccessible for ultrasound waves applied from an anterior chest wall transducer position (as in particular the right paracardial areas). This disadvantage of the transthoracic echocardiographic approach seems to be at least partially overcome when the imaging is performed using an esophageal transducer position.

Two recent studies [8, 29] have compared the value of transthoracic and

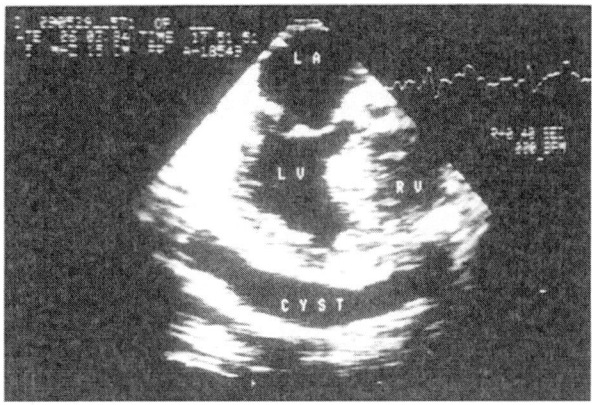

Fig. 14. Transesophageal echocardiogram of a patient with a pericardial cyst surrounding the left (LV) and right (RV) ventricle. LA = left atrium.

transesophageal echocardiography for identification of extracardiac masses. Engberding et al. [29] found in a series of 12 patients with peri- or paracardiac tumors four cases where a tumor visualization could only be achieved from the esophagus. In our own collective [8] of eight patients with extracardiac masses, five tumors were identified with the transesophageal technique alone; in four of them, the tumor was localized in the right paracardial region (Fig. 15).

In summary, transesophageal echocardiography improves the visualization of the left atrial appendage and the vena cava superior, seems to add additional information concerning acoustic properties, mobility and wall adherence of intracardiac masses, allows an easy detection of intracardiac spontaneous echo contrast and the technique may be helpful for the diag-

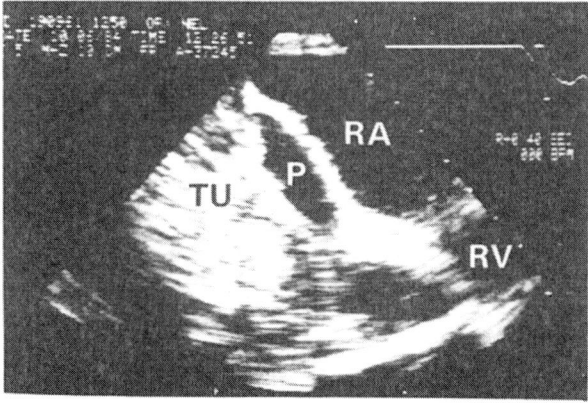

Fig. 15. Transesophageal echocardiogram of a patient with a right paracardial tumor (TU) and a small pericardial effusion (P). RA = right atrium, RV = right ventricle.

nosis of extracardiac masses, in particular, in cases where the tumor is localized in areas difficulty or not accessible by the transthoracic approach.

References

1. Effert S, Domanig E: The diagnosis of intraatrial tumors and thrombi by the ultrasound echo method. Ger Med Monthly 84: 1, 1959.
2. Bommer JW: Echocardiographic detection of cardiac masses. 2-D or not 2-D? Chest 78: 675, 1980.
3. Schmaltz A, Schweizer P: Echokardiographische Diagnostik von Herztumoren. Internist und Praxis 22: 407, 1982.
4. Fyke FE, Seward JB, Edwards WD, Miller FA, Reeder GS, Schattenberg TT, Shub C, Callahan JA, Tajik AJ: Primary cardiac tumors. Experience with 30 consecutive patients since the introduction of two-dimensional echocardiography. J Am Coll Cardiol 5: 1465, 1985.
5. Mazer MS, Harrigan PR: Left ventricular myxoma. M-mode and two-dimensional echocardiographic features. Am Heart J 104: 875, 1982.
6. Bogren HG, DeMaria AN, Mason DT: Imaging procedures in the detection of cardiac tumors, with emphasis on echocardiography: a review. Cardiovasc Intervent Radiol 3: 107, 1980.
7. Ennker J, Daniel W, Doehring W, Oelert H: Surgical experience with left atrial myxomas. Herz 8: 227, 1983.
8. Nellessen U, Daniel WG, Lichtlen PR: Bedeutung der transösophagealen Echokardiographie in der Diagnostik kardialer und parakardialer raumfordernder Prozesse. Z Kardiol 75: 91, 1986.
9. Ezekowitz MD, Smith EO, Rankin R, Harrison LG, Kraus HF: Left atrial mass: diagnostic value of transesophageal 2-dimensional echocardiography and indium-111 platelet scintigraphy. Am J Cardiol 51: 1563, 1983.
10. Nellessen U, Daniel WG, Matheis G, Oelert H, Depping K, Lichtlen PR: Impending paradoxical embolism from atrial thrombus: correct diagnosis by transesophageal echocardiography and prevention by surgery. J Am Coll Cardiol 5: 1002, 1985.
11. Thier W, Schlüter M, Kremer P, Polonius MJ, Klöppel G, Becker K, Hanrath P: Cysts in left atrial myxomas identified by transesophageal cross sectional echocardiography. Am J Cardiol 51: 1793, 1983.
12. Herzog CA, Bass D, Kane M, Asinger R: Two-dimensional echocardiographic imaging of left atrial appendage thrombi. J Am Coll Cardiol 3: 1340, 1984.
13. DePace NL, Soulen RL, Kotler MN, Mintz GS: Two-dimensional echocardiographic detection of intraatrial masses. Am J Cardiol 48: 954, 1981.
14. Come PC, Riley MF, Markis JE, Malagold M: Limitations of echocardiographic techniques in evaluation of left atrial masses. Am J Cardiol 48: 947, 1981.
15. Aschenberg W, Schlüter M, Kremer P, Schröder E, Siglow V, Bleifeld W: Transesophageal two-dimensional echocardiography for the detection of left atrial appendage thrombus. J Am Coll Cardiol 7: 163, 1986.
16. Daniel WG, Nikutta P, Schröder E, Nellessen U: Transesophageal echocardiographic detection of left atrial appendage thrombi in patients with unexplained arterial embolism. Circulation 74 (supp II): II-391 (abstract), 1986.
17. Mikell FL, Asinger RW, Elsberger J, Anderson WR, Hodges M: Regional statis of blood

in dysfunctional left ventricle: echocardiographic detection and differentiation from early thrombosis. Circulation 66: 755, 1982.

18. Iliceto S, Antonelli G, Sorino M, Biasco G, Rizzon P: Dynamic intracavitary left atrial echos in mitral stenosis. Am J Cardiol 55: 603, 1985.

19. Beppu S, Nimura Y, Sakakibara H, Nagata S, Park YD, Izumi S, Uecka M, Masuda Y. Nakasone I: Some-like echo in the left atrial cavity in mitral valve disease: its features and significance. J Am Coll Cardiol 6: 744, 1985.

20. Daniel WG, Nellessen U, Nonnast-Daniel B, Lichtlen PR: Linksatriale Spontanechos bei Mitralstenose als Hinweis auf ein erhöhtes Thrombembolie-Risiko. Z Kardiol 74 (supp. 3): 57 (abstract), 1985.

21. Daniel WG, Nellessen U, Nonnast-Daniel B, Bednarski P, Lichtlen PR: Left atrial spontaneous echo contrast in mitral valve disease – an indicator of increased thrombembolic risk. J Am Coll Cardiol 7: 31A (abstract), 1986.

22. Panidis IP, Kotler MN, Mintz GS, Ross J: Intracavitary echoes in the aortic arch in type III aortic dissection. Am J Cardiol 54: 1159, 1984.

23. Farooki ZQ, Adelman S, Green EW: Echocardiographic differentiation of a cystic and a solid tumor of the heart. Am J Cardiol 39: 107, 1977.

24. Chandraratna PAN, Littmann BB, Serafini A, Whayne T, Robinson H: Echocardiographic evaluation of extracardiac masses. Brit Heart J 40: 741, 1978.

25. Chandraratna PAN, Aronow W: Detection of pericardial metastases by cross-sectional echocardiography. Circulation 63: 197, 1980.

26. Daniel WG, Döhring W, Frank G, Gahl K, Lichtlen PR: Non-invasive diagnosis of a pericardial cyst. Combined use of M-mode echocardiography and computed tomography. Eur Heart J 1: 201, 1980.

27. Bluschke V, Köhler E, Kuhn H, Körfer R: Diagnostik einer kardialen Fibrosarkommetastase mittels zweidimensionaler Echokardiographie. Z Kardiol 70: 492, 1981.

28. Engberding R, Dittrich H, v. Bassewitz DB, Most E, Pfefferkorn J, Reich G: Klinische und echokardiographische Befunde bei 12 Patienten mit Herztumoren. Herz/Kreislauf 4: 171, 1985.

29. Engberding R, Schulze-Waltrup N, Große-Heitmeyer W, Stoll V: Transthorakale und transösophageale 2-D-Echokardiographie in der Diagnostik peri- und parakardialer Tumoren. Dtsch Med Wschr 112: 49, 1987.

4.5. Diagnosis of infective endocarditis by transesophageal echocardiography

WERNER G. DANIEL, ANDREAS MÜGGE & PAUL R. LICHTLEN

Since the initial reports by Dillon et al. [1] and Spangler et al. [2] in 1973, numerous studies have been published on the value of transthoracic M-mode and two-dimensional echocardiography for the assessment of valvular vegetations in patients with infective endocarditis. As a non-invasive bedside technique easily repeatable in the course of follow-up studies, echocardiography is the only method available today allowing a direct visualization of endocarditis-induced valvular lesions, otherwise being restricted to surgery or autopsy.

Conventional transthoracic echocardiography

Literature reviews [3, 4] including the studies with the largest numbers of patients with infective endocarditis report an average detection rate of valvular vegetations of about 55% when M-mode echocardiography is used alone; the combined use of the M-mode and two-dimensional approach increases the success rate up to 70–80%. In our own prospective studies [3, 5] on 196 consecutive patients with infective endocarditis proven by clinical signs as well as positive blood cultures and/or anatomical findings (surgery or autopsy), 134 patients with 149 diseased valves were investigated by M-mode echocardiography alone; in this group, vegetations could be identified on 103 valves (69.8%). Sixty-two patients with 74 infected valves were studied by the combined M-mode and two-dimensional approach; in this second group, vegetations were visualized on 58 valves (74.4%).

Transesophageal echocardiography

During the last years, the diagnostic potential of the echocardiographic technique could be further improved by the introduction of the transesophageal approach. This technique is of particular importance in cases where conventional transthoracic echocardiography fails due to a poor imaging quality

J. Cikes (ed.), *Echocardiography in Cardiac Interventions*, 273–280, 1989.

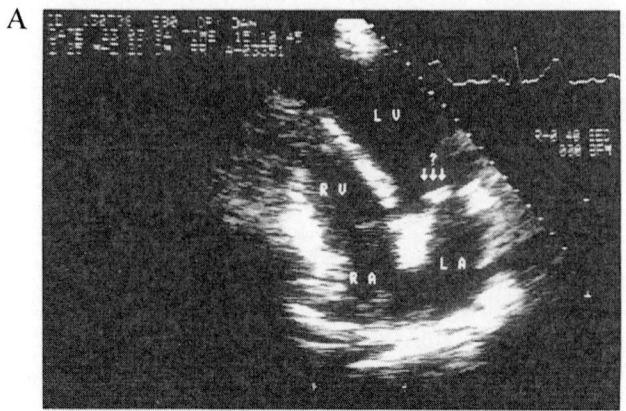

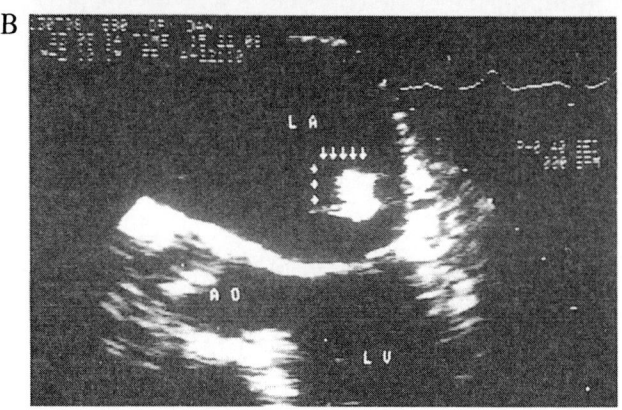

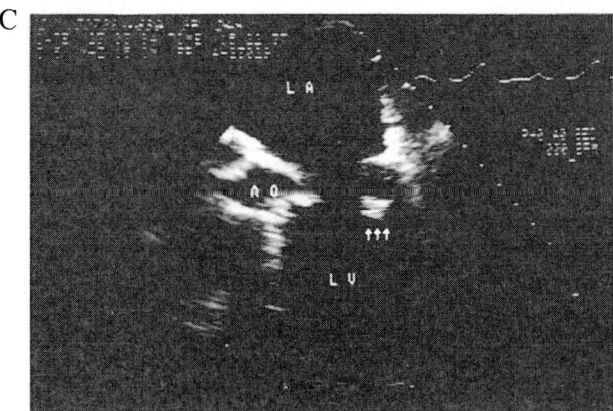

Fig. 1. Transthoracic (A) and transesophageal (B, C) 2D echocardiogram of a 76 years old patient with mitral valve endocarditis and heavy emphysema. Whereas on the transthoracic echocardiogram (four chamber view) vegetations could not be clearly identified (Fig. A: arrows with ?), the transesophageal imaging shows a large vegetation (arrows) pendulating in systole (Fig. B) into the left atrium (LA) and in diastole (Fig. C) into the left ventricle (LV). RV and RA = right ventricle and atrium, respectively. AO = aortic valve.

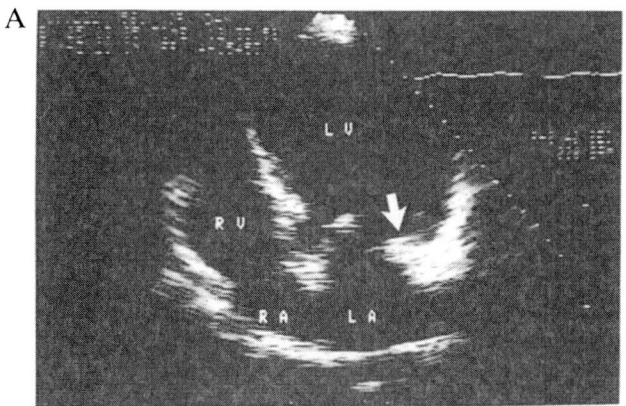

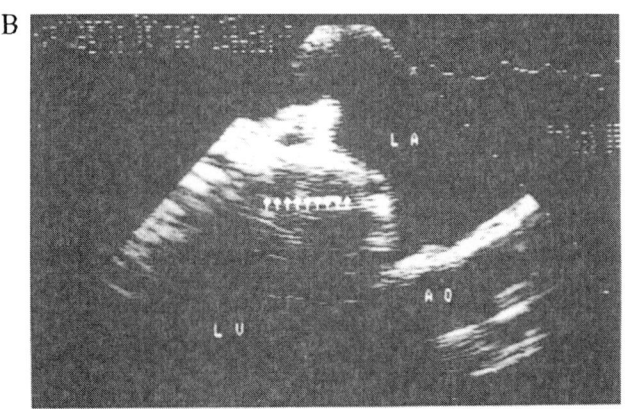

Fig. 2. Transthoracic (A) and transesophageal (B) echocardiogram of a patient with mitral valve endocarditis. In the transthoracic four chamber view (A), the posterior mitral leaflet (arrow) appeared thickened but did not show the typical configuration of a vegetation. The transesophageal image (B) revealed a large vegetation attached to the posterior mitral leaflet (arrows) with two large cavities subsequently identified as abscess areas during surgery. LA and LV = left atrium and ventricle. RA and RV = right atrium and ventricle. AO = aortic root.

as in patients with marked obesity, chest deformities, emphysema, early after thoracic surgery or under artificial respiration.

Recently, we evaluated 69 selected patients with infective endocarditis of 82 valves studied by transesophageal echocardiography (Diasonics Echoscope, 3.5 MHz phased array transducer mounted on the tip of a gastroscope) in addition to the conventional transthoracic approach [3, 6–9]. Endocarditis was proven in all cases by typical clinical signs (100%), positive blood cultures (67%) and/or surgery or autopsy findings (70%). Patients were selected on the basis of a poor imaging quality of the transthoracic studies possibly due to emphysema/obesity (13 patients), recently performed cardiac surgery (14 patients), preexisting valvular lesions (10 patients) and

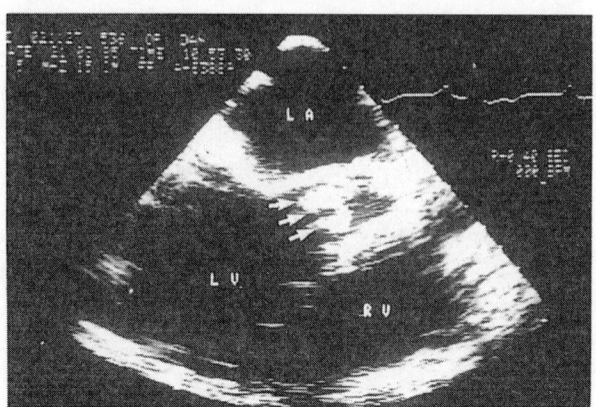

Fig. 3. Transesophageal echocardiogram of a patient with aortic valve endocarditis. The patient was studied during artificial respiration where the transthoracic approach failed to detect the aortic valve vegetations which could be clearly identified on the transesophageal image (arrows). LA and LV = left atrium and ventricle. RV = right ventricle.

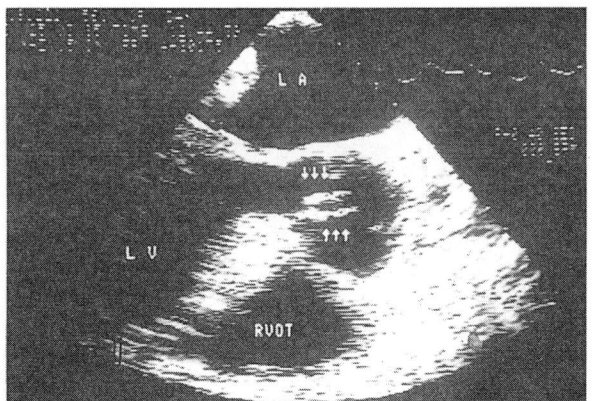

Fig. 4. Transesophageal echocardiogram of a patient with small vegetations at the aortic valve (arrows) which could not be detected on the transthoracic recording. LA and LV = left atrium and ventricle. RVOT = right ventricular outflow tract.

Table 1. Assessment of vegetations in infective endocarditis by transthoracic and transesophageal echocardiography.

		Transthoracic	Transesophageal
Vegetations	positive	33 (40.2%)	77 (93.9%)
	questionable	20 (24.4%)	5 (6.1%)
	negative	29 (35.4%)	–

patients (selected): n = 69
diseased valves: n = 82
(31 aortic, 30 mitral, 18 prosthetic, 3 tricuspid valves)

artificial respiration (3 patients), or the transesophageal technique was applied because an endocarditis associated perivalvular abscess was suspected. Figures 1–4 show typical examples of the transesophageal findings and the comparison with the visualization rate of vegetations or endocarditis induced valvular destructions obtained by the transthoracic technique is listed in Table 1. Due to the selection criteria of the patients in this group, transthoracic echocardiography was able to visualize vegetations on only 33 of the 82 diseased valves (40.2%). In contrast, the transesophageal approach revealed vegetations and related valve destructions in 93.9% (77 of 82 valves) with an interobserver variability of only 6.1% (5 of 82 valves). Similar favorable results are reported by Erbel et al. [10]. Independent on the imaging quality of the transthoracic echocardiogram, the transesophageal technique seems to be superior in the identification of small vegetations (Fig. 4) and those attached to prosthetic valves (see Chapter 4.6).

Endocarditis-associated abscesses

A problem which is still not satisfactorily solved by currently available transthoracic echocardiographic techniques is the reliable identification of endocarditis-associated perivalvular abscesses and, consequently, related reports in the literature are rare [11–13]. On the other hand, the clinical relevance of an early identification of patients with an abscess is obvious since these patients are usually threatened by an increased mortality risk.

According to the experience obtained in more than 900 transesophageal echocardiographic studies performed in our laboratory without complications during the last years, the valvular and perivalvular structures can regularily be visualized with an extremely high imaging quality when this technique is applied. We therefore performed a prospective study including 64 patients subsequently undergoing surgery due to an acute infective endocarditis of 76 valves (34 aortic, 23 mitral, 2 tricuspid, 17 prothestic valves) [14]. Surgery revealed abscesses in 22 of the 64 patients (34.4%). Abscesses were localized at the aortic root (9), in the interventricular septum (7), around a prosthetic valve ring (4) or at the mitral valve apparatus (2) (Figures 5–7). Whereas only four abscesses (18.2%) could be correctly diagnosed by transthoracic echocardiography (3 aortic root, 1 mitral valve apparatus), a correct preoperative diagnosis was possible in 18 cases (81.8%) on the transesophageal echocardiogram (Table 2) with an interobserver variability of 3.1% (2 of 64 patients). In two patients, however, a false-positive diagnosis was obtained. Thus, for the detection of endocarditis-associated abscesses a sensitivity of 81.8%, a specificity of 95.2%, and a positive and negative predictive value of 90.0% and 90.9%, respectively, were found.

278

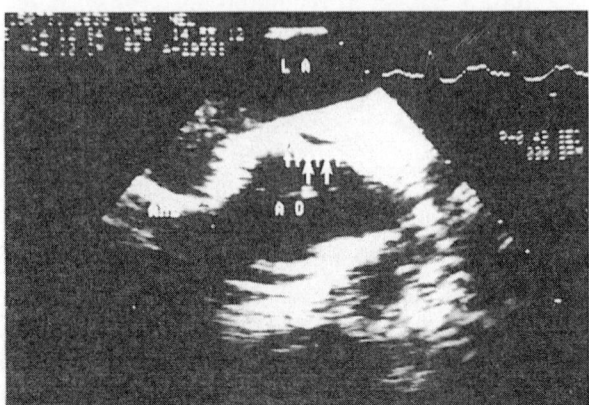

Fig. 5. Transesophageal echocardiogram of a patient with aortic valve endocarditis and an abscess cavity in the posterior aortic root (arrows). LA = left atrium. AO = aortic root. AML = anterior mitral leaflet.

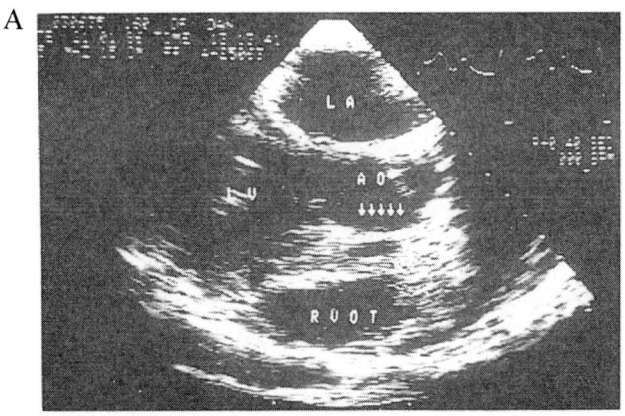

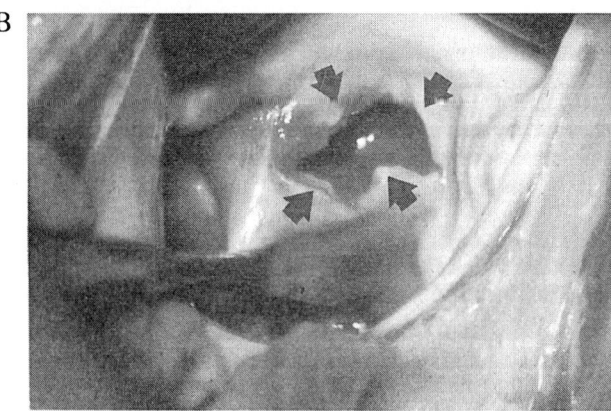

Fig. 6. Transesophageal echocardiogram (A) and intraoperative situs (B) of a patient with aortic valve endocarditis and a large abscess in the proximal part of the interventricular septum (arrows). LA and LV = left atrium and ventricle. AO = aortic root. RVOT = right ventricular outflow tract.

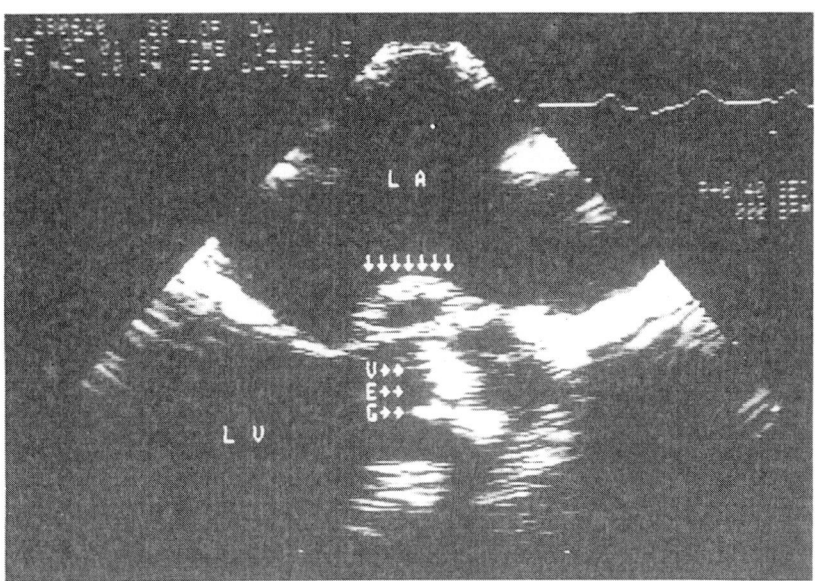

Fig. 7. Transesophageal echocardiogram of a patient with an aortic valve endocarditis showing vegetations (VEG) at the valve leaflets and an abscess at the posterior aortic root (arrows) proven by surgery. LA and LV = left atrium and ventricle.

Table 2. Diagnosis of endocarditis-associated abscesses.

	Surgery	TT-Echo	TE-Echo
Aortic root	9	3	6
Interventricular septum	7	–	7
Prosthetic valve ring	4	–	3
Mitral valve apparatus	2	1	2
Total	22	4 (18%)	18 (82%)

Numbers represent number of patients with abscesses found at surgery, conventional M-mode and 2D transthoracic echocardiography (TT-Echo) and transesophageal echocardiography (TE-Echo).

In summary, these data indicate that transesophageal echocardiography markedly improves the detection of valvular vegetations as well as the iden-tification of perivalvular abscesses in patients with infective endocarditis. Thereby, the transesophageal approach allows – at least in some cases – an earlier diagnosis and an earlier initiation of treatment in these patients who still have a considerable mortality risk.

280

References

1. Dillon JC, Feigenbaum H, Konecke L, Davis RH, Chang S: Echocardiographic manifesta-tions of valvular vegetations. Am Heart J 86: 698, 1973.
2. Spangler RD, Johnson MC, Holmes J, Blount G: Echocardiographic demonstration of bacterial vegetations in active infective endocarditis. J Clin Ultrasound 1: 126, 1973.
3. Daniel WG, Schröder E, Nonnast-Daniel B, Lichtlen PR: Conventional and transesoph-ageal echocardiography in the diagnosis of infective endocarditis. Eur Heart J 8, Suppl. 3: 287, 1987.
4. O'Brien JT, Geiser ES: Infective endocarditis and echocardiography. Am Heart J 108: 386, 1984.
5. Daniel W, Mügge A, Gahl K, Lichtlen PR: Echokardiographische Diagnostik. In: Gahl K, ed. Endokarditis. Dr. D. Steinkopff Verlag, Darmstadt, 108, 1984.
6. Daniel WG, Nellessen U, Nonnast-Daniel B, Lichtlen PR: Assessment of valvular vegeta-tions in infective endocarditis by transesophageal two-dimensional echocardiography. Europ Heart J 6: (Suppl. I): 28 (Abstract), 1985.
7. Daniel WG, Nellessen U, Nonnast-Daniel B, Lichtlen PR: Vergleich von M-mode, 2-dimensionaler transthorakaler und Oesophagus-Echokardiographie bei der Diagnostik der infektiösen Endokarditis. Z Kardiol 74: (Suppl. 5): 111, 1985.
8. Daniel WG, Nellessen U, Nonnast-Daniel B, Lichtlen PR: Ösophagusechokardiographie bei infektiöser Endokarditis. Z Kardiol 74: (Suppl. 3): 101 (Abstract), 1985.
9. Daniel WG, Nellessen U, Nonnast-Daniel B, Oelert H, Lichtlen PR: Oesophagusecho-kardiographie bei infektiöser Endokarditis. In: Erbel R, Meyer J, Brennecke, eds. Fort-schritte der Echokardiographie. Springer Verlag Heidelberg, 195–202, 1985.
10. Erbel R, Rohmann S, Drexler M, Mohr-Kahaly S, Meyer J: Diagnostic value of trans-esophageal echocardiography in infectious endocarditis. Circulation 74, Supp II, II-55 (Abstract), 1986.
11. Mardelli TJ, Ogawa S, Hubbard FE, Dreifus LS, Meixell LL: Cross-sectional echocardio-graphic detection of aortic ring abscess in bacterial endocarditis. Chest 74: 576, 1978.
12. Scanlan JG, Seward JB, Tajik AJ: Myocardial abscess: direct visualization with wide angle two-dimensional sector echocardiography. Circulation 60: (Suppl. II): II-37, 1979.
13. Ellis SG, Goldstein J, Popp RL: Detection of endocarditis-associated perivalvular abscesses by two-dimensional echocardiography. J Am Coll Cardiol 5: 647, 1985.
14. Daniel WG, Nellessen U, Schröder E, Nikutta P, Nonnast-Daniel B, Mügge A: Trans-esophageal echocardiography as the method of choice for the detection of endocarditis-associated abscesses. Circulation 74, Supp II, II-55 (Abstract), 1986.

4.6. Detection of prosthetic valve malfunction by transesophageal echocardiography

WERNER G. DANIEL, ULRICH NELLESSEN, ANDREAS MÜGGE,
EBERHARD SCHRÖDER, DIRK HAUSMANN & PAUL R. LICHTLEN

The assessment of the normal and abnormal function of prosthetic valves by echocardiography is known to be more difficult than the echocardiographic evaluation of native cardiac structure. This is in particular true for mechanical devices which are composed of highly echo-reflecting material leading to considerable artifacts which prevent an imaging quality sufficient to establish an unequivocal diagnosis in many cases. Therefore, in the evaluation of mechanical prostheses, the combined M-mode echo-phonocardiographic recording minimizing the amount of spurious echos is sometimes more helpful than the two-dimensional approach [1–4]. In contrast, bioprostheses can usually more easily be evaluated by two-dimensional echocardiography since their leaflets show a motion pattern and reflectivity which is similar to native valves. The few studies reported in the literature [5–10] comparing echocardiographic and anatomical findings in patients with bioprosthesis malfunction show satisfying results provided that the transthoracic examination allows a clear imaging quality – a condition which is sometimes difficult to achieve in patients after cardiac surgery.

Although only a few reports are published on the role of transesophageal echocardiography for the diagnosis of prosthetic valve malfunciton [11–14] the transesophageal approach seems to overcome at least some of the problems associated with transthoracic imaging. Our own experience in this field is based on more than 300 patients with artificial valves studied by the conventional as well as the transesophageal technique. Fifty-five of these selected patients subsequently underwent reoperation; in these cases, echocardiographic findings could be compared with the anatomical situs. The results will be illustrated by the following examples.

Endocarditis

In bioprostheses studied by transesophageal echocardiograpy, a clear visualization of the prosthetic leaflets can be obtained in virtually all patients with a mitral prosthesis (Fig. 1) and in most cases with an aortic device. Vegetations attached to the leaflets and/or endocarditis induced valve destructions (i.e.

I. Cikes (ed.), *Echocardiography in Cardiac Interventions*, 281–290, 1989.

282

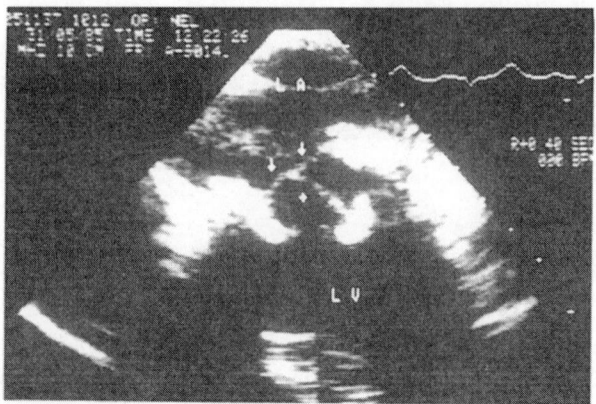

Fig. 1. Transesophageal echocardiogram of a normal Hancock bioprosthesis in mitral position. The three leaflets of the prosthesis (arrows) can clearly be visualized. LA/LV = left atrium/ventricle.

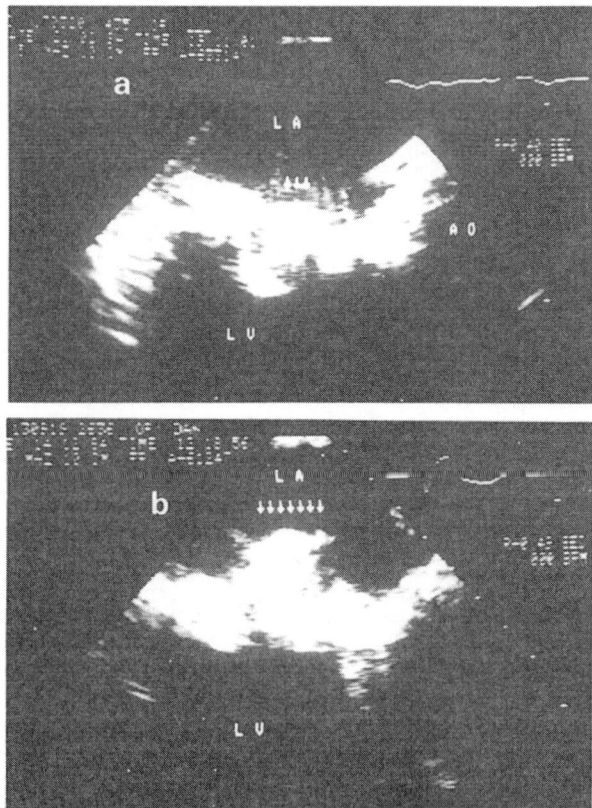

Fig. 2. Transesophageal echocardiogram of a Hancock (a) and Mitroflow (b) bioprsthesis in mitral position with large vegetations (arrows) at the leaflets. LA/LV = left atrium/ventricle.

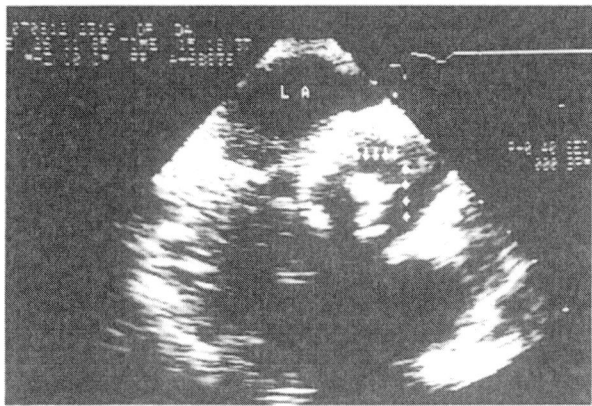

Fig. 3. Transesophageal echocardiogram of a Carpentier-Edwards bioprosthesis in aortic position with vegetations (arrows) at the leaflets. LA = left atrium.

partial leaflet rupture) can usually be differentiated without problems (Fig. 2, 3). In our series of selected patients who subsequently underwent reoperation, 12 bioprostheses were diseased by infective endocarditis; in ten cases (83%), the correct preoperative diagnosis could be established by transesophageal echocardiography (two valves were considered as 'negative') compared to only four patients (33%) where an unequivocal diagnosis was possible by the transthoracic approach (four 'questionable' and four 'negative' cases).

The identification of vegetations attached to mechanical devices seems also to be easier when patients are studied by the transesophageal technique. Whereas conventional transthoracic echocardiography was able to detect vegetations in only one of seven (14%) mechanical prosthesis (two cases with 'questionable' and four with 'negative' results) which had to be replaced due to endocarditis proven by subsequent surgery, the transesophageal approach allowed a clear visualization of vegetations at five prosthesis (71%) (one 'questionable' and one 'negative' case). A typical example is shown in Fig. 4.

Valve degeneration

During the last years, several studies could show an increasing rate of Hancock porcine valve malfunction due to primary tissue degeneration or calcification of the leaflets [10, 15–18]. Since this type of prosthesis has been extensively used because of the initially promising hemodynamic qualities and its low rate of thrombembolic complications a large number of patients may be considered as candidates for a necessary reoperation in the near future. Although leaflet degeneration is usually associated with a slow gradual pros-

284

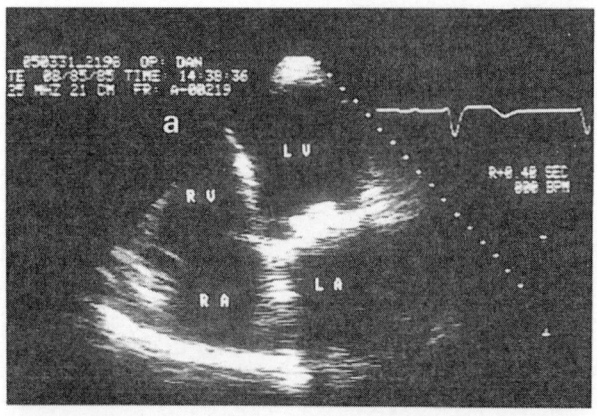

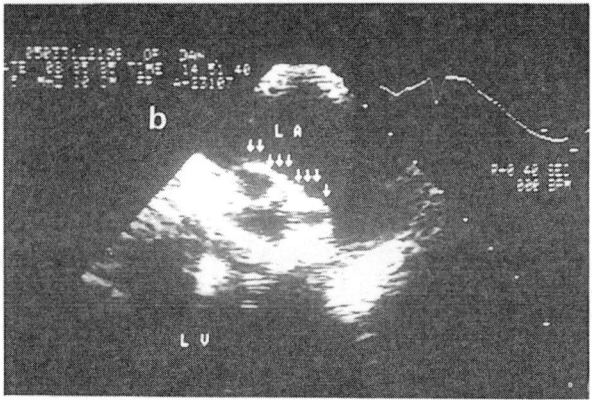

Fig. 4. Transthoracic (a) (four chamber view) and transesophageal (b) echocardiogram of a patient with Starr-Edwards disc prosthetic valve endocarditis in mitral position. In contrast to the transthoracic view, the transesophageal image clearly shows large vegetations (arrows) at the atrial surface of the prosthesis. RV/RA = right atrium/ventricle; LA/LV = left atrium/ventricle.

thetic valve malfunction, sudden valve rupture leading to severe heart failure is known [19]. Therefore, a close follow up of these patients and a reliable technique for early diagnosis of leaflet degeneration are mandatory. In this context, conventional transthoracic two-dimensional echocardiography is the method of choice [5–10]. In cases, however, where the transthoracic imaging quality does not allow a conclusive interpretation of the recordings, the transesophageal approach may provide additional information [15]. In the present series of patients, 24 bioprostheses had to be replaced because of advanced leaflet degeneration which was correctly diagnosed by transesophageal echocardiography in 79% (19 prostheses, including all devices in mitral position) (Fig. 5, 6); in four cases degeneration was missed, one prosthesis showed 'questionable' changes. In contrast, the transthoracic echocardiogram

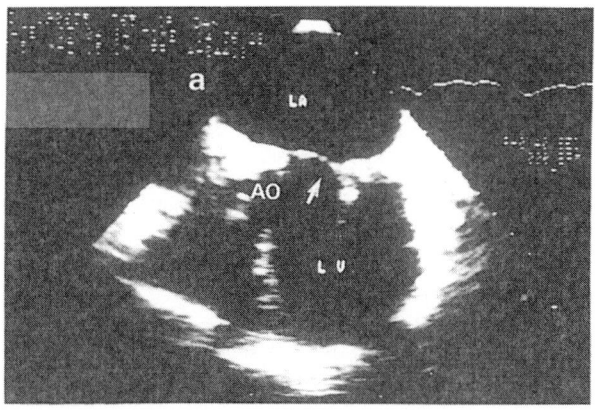

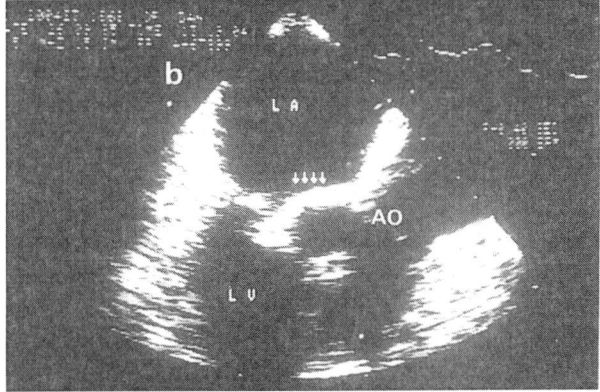

Fig. 5. Transesophageal echocardiogram of a monocusp (one leaflet) bioprosthesis in mitral position early after surgery (a) and 15 months later (b). The leaflet shows marked thickening on the second recording (b) and the prosthesis had to be replaced a few weeks later due to heavy degeneration associated with advanced hemodynamic impairment. LA/VA = left atrium/ventricle; AO = aortic outflow tract.

allowed a correct diagnosis in only 13 prostheses (54%), five cases were considered as 'questionable', six as 'negative' partially due to an insufficient imaging quality.

Thrombi

Thrombotic material attached to an arteficial valve usually results in an inhibited motion of the valve leaflets or of the occluder. In some cases, this abnormal motion pattern may be detected and correctly interpreted by M-mode and two-dimensional echocardiography – in particular, when combined with a phonocardiogram [4, 6, 20–26]. A reliable echocardiographic

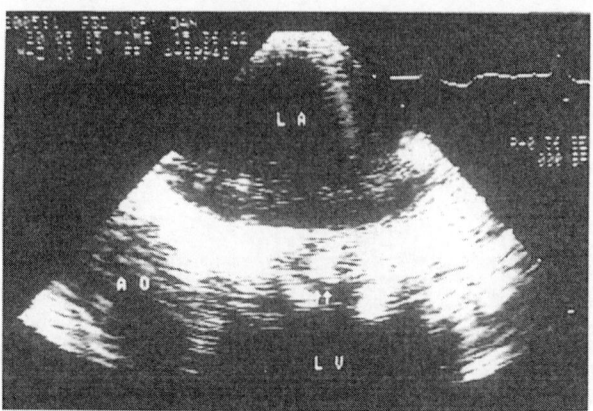

Fig. 6. Transesophageal echocardiogram of a Hancock bioprosthesis in mitral position. One leaflet is markedly thickened (arrows) due to degeneration. LA/VA =left atrium/ventricle; AO = aortic outflow tract.

differentiation between a thrombus and an endocarditis associated vegetation is, of course, usually not possible and in many patients with a mechanical device, the valve induced echocardiographic artifacts prevent an imaging quality sufficient to allow an unequivocal diagnosis (Fig. 7a).

In the series of cases presented here, four patients had a mechanical device in mitral position found to be partially thrombosed at reoperation. In all four cases, the thrombus could be correctly identified prior to surgery by transesophageal echocardiography (Fig. 7b). In contrast, transthoracic echocardiography allowed the correct diagnosis in only one patient whereas in two cases the thrombus was missed and in one case the findings were considered as 'questionable'.

Paravalvular leak

Prosthetic valve dehiscence is usually suspected when an abnormal rocking of the prosthesis is found in the two-dimensional echocardiogram [1, 27, 28] and/or an early diastolic hump of the occluder or the prosthesis ring in the M-mode recording [3, 29]. However, these findings are nonspecific and may be misleading (30). In any way, the direct visualization of a paravalvular leak (Fig. 8) remains a rare exception. Accordingly, in five patients of our series with proven paravalvular leaks, the dehiscending region of the circumference was correctly identified by transthoracic as well as transesophageal echocardiography in only one patient; the other four cases remained undetected or the echocardiographic findings were considered as 'questionable'. The detection rate of paravalvular leaks, however, may be markedly improved when

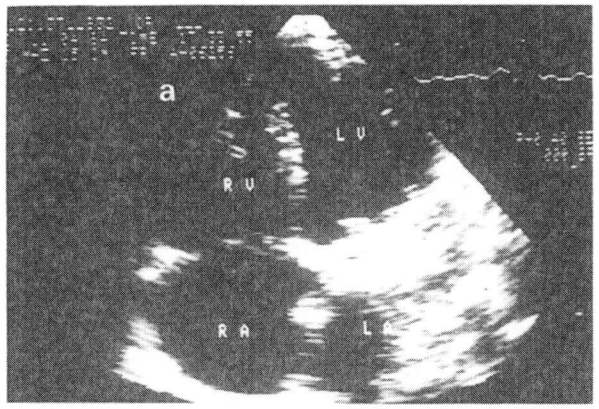

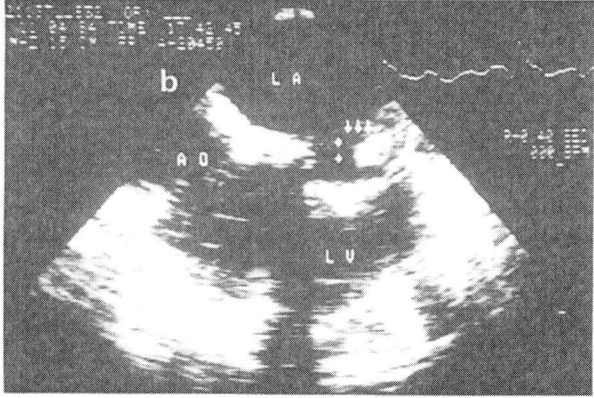

Fig. 7. Transthoracic (a) (four chamber view) and transesophageal (b) echocardiogram of a Starr-Edwards disc prosthesis (mitral position) infected by endocarditis. The transesophageal image clearly shows a large mass (arrows) within the prosthesis which was found to be a thrombus with vegetations during surgery; due to the usually seen artifacts of mechanical devices, vegetations could not be identified on the transthoracic echocardiogram. RA/RV = right atrium/ventricle; LA/LV = left atrium/ventricle; AO = aortic outflow tract.

colour coded Doppler is applied from the esophageal view (Fig. 9, 10).

Our preliminary experience with the use of transesophageal echocardiography in patients with prosthetic valves indicates that transesophageal Doppler in combination with the transesophageal two-dimensional echocardiogram may be considered as the diagnostic technique of choice for the assessment of prosthetic valve malfunction – not only as far as the differentiation between trans- and paravalvular regurgitation is concerned but also with regard to the etiology of the malfunction and in particular in devices in mitral position.

288

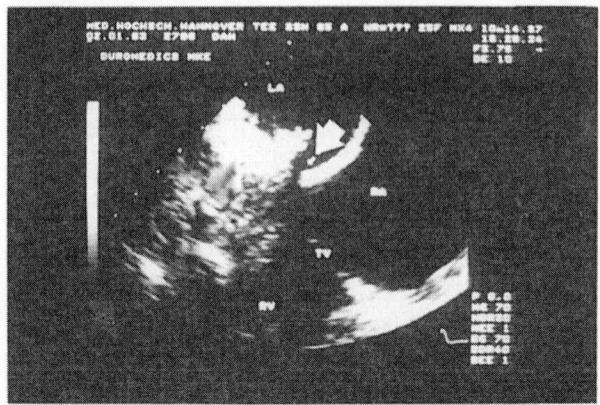

Fig. 8. Transesophageal echocardiogram of a Duromedics prosthesis in mitral position with a paravalvular leak (arrow) close to the interatrial septum. LA/RA = left/right atrium; RV = right ventricle; TV = tricuspid valve.

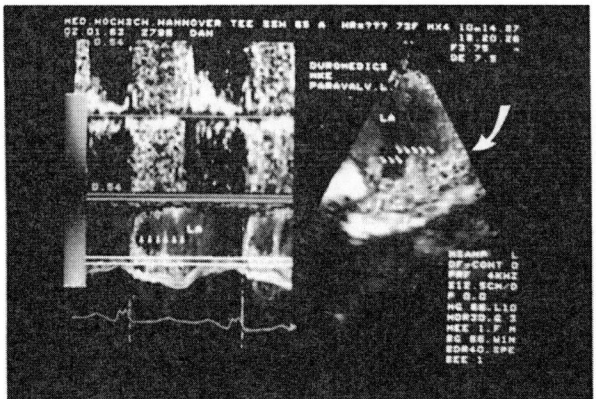

Fig. 9. Transesophageal colour coded Doppler echocardiogram of a Duromedics prosthesis in mitral position with a paravalvular leak (same patient as in fig. 8). The regurgitant jet through the dehiscence can clearly be identified by the mosaic pattern (arrows). The left side of the panel shows the pulsed Doppler signal and the colour coded M-mode recording. LA = left atrium.

References

1. Berndt TB, Goodman DJ, Popp RL: Echocardiographic and phonocardiographic confirmation of suspected caged mitral valve malfunctions. Chest 70: 221, 1976.
2. Mills P, Craige E: Echophonocardiography. Progr Cardiovasc Dis 20: 337, 1978.
3. Lehrer E, Motro M, Schneeweiss A, Neufeld HN: Combined echo-phonocardiographic diagnosis of mitral perivalvular leak with Björk-Shiley and Starr-Edwards prostheses. Am Heart J 106: 762, 1983.

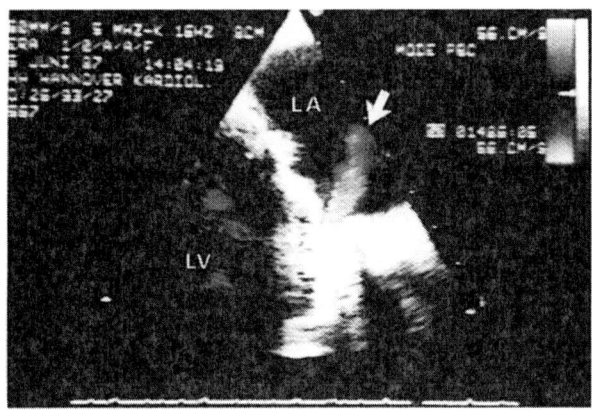

Fig. 10. Transesophageal Doppler echocardiogram of a Duromedics mitral prosthesis with a paravalvular leak; the regurgitant jet can clearly be identified (arrow). LA/LV = left atrium/ventricle.

4. Assanelli A, Aquilina M, Marangoni S, Morgagni GL, Visioli S: Echo-phonocardiographic evaluation of the Björk-Shiley mitral prosthesis. Am J Cardiol 57: 165, 1986.
5. Bloch WN, Felner JM, Wickliffe C, Symbas PN, Schlant RC: Echocardiogram of the porcine aortic bioprosthesis in mitral position. Am J Cardiol 38: 293, 1976.
6. Grube E, Richter R, Simon H, Bernhard A, Schaede A: Funktionskontrolle von Bioprothesen in der Mitralposition mit Hilfe der M-Mode und zweidimensionalen Sektorechokardiographie. Thoraxchirurgie 26: 74, 1978.
7. Harston WE, Roverston RM, Friesinger GC: Echocardiographic evaluation of porcine heterograft valves in the mitral and aortic positions. Am Heart J 96: 448, 1978.
8. Alam M, Madrazo AC, Magilligan DJ, Goldstein S: M-mode and two dimensional echocardiographic features of porcine valve dysfunction. Am J Cardiol 43: 502, 1979.
9. Shapira JN, Martin RP, Fowles RE, Rakowski H, Stinson EB, French JW, Shumway NE, Popp RL: Two dimensional echocardiographic assessment of patients with bioprosthetic valves. Am J Cardiol 43: 510, 1979.
10. Forman MB, Phelan BK, Robertson RM, Virmani R: Correlation of two-dimensional echocardiography and pathologic findings in porcine valve dysfunction. J Am Coll Cardiol 5: 224, 1985.
11. Nellessen U, Daniel WG, Bednarski P: Value of transesophageal echocardiography in the assessment of bioprosthetic valve malfunction. Circulation 72, Supp III: III-207 (abstract), 1985.
12. Nellessen U, Daniel WG, Hecker H. Hetzer R, Schleberger J, Lichtlen PR: Nachweis einer Malfunktion von Herzklappenprothesen mittels zweidimensionaler transösophagealer Echokardiographie. In: Erbel R, Meyer J, Brennecke R (eds): Fortschritte der Echokardiographie. Springer Verlag Berlin, Heidelberg, New York, Tokyo, p. 203–210, 1985.
13. Erbel R, Mohr-Kahaly S, Rohmann S, Schuster S, Drexler M, Wittlich N, Pfeiffer C, Schreiner G, Meyer J: Diagnostische Wertigkeit der transösophagealen Doppler-Echokardiographie. Herz 12: 177, 1987.
14. Krüger W, Plettenberg A, Poppele G, Langenstein BA, Hanrath P: Funktionsbeurteilung von Mitralklappenprothesen durch transösophageale Farbdopplerechokardiographie. Z Kardiol 76: 51 (abstract), 1987.

290

15. Nellessen U, Daniel W, Bednarski P, Lichtlen PR: Degenerationsrate bei Hancock-Bioprothesen jenseits von 5 Jahren: Eine echokardiographische Studie. Z. Kardiol 75, Supp 1: 55 (abstract), 1986.

16. Lakier JB, Khaja F, Magilligan DJ, Goldstein S: Porcine xenograft valves. Long term (60–89 month) follow-up. Circulation 62: 313, 1980.

17. Cohn LH, Mudge GH, Pratter F, Collins JJ Jr: Five to eight-year follow-up of patients undergoing porcine heart valve replacement. N Engl J Med 304: 258, 1981.

18. Goffin YA, Deuvaert F, Wellens F, Leclerc J-L, Kiehm J-L, Primo GC: Normally and abnormally functioning left-sided procine bioprosthetic valves after long-term implantation in patients: distinct spectra of histologic and histochemical changes. J Am Coll Cardiol 4: 324, 1984.

19. Alam M, Carcia R, Goldstein S: Echo-phonocardiographic features of regurgitant porcine mitral and tricuspid valves presenting with musical murmur. Am Heart J 105: 456, 1983.

20. Ben-Zvi J, Hildner FJ, Chandraratna PAN, Samet P: Thrombosis on Björk-Shiley aortic valve prosthesis. Am J Cardiol 34: 438, 1974.

21. Chandraratna PAN, Lopez JM, Hildner FJ, Samet P, Ben-Zvi J: Diagnosis of Björk-Shiley aortic valve dysfunction by echocardiography. Am Heart J 91: 318, 1976.

22. Srivastava TN, Hussain M, Gray LA, Flowres NC: Echocardiographic diagnosis of a stuck Björk-Shiley aortic valve prosthesis. Chest 70: 94, 1976.

23. Daniel W, Klein H, Oelert H, Gahl K, Lichtlen P: Echokardiographische Diagnose einer post-endokarditisch thrombosierten Hancock-Bioprothese in Mitralposition. Thoraxchirurgie 26: 413, 1978.

24. Amann FW, Burckhardt D, Jenzer H-R, Stulz P, Hasse J, Grädel E: Echocardiographic findings in prosthetic mitral valve dysfunction. Am Heart J 108: 1573, 1984.

25. Horowitz MS, Goodman DJ, Hancock EW, Popp RL: Noninvasive diagnosis of complications of mitral bioprosthesis. J Thorac Cardiovasc Surg 71: 450, 1976.

26. Waggoner AD, Quinones AM, Young JB, Nelson JG, Winters WL Jr, Peterson PK, Miller RR: Echo-phonocardiographic evaluation of obstruction of prosthetic mitral valve. Chest 78: 60, 1980.

27. Metha A, Kessler KM, Tamer D, Pefkaros K, Kessler RM, Myerburg RJ: Two-dimensional echographic observations in major detachment of a prosthetic aortic valve. Am Heart J 101: 231, 1981.

28. Kotler KM, Mintz GS, Panidis I, Morganroth J, Segal BL, Ross J: Noninvasive evaluation of normal and abnormal prosthetic valve function. J Am Coll Cardiol 2: 151, 1983.

29. Busch UW, Mathur VS, Garcia F, Hall RJ: Echocardiography and prosthetic valve malfunction. (Letter to the editor). Am J Cardiol 42: 690, 1978.

30. Kinney EL, Manasa M, Kessler KM, Matzer L, Cortada X, Zakharia A, Myerburg RJ, Chahine RA: Two-dimensional echocardiographic appearance of pseudo-dehiscence of Hancock aortic prosthesis. Am Heart J 109: 169, 1985.

4.7. Transesophageal Doppler color flow mapping: initial experience

NORBERT P. DE BRUIJN, FIONA M. CLEMENTS &
JOSEPH A. KISSLO

As has been explained elsewhere in this book (Chapter 4.1), esophageal transducers were developed by echocardiographers who were frustrated in their efforts to obtain images through the chest wall in obese and emphysematous patients. The avoidance of adipose tissue, lung and ribs, intervening between the transducer and the heart by positioning the transducer in the esophagus immediately behind the heart results in much better definition of cardiac structures (Fig. 1). The left atrium and left ventricle, are particularly well imaged from an esophageal approach with conventional Doppler echocardiography or Doppler color flow mapping (DCFM). A further advantage of the esophageal approach becomes apparent with Doppler studies when the esophageal transducer is positioned behind the left atrium and directed towards the cardiac apex. This provides a four chamber long axis view in which the ultrasound beam is aligned almost

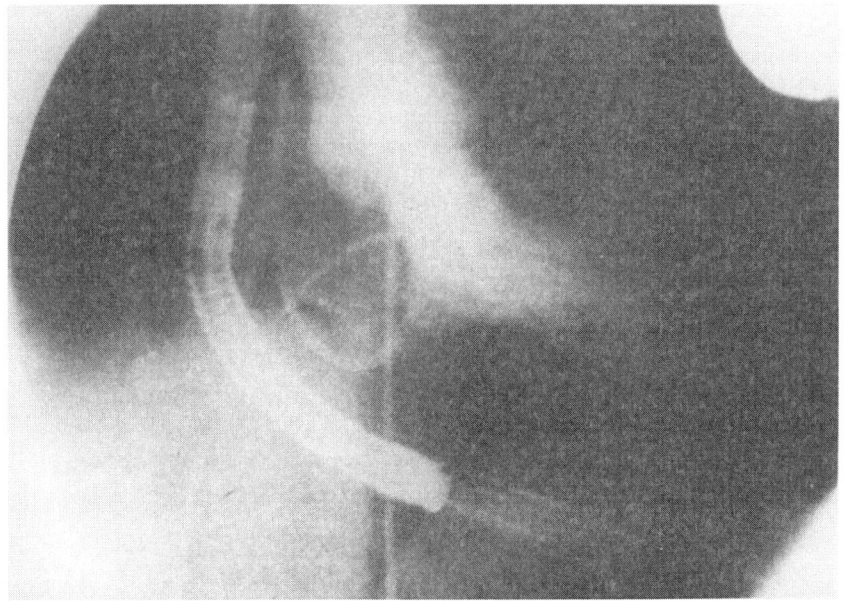

Fig. 1. Transesophageal ultrasound transducer in situ during ventriculography.

J. Cikes (ed.), *Echocardiography in Cardiac Interventions*, 291–297, 1989.
© 1989 *Kluwer Academic Publishers*.

parallel with the majority of normal intracardiac blood flow and provides excellent conditions for the detection of abnormal flow across the mitral valve. Esophageal approaches are also useful for evaluation of flow across the aortic valve. Although transesophageal M-mode and 2D transducers have been available for a number of years [1, 2, 3], the use of Doppler techniques with the esophageal approach is a relatively new development. In 1982, Schlüter and coworkers first reported the use of 2-dimensional imaging with a phased array transducer in 26 awake patients, leading several other investigators to explore the clinical value of transesophageal imaging [4]. Later Schlüter et al. [5] demonstrated, using conventional pulsed Doppler echocardiography, that the sensitivity and specificity of transesophageal imaging for the detection of mitral regurgitation is far superior to that of the transthoracic approach. They evaluated six patients with competent mitral valves and 12 patients with angiographically proven mild-to-moderate mitral regurgitation. The transesophageal approach detected regurgitation in 100% of cases whereas the transthoracic approach was successful in only 58%.

The following describes our initial experience with intraoperative transesophageal Doppler color flow mapping.

Mitral regurgitation

Many patients with coronary artery disease have mitral regurgitation at angiography. Often this is felt to be catheter-induced and not clinically significant. We found, in five of seven patients having coronary artery bypass grafting, at least some evidence of mitral regurgitation by transesophageal

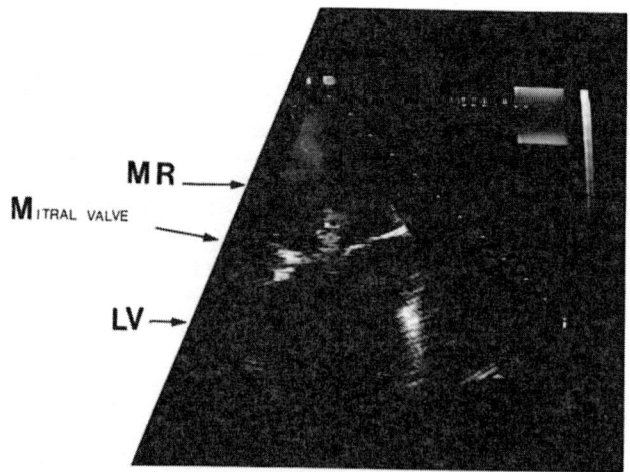

Fig. 2. 'Four-chamber' view during systole showing mitral regurgitation.

Doppler color flow mapping (Fig. 2). In all of these cases mitral regurgitation was not a preoperative diagnosis and had not been observed at angiography. No patient had a v-wave on the pulmonary artery wedge pressure tracing at the time of intraoperative imaging.

It appears therefore that Doppler Color Flow Mapping is extremely sensitive and may detect mitral regurgitation in many patients in whom it is clinically insignificant. Indeed, it has been reported that regurgitation through a 1 mm oriface can be detected by Doppler Color Flow Mapping [6]. Clinically significant mitral regurgitation appears as a narrow, mosaic colored jet of blood flow extending far back into the left atrium, sometimes into the pulmonary veins. This is in sharp contrast to the appearance of para-valvular leaks which we have seen following mitral valve replacement where a small jet of flow may appear intermittently arising from the mitral valve annulus, adjacent to the prosthetic valve (Fig. 3). Omoto has found that such leaks, apparent immediately after surgery, disappeared by two weeks postoperatively, suggesting that small suture line leaks are obliterated during the healing process and do not necessarily constitute grounds for revision of the annular attachment of the valve (personal communication).

Left atrial myxoma

In one patient with a large left atrial myxoma, intraoperative transesophageal imaging revealed some mitral regurgitation occurring around the myxoma, which abutted against the anterior mitral valve leaflet. It was also densely adherent to the interatrial septum which required repair with a pericardial

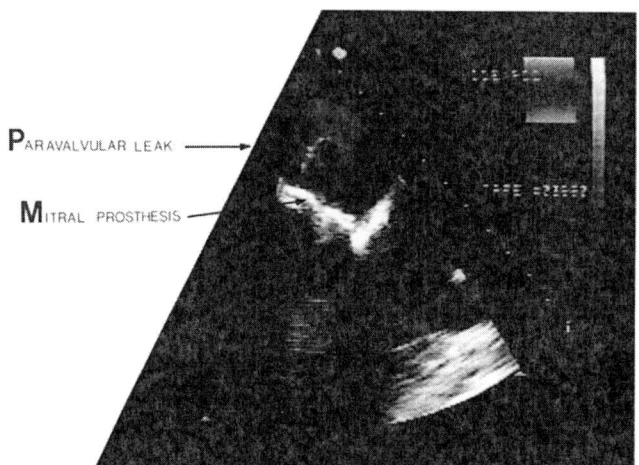

Fig. 3. Small paravalvular leak, adjacent to a freshly inserted mitral valve prosthesis.

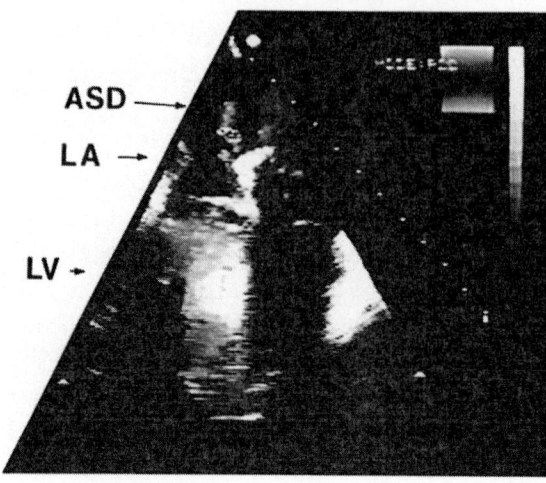

Fig. 4. Jet of blood flow crossing the interatrial septum from the right atrium to the left atrium, representing a small iatrogenic atrial septal defect at the suture line of a pericardial patch.

patch graft. Following resection of the myxoma, significant mitral regurgitation persisted, suggesting that valvular plication might be necessary as an additional procedure. There was also evidence of a small jet of blood flow crossing the interatrial septum from right to left (Fig. 4). This probably represented a small iatrogenic atrial septal defect arising at the suture line where the pericardial patch was grafted onto the interatrial septum. Such small suture line leaks may occur more often than has been recognized previously.

Type I ascending aortic aneurysm with aortic regurgitation

Figure 5A illustrates the transesophageal image of a patient with a Type I ascending aortic aneurysm in which the ascending aorta can be seen to be massively dilated. The intimal flap is clearly seen, separating the true lumen from the false lumen, and the defect in the intimal flap suggests a possible entrance side of the dissection. Color imaging confirmed extravasation of blood flow across the intimal tear identified on the black and white image (Fig. 5B). The mosaic of color in the true lumen reflects the turbulence of flow and in diastole, regurgitant flow can be seen extending back as far as the apex of the left ventricle because of massive aortic insufficiency (Fig. 5C). The consistently excellent quality of transesophageal images of aortic dissection promises not only to guide surgical therapy intraoperatively, but to become the diagnostic method of choice instead of the much more invasive angiography.

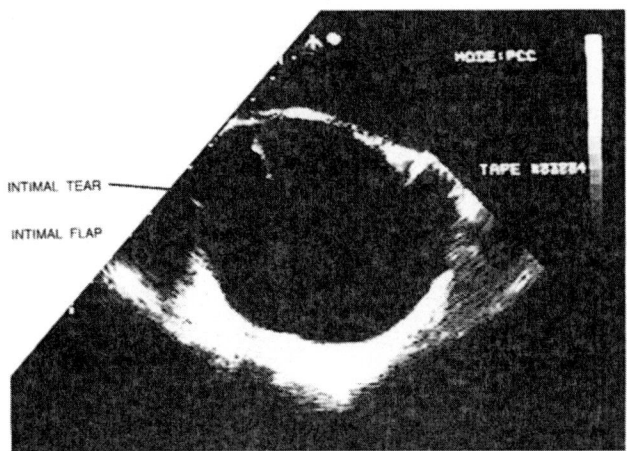

Fig. 5A. Image of the ascending aorta showing the intimal flap of a type one ascending aortic aneurysm.

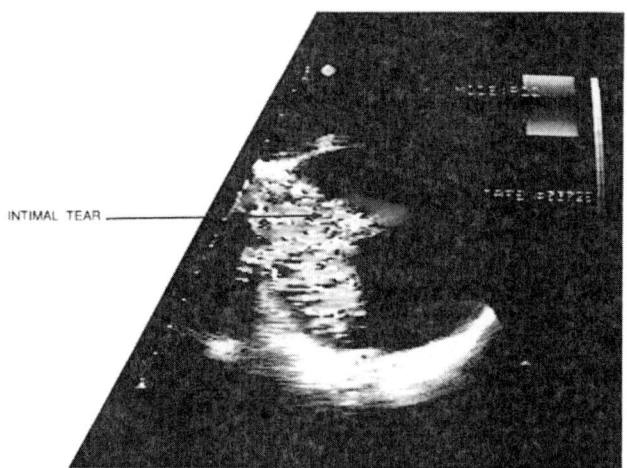

Fig. 5B. Transesophageal DCFM of the same patient confirming blood flow across the intimal tear.

Conclusions

The incorporation of Doppler color flow mapping in a transesophageal imaging system facilitates its use in the Operating Room for the intraoperative evaluation of anatomic lesions and surgical repairs; it also becomes available to the anesthesiologist to guide hemodynamic management. Thus, the effects of vasoactive drugs on valvular regurgitation or intracardiac shunting can be seen instantaneously, for example. This will be particularly helpful in

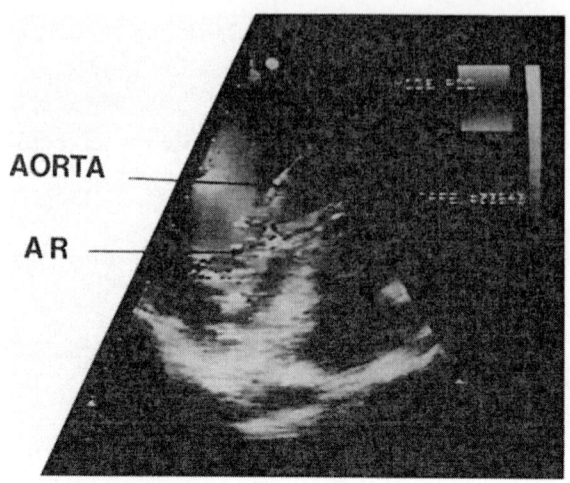

Fig. 5C. Aortic regurgitant flow extending far back into the left ventricular cavity.

patients with congenital heart disease. Our initial experience with this technique suggests that it will be relatively easy to learn, although a number of validation studies need to be done. In particular, more quantitative evaluations of Doppler flow are needed. Several investigators [6, 7] have noted that the linear dimensions of regurgitant flow, for example, generally correlated with the severity of regurgitation by cineangiography. In our own experience several patients, including a number of patients undergoing coronary artery bypass grafting, showed some degree of mitral regurgitation; this may not always be clinically significant. In addition, the technique allows the spatial orientation of flow to be determined. In two patients we observed evidence of blood flow originating from the site of surgical repair: in one patient it suggested a paravalvular leak at the mitral valve annulus and in another patient repair of the interatrial septum was followed by the development of a small right-to-left shunt.

Small leaks along suture lines may prove to be frequent occurrences detectable by Doppler color flow mapping but of little clinical significance. However, with experience, surgically unacceptable repairs my be identified and corrected promptly, to the benefit of the patient.

In addition transesophageal ultrasound techniques provide superior images compared with transthoracic techniques in patients undergoing re-operation and in the early postoperative phase after cardiac surgery.

The diagnostic potential of transesophageal DCFM in awake patients with valvular disease and in thoracic aortic dissection is largely unexplored but our initial experience indicates that it will provide an exciting extension to the cardiologist's diagnostic capabilities.

In conclusion, the development of transesophageal Doppler color flow mapping holds considerable promise for the understanding of blood flow in normal and pathological conditions, which will find clinical application in the management of patients under the care of cardiologists, anesthesiologists and surgeons.

References

1. Frazin L, Talano JV, Stephanides L, Loeb HS, Kopel L, Gunnar RM: Esophageal echo-cardiography. Circulation 54: 102–108, 1976.
2. Matsumoto M, Hanrath P, Kremer P, Tamo C, Langenstein BA, Schlüter M, Weiter R, Bleifeld W: Evaluation of left ventricular performance during supine exercise by trans-esophageal M-mode echocardiography in normal subject. Br Heart J 48: 61–66, 1982.
3. Matsumoto M, Oka Y, Strom J, Frishman W, Kadish A, Becker RM, Frater RWM, Soneblich EH: Application of transesophageal echocardiography to continuous intra-operative monitoring of left ventricular performance. Am J Cardiol 46: 95–105, 1980.
4. Schlüter M, Langenstein BA, Polster J, Kremer P, Souquet J, Engel S, Hanrath P: Trans-esophageal cross-sectional echocardiography with a phased array transducer system: technique and initial clinical results. Br Heart J 48: 67–72, 1982.
5. Schlüter M, Langenstein BA, Hanrath P, Kremer P, Bleifeld W: Assessment of transesoph-ageal pulsed Doppler echocardiography in the detection of mitral regurgitation. Circulation 66: 784–789, 1982.
6. Switzer DF, Nanda NC: Doppler color flow mapping. Ultrasound in Med and Biol 11: 403–416, 1985.
7. Myatake K, Okamoto M, Kinoshita N, Tzumi S, Owa M, Takao S, Sakakibara H, Nimura Y: Clinical applications of a new type of real-time two-dimensional flow imaging system. Am J Cardiol 54: 857–864, 1984.

PART 5: Intraoperative Echocardiography

5.1. Intraoperative evaluation of valvular disease

MARTIN E. GOLDMAN, THERESA GUARINO &
BRUCE P. MINDICH

Introduction

Routine methods for evaluation of valvular regurgitation and insufflation intraoperatively are primarily indirect and nonphysiological: inspection of the flaccid heart, digital palpation of the cardiac chambers following discontinuation of cardio-pulmonary bypass, dye curves, and hemodynamic evaluation (regurgitant 'V' waves). However, a new, more accurate technique, *intraoperative two-dimensional echocardiography* (with either contrast or real-time color-flow Doppler), can evaluate the presence and quantify the severity of residual regurgitation before and immediately following valve surgery.

Recently, the superiority of mitral valve repair over valve replacement for mitral regurgitation for both short and long term survival has been established [1, 2]. In a study by Perier, 100 mitral valve repair operations were compared to a 300 valve replacements (100 each for Starr Edwards, a disc valve, and porcine heterograft prostheses). The results demonstrated a significantly improved long-term survival in patients with valve repair [1]. However, a significant problem in valve repair surgery remains the lack of an accurate method to evaluate intraoperative regurgitation. Importantly, intraoperative echocardiography can reduce the necessary surgical learning curve for valve repair operations as well as facilitate a more aggressive approach in potentially salvaging abnormal valves [3].

Methodology

Intraoperative echocardiography can be performed with routine echocardiographic equipment. The most important aspect of the procedure is the participation and cooperation of the surgeons, cardiologists, nurses and support personnel involved in the operation. Echocardiography is best performed by the surgeon under the guidance of an echocardiographer (either a cardiologist experienced in echocardiography or a trained physician, technician, or nurse). The transducer itself is either gas sterilized or sterilely prepared by enclosing the head of the transducer (either mechanical or phased array) in a

I. Cikes (ed.), *Echocardiography in Cardiac Interventions*, 301–311, 1989.
© 1989 *Kluwer Academic Publishers*.

302

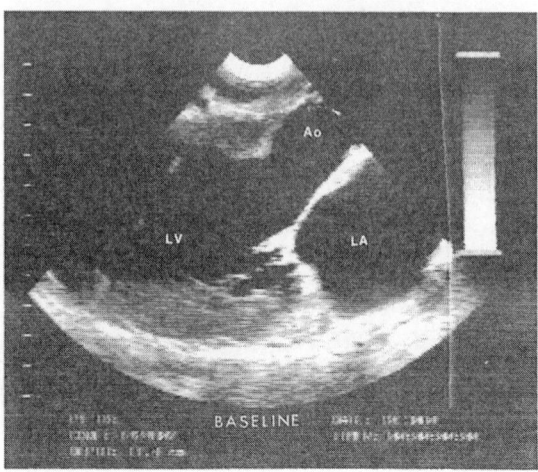

Fig. 1. Baseline Intraoperative (Long Axis View): Systolic frame (Ao = aorta, LA = left atrium, LV = left ventricle).

sterile plastic sheath and the transducer cord is enclosed in a long, sterile sheath (which can be obtained commercially or from the orthopedic suite). Though phased array transducers can be gas sterilized, the transducer elements may be damaged and the manufacturer should be consulted. Additionally, no infectious problems have been encountered by sterile draping alone. The transducer is then placed directly on the free wall of the right ventricle and minimal manipulation of the transducer can easily obtain a modified long axis, complete short axis sweep from the base to the apex, right ventricular inflow and outflow views (Fig. 1). With special phased array transducers, an apical approach may be possible. All four cardiac valves and cardiac chambers can be assessed.

The intraoperative echocardiographic appearance of the mitral valve assists the surgeon in determining whether the valve is appropriate for repair or the excessive calcification or fibrosis necessitates valve replacement. Additionally, by visualizing the aortic valve, the surgeon can assess the extent of the aortic excursion and degree of calcifications. The entire tricuspid valve apparatus can be viewed in a modified right ventricular inflow plane to assess coaptation of the tricuspid leaflets. All this is performed after the patient has been cannulated yet still in sinus or baseline rhythm. This is the most physiological evaluation of valvular function possible in the operating room.

Intraoperative contrast echocardiography

Contrast is generated by insertion of a long spinal needle through the inter-ventricular septum into the left ventricle or right ventricle. 5cc of agitated D_5W or normal saline is cleared of all visible bubbles and injected rapidly generating microbubbles of approximately 5 to 100 microns in diameter which are easily visible echocardiographically. Parenthetically, a similar volume of microbubbles is occasionally visualized spontaneously during open heart surgery and is probably related to sequestered air in the emptied heart or opened atria [4]. Importantly, both spontaneous and injected micro-bubbles produce no neurological complications as evidenced by more than 600 intraoperative contrast echocardiograms performed in our institution.

The extent of regurgitation can easily be assessed by the injection of contrast into a particular chamber and visualizing either normal, antegrade exiting of the microbubbles or retrograde reflux in the presence of regurgita-tion. For evaluation of mitral regurgitation, contrast is injected into the left ventricle which normally exits out the aorta (Figs. 2, 3). However, with mitral regurgitation, there is reflux into the left atrium of varying amounts of micro-bubbles which can be quantified depending upon the extent and severity of mitral regurgitation: 0 is no reflux, 1 to 2+ is minimal degree, 3 to 4+ is significant regurgitation, with a similar density of microbubbles in left atrium as in the left ventricle, as well as a long duration for total clearance of the left atrium of microbubbles. For evaluation of the tricuspid regurgitation, micro-

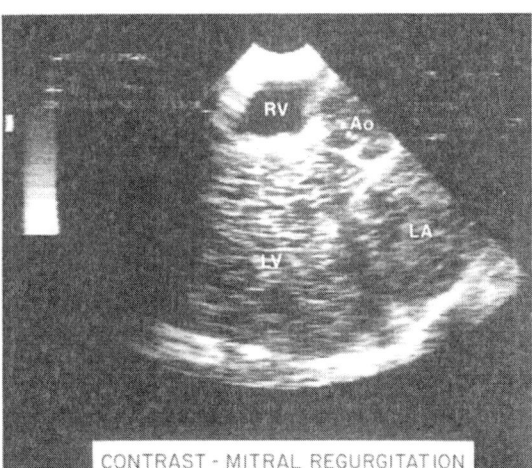

Fig. 2. Contrast Injection (Long Axis, Mitral Regurgitation): Microbubbles injected into the left ventricle completely fill the left atrium as well, consistent with severe mitral regurgitation (RV = right ventricle).

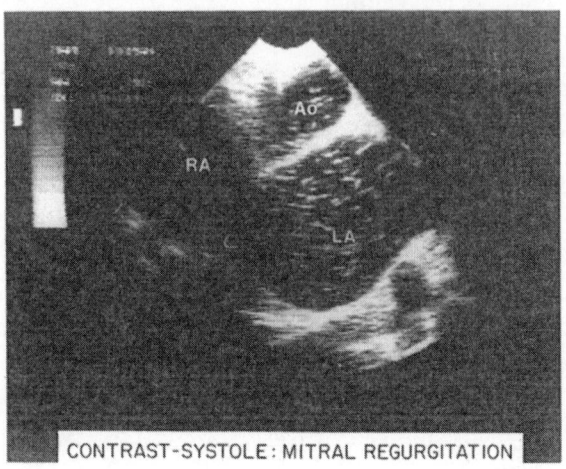

CONTRAST-SYSTOLE: MITRAL REGURGITATION

Fig. 3. Contrast Injection (Short Axis, Mitral Regurgitation): Microbubbles injected into the left ventricle are seen exiting out the aorta (Ao) as well as refluxing into the left atrium (LA).

bubbles are injected into the right ventricle with normal flow exiting antegrade out the pulmonary artery with reflux into the right atrium occuring with tricuspid regurgitation. A similar grading system is used as in mitral regurgitation. Assessment of aortic regurgitation is more difficult since aortic reflux is difficult to assess with routine injections. Therefore, larger infusions via the aortic cannula may be of benefit in assessing the reflux; however, quantification may be more difficult and require more experience than the atrio-ventricular valves. Pulmonic insufficiency is also assessible by this contrast technique. If microbubbles dissipate after two to three injections, continued agitation or new syringe and tubing system may be necessary to create additional contrast. Also, the mixing of the injectate with a few cc's of blood is valuable in increasing the echogenecity of the bubbles.

There are several technical limitations of intraoperative echocardiography. Caution must be applied to avoid too vigorous an injection of contrast wich may cause ventricular irritability and subsequent arrhythmias which may yield false positive evidence of valvular regurgitation. The most difficult technical aspect of the procedure is to continuously visualize the heart throughout the cardiac cycle. The transducer, being placed directly on the free wall of the right ventricle, is prone to significant rocking motion. However, if there is an adequate gel interface, and the surgeon has a light touch with the transducer and rides the heart, the entire cardiac cycle can be seen. A pericardial water bath (the filling of the pericardial sac with fluid) may provide an imaging medium for improved visualization of the heart without requiring direct epicardial contact.

Color flow (real-time) Doppler echocardiography

Valvular regurgitation can also be evaluated intraoperatively with color flow (real-time) echocardiography. In this technique, ultrasound information is analyzed along two circuits: one for the real-time anatomical information presented in black and white and the second for the color-coded Doppler flow information over a wide sector presented in superimposition over the anatomical image [5]. Blood flow moving towards the transducer is displayed in shades of red and blood flow away from the transducer is in shades of blue. Lighter shades represent higher velocities while mosaic or multi-color shading represents turbulent flow. Routine pulsed or continuous wave Doppler analyzes frequency shifts along a single beam, but is extremely tedious, time-consuming, technically difficult and potentially inaccurate in the operating room because of the limited angles available to interrogate the specific chambers. However, color flow Doppler accurately displays flow within 3° of the perpendicular plane. Therefore, even in the limited views available intraoperatively, color flow Doppler can be used to evaluate valvular regurgitation (Fig. 4). The major limitation of color-flow is the cost of the equipment, the greater technical skill required for the more complex instrumentation, and importantly the large size of the machine. Color flow intraoperatively avoids the necessity for contrast injections and the potential for false positives from that technique. Also, with real-time Doppler echocardiography intraoperatively, every single beat can be assessed not only those with injected contrast.

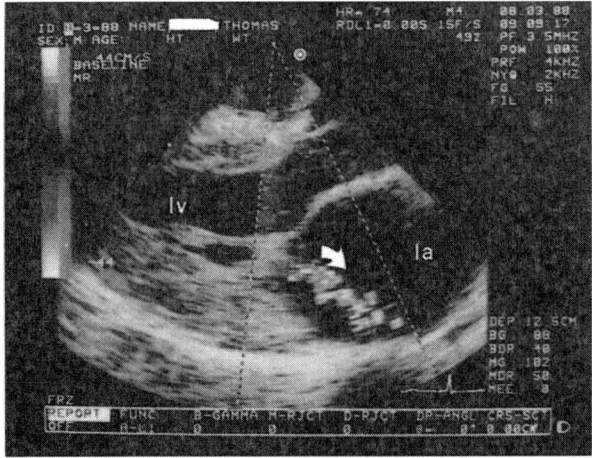

Fig. 4. Intraoperative Color Flow Doppler (Long Axis, Mitral Regurgitation): Systolic jet is seen in left atrium.

Mitral regurgitation

Our experience in intraoperative echocardiography began with the evaluation of mitral regurgitation and we have thus far performed over 300 intraoperative evaluations for the presence or absence of mitral regurgitation [3]. We have not had any untoward reactions (specifically CNS nor infectious problems). When intraoperative echocardiography was compared to preoperative angiography for the detection of the presence or absence of mitral regurgitation the yield was excellent (sensitivity = 100%, specificity = 100%). More importantly, intraoperative echocardiography compared favorably with preoperative catheterization, for quantification of mitral regurgitation of the severity on a scale of 0 to 4+ (r = .93 in 125 patients). Following either valve replacement or repair, the mitral valve can be reassessed after the patient is weaned from cardio-pulmonary bypass, but still cannulated (Fig. 5). If the systemic pressure is low, a vasopressor may be utilized to more accurately simulate physiological circumstances in evaluation of valve function. However, if there is significant valve dysfunction, it can usually be detected even at lower pressures. Mitral annular ring prostheses are an important aspect of valve repair for maintaining valve competency and may be valuable in the long term function of the valve to reduce subsequent dilatation and prolapse.

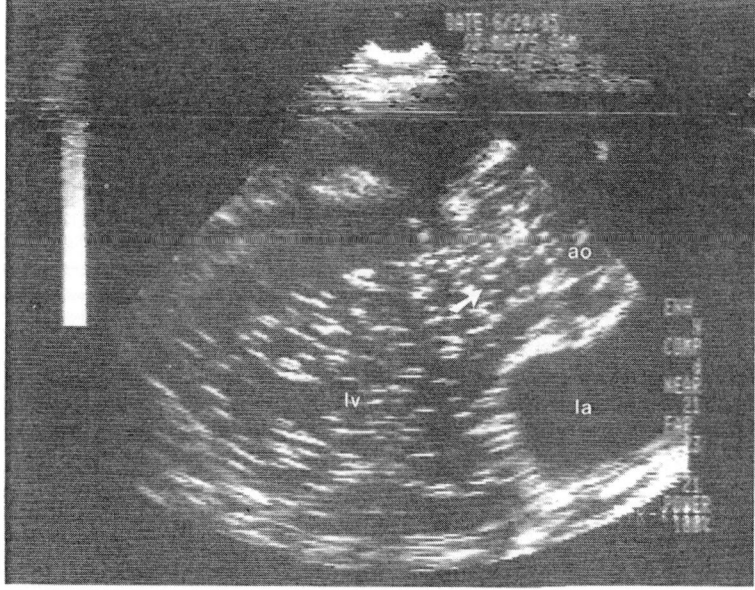

Fig. 5. Post-procedure Contrast Injection (Long Axis): All microbubbles exit out the aorta and none reflux into the left atrium, confirming a good mitral repair.

We have found intraoperative echocardiography extremely useful in evaluating both valve repair and replacement. Specifically, we have had several instances in which malfunction of disc or ball prosthetic valves have been detected immediately following weaning of the patient off cardiopulmonary bypass. In these situations, residual strands of chordae tendineae have been wedged through the valve, the valve has been mis-seated or the valve itself was malfunctioning. However, this was detected before decannulation and was promptly revised. Additionally, continued significant regurgitation, occasionally due to mitral valve prolapse, has been detected following valve repair. Using the short axis view at the level of the aorta and left atrium, the specific location of the regurgitation can be detected. The patient, who is still cannulated, can be replaced on bypass and the valve re-repaired or replaced.

Because of the improved long-term survival of patients with mitral valve repair compared to replacement in pure mitral regurgitation, intraoperative echocardiography can reduce the learning curve as well as improve long-term results in those patients undergoing mitral repair.

Tricuspid valve disease

Tricuspid regurgitation can be due to either primary abnormalities of the valve (rheumatic, carcinoid) in which the valve leaflets and apparatus are fibrosed and calcified, or in the majority of cases, secondary to right ventricular volume or pressure overload. The preoperative evaluation of the extent of the tricuspid regurgitation clinically or angiographically is difficult. Color flow Doppler used in the echocardiography lab may be the most accurate method for quantifying tricuspid regurgitation. However, the expense of this technique may preclude its widespread intraoperative application.

In our experience, intraoperative echo has had an excellent sensitivity and specificity compared to preoperative Doppler and cardiac catheterization for detection of tricuspid regurgitation [6]. More important, however, is the correlation of dilated tricuspid annuli with the severity of tricuspid regurgitation [7]. Secondary tricuspid regurgitation is due to dilatation of the annulus secondary to dilatation of the right ventricle. The persistence of tricuspid regurgitation following left-sided heart operation may be dependent upon two factors: severity of pulmonary hypertension, and its rate of reduction following surgery and the degree of tricuspid annular dilatation. If on the baseline intraoperative evaluation, pulmonary pressures are elevated and the annulus is markedly dilated with significant tricuspid regurgitation, the surgeon should consider repairing the tricuspid valve at the same time as the initial mitral operation. However, if the surgeon considers the tricuspid regurgitation to be a secondary finding which may decrease precipitously following repair of the left-sided lesion, he can reassess the tricuspid valve once the left-sided lesion has been repaired and the patient is weaned off cardio-pulmonary bypass.

In our experience, markedly dilated annuli rarely shrink significantly post-operatively and persistent tricuspid regurgitation persists as a major post-operative problem. Additionally, studies have shown that persistent severe tricuspid regurgitation increases the long term morbidity and mortality in patients undergoing mitral operations. Therefore, intraoperative assessment of tricuspid regurgitation by either contrast two-dimensional echocardiography or color flow intraoperatively may be very useful in detecting those patients in whom the tricuspid valve should be repaired.

Aortic valve disease

As mentioned previously, aortic regurgitation is more difficult to assess and quantify with contrast echocardiography than the atrio-ventricular valves. However, those patients with 3 to 4+ aortic regurgitation can usually be identified quite easily with either color flow imaging or contrast injections directly into the aortic root with larger volumes infused through the aortic cannula (Fig. 6). Echocardiography can also detect residual aortic regurgitation intraoperatively following aortic valve or root repair [8].

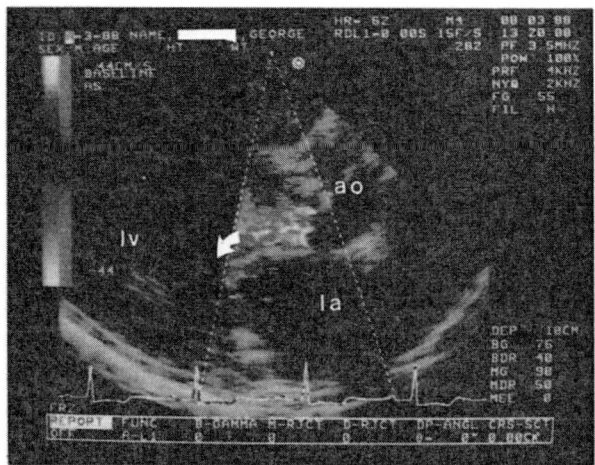

Fig. 6. Intraoperative Color Flow Doppler (Long Axis, Aortic Regurgitation): Though the aortic valve is closed, the LV outflow tract is entirely colored in greenish hues, indicating significant AR.

Myocardial function

The assessment of ventricular function is one of the most important applications of intraoperative echocardiography [9]. This is invaluable in valvular heart disease when assessing the patient coming off cardiopulmonary bypass. If there is difficulty in weaning the patient, echocardiography can be introduced to differentiate between myocardial dysfunction and residual valve malfunction. As we have previously reported, ventricular function is maintained following mitral valve repair for mitral regurgitation, however, it declines immediately following mitral valve replacement. Ventricular function is stable following valve repair or valve replacement if the papillary muscles are spared.

Mitral stenosis

Intraoperative echocardiography can easily assess the valve area and severity of the regurgitation in mitral stenosis both immediately before and following commissurotomy or valve replacement. Using intraoperative echocardiography, the mitral valve apparatus can be assessed and the potential for valve repair can be determined. The post cardiopulmonary bypass echocardiogram can localize areas of residual regurgitation along commissure lines both in the long and short axis views.

Hypertrophic cardiomyopathy, myxomas

Patients with hypertrophic cardiomyopathy have left ventricular outflow obstruction due to the apposition of the anterior leaflet of the mitral valve against the septum (several authors believe that this is dynamic, not a physical obstruction) which can also generate mitral regurgitation. Following myomectomy, there may be continued mitral regurgitation if there has been damage to the underlying mitral apparatus. Therefore, intraoperative echocardiography facilitates intraoperative evaluation of both ventricular function following myomectomy as well as the severity of any residual mitral regurgitation.

Left atrial myxomas may sometimes cause damage of the mitral valve and the potential residual regurgitation following excision of the myxoma can be assessed with intraoperative 2D echo [10].

Comparison of intraoperative contrast vs. color flow echocardiography

Both intraoperative contrast and color flow echocardiography can detect the presence and relative severity of regurgitation. However, while contrast echocardiography requires injection of agitated fluid into a cardiac chamber and has the potential for false positive results, color flow echocardiography requires no injections and can detect beat to beat changes in severity of regurgitation. Though intraoperative echocardiography with contrast can be performed with any two-dimensional instrument, color flow requires much more expensive, elaborate, and technically difficult equipment.

Transesophageal echocardiography

Transesophageal echocardiography incorporates a small phased array transducer on the tip of a routine gastroscope, which is then inserted through the oropharynx into the esophagus and positioned in a retrocardiac position [11, 12]. The echocardiographic views available transesophageally are similar to those obtained by epicardial intraoperative echocardiography. Additionally, a modified four-chamber view is also possible which allows the potential use of routine pulsed Doppler echocardiography as well as contrast or color flow echocardiography. Transesophageal echocardiography is usually performed by the anesthesiologist. The advantages are that it does not require the surgeon to perform echocardiography and allows surgery to continue uninterrupted. Transesophageal echocardiography can perform similar valvular evaluations for regurgitation and stenosis as epicardial echocardiography.

Conclusion

Intraoperative echocardiography allows improved assessment of valve function and allows closer inspection of the valve apparatus under physiological circumstances. The possibility of valve repair can be determined before the patient has gone on cardiopulmonary bypass and valve function can be visualized immediately following repair or replacement following weaning from cardiopulmonary bypass. Intraoperative echocardiography will allow surgeons to be more aggressive in attempts at salvaging native valves and potentially reduce morbidity and mortality from valvular surgery.

References

1. Perier P, Deloche A, Chauvaud S, Fabiani JN, Rossant R, Beesou JP, Relland J, Bourezak H, Gomez F, Bloudeau P, D'Allaines C, Carpentier A: Comparative evaluation of mitral valve repair and replacement with Starr, Bjork, and porcine valve prostheses. Circulation 70 (suppl. I) I; 187–1982, 1984.
2. David TE, Uden De, Strauss HD: The importance of the mitral apparatus in left ventricular function after correction of mitral regurgitation. Circulation 68 (suppl. II) II: 76–82, 1983.
3. Goldman ME, Mindich BP, Stavile K, Teichholtz LE, Fuster VF: Intraoperative contrast two-dimensional echocardiography to assess mitral valve operations. J Am Coll Cardiol 4: 1035–40, 1984.
4. Rodigas PC, Meyer JM, Haasler GB, Dubroff JM, Spotnitz HM: Intraoperative two-dimensional echocardiography: ejection of microbubbles from the left ventricle after cardiac surgery. Am J Cardiol 50: 1130–1132, 1982.
5. Miyatake K, Okamoto M, Kinoshita N, et al.: Clinical applications of a new real-time two-dimensional Doppler flow imaging system. Am J Cardiol 54: 857–868, 1984.
6. Goldman ME, Mindich BP, Guarino T, Fuster V: Intraoperative contrast echo: a new method to evaluate tricuspid regurgitation (abstr.) J Am Coll Cardiol 5: 459, 1985.
7. Goldman ME, Guarino T, Fuster V, Mindich B: The necessity for tricuspid valve repair can be determined intraoperatively by two-dimensional echocardiography. The Journal of Thoracic and Cardiovascular Surgery 94: 542–50, 1987.
8. Mindich BP, Guarino T, Goldman ME: Aortic valvuloplasty for acquired aortic stenosis. Circulation 74 (supp. I): 1130–1135.
9. Dubroff JM, Clark MB, Wong CYH, Spotnitz AJ, Collins RH, Spotnitz HM: Left ventricular ejection fraction during cardiac surgery: a two-dimensional echocardiographic study. Circulation 68: 95–103, 1983.
10. Mora F, Mindich BP, Guarino T, Goldman ME: Improved surgical approach to cardiac tumors with intraoperative two-dimensional echocardiography. Chest 91: 142–44, 1987.
11. Beaupre PN, Kremer PF, Cahalan MK, Lurz FW, Schiller NB, Hamilton WK: Intraoperative detection of changes in left ventricular segmental wall motion by transesophageal two-dimensional echocardiography. Am Heart J 107: 1021–1023, 1984.
12. Konstadt SN, Thys D, Mindich BP, Kaplan JA, Goldman ME: Validation of quantitative intraoperative transesophageal echocardiography. Anesthesiology 65: 418–21, 1986.

5.2. Intraoperative echocardiography in valvular heart disease — quantitative study of left ventricular properties

HENRY M. SPOTNITZ, MARIA L. ANTUNES, MICHAEL B. CLARK, CALVIN Y. H. WONG & ROBERT C. ROBBINS

Our experience with intraoperative studies in valvular heart disease began with M-mode studies of left ventricular compliance [1]. In the course of those studies, dramatic reductions in left ventricular ejection fraction during valve replacement became apparent [2]. Subsequently, we applied phased-array technology intraoperatively, using gas-sterilized transducers applied gently to the anterior surface of the right ventricle in patients cannulated for cardio-pulmonary bypass (Fig. 1) to produce high-quality short axis views and partial long-axis sections as well (Fig. 2). This early work demonstrated that two-dimensional echocardiography employed in this way is safe and can provide images useful for both qualitative and quantitative purposes [3].

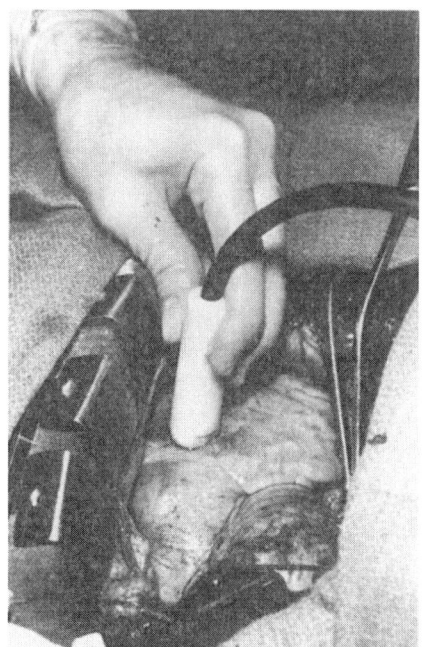

Fig. 1. Gas-sterilized phased-array transducer applied gently to the anterior surface of the right ventricle permits intraoperative two-dimensional echocardiography without significant ar-rhythmias.

I. Cikes (ed.), *Echocardiography in Cardiac Interventions*, 313–330, 1989.
© 1989 *Kluwer Academic Publishers.*

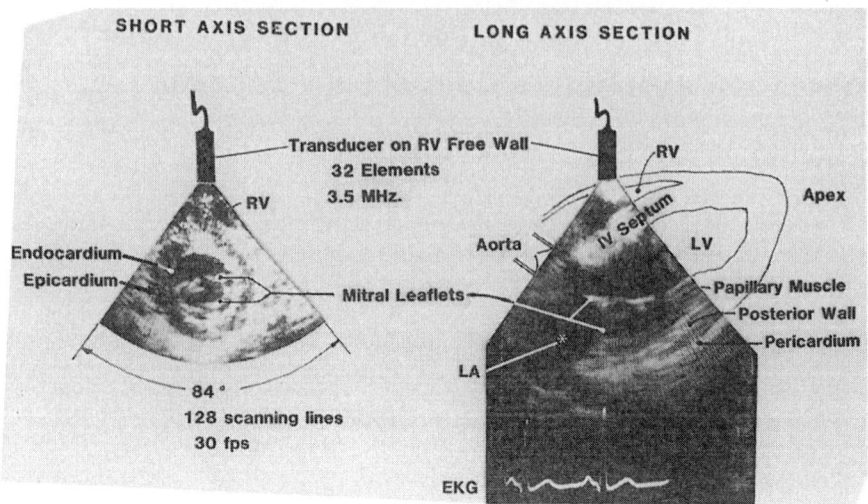

Fig. 2. Representative two-dimensional echocardiograms. Use of the right ventricle as a stand-off enhances echo sections of the left ventricle. Short axis views are readily obtained at multiple levels, but interference from the sternum prevents quantitatively useful images encompassing the entire long axis.

Subsequently, transesophageal echocardiography has been shown to be useful for these purposes as well [4], with the additional benefits of continuous imaging and applicability during high-risk surgery which does not provide exposure of the heart (e.g., abdominal aortic aneurysm resection). The morbidity resulting from insertion of an esophageal probe in anesthetized patients apparently has been minimal, though consequences of a perforated esophagus could be grave. The benefits of echo contrast for assessing integrity of valve repair have also been demonstrated in studies based on mechanical scanners contained by a sterile sleeve [5]. Color-flow doppler also may be useful at surgery [6]. Techniques for echo visualization of the coronary arteries have also been reported [6a]. We will limit the present discussion to our quantitative studies of ventricular properties in patients undergoing valve replacement surgery, as other related material is covered elsewhere in this book. Our experience has demonstrated that two-dimensional echocardiography is valuable for studies of ejection fraction, mass, compliance, and (in combination with other data) systolic mechanics of the left ventricle during valve replacement surgery.

Technical notes

Consoles brought into the operating room must be disinfected to meet local epidemiologic standards, and equipment must be cleaned to avoid accidental release of dust from within the equipment by cooling fans. All equipment must be periodically tested for electrical leaks. Extender cables, permitting the equipment to be placed 12 feet from the surgical field are advantageous. Finally, the transducers must be sterilized. The choices are soaking in bactericides, gas sterilization, or encasing the transducer in a sterile sleeve. We prefer gas sterilization, but this is associated with accelerated degradation of transducer elements. It is also hazardous to mechanical transducers with liquid lenses or water paths, since the uptake of gas bubbles will degrade the image and require first aid at the operating table. Sterile sleeves can degrade image quality and must be water tight to ensure sterility.

The merits of phased-array vs. mechanical scanning technology are open to debate. Phased-array offers the theoretical benefit of custom-made, low-profile, right-angle transducers, which can provide special views from the lateral or posterior aspects of the heart when required. Phased-array equipment is also preferable for transesophageal work and has advantages for research studies as well, though the increased cost is a major disadvantage.

Ejection fraction

Our intraoperative measurements of alterations in ejection fraction are based on data obtained immediately prior to cardiopulmonary bypass and immediately after the conclusion of bypass, before protamine administration. Data reported here reflect studies in stable patients not requiring infusions of vasoactive drugs at the time of study. All operations were performed with myocardial protection by hyperkalemic, albumin-fortified crystalloid cardioplegia. Most measurements of ejection fraction are based on end-diastolic area (EDA) and end-systolic area (ESA) provided by computerized light-penning of videotaped images, with 'EF' = (EDA-ESA) $\times$ 100%/EDA. Ejection fraction measured in this way has proven sufficiently accurate ($r = .80$ vs, RAO angography) and reproducible in patients with valvular heart disease, although we prefer the multiple-section method of Quinones (7) ($r = .89$ vs RAO angriography) in patients with significant asymmetry of LV wall motion. Our results in valve replacement surgery for mitral valve disease are presented in Fig. 3 and for aortic valve disease in Fig. 4. These data are consistent with our earlier observations [3, 8] and indicate that most patients undergoing valve replacement for aortic or mitral regurgitation experience substantial decreases in intraoperative ejection fraction, while the opposite is true for relief of valvular stenosis. Decreased preload may be contributory in some patients. These differences are consistent and cannot be explained by differences in surgical technique, valves used, operative time or other systematic differences between groups. Late follow-up in mitral

316

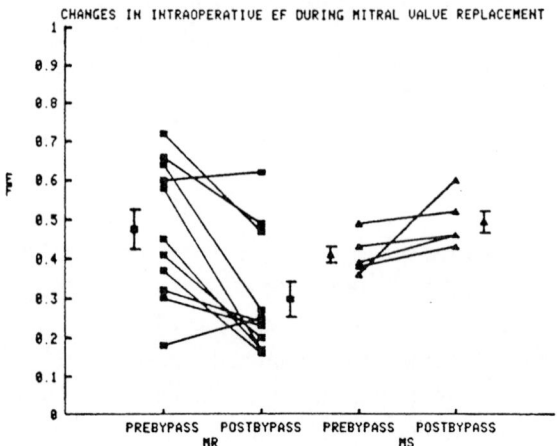

Fig. 3. Effects of mitral valve replacement on prebypass and postbypass echocardiographic EF. Intraoperative EF decreased (left) in 9/11 patients with mitral regurgitation and increased in 5/5 with mitral stenosis (right). Mean values are also plotted with standard error bars.

regurgitation patients indicates that the intraoperative measurements are generally predictive of late ejection fraction, although ejection fraction is somewhat improved in late studies (Fig. 5). These observations are similar to other studies of valve replacement surgery [9, 10] which have stimulated reports, as yet inconclusive, that depressed postoperative ejection fraction in mitral regurgitation can be avoided by valve repair [11], earlier intervention in class II patients [12], or innovative methods of valve replacement [13]. Our studies in the absence of altered loading conditions suggest that ejection fraction of the undamaged LV increases slightly intraoperatively, apparently due to catecholamine release.

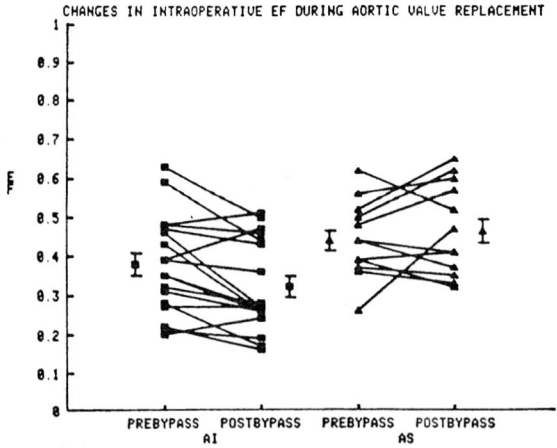

Fig. 4. Similar to Fig. 3, intraoperative EF decreased in 15/18 patients during valve replacement for aortic regurgitation but increased in 6/12 during valve replacement for aortic stenosis.

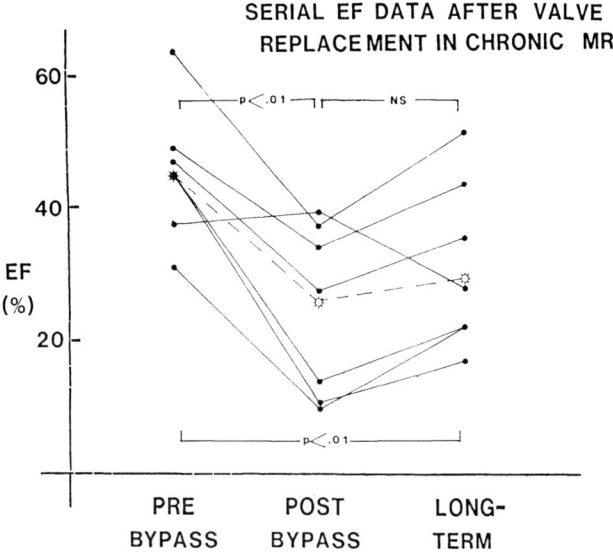

Fig. 5. Prebypass, postbypass, and long-term (6–18 months postoperative) EF in 7 patients after valve replacement for chronic mitral regurgitation. Mean results are indicated by open symbols and the dashed line. In 6/7 patients, intraoperative EF was predictive of EF at late follow-up, which increased but remained lower than the preoperative value.

Left ventricular mass

Our echo methods are based on echocardiographic detection of the endocardial border of the left ventricle, used to define end-diastolic volume, and of the epicardial border, which allows LV mass to be designated as the geometric space between the epicardium and endocardium [14,15]. Echo studies are videotaped and later analyzed using stop-motion, freeze-frame techniques and a computerized light pen. Human intelligence is used for definition of echo boundaries. In dogs we use a gel-filled pericardial well and three echo sections. The sections are paired for analysis by a Simpson's rule algorithm, and results are subsequently averaged. This method has proven quite accurate for mass studies in dogs, as demonstrated by a correlation coefficient of .95 for the relation of echocardiographic mass in vivo to true postmortem weight of the trimmed left ventricle in the last twenty-eight studies done in our laboratory by three blinded investigators working independently.

Global ischemic injury and reperfusion in dogs (Fig. 6) increases LV mass 18–30% [14–17]. The increased mass is quantitatively consistent with increases in myocardial water content of 2–4% measured concurrently [14] and is accompanied by decreased left ventricular compliance [16] and a 10% mean increase in wall thickness [14]. However, the relevance of these obser-

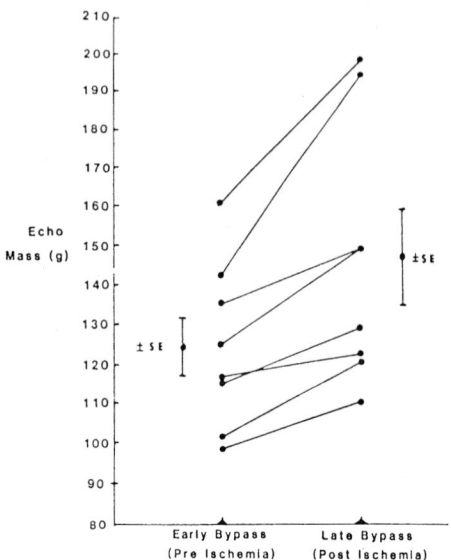

Fig. 6. Effect of severe global ischemic injury (45 minutes at normothermia) during cardio-pulmonary bypass on echocardiographic LV mass in eight dogs. Preischemic and post-reperfusion data are displayed. Mass increased in every experiment, with an overall mean increase of 18%. Two-thirds of this mass increase were accounted for by a 2% increase in myo-cardial water content. The edema reflects impaired volume regulation associated with ischemic injury and is easily detectable by the two-dimensional echo methods used.

vations to human surgery is dimished somewhat by the observation that close experimental simulation of the conditions of human surgery is still associated with a 14% increase in left ventricular mass in dogs [18], while studies during routine human surgery demonstrate no mass increase [17].

Our algorithms for human left ventricular mass intraoperatively are based on one (r = .76 vs. RAO angiography) or three (r = .81 vs. RAO angiography) short axis sections and do not appear substantially preload dependent for limited changes in preload observed intraoperatively in the working human heart. Our studies in humans suggest that mass changes, when they occur, are considerably less than observed in dogs. Furthermore, our ability to detect changes may be affected by our inability to obtain accurate long axis views.

Our studies during valve replacement surgery suggest that mass increases do occur in patients undergoing correction of valvular regurgitation and that depressed preoperative ejection fraction is associated with increased suscep-tibility to increasing mass at surgery. Relevant data are illustrated in Fig. 7 for 34 patients during valve replacement for aortic or mitral regurgitation. Patients were divided into 'high' and 'low' groups on the basis of pre-bypass intraoperative ejection fraction, and relevant data are presented in Table 1. While observed alterations in left ventricular mass were not statistically sig-

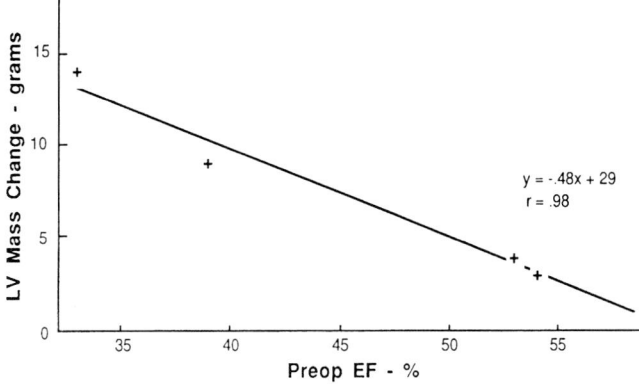

Fig. 7. Relation of prebypass EF in four groups of patients with mitral or aortic regurgitation to mean intraoperative change in LV mass. Largest increases in mass are seen in patients with lowest preoperative EF (see Table 1).

nificant within individual groups, the relation of alterations in mass to EF is striking and suggests an increased susceptibility to increased mass in patients with decreased EF. The underlying hypothesis of this analysis is that increasing mass at surgery reflects ventricular injury and that chronic volume overload increases susceptibility to ischemic damage et surgery.

Another approach to the same issue is based on the segregation of patients according to alterations of end-diastolic volume (derived from EDA)

Table 1. Mean results – aortic/mitral regurgitation study.

	Mitral hi	Mitral low	Aortic hi	Aortic low
Number of patients	7	5	11	11
EF pre (%)	0.54 ± .03*#	0.39 ± .02	0.53 ± .02*	0.33 ± .01
EF post (%)	0.36 ± .04*	0.33 ± .02	0.45 ± .02*	0.30 ± .02
LVM pre (g)	200 ± 13	216 ± 17	227 ± 12	241 ± 16
LVM post (g)	203 ± 12	225 ± 21	231 ± 12	225 ± 15
EDV pre (ml)	148 ± 11*	131 ± 7	153 ± 10*	162 ± 12*
EDV post (ml)	129 ± 09*	135 ± 6	130 ± 07*	150 ± 10*
ESV pre (ml)	68 ± 8*	81 ± 6*	71 ± 4	109 ± 9
ESV post (ml)	84 ± 10*	90 ± 4*	71 ± 5	106 ± 9
ESWS/ESV pre	0.71 ± .04	0.71 ± .03*	0.79 ± .04*	0.61 ± .07*
ESWS/ES post	0.69 ± .03	0.63 ± .04*	0.63 ± .04*	0.50 ± .05*

Mean ± S.E.M.

* $p < .05$, pre vs. post.

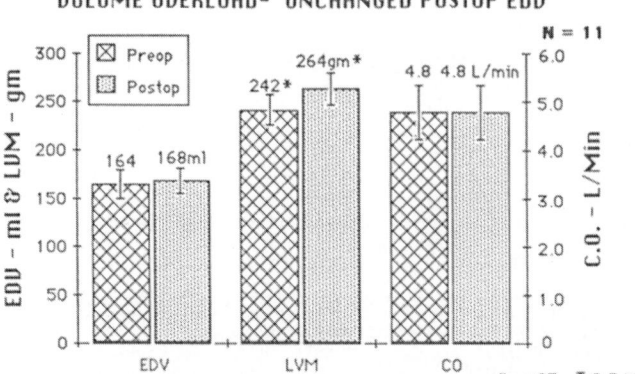

Fig. 8. Mean values for pre- and postbypass end-diastolic volume, LV mass, and cardiac output in 11 patients during valve replacement for aortic or mitral regurgitation. Patients were selected for minimal effects of surgery on end-diastolic volume. Mean EDV and cardiac output are unchanged, and a statistically significant 10% increase in LV mass is apparent.

measured at surgery. In eleven patients selected because end-diastolic volume did not change after valve replacement (Fig. 8), no improvement in cardiac output occurred postoperatively and left ventricular mass increased. In six patients in whom end-diastolic volume decreased during valve replacement for aortic or mitral regurgitation (Fig. 9), end-diastolic volume decreased significantly from 203 to 154 ml, and cardiac output increased significantly from 4.1 to 5.6 l/min. No change in left ventricular mass was observed. This suggests that the failure to observe a decrease in end-diastolic

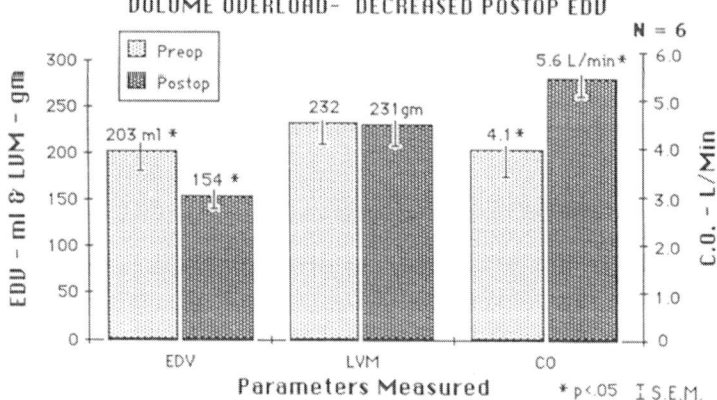

Fig. 9. In contrast to Fig. 8, these 7 patients, selected for a decrease in intraoperative end-diastolic volume, also demonstrate a significant increase in cardiac output and no change in LV mass.

volume or an increase in cardiac output during valve replacement for mitral or aortic regurgitation may reflect inadequate myocardial protection with edema formation and an increase in left ventricular mass.

Left ventricular compliance

Our studies of left ventricular compliance initially were based on M-mode echocardiography and utilized a low-profile 5 mHz transducer mounted in a silastic disk. This was placed in the posterior pericardium while left ventricular pressures were measured with a catheter-tip micromanometer during filling and emptying of the left ventricle on cardiopulmonary bypass. The relation between end-diastolic pressure and end-diastolic diameter was used to define changes in left ventricular compliance. These studies initially suggested that left ventricular injury could be detected as a decrease in left ventricular compliance in surgery performed prior to the availability of cardioplegia [1]. Presently, we no longer use unguided m-mode echo, but utilize an M-mode cursor visually guided in real time across the maximal diameter of the left ventricle using the corresponding two-dimensional image. End-diastolic pressure and diameter are digitized and analyzed by exponential curve-fitting (Fig. 10). With this technique, we have seen decreased compliance during valve replacement surgery (Fig. 11). Our M-mode

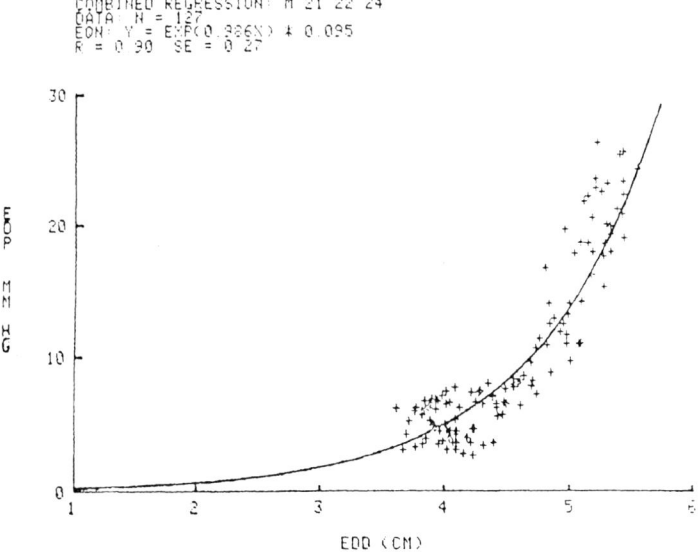

Fig. 10. Representative example of the relation between end-diastolic LV diameter (EDD) and LVEDP in 127 cardiac styles. A computer-fitted exponential curve is displayed.

322

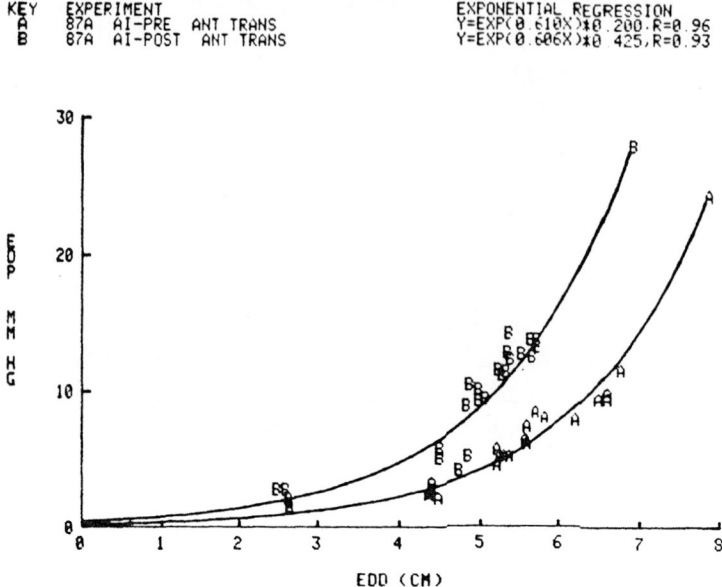

KEY   EXPERIMENT   EXPONENTIAL REGRESSION
 A   87A   AI-PRE   ANT TRANS   Y=EXP(0.610X)*0.200,R=0.96
 B   87A   AI-POST ANT TRANS   Y=EXP(0.606X)*0.425,R=0.93

Fig. 11. Similar to fig. 11, EDP-EDD curves before (A) and after (B) valve replacement for aortic regurgitation are illustrated. Excellent hemodynamics and increased intraoperative EF suggested that the observed decrease in compliance represent effects of edema, rather than ischemic ventricular injury.

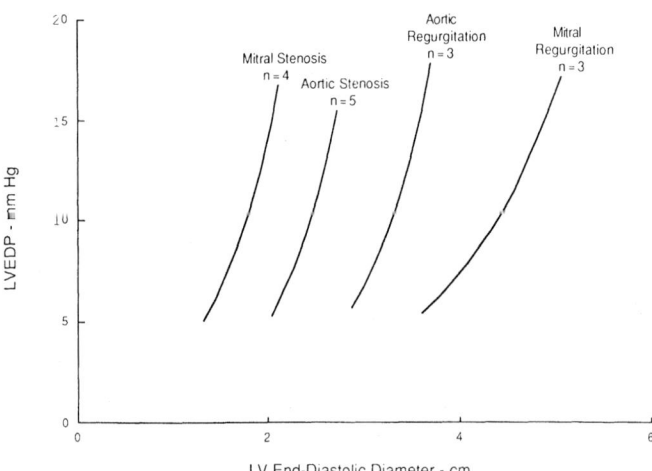

Fig. 12. Mean intraoperative EDP-EDD relations measured by M-mode echocardiography in patients undergoing valve replacement for mitral stenosis, aortic stenosis, aortic regurgitation, and mitral regurgitation. Curves were derived by exponential curve fitting to initial EDP-EDD data, followed by averaging of base constants and exponents. Despite the small number of patients, increased LV diameter and decreased slope in valvular regurgitation are apparent.

studies provided a view of the relation between various forms of surgical heart disease and the shape of the end-diastolic pressure diameter curve which is presented in Fig. 12. The diameters are somewhat compressed by the nature of the retrocardiac M-mode data, and while an analysis based on recent methods is still in progress, these earlier results appear qualitatively correct.

Left ventricular mechanics

In addition to intraoperative two-dimensional echocardiography, recordings of left ventricular pressure, aortic flow, and dp/dt provide a data base for study of ventricular mechanics. Thse data are obtained intraoperatively with patient consent by positioning a dual-sensor aortic and left ventricular pressure micromanometer across the aortic valve via the cardioplegia injection site and adding a scissors type electromagnetic flow probe to the aortic root. Representative tracings are illustrated in Fig. 13, and representative tracings of the time course of left ventricular wall stress before and after valve replacement surgery for representative lesions are presented in Figs. 14–18. The changes observed reflect significant ventricular unloading in both aortic stenosis and regurgitation, while increased afterload commonly occurs in

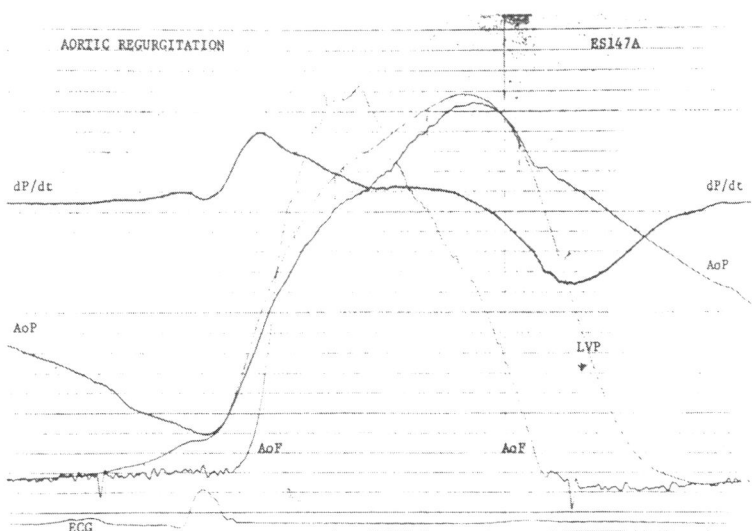

Fig. 13. Analog tracings of LV (LVP) and aortic (AoP) pressures and dP/dt by micromanometer are plotted with electromagnetic flow (AoF) and the electrocardiogram (ECG) during surgery immediately prior to valve replacement for aortic regurgitation.

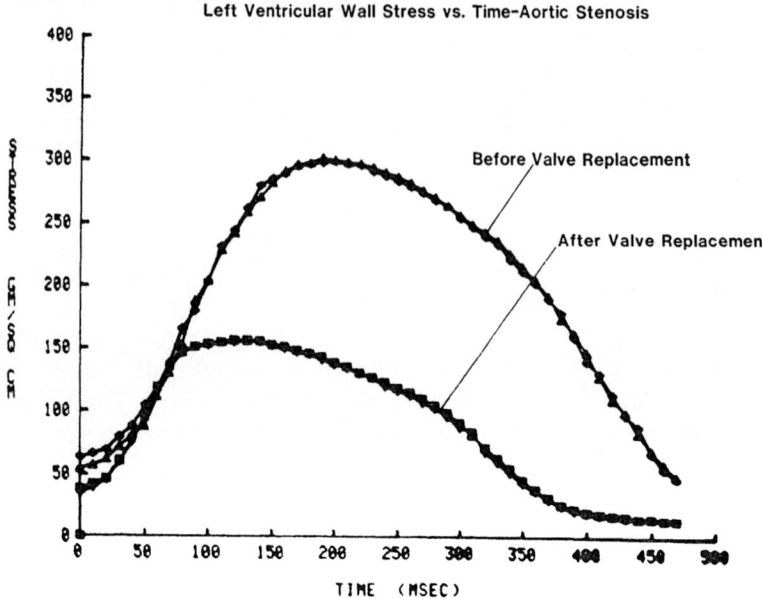

Fig. 14. Representative illustration of time course of LV wall stress reveals substantial unloading after valve replacement for aortic stenosis.

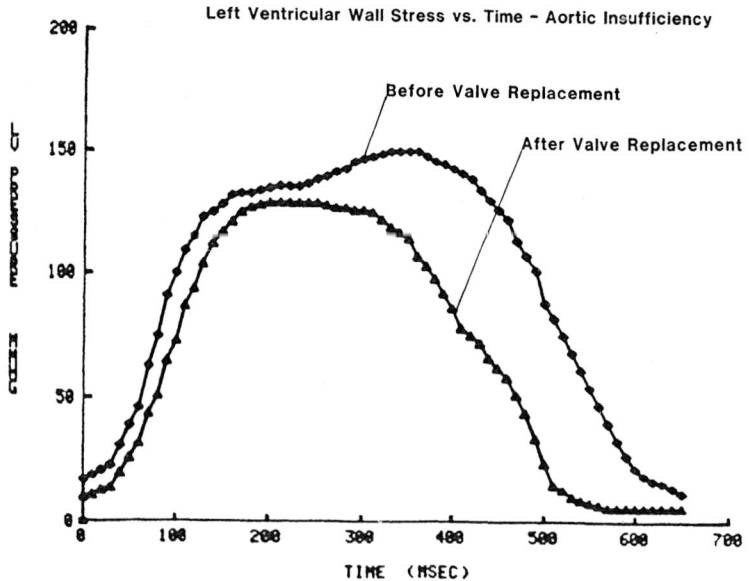

Fig. 15. Similar to fig. 15, these data illustrate decreased LV wall stress after valve replacement for aortic regurgitation, in part due to decreased postoperative EDV.

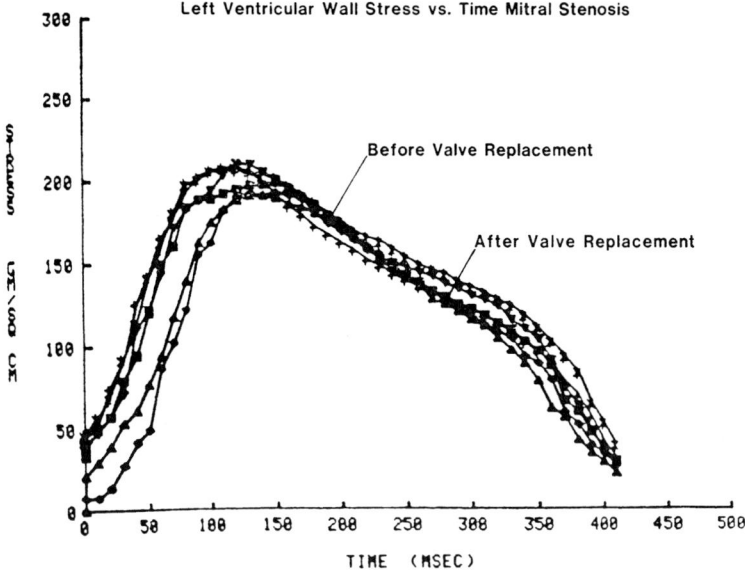

Fig. 16. Wall stress plot during valve replacement for mitral stenosis reveals little effect of surgery.

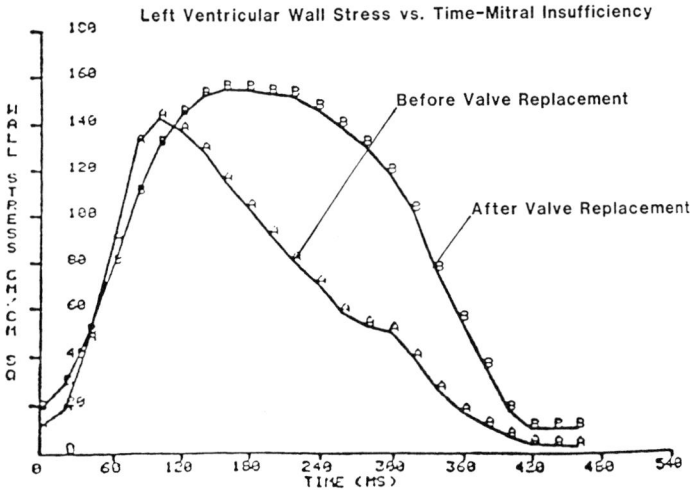

Fig. 17. Representative effect of valve replacement for chronic mitral regurgitation on the time course of wall stress. In contrast to figs. 15–17 (AS, AI, MS) wall stress increases after surgery.

326

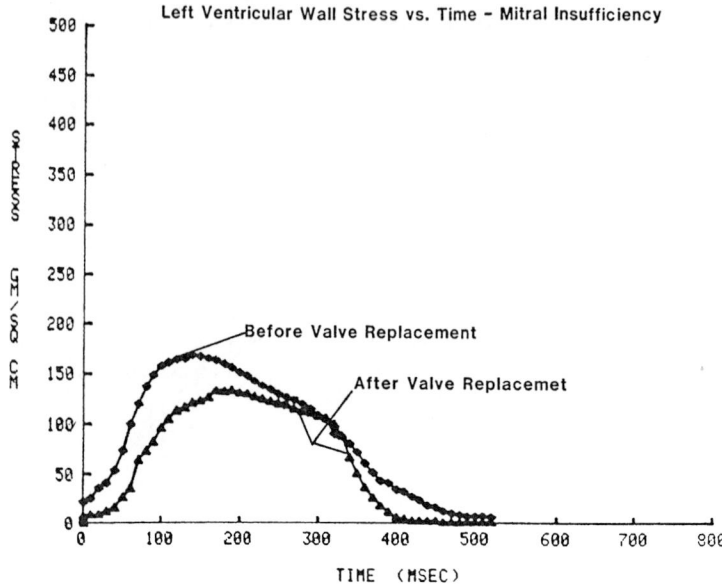

Fig. 18. In contrast to fig. 18, wall stress decreased in this patient following valve replacement for mitral regurgitation, the result of a substantial decrease in end-diastolic volume.

mitral regurgitation. A statistically significant increase in the integral of wall stress after correction of mitral regurgitation was reported in a previous study from our laboratory [2] and was implicated as a major cause of decreased postoperative ejection fraction. However, it is now apparent that an increase in wall stress is not obligatory with correction of mitral regurgitation, because a large intraoperative decrease in end-diastolic volume can effectively overcome the increased impedence resulting from elimination of the low resistance blowoff into the left atrium (Fig. 18).

While mechanical factors (increased impedence in mitral regurgitation and decreased preload in aortic regurgitation) are clearly implicated in the decreased intraoperative ejection fraction accompanying surgery for both aortic and mitral regurgitation, it is clear that depressed contractility must also be implicated. Evidence for this includes improved ejection fraction at late followup compared to intraoperative observations, as well as numerous reports of higher ejection fraction at late followup than we have observed at surgery [9, 10, 19]; furthermore, ejection fraction in aortic regurgitation frequently improves after surgical correction. Our own data also include serial observations in an echogenic patient of improving ejection fraction over 12 days after correction of mitral regurgitation in the absence of changes in heart rate or end-diastole volume (Fig. 19).

The definition of alterations in contractility in this setting is fraught with difficulty, but we have found that the end-systolic stress/end-systolic volume

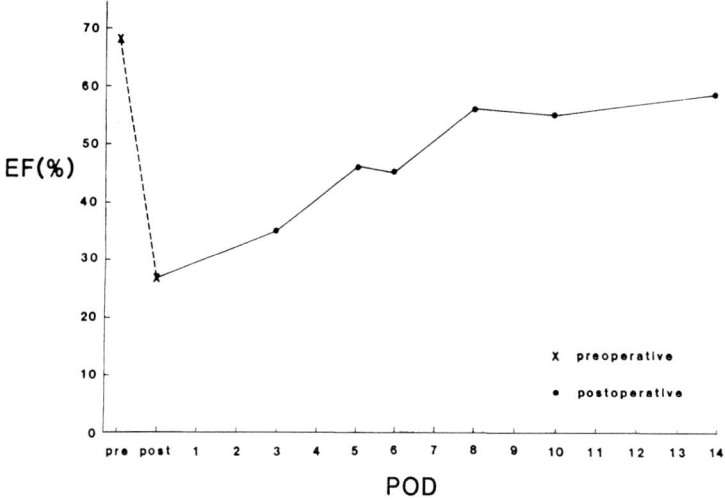

Fig. 19. EF vs. time following valve replacement for mitral regurgitation. EF returns toward preoperative value over 14 days in hospital. Changes in heart rate and end-diastolic volume were minimal in this patient.

index indicates decreased intraoperative contractility in 3/4 subgroups of our patients undergoing correction of valvular regurgitation (Fig. 20, Table 1). The only exception to this in our data is the subgroup of patients with mitral regurgitation and EF > 45%. Paradoxically, however, the largest

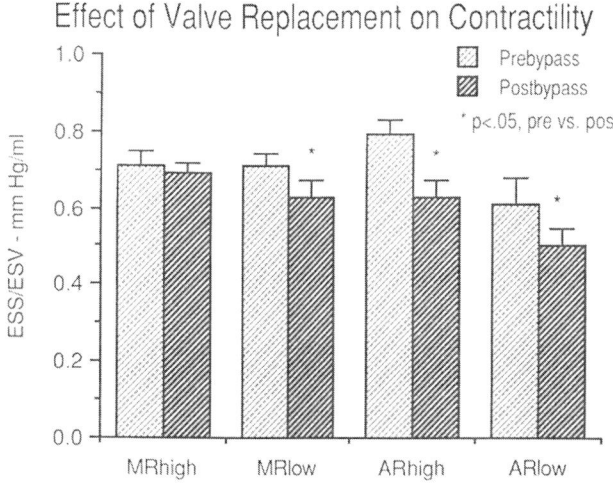

Fig. 20. Effects of valve replacement on contractility evaluated as end-systolic stress/volume ratio in patients undergoing valve replacement for aortic or mitral regurgitation. Groups are divided into high and low subgroups according to EF (see Table 1). All subgroups except 'MRhigh' demonstrate decreased contractility, though effects of edema may undermine validity of stress calculations in this setting. Brackets indicate standard errors.

328

decrease in intraoperative ejection fraction also occurs in patients with high preoperative ejection fractions (Fig. 21). Furthermore, the highest postoperative ejection fractions (and presumably best prognosis for long term LV function) occur in patients with high preoperative ejection fraction (Fig. 22). Difficulties in interpreting these results are added by an apparent correlation between decreasing intraoperative ejection fraction and increasing preoperative end-diastolic volume (Fig. 23).

In this setting, and with consideration of the perioperative clinical course of these patients, it is difficult to avoid the conclusion that falling ejection fraction during valve replacement for mitral or aortic regurgitation is frequently a misleading index of effects of surgery on contractility. Clinical history, combined with our studies of mass and contractility, however, suggest

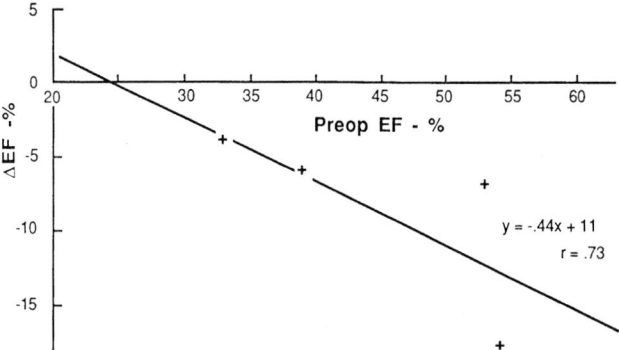

Fig. 21. The relation between mean preoperative EF for the four subgroups presented in Table 1 is plotted against the mean intraoperative change in EF. Results suggest that a preoperative EF > 45% is likely to be associated with a decrease in EF > 10% during valve replacement.

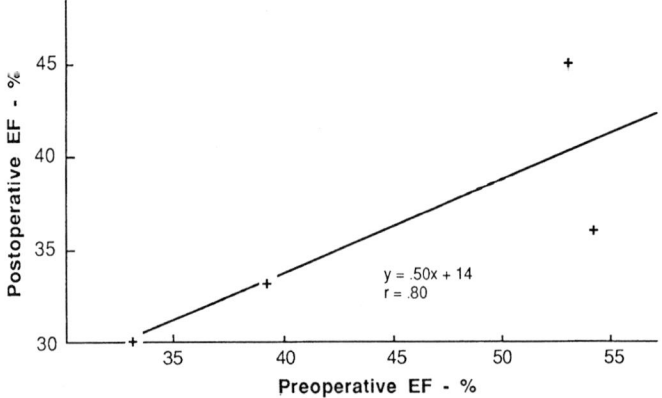

Fig. 22. Prebypass EF vs. Postbypass EF for the four patient groups also described in Figs. 7, 21, and 22. The largest values for postoperative EF are seen in patients with high initial EFs, although these patients also experience the largest absolute decrease in EF (Fig. 22).

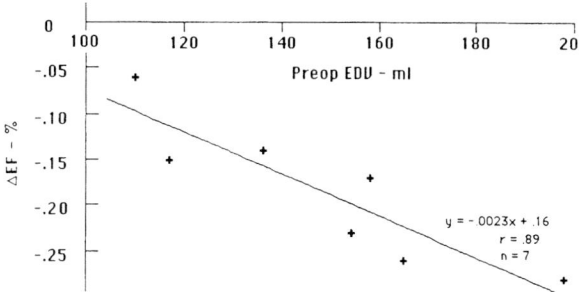

Fig. 23. Effect of valve replacement for mitral regurgitation on EF in patients with high initial EFs (Table 1) is plotted against prebypass end diastolic volume. The r value of .89 indicates a strong negative correlation between increased preoperative end-diastolic volume and decreased intraoperative EF. Both high initial EF and large end-diastolic volume predicted a large drop in intraoperative EF in our series.

to us that patients with severe regurgitation, LV hypertrophy, and depressed preoperative ejection fraction have increased susceptibility to intraoperative injury and that improved methods of caring for these patients are needed.

Acknowledgement

The authors gratefully acknowledges the technical assistance of Mr. Meyer Steinhardt, Dr. James Vayda, Mr. Edward Shadiack, Mr. Anthony Cuffy, and Mr. Reynal von Muchow.

References

1. Spotnitz HM, Bregman D, Bowman FO Jr, Edie RN, Reemtsma K, King DL, Hoffman BF, and Malm JR: Effect of open heart surgery on end-diastolic pressure-diameter relations of the human left ventricle. Circulation 59: 662–670, 1979.
2. Wong CYH and Spotnitz, HM: Systolic and diastolic properties of the human left ventricle during valve replacement for chronic mitral regurgitation. Am J Cardiol 47: 40-50, 1981.
3. Spotnitz HM: Two-dimensional ultrasound and cardiac surgery. J Thorac Cardiovasc Surg 83: 43–51, 1982.
4. Topol EJ, Weiss JL, Guzman PA, Dorsey-Lima S, Blanck TJJ, Humphrey LS, Baumgartner WA, Flaherty JT, Reitz BA: Immediate improvement of dysfunctional myocardial segments after coronary revascularization: Detection by intraoperative transesophageal echocardiography. JACC 4: 1123–34, 1984.
5. Goldman ME, Mindich BP, Teicholz LE, Burgess N, Steville K, Fuster V: Intraoperative contrast echocardiography to evaluate mitral valve operations. J Am Coll Cardiol 4: 1035–1040, 1984.
6. Takamoto S, Kyo S, Adachi H, Matsumura M, Yokote Y, Omoto R: Intraoperative color flow mapping by real-time two-dimensional Doppler echocardiography for evaluation of

330

valvular and congenital heart disease and vascular disease. J Thorac Cardiovasc Surg 90: 802–812, 1985.

6a. Sahn DJ, Barratt-Boyes BG, Graham K, Kerr A, Roche A, Hill D, Brandt PWT, Copeland JG, Mammana R, Temkin LP, Glenn W: Ultrasonic imaging of coronary arteries in open-chest humans. Evaluation of coronary atherosclerotic lesions during cardiac surgery. Circulation 66: 1034–1044, 1982.

7. Quinones MA, Waggoner AD, Reduto LA, Nelsson JF, Young JB, Winters WL, Ribeiro LG, Miller RR: A new simplified and accurate method for determining ejection fraction with two-dimensional echocardiography. Circulation 64: 744, 1981.

8. Dubroff JM, Clark M, Wong CYH, Spotnitz AJ, Collins RH, Spotnitz HM: Left ventricular ejection fraction during cardiac surgery: a two-dimensional echocardiographic study. Circulation 68: 95–103, 1986.

9. Schuler G, Peterson KL, Johnson A, Francis G, Dennish G, Utley J, Daily PO, Ashburn W, Ross J Jr: Temporal response of left ventricular performance to mitral valve surgery. Circulation 59: 1218–1231, 1979.

10. Kennedy JW, Doces JG, Stewart DK: Left ventricular function before and following surgical treatment of mitral valve disease. Am Heart J 97: 592–598, 1979.

11. Bonchek LI, Olinger GN, Sieger R, Tresh DD, Keelan MH Jr: Left ventricular performance after mitral reconstruction for mitral regurgitation. J Thorac Cardiovasc Surg 88: 122–127, 1984.

12. Peter CA, Austin EH, Jones RH: Effect of valve replacement for chronic mitral insufficiency on left ventricular funtion during rest and exercise. J Thorac Cardiovasc Surg 82: 127–135, 1981.

13. David TE, Burns RJ, Bacchus CM, Druck MN: Mitral valve replacement for mitral regurgitation with and without preservation of chordae tendineae. J Thorac Cardiovasc Surg 88: 718–725, 1984.

14. Haasler GB, Rodigas PC, Colins RH, Wei J, Meyer FJ, Spotnitz AJ, Spotnitz HM: Two-dimensional echocardiography in dogs: Variation of LV mass, geometry, volume, and ejection fraction on cardiopulmonary bypass. J Thorac Cardiovasc Surg 90: 430–440, 1985.

15. Collins RH, Haasler GB, Krug JH Jr, Martin EC and Spotnitz HM: Canine left ventricular volume and mass during thoracotomy by two-dimensional echocardiography. Increased ventricular mass after ischemia and reperfusion. J Surg Res 33: 294–304, 1982.

16. Lazar HL, Haasler GB, Collins RH, Dubroff JM, Meisner J, Spotnitz HM: Compliance, mass, and shape of the canine left ventricle after global ischemia analyzed with two-dimensional echocardiography. J Surg Res 39: 199–208, 1985.

17. Spotnitz WD, Clark MB, Rosenblum HM, Haasler GB, Lazar HL, Collins RH, Spotnitz AJ, and Spotnitz HM: Effect of cardiopulmonary bypass and global ischemia on human and canine left ventricular mass: Evidence for interspecies differences. Surgery 96: 230–239, 1984.

18. Rosenblum HM, Haasler GB, Spotnitz WD, Lazar HL, and Spotnitz HM: Effects of simulated cardiopulmonary bypass and cardioplegia on mass of the canine left ventricle. Ann Thorac Surg 39: 139–148, 1985.

19. Borer JS, Rosing DR, Kent KM, Bacharach SL, Green MV, McIntosh CJ, Morrow AG, Epstein SE: Left ventricular function at rest and during exercise after aortic valve replacement in patients with aortic regurgitation. Am J Cardiol 44: 1297, 1979.

5.3. Intraoperative two-dimensional echocardiography in congenital heart disease

W. J. GUSSENHOVEN, L. A. VAN HERWERDEN, H. K. THE, E. BOS, J. ROELANDT, M. A. TAAMS, M. WITSENBURG & N. BOM

Introduction

In the past decade much has been achieved regarding the understanding of congenital heart disease. The sequential analysis of the congenitally malformed heart has been widely accepted as a most useful method, particularly in cases of complex anomalies. The crux of this approach is the analysis of the cardiac junctions. It is here that echocardiography comes in to its own, since two-dimensional techniques demonstrate the actual connections and valve morphology at both atrioventricular and ventriculo-arterial junctions. The technique is non-invasive and in addition yields qualitative as well as quantitative information regarding anatomy and function. Thus two-dimensional echocardiography has become an established tool in the complete assessment of congenital heart disease [1]. Recently it has been introduced in the cardiac surgery department [2–9].

This chapter presents our experience in 250 patients referred to the Thorax-center for correction of congenital heart disease since January 1, 1984. They included newborns and patients up to 73 years. Ninety percent were younger than 16 years; thirty percent of them were under 1 year of age. The preoperative diagnosis was jointly established in the customary fashion by reviewing the medical history, physical examination, the chest X-ray, electrocardiogram, M-mode and two-dimensional echocardiograms, Doppler studies and cardiac catheterization data.

One of the questions to be considered is how frequently does this technique contribute to a more sophisticated surgical treatment than initially planned on the basis of the preoperative review of the available cardiovascular data. Another question concerns the benefit of the method for the immediate assessment of the surgical repair.

Echocardiographic investigation

A mechanical 5 MHz imaging system was used (ATL-Mark 300 LX) (Fig. 1). The transducer assembly and cable carefully cleansed with chlorhexidine

I. Cikes (ed.), *Echocardiography in Cardiac Interventions*, 331–342, 1989.
© 1989 *Kluwer Academic Publishers.*

332

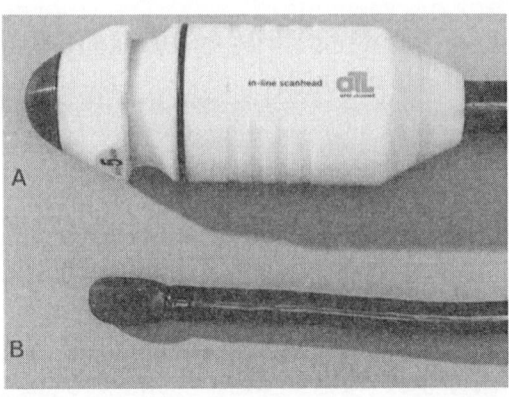

Fig. 1. For the intraoperative studies 2 systems were used: a 5 MHz mechanical scanner (A) and a 5 MHz phased array hand-held finger tip transducer (B). Note that the size of the mechanical transducer may hamper appropriate imaging of the heart, particularly in small infants. This problem can be solved by using the finger tip transducer.

0.1% were placed in a 2 metres-long gas sterilized plastic bag. To achieve good ultrasound coupling sterile gel was placed within the plastic bag and warm saline was poured over the heart. A damping resistor (50 Ohm) was switched in parallel with the transducer element in order to prevent overloading of the receiver, which considerably improved the image quality. Initial echocardiograms were obtained after sternotomy and pericardiotomy, prior to cardiopulmonary bypass. A second set of echocardiograms was made before closure of the chestwall.

The image quality of the near field, approximately 10 mm of depth, however, proved inadequate for obtaining detailed information in the infants. To avoid this problem, recordings can be made before opening the pericardium, which facilitates the filling of the chest with warm saline. A second solution is the use of a miniaturized phased array fingertip transducer. We used a 64-elements; 5.6 MHz; 1.5 × 1.0 cm in size and only 5 mm thick transducer, based on the esophageal device developed at our institution (Fig. 1). With this small transducer, the heart can be imaged through the right atrial lateral wall. From this position, the right ventricular outflow tract can be visualized in detail, which is impossible with the larger mechanical scanner in the young infants (Fig. 2).

The handling of the probe was carried out by the surgeon in charge, while the ultrasound equipment was adjusted by the echocardiographer. The mechanical scanhead was placed on the right ventricular surface. From this position the actual connections and the valve morphology at both atrioventricular and ventriculo-arterial connections were identified. Table 1 shows the preoperative diagnoses of the 250 patients studied. The results and

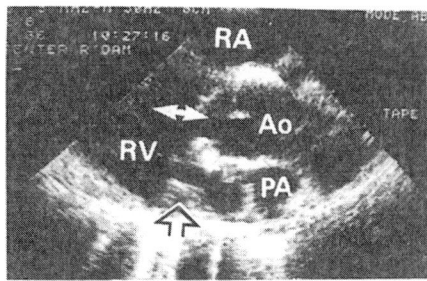

Fig. 2. Intraoperative two-dimensional image obtained in a 3-months-old child with tetralogy of Fallot. The right atrial lateral wall served as acoustic window. The image shows in the following sequence first the right atrium (RA), the aorta (Ao) and then the pulmonary artery (PA). The ventricular septal defect (arrow) gives direct communication between the right ventricle (RV) and the aorta. Note the narrowed right ventricular outflow tract (open arrow).

Table 1. Preoperative morphologic diagnosis in 250 patients with congenital heart disease studied with intraoperative two-dimensional echocardiography.

· Aortic and/or mitral valve lesion	53
· Atrial septal defect (ASD II; ASD I)	46
· Ventricular septal defect (VSD)	40
· Pulmonary stenosis (PS)	7
· VSD + PS	7
· Tetralogy of Fallot	37
· Double outlet right ventricle	11
· Complete transposition of the great arteries	26
· Single outlet heart	6
· Heart with univentricular connection	6
· Miscellaneous	11

Table 2. Results of intraoperative two-dimensional echocardiography in 250 patients.

Preoperative		Postoperative	
No new information	88%	No new information	91%
Altered surgical approach	10%	Contributed to surgical management	9%
Refined surgical approach	2%		

the significance of the intraoperative echocardiography are shown in Table 2. The findings are discussed in more detail according to the step-by-step analysis of the intracardiac structures [10].

334

Atrial level

With the right ventricle as contact point both the left and right atrium were identified using the four-chamber view. In this section the entrance of the inferior caval vein is readily seen, sometimes bordered by an Eustachian valve. In the same echoplane the entrance of the coronary sinus is visualized, indicating the lowermost portion of both atria.

When necessary, the right atrial appendage can also be used as the point of entrance. These cross-sections are valuable to locate an atrial septal defect, to demonstrate an enlarged coronary sinus caused by a persistent superior left caval vein or to evaluate the intracardiac repair in case of a total anomalous pulmonary venous drainage, complete transposition of the great arteries. The patency of the anastomosis between right atrium and pulmonary artery following a Fontan's procedure can be checked (Fig. 3).

In patients referred for correction of an interatrial septal communication the technique enabled us to precisely locate the defect. In a patient referred with a secundum type atrial septal defect a sinus venosus was found instead. In another patient, who was diagnosed to have a primum type atrial septal defect, a secundum type defect was identified. In itself, this information may not be so important for the surgeon. However, their experience in identifiying these anatomical structures in detail did result in the determination of an optimal site of atriotomy and, what is more important, it facilitated their decision in emergency conditions. This is illustrated in a newborn referred for severe aortic stenosis. After surgery the infant remained hypotensive. Intraoperative echocardiography revealed an unsuspected secundum type atrial septal defect (Fig. 4). Cardiopulmonary bypass was restarted and the defect was closed in the same session.

Intraoperative echocardiography was most important in patients in whom

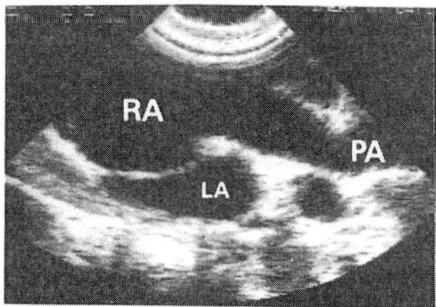

Fig. 3. Intraoperative two-dimensional echocardiogram obtained with the 5 MHz mechanical sector scanner in a patient with univentricular heart, following Fontan's correction. The transducer was placed onto the right atrial surface. Patency of the anastomosis between the right atrium (RA) and the pulmonary artery (PA) can readily be seen. LA = left atrium.

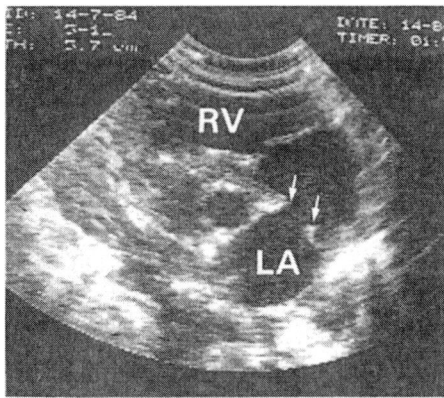

Fig. 4. Intraoperative two-dimensional echocardiogram obtained in an infant referred for critical aortic stenosis. The echocardiographic study following commissurotomy for which the right ventricle (RV) was used as acoustic window, revealed an unsuspected large secundum type atrial septal defect (arrows). LA = left atrium.

the surgeon found an unsuspected external cardiac geometry which did not correspond with the preoperative diagnosis. In 2 patients, one with a tetralogy of Fallot and the other with a complete transposition of the great arteries, an unsuspected juxtaposition of the atrial appendages was seen on external inspection. The possibility of additional complex intracardiac pathology, frequently associated with this disorder, could be excluded with intraoperative echocardiography [11, 12].

Atrioventricular level

The connection between atrium and ventricle is identified from the four-chamber view which further allows a detailed analysis of both the mitral and tricuspid valve morphology and a precise delineation of the size and position of a ventricular septal defect. As a result of the high resolution of the ultrasound device, we never encountered problems in interpretation of a ventricular septal defect in the perimembranous ventricular septum as a result of drop-outs. In a 2-year-old patient with severe mitral valve insufficiency, intraoperative echocardiography revealed an unsuspected communication between right atrium and left ventricle (Fig. 5). Thus the child had mitral valve replacement and could have, in addition, closure of the ventricular septal defect.

After termination of cardiopulmonary bypass injection of saline echo contrast was used to test for valve incompetence or residual shunts. In the majority of patients those studies confirmed an adequate cardiac repair.

336

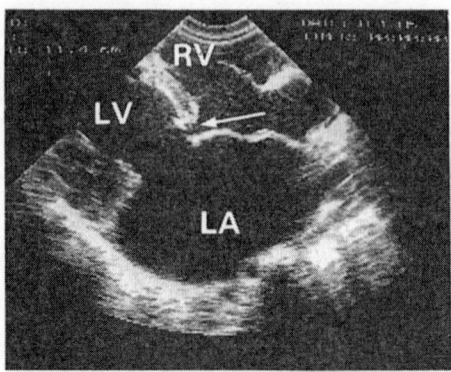

Fig. 5. Intraoperative two-dimensional echocardiogram obtained in a child with severe mitral valve incompetence. The four-chamber view revealed a large left atrium (LA) and left ventricle (LV). In addition, a communication was identified between left and right heart cavities, just underneath the septal mitral valve leaflet (arrow). RV = right ventricle. (Reproduced from Gussenhoven W. J. et al.: Intraoperative two-dimensional echocardiography in congenital heart disease. J Am Coll Cardiol 9: 565, 1987, with permission of the American College of Cardiology.)

Small amounts of contrast passing the mitral valve after left ventricular injection, or the interventricular septal defect patch after left atrial injection, were considered without consequences. This is probably due to normal patch and interstitch permeability during the first 24 hours after repair. When a large ventricular septal defect patch was used for intracardiac repair, however, we

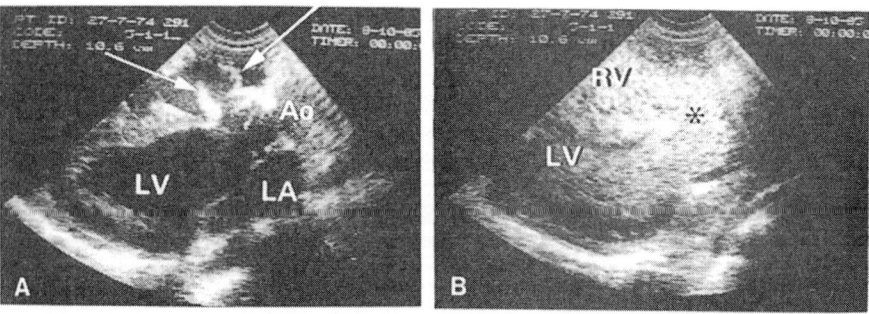

Fig. 6. Intraoperative two-dimensional echocardiograms obtained in a child after correction of a tetralogy of Fallot. Although the hemodynamic parameters did not present evidence of an intracardiac problem, the echocardiographic study revealed an exaggerated and floppy motion of the ventricular septal defect patch (A: arrows). Contrast injected via the left atrial monitoring line resulted in an equal opacification of left (LV) and right (RV) ventricle. The asterisk indicates the level of the defect. It was decided to reinstitute bypass. A partially disrupted patch was seen that had to be resecured. Postoperative period was uneventful. LA = left atrium; Ao = aorta. (Reproduced from Gussenhoven W. J. et al.: Intraoperative two-dimensional echocardiography in congenital heart disease. J Am Coll Cardiol 9: 565, 1987, with permission of the American College of Cardiology.)

experienced that large amounts of the contrast material could be noted within the right ventricle. The same accounts for the contrast studies in patients who underwent a Mustard's procedure for complete transposition of the great arteries: a significant amount of contrast could be seen in the right ventricle after a venous injection. In order to discriminate between physiologic and pathognomonic leakage particularly in this category of patients, it is important to focus on the patch itself. Floppy patch motion points to patch dehiscence. This occurred in a child operated upon for a tetralogy of Fallot. Dehiscence of the ventricular septal defect patch was proven echocardiographically with contrast injection. Both ventricles opacified with equal intensity (Fig. 6). A patch, on the other hand, that is properly secured will not show such exaggerated and floppy motion. In those instances where a significant leakage is noted, we recommend an oxygen saturation test to be performed in addition.

Ventriculo-arterial level

Left ventricular and right ventricular long-axis views are used for a detailed analysis of the size of both outflow tracts, the level of outflow tract obstruction, the position of the great arteries relative to the ventricular septum and the presence or absence of the infundibular septum. This information is particularly useful in patients with tetralogy of Fallot, double outlet right ventricle and complete transposition of the great arteries.

In these patients the intraoperative echocardiographic information is extremely important. So is the step-by-step analysis of all cardiac junctions. This is illustrated by 2 patients referred with tetralogy of Fallot in whom the surgeon disclosed an abnormal cardiac geometry that dit not correspond with the preoperative diagnosis and cardiac pathology. Intraoperative echocardiography was used to exclude the possibility of additional intracardiac pathology. In both patients, a deep atrioventricular sulcus was noted on external inspection. In one patient with a preoperatively diagnosed secundum type atrial septal defect an additional primum type atrial septal defect was found. Regular atriotomy was performed and both defects were closed. In the second patient, the tricuspid valve diameter appeared to be half of the mitral valve diameter, which prevented the surgeon from performing the planned correction and a palliative procedure was done.

Furthermore, the planned surgical procedure was cancelled in another patient with tetralogy of Fallot, in whom an unsuspected transposition of the great arteries was noted on external inspection. Intraoperative echocardiography revealed a double outlet right ventricular connection with a significant subpulmonary valve obstruction. It was decided to perform a Waterston shunt.

338

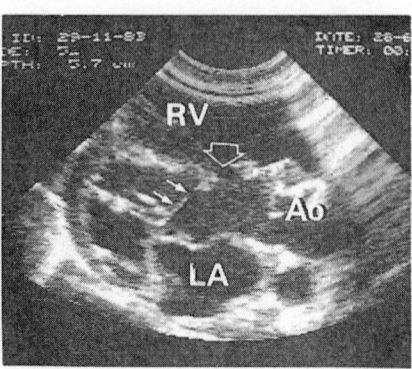

Fig. 7. Intraoperative two-dimensional echocardiogram obtained in a child operated for a ventricular septal defect (open arrow). The left ventricular long-axis view obtained using the right ventricle (RV) as contact area revealed an anomalous chord connecting the anterior mitral valve leaflet to the interventricular septum (arrows). Part of this chord was seen by the surgeon through the ventricular septal defect. As the chord gave no obstruction, it was decided not to do anything to it. LA = left atrium; Ao = aorta.

Delineation of the precise nature of right or left ventricular outflow tract using intraoperative echocardiography was of significance in several patients. For example, an unsuspected multileveled subaortic obstruction in a patient with idiopathic hypertrophic subaortic stenosis necessitated not only planned myectomy but also relief of the distal subaortic obstruction (see also Chapter 5.4.). In another patient with a ventricular septal defect an anomalous chord was noted connecting the mitral valve with the interventricular septum. In this patient, however, the anomalous chord did not give obstruction to the left ventricular outflow tract (Fig. 7) and no extra surgical intervention was felt to be indicated.

Knowing the precise morphology of the right ventricular outflow tract obstruction by intraoperative echocardiography, the surgeon could decide to perform a transverse right ventriculotomy, which is the best possible and least traumatic approach for relief of obstruction (Fig. 8A). On the other hand, when intraoperative echocardiography did not reveal significant right ventricular outflow tract obstruction right ventriculotomy could be avoided (Fig. 8B).

Direct assessment with intraoperative two-dimensional echocardiography following surgical repair and before chest closure is of advantage in many patients. Residual obstruction in the ventricular outflow tract was found with intraoperative echocardiography in 4 patients, 3 with a double outlet right ventricular connection and 1 patient with a tetralogy of Fallot. Cardiopulmonary bypass was restarted and the obstruction relieved.

A second application of the contrast technique in this category of patients is to discriminate between residual elevated right ventricular pressure due to

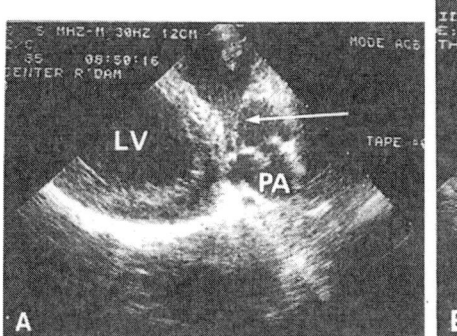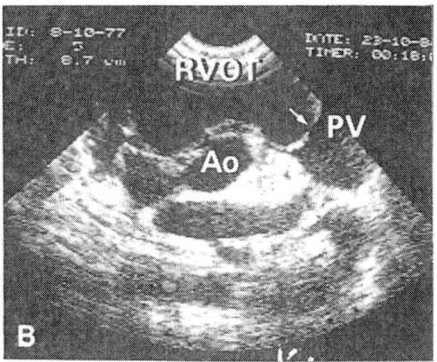

Fig. 8. Intraoperative two-dimensional echocardiograms obtained in patients known to have right ventricular outflow tract (RVOT) obstruction. The transducer is placed onto the right ventricular outflow tract. A: A small trabecle (arrow) was seen in the distal part of the right ventricular outflow tract adjacent to the pulmonary artery (PA). Transverse ventriculotomy was performed. B: No evidence of right ventricular outflow tract obstruction was found in this patient. Consequently no ventriculotomy was performed. Note the pinhole opening (arrow) within the doming of the stenotic pulmonary valve (PV). Ao = aorta.

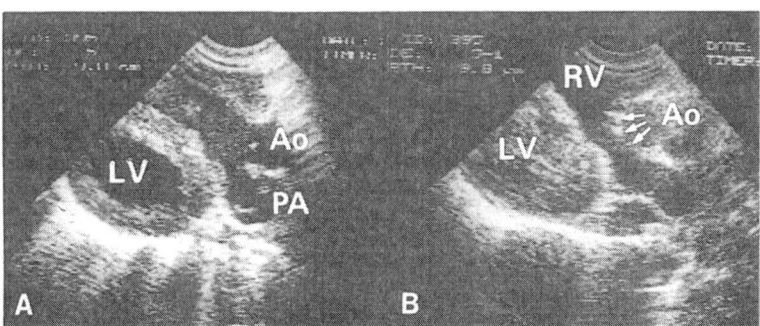

Fig. 9. Intraoperative two-dimensional echocardiograms showing an alternative right ventricular long-axis view. The images are obtained before (A) and after (B) repair of a tetralogy of Fallot. Hemodynamic measurements after repair had shown an elevated right ventricular pressure Contrast injection into the left atrium resulted in opacification of the left ventricle (LV) and aorta (Ao). Not a trace of bubbles was noted in the right ventricular cavity (RV). These images reveal that the ventricular septal defect patch (arrows) gave obstruction to the right ventricular outflow tract. PA = pulmonary artery.

inadequate relief of right ventricular outflow tract obstruction (Fig. 9) or due to a residual ventricular shunt (see also Fig. 6).

Arterial level

Imaging of the ascending aorta with the transducer immediately placed onto the aorta allowed demonstration of the size of the aortic root and pulmonary

340

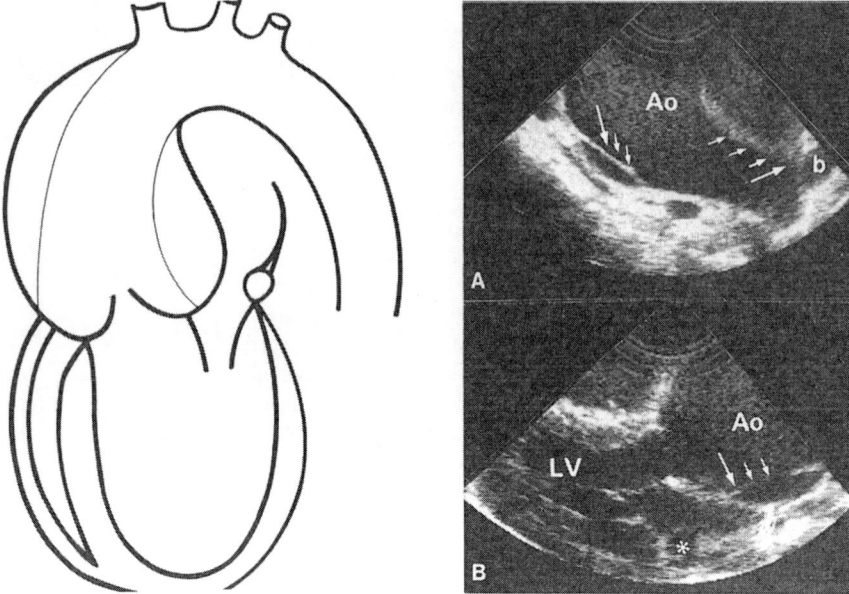

Fig. 10. Intraoperative two-dimensional echocardiogram obtained in a patient known to have a saccular aneurysm. An unsuspected dissection was noted in the aorta (Ao). This dissection started just above the aortic annulus (arrows) and ended before the take-off of the brachiocephalic artery (b). For this study the transducer was placed first onto the right ventricular surface (A), thereafter onto the ascending aorta (B). The coronary sinus is indicated by an asterisk. LV = left ventricle. (Reproduced from Gussenhoven W. J. et al.: Intraoperative two-dimensional echocardiography in congenital heart disease. J Am Coll Cardiol 9: 565, 1987, with permission of the American College of Cardiology.)

arteries. Images of a dilated ascending aorta in one patient showed an unsuspected aortic dissection (Fig. 10). This kind of information may alter the surgical procedure including femoral artery cannulation for extracorporeal circulation. Moreover, this approach has been useful for measurement of the right pulmonary artery internal diameter in patients in whom a Waterston anastomosis was closed. It is not uncommon that the pulmonary artery internal diameter is obstructive following this type of correction [13].

Conclusion

Excellent intraoperative echocardiographic imaging was possible in almost all 250 patients. None of them had complications that were related to the intraoperative echocardiographic procedure. We experienced that intraoperative two-dimensional echocardiography provided relevant information for surgical decision-making. Before extracorporeal circulation ·this technique allowed us to verify the preoperative diagnosis and to detect additional and important information for subsequent surgical management. The echographic investigation was particularly helpful when the surgeon found an abnormal cardiac geometry not corresponding to the preoperative diagnosis. Most frequently (88%) intraoperative echocardiographic imaging confirmed the preoperative diagnosis. In 2% of the patients studied, the technique revealed unsuspected intracardiac morphologic findings which altered the originally assessed preoperative diagnosis. These findings necessitated a modification of the planned surgical procedure. In 10% of the patients the intraoperative echocardiographic information was judged as pertinent and helpful for surgical management. In this particular group of patients the preoperatively established diagnosis was correct but the additional morphologic information contributed to the refinement of the surgical approach. One may wonder why in so many patients new morphologic information was found despite careful preoperative investigation.

Preoperative studies have shortcomings which result from the complexity of the pathology or are inherent to the diagnostic methods, e.g. angio superimposes structures and the crux cordis and atrioventricular valves cannot be evaluated [14–16].

Intraoperative echocardiography has the advantage of high resolution images not hampered by intervening tissues. The entire anterior cardiac surface can be used as acoustic window. Intraoperative echocardiography would further be facilitated and improved by a small high resolution hand-held finger tip transducer. Such a transducer would permit to use the lateral surface of the heart as acoustic entrance and increase the versatility of imaging the right ventricular outflow tract pathology in the very young.

After the completion of the operation intraoperative echocardiography permits assessment of the surgical result and critical problems which may occur are readily solved. In 9% the intraoperative echocardiographic information contributed to the problem-solving and to subsequent surgical management (vide supra).

The experience of the surgeons in performing echocardiographic studies increased rapidly. This was facilitated by the permanent availability of the ultrasound equipment in the operating theatre.

Contrast studies became a routine for the postoperative analysis. Recently we started to use colour-coded Doppler echocardiography intraoperatively. The major advantage of the colour information over that obtained with continuous wave or pulsed Doppler techniques is its easiness as to performance and interpretation.

342

References

1. Gussenhoven WJ, Becker AE: Congenital Heart Disease. Morphologic echocardiographic correlations. Edinburgh, Churchill Livingstone, 1983.
2. Sahn DJ: Intraoperative applications of two-dimensional and contrast two-dimensional echocardiography for evaluation of congenital, acquired and coronary heart disease in open-chested humans during cardiac surgery. In Rijsterborgh H, ed. Echocardiology, The Hague/Boston/London: Martinus Nijhoff Publishers, pp. 9–23, 1981.
3. Sahn DJ: Application of two-dimensional echocardiography during open heart surgery in humans for evaluation of acquired and coronary heart disease. In: Hanrath P, Bleifeld W, Souquet J, eds. Cardiovascular Diagnosis by Ultrasound. The Hague/Boston/London: Martinus Nijhoff Publishers, pp. 294–307, 1982.
4. Goldman ME, Mindich BP: Intraoperative two-dimensional echocardiography: new application of an old technique. J Am Coll Cardiol 7: 374–82, 1986.
5. Mindich BP, Goldman ME, Fuster V et al.: Improved intraoperative evaluation of mitral valve operations utilizing tow-dimensional contrast echocardiography. J Thorac Cardiovasc Surg 90: 112–8, 1985.
6. Gussenhoven WJ, Van Herwerden LA, Roelandt J, Ligtvoet CM, Bos E, Witsenburg M: Intraoperative two-dimensional echocardiography in congenital heart disease. J Am Coll Cardiol 9: 565–572, 1987.
7. Van Herwerden LA, Gussenhoven WJ, Roelandt J, Bos E, Ligtvoet CM, Haalebos MM, Mochtar B, Leicher F, Witsenburg M: Intraoperative epicardial two-dimensional echocardiography. Eur Heart J 7: 386–395, 1986.
8. Van Herwerden LA, Gussenhoven WJ, Roelandt JRTC, Haalebos MMP, Mochtar B, Ligtvoet CM, Bos E: Intraoperative two-dimensional echocardiography in complicated infective endocarditis of the aortic valve. J Thorac Cardiovasc Surg 93: 587–591, 1987.
9. Eguaras MG, Pasalodos J, Gonzales V et al.: Intraoperative contrast two-dimensional echocardiography. J Thorac Cardiovasc Surg 89: 573–79, 1985.
10. Becker AE, Gussenhoven WJ: Segmental analysis of congenital heart disease. A correlation between pathology and echocardiography. In: Rijsterborgh H (ed.) Echocardiology. The Hague, Martinus Nijhoff Publishers, p. 307–321, 1981.
11. Melhuish BPP, Van Praagh R: Juxtaposition of the atrial appendages – A sign of severe cyanotic congenital heart disease. Brit Heart J 30: 269–84, 1968.
12. Anderson RH, Smith A, Wilkinson JL: Right juxtaposition of the auricular appendages. Eur J Cardiol 4: 495–503, 1976.
13. Stark J, De Leval M: Surgery for congenital heart defects. London New York, Grune & Stratton: pp. 180–182, 1983.
14. Pestana C, Weidman WH, Swan HJC, McGoon DC: Accuracy of preoperative diagnosis in congenital heart disease. Am Heart J 74: 446–50, 1966.
15. Maron BJ, McIntosh CL, Wesley YE, Arce J: Application of intraoperative two-dimensional echocardiography to patients with obstructive hypertrophic cardiomyopathy undergoing ventricular septal myotomy-myectomy. J Am Coll Cardiol 3: 565 (abstr.), 1984.
16. Takamoto S, Kyo S, Adachi H, Matsumura M, Yokote Y, Omoto R: Intraoperative color flow mapping by real-time two-dimensional Doppler echocardiography for evaluation of valvular and congenital heart disease and vascular disease. J Thorac Cardiovasc Surg 90: 802–12, 1985.

5.4. Intraoperative two-dimensional echocardiography for guiding surgical correction in subvalvular aortic obstruction

L. A. VAN HERWERDEN, W. J. GUSSENHOVEN, O. A. SCHIPPERS, E. BOS & F. J. TEN CATE

Introduction

Congenital obstructive lesions of the left ventricular outflow tract vary in nature and often are complex [1, 2]. Although the hemodynamic features are resemblant, the anatomy between the different types varies and so does the prognosis after surgical intervention.

The best known type of fixed subaortic stenosis is the membranous type. The membrane closely adjacent to the right coronary cusp extends from the surface of the ventricular septum onto the base of the anterior mitral leaflet as a U-shaped diaphragm. The second type is an obstruction caused by a fibromuscular ridge, usually more inferiorly from the aortic valve. The third type of fixed subaortic stenosis is the so-called diffuse tunnel stenosis. The obstruction forms a narrow channel. Usually the interventricular septum in the outflow tract is grossly hypertrophied and covered by a thick layer of fibrous tissue. Subaortic obstruction caused by hypertrophic cardiomyopathy is mainly characterized by a distinct thickening of the septal myocardium causing a subaortic gradient due to abnormal mitral valve motion. This gradient is not fixed but functional in nature.

Precordial M-mode, two-dimensional and Doppler echocardiography, cardiac catheterization and angiography are established methods to confirm the diagnosis and to define the nature, level and severity of the obstruction [3]. The main indications for surgery in fixed subaortic stenosis are congestive heart failure, cardiomegaly, a systolic gradient across the obstruction of more than 50 mmHg or the development of a strain pattern on the electrocardiogram in childhood. However, due to the complexity of the surgical correction, the indications for treatment of diffuse tunnel stenosis are less well-defined. In cases of hypertrophic obstructive cardiomyopathy surgical intervention must be considered when disabling symptoms persist despite medical treatment. Relief of obstruction can be achieved by excision of the membrane or by ventricular septal myotomy/myectomy.

Precise knowledge of the anatomy of the left ventricular outflow tract is crucial for the surgeon as the aortotomy in itself is restrictive in that it prevents the surgeon from inspecting all sites of obstruction.

I. Cikes (ed.), *Echocardiography in Cardiac Interventions*, 343–350, 1989.
© 1989 *Kluwer Academic Publishers*.

Recently, we introduced the application of two-dimensional echocardiography in the operating room [4]. Initially, the main purpose was to study patients with congenital heart disease (see also Chapter Gussenhoven et al.). Subsequently, patients with an acquired heart disease were included in the study. Unsuspected additional morphologic lesions were found not uncommonly, which in some patients had major significance for the surgical intervention [4–6]. The magnitude of inaccurate preoperative diagnoses in the setting of left ventricular outflow tract obstruction is not known. Maron and coworkers [7] were the first to document that preoperative echocardiography may not provide an accurate assessment of the interventricular septal thickness. Application of intraoperative two-dimensional echocardiography on the other hand proved to be a more sophisticated method.

We have studied 20 consecutive patients known to have a subvalvular obstructive lesion. The role of intraoperative two-dimensional echocardiography before and immediately after surgical relief of the obstruction is described in this chapter.

Procedure

The intraoperative two-dimensional study was performed with a 5 MHz mechanical sector scanner (ATL Mark 300LX). The transducer was wrapped in a gas sterilized plastic bag. After sternotomy and pericardiotomy, warm saline was poured over the heart to optimize contact between transducer and heart. The surgeon in charge performed the echocardiographic investigation. The right ventricular surface was most commonly used for the study of the left ventricular outflow tract. Left ventricular long axis view as well as short axis view were obtained in the same way as the precordial images. Immediately after termination of cardiopulmonary bypass, and as soon as the patient's condition was stable, a second set of echocardiograms – including a contrast echocardiogram – were made to test the outcome of the surgical repair.

Patients

The study applies to 20 patients in whom the diagnosis of a subvalvular aortic obstruction and gradients had preoperatively been established. All patients had preoperative investigations including precordial echocardiography as well as hemodynamic evaluation and cineangiocardiography. Fifteen patients had fixed subaortic stenosis. This was due to a membrane in 14 patients and in one patient a fibromuscular tunnel obstruction together with a ventricular septal defect was involved. Five patients had hypertrophic obstructive cardiomyopathy. There was an equal sex distribution. The age of the patients ranged from 2 months up to 66 years.

Results before repair

In 13 patients intraoperative echocardiography and surgical inspection were consistent with the preoperative diagnosis. In 7 patients the intraoperative study revealed additional morphologic abnormalities. The surgical procedure was influenced by these findings in 3 patients. In one patient with hyper-

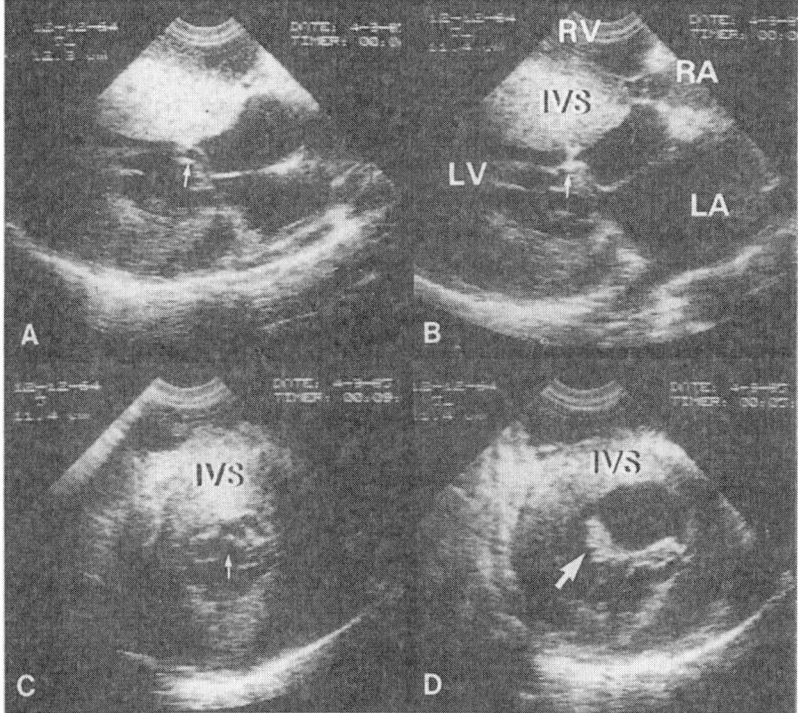

Fig. 1. Intraoperative two-dimensional echocardiograms obtained in a patient with hypertrophic obstructive cardiomyopathy. The transducer was placed onto the right ventricular (RV) surface. The left ventricular long-axis view (A) and the modified four-chamber view (B) both revealed the hypertrophied interventricular septum (IVS) of approximately 30 mm thickness. The systolic anterior motion of both the anterior and posterior mitral valve leaflet is recognized in these images as well as in the short-axis view (C; small arrow). The left ventricular short-axis view obtained at a somewhat lower level (D) shows that the ventricular septal thickness was reduced (± 18 mm). In addition, in this cross-section a second obstruction was noted that was represented by an anomalous chord connecting the interventricular septum with the anterior mitral valve leaflet (solid arrow). RA = right atrium; LA = left atrium; LV = left ventricle.

trophic obstructive cardiomyopathy, a second level of obstruction was identified, situated 4 cm proximal from the aortic valve (Fig. 1). Excision of this obstruction was performed. In the 2 other patients, the precise underlying pathology remained uncertain after preoperative evaluation. Both had a subaortic membrane with secondary muscular hypertrophy. The likelihood of a co-existing hypertrophic obstructive cardiomyopathy had been suggested by the preoperative echocardiographic findings. With intraoperative echocardiography only a subvalvular aortic membrane was seen which was subsequently excised (Fig. 2). In 4 of the 7 patients the additional morphologic information, albeit without surgical consequences, was judged as valuable. In one patient, a subvalvular aortic membrane actually was of fibromuscular nature. Although direct intracardiac inspection by an experienced surgeon would have been sufficient to establish the type of obstruction, intraoperative echocardiography helped to define the way in which to perform the myectomy. In the other patients intraoperative echocardiography did provide more detailed information on the mitral valve apparatus without influencing the surgical procedure. This information included a redundant mitral valve chorda in one patient and a papillar structure in the left ventricle seen in 2 patients, which on the precordial echocardiograms mimicked a false tendon.

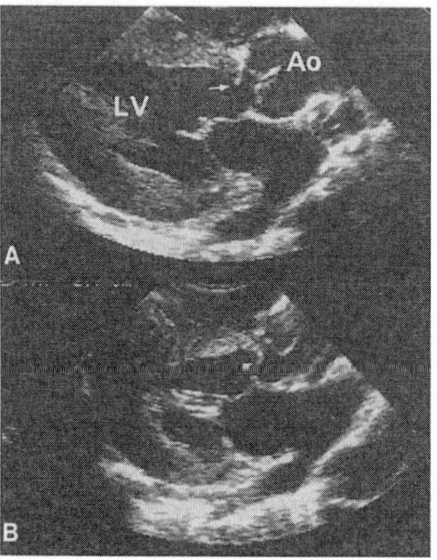

Fig. 2. Left ventricular long-axis views (A, B) obtained intraoperatively with the transducer placed onto the right ventricular surface. The patient was known to have a subaortic membrane. Preoperative echocardiographic investigation, however, had left doubt whether the interventricular septum showed characteristics of a hypertrophic obstructive cardiomyopathy. The echocardiographic images revealed left ventricular hypertrophy and a discrete subaortic membrane closely to the right aortic valve (arrow). No evidence was found of hypertrophic cardiomyopathy. Ao = aorta; LV = left ventricle.

Results after repair

All patients were studied intraoperatively immediately after termination of cardiopulmonary bypass. In 9 of the 14 patients with a subaortic membrane the remnants of the membrane were still visibile near its attachment to the interventricular septum and/or to the anterior mitral valve. The systolic anterior motion of the mitral valve if present before repair, persisted in all patients after relief of the obstruction, but its magnitude decreased (Fig. 3). In patients with hypertrophic obstructive cardiomyopathy, intraoperative echocardiography assessed the extent of the septal myectomy (Fig. 4). Finally, when necessary, left-sided echo contrast studies were used in order to exclude significant aortic or mitral valve regurgitation (Fig. 5).

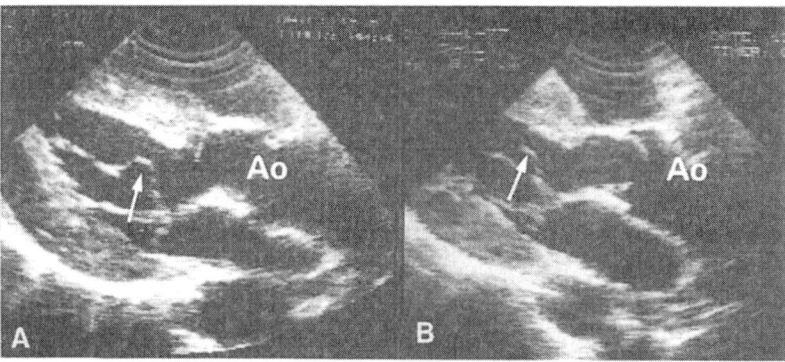

Fig. 3. Intraoperative two-dimensional left ventricular long-axis views obtained in a patient with subaortic stenosis due to a membrane. The systolic anterior motion of the mitral valve (arrow) was present before (A) and after (B) surgical repair. Ao = aorta.

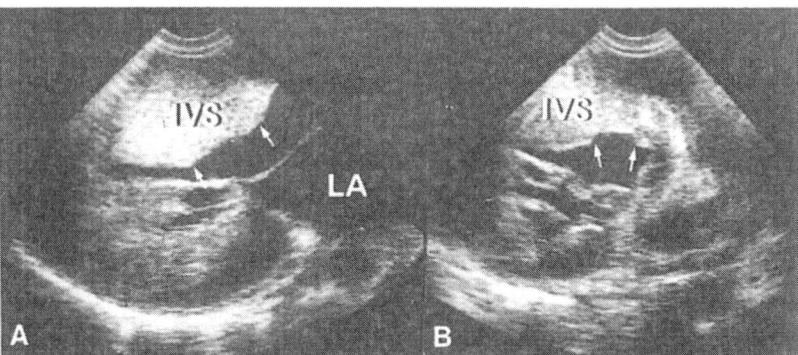

Fig. 4. Intraoperative two-dimensional echocardiograms showing the results of left ventricular outflow tract myectomy in a patient with hypertrophic obstructive cardiomyopathy. The length (arrows) of the myectomy is seen in the left ventricular long-axis view (A). The short-axis view (B) indicates its width and depth within the interventricular septum (IVS) (arrows). LA = left atrium.

348

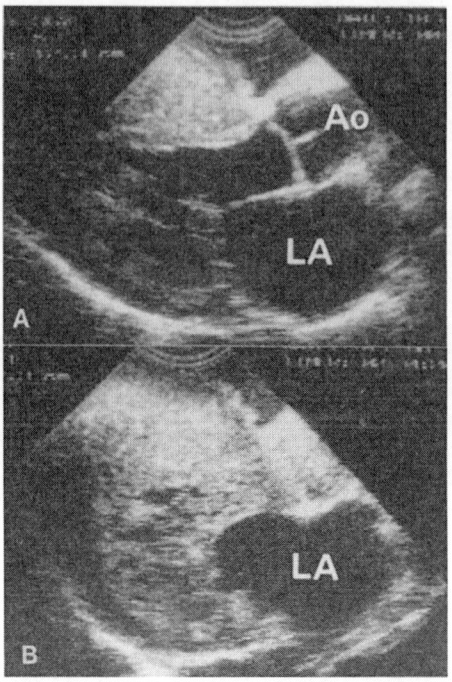

Fig. 5. Intraoperative two-dimensional left ventricular long-axis views (A, B) in a patient with hypertrophic obstructive cardiomyopathy and mitral valve incompetence. Following myectomy the contrast study with saline injected in the left ventricle (B) did not reveal a trace of bubbles entering the left atrium (LA). Ao = aorta.

Conclusion

The value of the intraoperative echocardiographic findings in relation to their surgical consequences, is a matter of debate. Nonetheless, an intraoperative echocardiographic study that confirms the preoperatively assessed morphologic diagnosis, is important. Moreover, the technique is the examination of choice in eliminating doubts, if any, after the preoperative clinical diagnosis. If the surgeon finds additional unsuspected morphology, his experience enables him to judge whether this finding is of importance. This is best illustrated in 4 patients not known to have left ventricular outflow tract abnormalities. In one patient referred with mitral and aortic valve incompetence, an unsuspected fixed subvalvular aortic obstruction of fibromuscular nature was noted on the intraoperative echocardiogram (Fig. 6). This obstruction could otherwise have been missed but was now resected via an aortotomy. Thus a second operation could be prevented. In 3 other patients with mitral valve and/or aortic valve disease a highly reflective bar of echoes

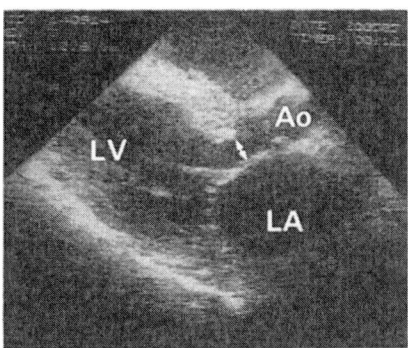

Fig. 6. Intraoperative two-dimensional echocardiogram of the left ventricular outflow tract obtained in a patient referred for correction of mitral and aortic valve insufficiency. Unexpectedly discrete subvalvular aortic stenosis of fibromuscular nature was seen (arrow). Note the enlarged left atrium (LA) and left ventricle (LV). Ao = aorta.

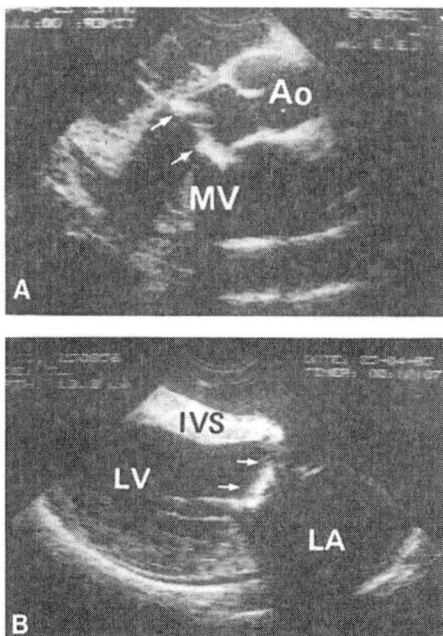

Fig. 7. A modified left ventricular long-axis (A) and four-chamber (B) view obtained in a patient referred for aortic valve replacement because of insufficiency. Unexpectedly the images showed highly reflective echoes upstream (arrows) in the left ventricular outflow tract, apparently connecting the anterior mitral valve leaflet (MV) to the interventricular septum (IVS). Intracardiac inspection revealed a significant bar of calcium in the posterior wall of the left ventricular outflow tract which did not give obstruction. LA = left atrium; Ao = aorta; LV = left ventricle.

was seen in the left ventricular outflow tract 2 cm beneath the aortic valve (Fig. 7). This phenomenon was due to a local concentration of calcium on the posterior surface of the left ventricular outflow tract which, however, needed no surgical intervention.

It is noteworthy that 2 of the 14 patients with a subvalvular aortic membrane discussed in this chapter had surgical correction for a ventricular septal defect in childhood. This underlines the importance of intraoperative echocardiography. One should realize that patients referred for surgery may have a preoperatively undiagnosed abnormality (vide supra). Intraoperative echocardiographic detection of such abnormality renders the facility to perform the repair in the same session and thus a reoperation can be prevented.

Thus, intraoperative two-dimensional echocardiography is a safe, accurate and easy technique. The procedure is not time-consuming. Based on a large population of patients studied the cardiac surgeons have gained experience both in obtaining diagnostic images and in the interpretation thereof. It is this experience that enabled them to use the intraoperative echocardiographic information in an optimal way.

References

1. Gussenhoven WJ, Becker AE: Congenital Heart Disease. Morphologic echocardiographic correlations. Edinburgh 1983, Churchill Livingstone, 1983.
2. Stark J, De Leval M: Surgery for congenital heart defects. London New York 1983, Grune & Stratton, 1983.
3. Ten Cate FJ (ed.): Hypertrophic cardiomyopathy. New York 1985, Marcel Dekker Inc., Chapter 6.
4. Van Herwerden LA, Gussenhoven WJ, Roelandt J et al.: Intraoperative epicardial two-dimensional echocardiography. Eur Heart J 7: 386–95, 1986.
5. Van Herwerden LA, Gussenhoven WJ, Roelandt JRTC et al.: Intraoperative two-dimensional echocardiography in complicated infective endocarditis of the aortic valve. J Thorac Cardiovasc Surg 93: 587–591, 1987.
6. Gussenhoven WJ, Van Herwerden LA, Roelandt J, Ligtvoet CM, Bos E, Witsenburg M: Intraoperative two-dimensional echocardiography in congenital heart disease. J Am Coll Cardiol 9: 565–572, 1987.
7. Maron BJ, McIntosh CL, Wesley YE, Arce J: Application of intraoperative two-dimensional echocardiography to patients with obstructive hypertrophic cardiomyopathy undergoing ventricular septal myotomy-myectomy. J Am Coll Cardiol 3: 565 (abstr.), 1984.

5.5. Intraoperative assessment of left ventricular performance

MORRIS N. KOTLER

Introduction

The immediate effects of surgery on left ventricular function for acquired heart disease have not been well defined until the era of intraoperative echocardiography. Left ventricular dysfunction is one of the major determinants of prognosis following coronary artery bypass surgery and valve replacement. The feasibility and ease of performing intraoperative echocardiography on patients undergoing open heart surgery provides the clinician with important data regarding therapeutic strategies especially in the high risk subset of patients.

Technique

Intraoperative two-dimensional echocardiography can generally be readily performed before cardiopulmonary bypass with the pericardium opened and immediately after bypass or valve replacement [1–3]. Ideally a 3.5 MHz non-

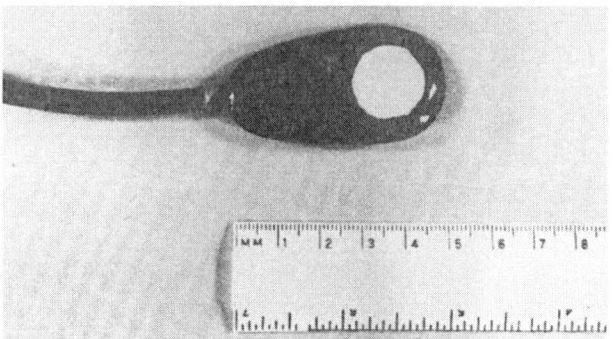

Fig. 1. The 3.5 MHz thin ceramic wafer transducer used for intraoperative two-dimensional echocardiographic studies is shown. Reproduced with permission Ren JF, Panidis IP, Kotler MN, Mintz GS, Goel I, Ross J. Effect of coronary bypass surgery and valve replacement on left ventricular function: Assessment by intraoperative two-dimensional echocardiography. Am Heart J 109: 281–289, 1985.

I. Cikes (ed.), *Echocardiography in Cardiac Interventions*, 351–362, 1989.
© 1989 *Kluwer Academic Publishers.*

352

commercially available thin ceramic wafer transducer can be used [2] (Fig. 1). The transducer is connected to a regular two-dimensional echocardiographic scanner. The hand held transducer can be directly applied to the right ventricular surface and left ventricular apex by the operator so that constant contact to the beating heart can be maintained. Several echocardiographic views can be performed depending on the type of formula used to calculate the two-dimensional volumes and ejection fraction. In our institution, we generally performed left ventricular short axis and apical two-chamber views [2, 3]. Once the images have been obtained and recorded on video-tape, individual views of the left ventricle can be visualized by the use of a video tape Sony recorder which provides slow speed and frame-by-frame forward

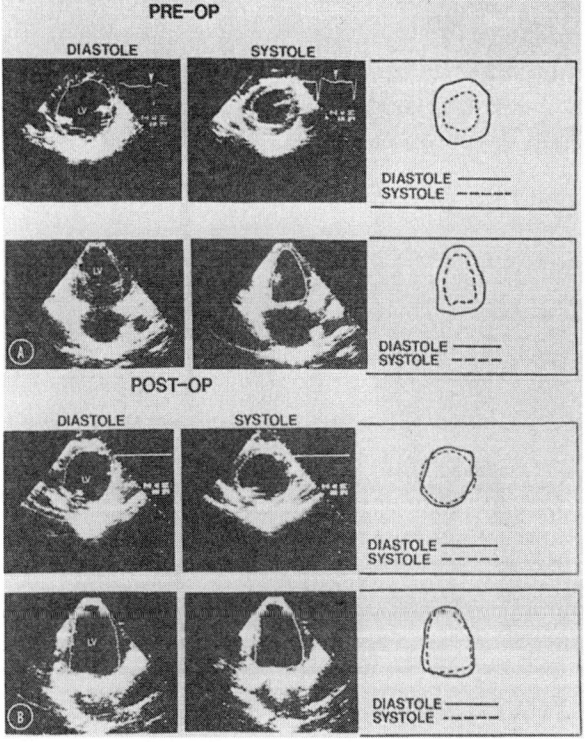

Fig. 2. Intraoperative two-dimensional echocardiography during mitral valve replacement for mitral regurgitation before (PRE-OP) and after (POST-OP) cardiopulmonary bypass. Upper, left ventricular (LV) short-axis view. Lower, Apical two-chamber view in diastole and systole with schematic diagram in right panel. A, Normal left ventricular contraction is present in the PRE-OP study. B, Severe diffuse left ventricular (LV) hypokinesis is apparent in the POST-OP study. Dottled lines indicate the tracing along the outermost edge of the endocardium.
Reproduced with permission Ren JF, Panidis IP, Kotler MN, Mintz GS, Goel I, Ross J. Effect of coronary bypass surgery and valve replacement on left ventricular function: Assessment by intraoperative two-dimensional echocardiography. Am Heart J 109: 281–289, 1985.

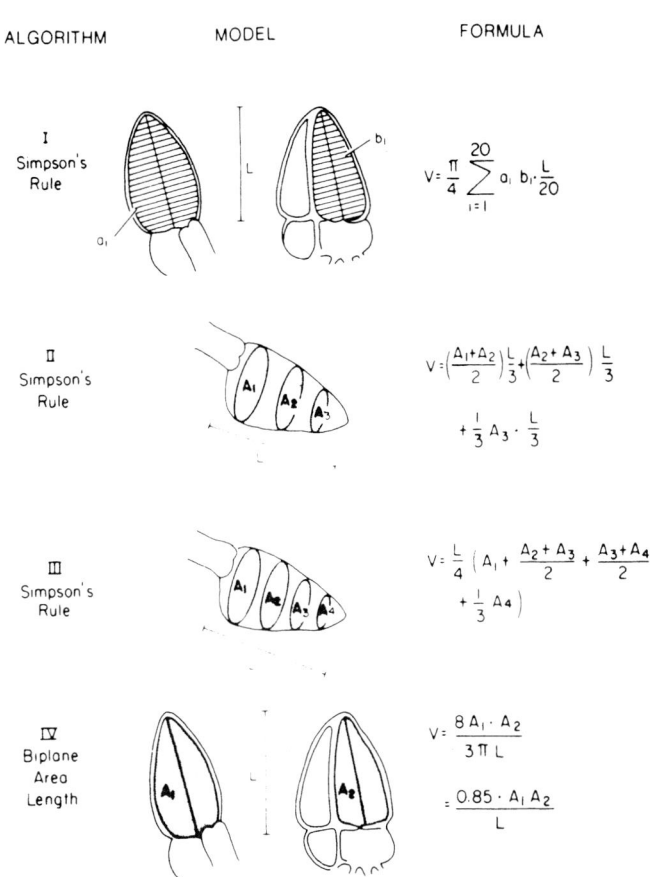

ALGORITHM   MODEL   FORMULA

I
Simpson's
Rule

$$V = \frac{\pi}{4} \sum_{i=1}^{20} a_i \cdot b_i \cdot \frac{L}{20}$$

II
Simpson's
Rule

$$V = \left(\frac{A_1 + A_2}{2}\right)\frac{L}{3} + \left(\frac{A_2 + A_3}{2}\right)\frac{L}{3} + \frac{1}{3} A_3 \cdot \frac{L}{3}$$

III
Simpson's
Rule

$$V = \frac{L}{4}\left(A_1 + \frac{A_2 + A_3}{2} + \frac{A_3 + A_4}{2} + \frac{1}{3} A_4\right)$$

IV
Biplane
Area
Length

$$V = \frac{8 A_1 \cdot A_2}{3 \pi L} = \frac{0.85 \cdot A_1 A_2}{L}$$

Fig. 3. Biplane and single plane algorithms calculating chamber volume from two-dimensional echocardiograms.

I. Simpson's rule method based on orthogonal planes from the apical two-chamber and apical four-chamber planes. The calculation is based on the summation of areas from diameters a1 and b1 of 20 equal cylinders or discs obtained by dividing the LV or LA longest length in 20 equal sections.

II. Simpson's rule using a summation of parasternal short-axis planes obtained from the apex to the base. The areas of A1, A2 and A3 are the planimetered areas in the parasternal short axis projection. L is derived from an apical projection, usually the apical two-chamber view.

III. An expansion of Method II that is even more difficult to use.

IV. Biplane area-length method of the traced area outlines (A1 and A2) obtained from the apical two-chamber and four-chamber planes. L is obtained from either the apical two-or four chamber view. This formula is frequently used in biplane cineangiography taking into account the ellipsoid configuration of the left ventricle.

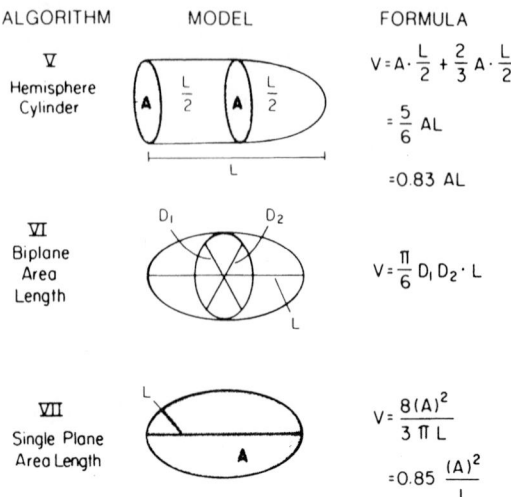

ALGORITHM	MODEL	FORMULA

V. The hemispheric cylinder model uses an area obtained from the parsternal short axis plane at the level of the papillary muscles (or mitral valve) and a length from an apical plane. This model is the arithmetic average of a cylinder and an ellipse and as such places the minor axis at the mid point of its long axis. In the human ventricle, the minor axis is considerably more basal.

VI. Ellipsoid biplane technique using the length obtained from an apical plane, usually the two-chamber apical plane, and a parasternal short axis plane at either the level of the tips of the papillary muscles or at the mitral valve level.

VII. Single plane area length method and is similar to the single plane method developed for angiography.

Reproduced from Reference 4 – Schiller NB, Botvinick EH. Non invasive quantitation of the left heart by echocardiography and scintigraphy. In 'Cardiac Imaging: New Technologies and Clinical Applications. Editors Kotler MN, Steiner RM. F. A. Davis Company, Philadelphia 1986, pp 45–93. With permission.

features. Left ventricular volumes are generally measured at end-diastole, (the largest chamber at the onset of the QRS complex) and at end-systole the smallest chamber at the end of the T wave from two orthogonal planes. As shown in Fig. 2, the feasibility of obtaining good quality intraoperative echocardiograms is easily reproducible. Left ventricular short axis views are generally obtained at the level between the mitral valve and papillary muscles.

By means of a microprocessor light pen system, or on-line computer analysis system, images from both views can be traced along the outermost edge of the endocardial echoes. Volume determinations can be calculated by a program computerized system using a bi-plane Simpson's rule: however a variety of formulae and algorithms can be employed (Fig. 3) [4]. Generally three consecutive beats are measured and averaged for determinations. Another group of investigators [1] utilizing intraoperative echocardiography have obtained short axis views that were recorded at four levels; namely, (1)

The base of the mitral valve, (2) The tip of the mitral valve. (3) The maximum diameter of the left ventricle and (4) at the level of the papillary muscle. The long axis views including the cardiac apex can be also recorded from the apical four or two-chambered view. In that particular study the left ventricular ejection fraction was calculated by two different methods. The short-axis area change (SAAC-EF) was defined as:

$$SAAC-EF = \frac{EDA - ESA}{EDA}$$

based on diastolic and systolic sections from level 3 (maximum cross-section). This formula may be misleading especially in ventricles with distorted geometry such as occurs in patients with large antero-apical aneurysms.

Another method of calculating ejection fraction utilized a modification of the Quinone's (Q) formula [5]

$$EFQ = ef + L(1 - ef)$$

where $ef = EDA - ESA/EDA$ and L is a correction factor for apical shortening.
EDA and ESA represented the average of the short axis sections 1, 2, and 4.

The correction factor for apical shortening is determined as follows: normal apical motion $L = 0.15$; hypokinetic apical motion $L = 0.05$; akinetic apical motion, $L = -0.05$; and dyskinetic motion, $L = -0.15$.

Thus, this indirect method of calculation of EF has been correlated with the EF obtained by angiography [1, 5]. However most investigators prefer to directly measure the length of the left ventricle by obtaining a technical adequate echocardiogram rather than using indirect assumptions.

Validity of intraoperative echocardiographic determination of left ventricular function

The validation of the echocardiographic determination of volumes and ejection fraction have been correlated with angiographic determinations using RAO cineangiography in patients who underwent cardiac catheterization within 24 hours prior to the surgery [1]. In our study, we correlated cardiac catheterization and intraoperative two-dimensional echo within one week prior to the measurements being taken [2, 3]. The correlation as determined by echocardiography correlated well with cineangiography with an R value of 0.91; however there was only fair correlation with regard to left ventricular end-diastolic volumes [2, 3].

Clinical utility of intraoperative echocardiography

Effects of coronary artery by-pass grafting on left ventricular function

In patients who underwent coronary artery bypass surgery, there was no significant change in left ventricular volumes immediately after coronary artery bypass grafting (CABG) (Fig. 4). The left ventricular ejection fraction also remained unchanged in patients without intraoperative complications, i.e. in those patients without new Q waves or enzyme elevation following coronary artery bypass surgery (Fig. 4). This compares favorably with other studies using contrast angiography or radionuclide techniques which have also shown lack of improvement in ejection fraction [6–9]. In one study a decrease in left ventricular ejection fraction was found at 1 week after CABG: however improvement occurred at 2 months and no change over 1 year was noted [10]. In patients in the immediate post CABG period, who develop new Q waves or evidence of MB-CPK isoenzymes to total CPK elevation greater than 5%, there was a decrease in the intraoperative ejection fraction (Fig. 5). In those patients who developed intraoperative myocardial infarction, prolonged cardiopulmonary bypass and aortic cross clamp time

CABG

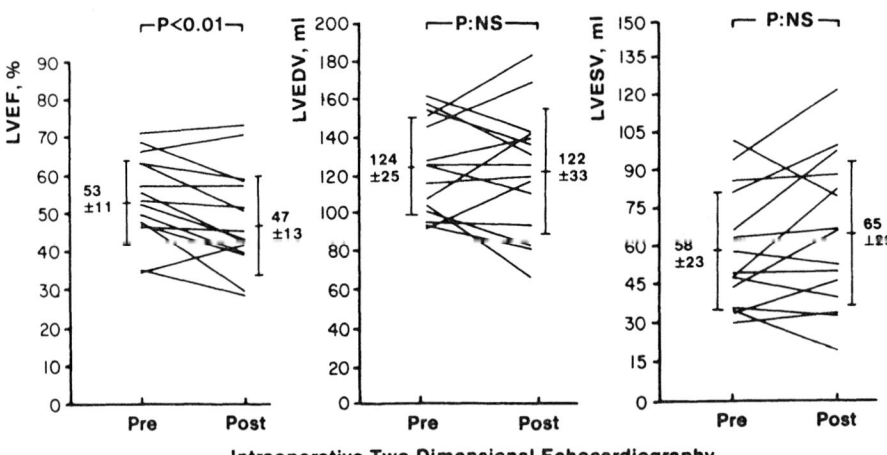

Fig. 4. Left ventricular ejection fraction (LVEF), end-diastolic (LVEDV), and end-systolic volume (LVESV) in patients undergoing coronary artery bypass grafting (CABG) before (Pre) and after (Post) cardiopulmonary bypass.

Reproduced with permission Ren JF, Panidis IP, Kotler Mn, Mintz GS, Goel I, Ross J. Effect of coronary bypass surgery and valve replacement on left ventricular function: Assessment by intraoperative two-dimensional echocardiography. Am Heart J 109: 281–289, 1985.

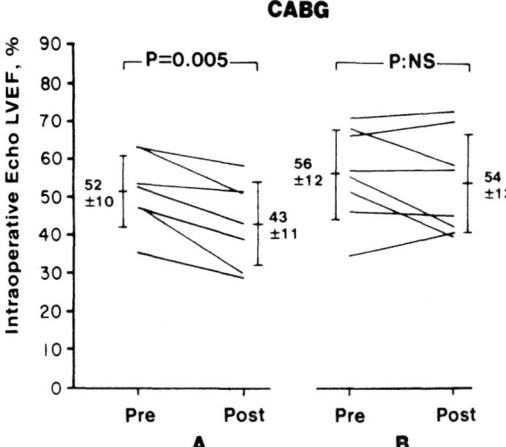

Fig. 5. Intraoperative echocardiographic left ventricular ejection fraction (LVEF) before (Pre) after (Post) cardiopulmonary bypass in patients with elevated (MB/CPK) ratio or development of new Q waves after coronary artery bypass grafting (CABG) (A) and patients without these changes (B).
Reproduced with permission. Ren JF, Panidis IP, Kotler MN, Mintz GS, Goel I, Ross J. Effect of coronary bypass surgery and valve replacement on left ventricular function: Assessment by intraoperative two-dimensional echocardiography. Am Heart J 109: 281–289, 1985.

was noted. Other investigators have also reported that prolonged cardiopulmonary bypass time can be associated with an increase risk of perioperative infarction [11–14]. In our study, only three patients demonstrated new wall motion abnormalities after CABG. However abnormal septal motion which commonly occurs after open heart surgery can be confused with new wall motion abnormalities.

Effects of valve surgery on left ventricular function

In another study, intraoperative two-dimensional echocardiography was performed in 31 patients during aortic or mitral valve replacement using similar intraoperative echocardiographic techniques [3]. In patients with mitral regurgitation the left ventricular ejection fraction decreased from 64 ± 10 to $46 \pm 20\%$. Similarly, decreases in left ventricular end-diastolic volume occurred from 162 ± 38 ml to 142 ± 39 ml. In patients with aortic regurgitation, the left ventricular ejection fraction decreased from 52 ± 13 to $37 \pm 16\%$ and left ventricular end-diastolic volume from 183 ± 68 to 157 ± 67 mls. (Figs. 6 & 7). In that study there were 7 patients with aortic and mitral regurgitation who remainded normotensive (Group A) and they were compared with 8 patients who developed hypotension after valve surgery Group

358

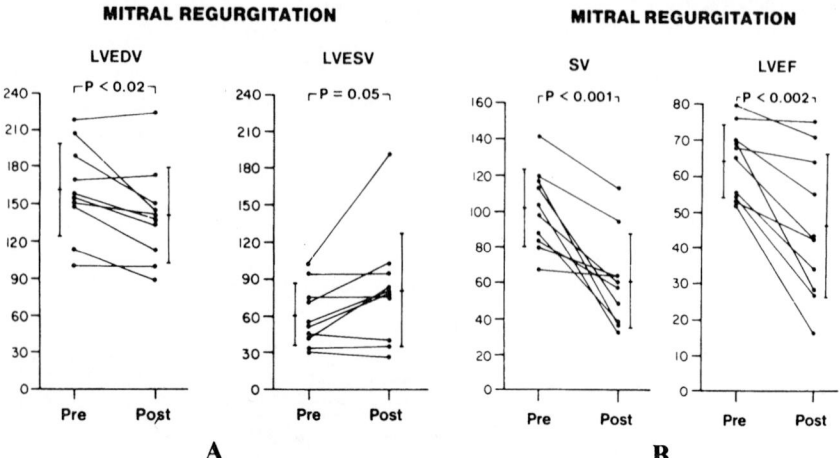

Fig. 6. (A) Left ventricular end-diastolic volume (LVEDV), end-systolic volume (LVESV); and (B) stroke volume (SV) and ejection fraction (LVEF) before (pre) and after (post) cardiopulmonary bypass during valve replacement for mitral regurgitation as assessed by intraoperative 2-D echo. A significant decrease in LVEDV, SV, and LVEF, and a significant increase in LVESV, are shown.

Reproduced with permission. Panidis IP, Ren JF, Mintz GS, Kotler MN, Goel I, Ross J. Effects of prosthetic valve replacement on left ventricular function assessed intraoperatively by two-dimensional echocardiography. J Cardiovascular Ultrasonography 5: 135–142, 1986.

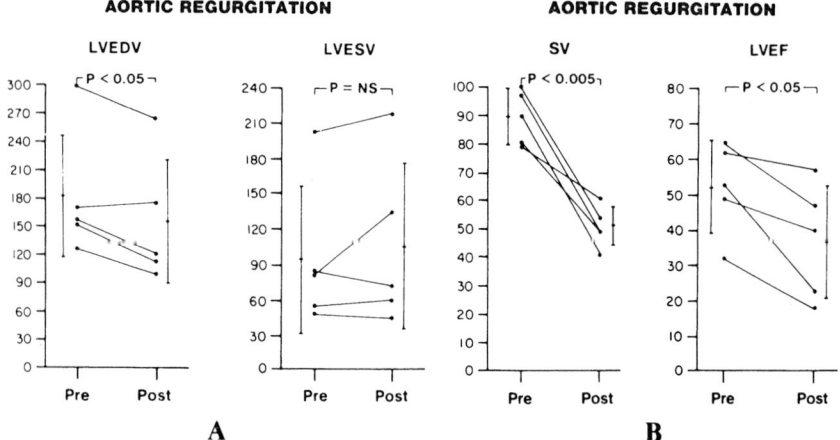

Fig. 7. (A) Left ventricular end-diastolic volume (LVEDV), end-systolic volume (LVESV); and (B) stroke volume (SV) and ejection fraction (LVEF) before (pre) and after (post) cardiopulmonary bypass during valve replacement for aortic regurgitation as assessed by intraoperative 2-D echo. A significant decrease in LVEDV, SV and LVEF is shown.

Reproduced with permission. Panidis IP, Ren JF, Mintz GS, Kotler MN, Goel I, Ross J. Effects of prosthetic valve replacement on left ventricular function assessed intraoperatively by two-dimensional echocardiography. J Cardiovascular Ultrasonography 5: 135–142, 1986.

VALVE REPLACEMENT

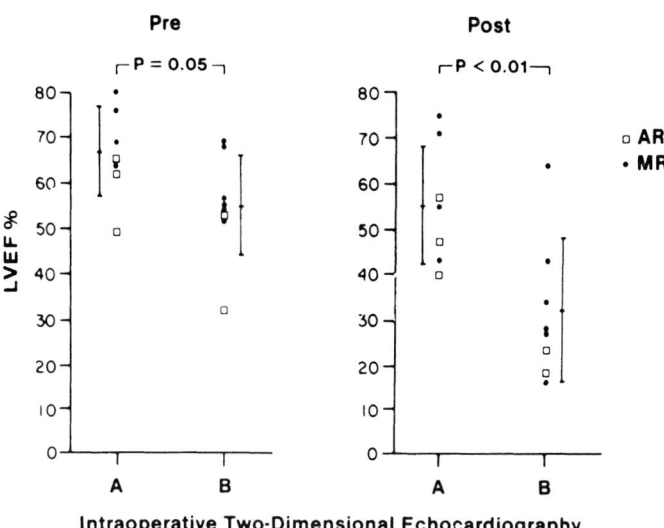

Fig. 8. Left ventricular ejection fraction (LVEF) before (pre) and after (post) cardiopulmonary bypass in 7 patients (A) with valve replacement for aortic regurgitation (AR) or mitral regurgitation (MR) and no postoperative hypotension as compared to the remaining 8 patients (B) with AR or MR and persistent postoperative hypotension. Pre- and post-LVEF as assessed by intraoperative 2-D echo are significantly lower in the later group.

Reproduced with permission. Panidis IP, Ren JF, Mintz GS, Kotler MN, Goel I, Ross J. Effects of prosthetic valve replacement on left ventricular function assessed intraoperatively by two-dimensional echocardiography. J Cardiovascular Ultrasonography 5: 135–142, 1986.

B (Figure 8). In Group A who remained normotensive a higher initial ejection fraction with less of a reduction postoperatively was present. However, in Group B (post operative hypotension) the initial ejection fraction was lower preoperatively and dropped to a greater extent than in Group A patients. These findings have been also confirmed by Dubroff and his group [1].

Reduction in stroke volume and ejection fraction and decrease in volumes following valve replacement for aortic and mitral regurgitation suggest that they occur immediately after valve replacement and may persist throughout the late postoperative period. In patients with aortic regurgitation, generally preload and afterload is increased. In our study, preoperative systolic volume was high and it increased slightly, although not significant after valve replacement. This may have occurred as a result of the insertion of aortic valve prosthesis and an increase in left ventricular outflow resistance. A drop in the ejection fraction immediately after valve replacement can be explained as a result of a decrease in the end-diastolic volume preload. Several studies have shown that although the ejection fraction in patients with aortic regurgitation is reduced postoperatively, it may require several months before improving [15, 16]. With regard to mitral regurgitation, generally there is a reduction of afterload due in part to ejection of the left ventricular stroke volume into a low pressure, low compliant left atrium. After valve replacement, the low resistance chamber is eliminated and the entire stroke volume is ejected against normal aortic resistance. In our study, a significant decrease in left ventricular ejection fraction and end-diastolic volume occurred, although there was a slight increase in left ventricular systolic volume, suggesting that latent left ventricular dysfunction can be unmasked by the surgical correction and removal of the low atrial compliance chamber [2, 3]. Other investigators have confirmed that patients with mitral regurgitation who have a decreased or even low normal ejection fraction may have a pronounced drop in left ventricular ejection fraction post-operatively [17, 18]. Thus, a super normal preoperative ejection fraction in patients with mitral regurgitation may have a better result postoperatively. The clinical implications of these studies suggest that those patients who have the most profound immediate drop in ejection fraction intraoperatively are most likely to develop low cardiac output states and hypotension in the immediate postoperative period. Thus, this subset of patients may require aggressive inotropic support and/or postoperative intraaortic balloon insertion to improve cardiac output and improve left ventricular dysfunction.

In patients with aortic stenosis undergoing valve replacement improvement in ejection fraction has occurred even in patients with impaired preoperative left ventricular function and clinically evident heart failure [19, 20].

Limitations of intraoperative echocardiography

There are factors that can depress ejection fraction in the immediate intraoperative and postoperative state which include: (1). Type of anesthesia (2), myocardial preservation techniques including hypothermia and crystalloid cardioplegia (3), cardiopulmonary bypass duration and cross-clamping time (4) changes in circulating hormone levels during and after surgery.

Virtually all anesthestic agents including Ketamine, Morphine and nitrous-oxide can depress myocardial contractility. Patients with a stunned myocardium occurring as a result of topical hypothermia and cold crystalloid cardioplegia and relative ischemia can account for depression of ejection fraction that may still improve in the late postoperative period. In addition, changes in circulating levels of norepinephrine, epinephrine, cortisol, antidiuretic hormone and renin have been shown to occur during and after surgery in patients undergoing open heart surgery [21]. However, these hormonal changes would tend to elevate ejection indices and would not account for the observed depression of ejection fraction in patients who have mitral or aortic regurgitation. Inability to record endocardial echoes when the transducer is not in constant contact with the epicardial surface during systole may account for some echo drop out and inability to obtain ideal volume determinations. Abnormal septal motion commonly seen after open heart surgery may also interfere with calculation of the ejection fraction.

In summary, intraoperative two-dimensional echocardiography studies is technically feasible and can be readily performed in patients undergoing open heart surgery. Generally ejection fractions and volumes are not significantly changed in the immediate postoperative coronary artery bypass patient. A significant decrease in intraoperative ejection fraction and/or new segmental wall motion abnormalities should be regarded as evidence of myocardial damage or intraoperative infarction occurring during CABG and these patients should be observed closely for signs of left ventricular decompensation. In patients with mitral or aortic regurgitation undergoing mitral valve or aortic valve replacement, left ventricular ejection fraction and left ventricular end-diastolic volume is significantly decreased. Those patients with the lowest ejection fractions generally have the greatest drop and are most likely to develop post operative hypotension. Thus, intraoperative two-dimensional echo may be helpful in identifying a subset of patients who may benefit from inotropic support or intraoperative balloon insertion after CABG or valve replacement.

References

1. Dubroff JM, Clark ME, Wong CYH, et al: Left ventricular ejection fraction during cardiac surgery: a two-dimensional echocardiographic study. Circulation 68: 95, 1983.
2. Ren JF, Panidis IP, Kotler MN, et al: Effect of coronary bypass surgery and valve replacement on left ventricular function: Assessment by intraoperative two-dimensional echocardiography. Am Heart J 109: 281, 1985.
3. Panidis IP, Ren JF, Mintz GS, et al: Effects of prosthetic valve replacement on left ventricular function assessed intraoperatively by two-dimensional echocardiography. J Cardiovascular Ultrasonography 5: 135, 1986.
4. Schiller NB, Botvinick EH: Noninvasive quantitation of the left heart by echocardiography and scintigraphy. In 'Cardiac Imaging: New technologies and Clinical Applications'. Editors Kotler MN, Steiner RM. Philadelphia, FA Davis Co, 1986, pp 45.
5. Quinones MA, Waggoner Ad, Reduto LA, et al: A new simplified and accurate method for determining ejection fraction with two-dimensional echocardiography. Circulation 64: 744, 1981.
6. Arbogast R, Solignac A, Bourassa MG: Influence of aorto coronary saphenous vein bypass surgery on left ventricular volumes and ejection fraction. Am J Med 54: 790, 1973.

7. Hammermeister KE, Kennedy JW, Hamilton GW, et al. Aorto-coronary vein bypass failure of successful grafting improve resting left ventricular function in chronic angina. N Engl J Med 290: 186, 1974.

8. Shepherd RL, Itscoitz SB, Glancy DL, et al: Deterioratiiong of myocardial function following aorto coronary bypass operation. Circulation 49: 467, 1974.

9. Ress G, Bristow JD, Kremkau EL, et al: Influence of aorto coronary bypass surgery on left ventricular performance. N Engl J Med 284: 1116, 1971.

10. Mintz LJ, Ingels NB, Daughters GT, et al: Sequential studies of left ventricular function and wall motion after coronary arterial bypass surgery. Am J Cardiol 45: 210, 1980.

11. Langou RA, Wiles JC, Cohen LS: Coronary surgery for unstable angina pectoris. Incidence of mortality of perioperative myocardial infarction. Br Heart J 40: 767, 1978.

12. Baur HR, Peterson TA, Amar O, et al: Predictors of perioperative myocardial infarction in coronary artery operation. Ann Thorac Surg 31: 36, 1981.

13. Chaitman BR, Alderman EL, Sheffield T, et al: Use of survival analysis to determine the clinical significance of new Q waves after coronary bypass surgery. Circulation 67: 302, 1983.

14. Gray RJ, Matloff JM, Conkin CM, at al: Perioperative myocardial infarction. Late clinical course after coronary by-pass surgery. Circulation 66: 1185, 1982.

15. Boucher CA, Bingham JB, Osbakken MD, et al: Early changes in left ventricular size and function after correction of left ventricular volume overload. Am J Cardiol 47: 991, 1981.

16. Gaasch WH, Andrias CW, Levine H: Chronic aortic regurgitation: The effect of aortic valve replacement on left ventricular volume, mass and function. Circulation 58: 825, 1978.

17. Schuler G, Peterson KL, Johnson A, et al: Temporal response of left ventricular performance to mitral valve surgery. Circulation 59: 1218, 1979.

18. Kennedy JW, Doces JG, Stewart DK: Left ventricular function before and following surgical treatment of mitral valve disease. Am Heart J 97: 592, 1978.

19. Murphy ES, Lawson RM, Starr A, et al: Severe aortic stenosis in patients 60 years of age and older. Left ventricular function and 10 year survival after valve replacement. Circulation 64: Suppl II 184–188, 1981.

20. Smith N, McAnulty JH, Rahimtoola SH: Severe aortic stenosis with impaired left ventricular function and clinical heart failure. Results of valve replacement. Circulation 58: 255, 1978.

21. Landymore RW, Murphy DA, Kinley CE, et al: Does pulsatile flow influence the incidence of postoperative hypertension? Ann Thoracic Surg 28: 261, 1978.

5.6. Intraoperative contrast echocardiography can directly assess myocardial perfusion

MARTIN E. GOLDMAN, THERESA GUARINO &
BRUCE P. MINDICH

Despite improved surgical techniques, institution of hyperkalemic, hypothermic cardioplegia and more modern postoperative care, perioperative infarction is still an important complication of open heart surgery [1]. Therefore, techniques to better identify myocardial regions at ischemic risk and development of techniques for improved myocardial protection is a priority in cardiac surgery.

At present, most institutions utilize cold potassium cardioplegic solutions for myocardial protection [2]. However, if significant coronary disease is present, routine aortic root perfusion of the cardioplegia may not reach regions of greatest risk. Surgeons now use temperature probes and direct visualization of the epicardium to determine if cardioplegia has been effective in cooling and arresting the heart [3]. However, areas of the septum which are at greatest risk for intraoperative ischemia cannot be easily evaluated.

Intraoperative echocardiography is a relatively new technique which facilitates direct visualization of myocardial and valvular functions [4]. By placing the sterilely prepared transducer directly on the epicardium, the surgeon can directly visualize ventricular contractility. Interestingly, routine cardioplegic instillation generates a perfusion study when viewed with intraoperative echocardiography. Areas of the myocardium with normal flow can be seen slowly whiting out as the cardioplegia percolates through. Areas with inadequate perfusion secondary to significant proximal coronary stenoses continue to remain dark and may continue to finely fibrillate, indicative of persistent ischemia. Therefore, regions of myocardium at risk for intraoperative ischemia can potentially be identified and protected [5].

We evaluated intraoperative cardioplegic contrast echocardiography to detect areas of ischemic risk during open heart surgery. Forty-two patients undergoing various cardiopulmonary bypass procedures, were imaged during hypothermic, hyperkalemic cardioplegic instillation in the ascending aorta. The echocardiographic plane chosen was the short axis view at the tips of the papillary muscle since areas of the septum, antero-lateral wall and inferior wall can all be seen in this view which generally localize three different coronary perfusion beds: left anterior descending, left circumflex and right coronary, respectively. The transducer was maintained in the same position

I. Cikes (ed.), *Echocardiography in Cardiac Interventions*, 363–366, 1989.
© 1989 *Kluwer Academic Publishers*.

just prior to and throughout cardioplegic perfusion. Areas of gradual graying to whiting (therefore receiving cardioplegic protection) could be differentiated from those areas which did not lighten at all. Additionally, distinct areas of persistent fine fibrillation could also be identified. In patients with normal coronary arteries, the entire myocardium would uniformly and simultaneously whiten. In patients with significant proximal coronary disease, imaging demonstrated persistent dark areas, frequently with fine fibrillation.

An additional interesting finding was during aortic root cardioplegic infusion as well as with subselective coronary injections, microbubbles could be visualized perfusing through the microcapillary system of the myocardium. This was an irregular finding, but generally correlated with the perfusion distribution of the respective coronary arteries.

For analysis of the study, 126 myocardial segments were examined for the presence and rate of whiting out, and compared to preoperative cardiac catheterization for the ability to identify the most jeopardized myocardial segment. Sensitivity of contrast cardioplegia to detect significant coronary stenoses for the septal or left anterior descending region was 96% compared to 100% for the antero-lateral or circumflex region and only 58% for the inferior or right coronary area. The overall sensitivity and specificity for all regions was 83 and 92%, respectively, when comparing intraoperative contrast cardioplegia to preoperative cardiac catheterization. Also, persistent fine fibrillation was seen in 10 of 30 cases with coronary disease, 8 in the septal region, 1 each in the antero-lateral and inferior region.

Several factors may be implicated in the visualization of cardioplegic perfusion by echocardiography: the nature of the solution, agitation of the solution by roller pump prior to infusion, temperature, and rate of perfusion. Current studies have shown that the roller pump agitation of the cardioplegic solution just prior to aortic root installation is a very important factor in the generation of microbubbles. The cold temperature of the solution may be important in maintaining microbubble integrity as perfusion occurs down into the microcapillary system. Additionally, vasoregulatory mechanisms, such as the accumulation of local and anaerobic metabolites, prostaglandins, and bradykinin may play a significant role in mediating vasodilatation in response to intraoperative hypoxia during aortic cross-clamping [6]. Preoperative and intraoperative pharmacologic interventions may also effect coronary flow.

There are obvious limitations of intraoperative cardioplegic contrast for evaluation of myocardial perfusion. The heart is profoundly ischemic, nonperfused, quickly cooling, which therefore makes this a poor physiologic model system. Another important consideration of intraoperative perfusion techniques is the mode of microbubble delivery; uniform and equal microbubble distribution to all coronary beds is a vital assumption if myocardial regions are to be compared. Aortic root delivery does not provide a true mixing chamber and the cardioplegic needle may direct more flow down one vessel, causing preferential flow to one region. However, results of cardioplegic perfusion correlated well with actual coronary anatomy. The right coronary system is harder to assess since the particular echo view at the short axis papillary muscle level may reflect mixed flow to the posterior myocardium. Therefore, right coronary stenoses were not as accurately predicted as the left system. Additionally, collateral flow which may develop during the acute ischemia induced by aortic cross-clamping could not be fully evaluated, except by subselective injections.

Other contrast techniques have been described which potentially could be applied intraoperatively to evaluate myocardial perfusion. Sonicated albumin microbubbles, developed by Feinstein, are small ($\leqslant$10 microns), and do not appear to cause myocardial depression as seen with larger, non-uniform microbubbles which may clog the microcapillary bed with subsequent ischemia. However, logistics of microbubbles preparation and their very short half life, do not make them feasible for routine intraoperative application. Therefore, imaging of cardioplegic perfusion is attractive because it is an integral part of the operative procedure, requiring no additional intervention.

Intraoperative cardioplegic contrast echocardiography could have more practical application if uniform microbubbles or a stable contrast agent could be introduced into the cardioplegia. This would facilitate frequent assessment of myocardial perfusion at various times during the operative procedure. Potentially, this method could help the surgeon identify myocardial regions at greatest intraoperative ischemic risk on line; thereby, allowing subselective myocardial protection which could potentially reduce morbidity and mortality from open heart surgery.

References

1. Hilton CJ, Teubl W, Acker M, et al.: Inadequate cardioplegic protection with obstructed coronary arteries. Ann Thorac Surg 28: 323–334, 1979.
2. Stiles QR, Kirklin JW: Myocardial preservation symposium. J Thorac Cardiovasc Surg 870–877, 1981.
3. Chiu RCJ, Blundell PE, Scott HJ, Cain S: The importance of monitoring intramyocardial temperature during hypothermic myocardial protection. Ann Thorac Surg 28: 317–322, 1978.
4. Goldman ME, Mindich BP: Intraoperative two-dimensional echocardiography: new application of an old technique. JACC 7: 374–382, 1986.
5. Goldman ME, Mindich BP: Intraoperative cardioplegic contrast echocardiography for assessing myocardial perfusion during open heart surgery. JACC 4: 1029–1034, 1984.
6. Gould KI, Lipscomb K, Hamilton GW: Physiologic basis for assessing critical coronary

stenosis: instantaneous flow response and regional distribution during coronary hyperemia as measures of coronary flow reserve. Am J Cardiol 33: 87–94, 1974.

5.7. Intraoperative epicardial echocardiography in recognizing acute myocardial ischemia

K. CHANDRASEKARAN, J. F. GREENLEAF, J. B. SEWARD & A. J. TAJIK

Cardiovascular morbidity and mortality of cardiac surgery is often due to failure to recognize underlying myocardial ischemia intraoperatively [1–2]. Perioperative myocardial infarction is an important complication whose incidence varies from 5–23% [3] and has a direct bearing on subsequent cardiac morbidity [3–7]. Several techniques have been used in an attempt to diagnose perioperative and intraoperative myocardial injury [8–18]. However to date there is no *in vivo* method which reliably identifies ischemic myocardium.

Various approaches to detecting myocardial ischemia intraoperatively are shown in Table I. Some are experimental, nevertheless they address the same issue. We will discuss the merits and pitfalls of each method briefly.

Electrocardiographic monitoring

ST-segment displacement on the surface ECG is considered to be a sensitive indicator of myocardial ischemia. However, it is not specific for ischemia [19],

Table 1. Approaches to detect myocardial ischemic intraoperatively.

1. Electrocardiographic Monitoring

2. Serum Markers
   Creatine Kinase
   Myoglobin

3. Myocardial Metabolism
   Thermocardiography
   Laser Fluorometry

4. Echocardiography – Doppler
   M-mode
   2D Echo
       Transesophageal Echocardiography
       High-frequency Epicardial Echocardiography
   Doppler Assessment of Coronary Blood Flow

I. Cikes (ed.), *Echocardiography in Cardiac Interventions*, 367–378, 1989.
© 1989 *Kluwer Academic Publishers*.

as false negative and false positive findings have been reported [20–22]. Although intraoperative ECG provides information about heart rate and rhythm, the single standard surface ECG lead is not suitable for diagnosing episodes of myocardial ischemia that result in sublte ST-segment changes [23] and at times transmural ischemia [24]. This is because of difficulties of displaying multiple leads. The low frequency response of the ECG amplifiers of monitors designed for operating room use, or any ECG in the monitor mode, is not adequate for assessing ST-segment changes [25–27]. Furthermore, during cardiac surgery, multiple precordial lead placement for monitoring is not feasible. Even though improved intraoperative ECG monitoring systems have been shown to result in an increased incidence of myocardial ischemia recognition [8, 28], it is still not good enough to detect myocardial ischemia when compared to modalities that identify changes in mechanical function and/or hemodynamics resulting from ischemia [15, 17, 29].

Serum markers

Creatine kinase (CK). Measurements of serum creatine kinase and specifically its MB enzyme have been very useful in establishing the diagnoses of myocardial damage. Some investigators feel that CK MB is specific for myocardium and hence its appearance in the serum is indicative of myocardial damage [30]. Although it is generally true that elevated CK MB indicates myocardial injury, in surgical patients, several factors can cause an elevation of this enzyme. Atrial myocardium is also rich in CK MB as is ventricular myocardium [31]. Hence, surgical manipulation of the atria, including the placement of purse-string sutures or a small atriotomy for insertion of venus cannula or both can cause release of sufficient CK MB to suggest myocardial injury [9]. Serum CK MB has been found to be elevated in the early postoperative period to suggest myocardial injury in patients who have had thoracotomy for pulmonary resection [32, 33]. Hence, serum CK MB by itself is not a reliable predictor of intraoperative or perioperative myocardial injury.

Serum myoglobin. Estimation of serum myoglobin appears to be a sensitive index of intraoperative myocardial injury [10, 11]. In experimental ischemia in dogs, myoglobin release was associated with tissue damage [34]. Although release of myoglobin may indicate myocardial injury, one has to realize that myoglobin is the largest reservoir of oxygen-binding capacity in the myocardium and has greater affinity than hemoglobin. Hence, theoretically, functional elimination and release of myoglobin can lead to myocardial ischemia. Furthermore, its elevation in other hypoxic conditions [35, 36] and further elevation with reperfusion questions its value as a reliable marker for myocardial injury.

Monitoring metabolism

Thermocardiography

Thermography is a technique by which images of the temperature are developed. Thermographs sense infrared radiation emitted by the surface of the heart. Regional myocardial ischemia causes changes in the temperature [37]. The decrease in temperature in the ischemic region is due to low metabolism and is seen as a cold region on the thermocardiographic (Fig. 1) [13]. Investigators have applied this technique intraoperatively to detect myocardial ischemia [12, 13]. Surface temperature mapping with thermograph has the following limitations:

1. Only anterior and lateral surfaces can be explored. Posterior surfaces cannot be explored without lifting the heart which may alter the temperature.
2. Epicardial fat and extensive scar tissue may mask the surface of the myocardium and may give rise to false values in the temperature map.

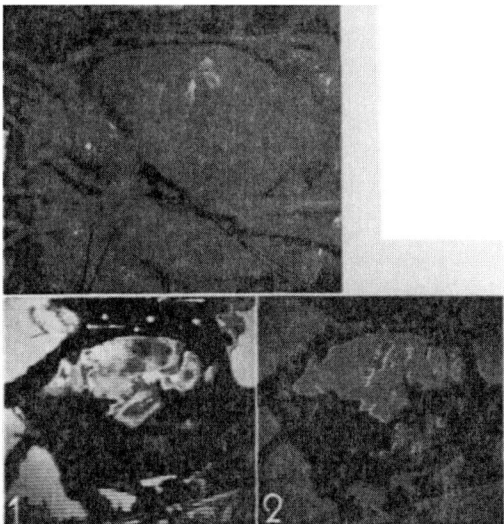

Fig. 1. The thermograms taken with two different sensitivities illustrates the ischemic area of the scar on the anterior surface of the left ventricle as a dark spot. (Reproduced with permission from [13].)

NADH laser fluorimetry

Myocardial metabolism depends on O_2 supply. Lack of O_2 or regional ischemia causes changes in regional myocardial metabolism. Nicotinamide Adenine Dinucleotide (NAD), a component of the intramitochondrial electron transport system is reduced to NADH with insufficient O_2. NADH fluoresces when excited by ultraviolet light and NAD does not. Based on these fluorescent characteristics of NAD, Barlow and associates developed the technique to assess myocardial O_2 supply [38, 39]. Investigators have applied this technique to evaluate the metabolic changes resulting from experimental ischemia [14].

These techniques are still experimental and are being developed for *in vivo* monitoring of myocardial metabolism thereby detecting myocardial ischemia.

Echocardiography

Acute myocardial ischemia produces abnormal movement of the involved myocardial segment. This was first demonstrated by Tennant and Wiggers in 1935 [40] and subsequently by other investigators [41–43]. These changes were sensitive to ischemia [44, 45] and appeared earlier than ECG changes [29]. Since echocardiography provides reliable estimates of wall thickening [46], investigators have used both M-mode echo mapping of left ventricle [16] and transesophageal assesment of segment wall motion abnormalities [17] to detect ischemia, intraoperatively. Although two-dimensional echocardio-graphic assessment provides important information regarding segmental wall thickening as well as wall motion patterns, experimental evidence suggest that these wall motion changes are seen *in normally perfused myocardium as well* [47] and in the normally perfused *myocardium adjacent to an infarct area* [48, 49]. Furthermore, technical limitations of transesophageal echo makes it difficult technique for detecting myocardial ischemia intraoperatively. There-fore, it appears that observation of segmental wall motion abnormality alone is not adequate for diagnosing myocardial ischemia.

Epicardial echocardiography using high-frequency (12 MHz) ultrasound provides high-resolution 2-D echo images [50, 51]. In an *in vivo* intra-operative experimental canine ischemic model we have used this technique to identify ischemic myocardium [51]. The two-dimensional echo images obtained from the anterior and posterior walls demonstrated smooth, uniform echoes from the myocardium with bright specular echoes from the endo- and epicardium (Figs. 2 and 3). The texture of myocardial echoes in the control state demonstrated a uniform change, i.e., the echoes became less

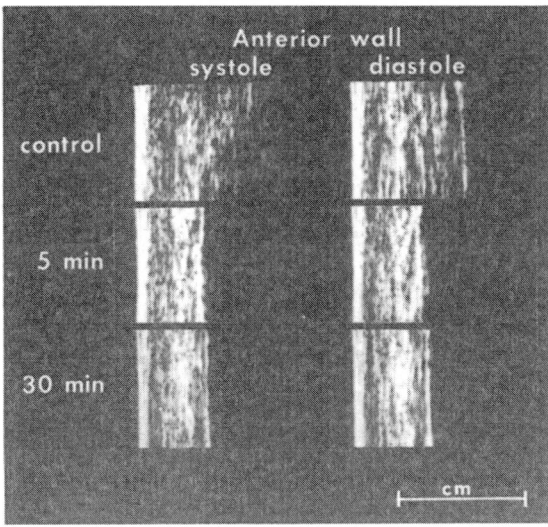

Fig. 2. End systolic and end diastolic frames of two-dimensional echo images in the control state and at 5 and 30 minutes during ischemia. *Anterior wall*. In the control state, the end diastolic image appears brighter compared to end-systolic image. During ischemia the end diastolic images appear somewhat brighter and blotchier than the corresponding control image. However, end systolic images have increased brightness with no appreciable change from end diastolic images. There is significant reduction in end systolic and end diastolic wall thicknesses during ischemia, more so in end systole. (Reproduced with permisson from [51].)

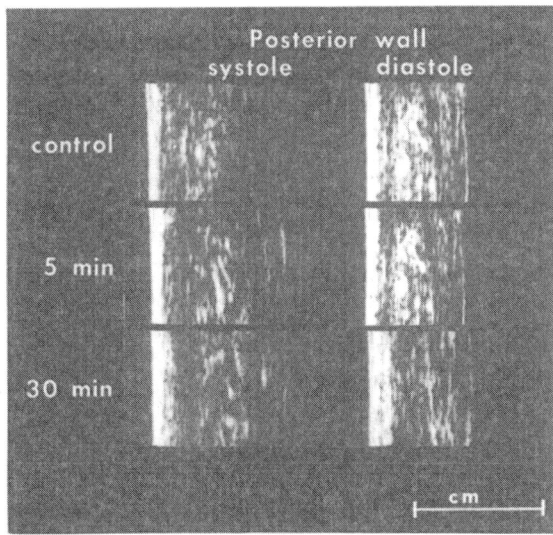

Fig. 3. *Posterolateral wall*. Normally perfused tissue produces uniformly distributed brightness of the images which are normally brighter at end diastole. No changes are visually apparent in the image texture or wall thickness during LAD ligation. (Reproduced with permission from [51].)

372

bright and somewhat separated from one another during systole and became more bright and approximated with each other during diastole. This cardiac cycle dependent change in the echo texture was more pronounced in end systole and end diastole. Following ischemia, the echo images from the anterior wall (Fig. 2) demonstrated three important features: 1) the echoes were brighter, coarser and blotchier during both systole and diastole compared to the control images, 2) the cyclic variation in the image texture observed in the control state was greatly diminished, and 3) the systolic decrease in echo intensity observed in the control state was no longer present, and there was no visually applicable difference in echo texture (echo intensity and its spatial distribution) between systolic and diastolic images. The nonischemic posterolateral wall showed no changes in image texture (Fig. 3). Similarly, the mean gray level value (MGL) (measure of echo intensity) estimated from the images demonstrated a cardiac cycle dependent decrease in echo intensity during systole and increase during diastole. This cardiac cycle dependent change in echo intensity was blunted in the anterior wall echo images obtained following ischemia (Fig. 4). The ischemic anterior wall

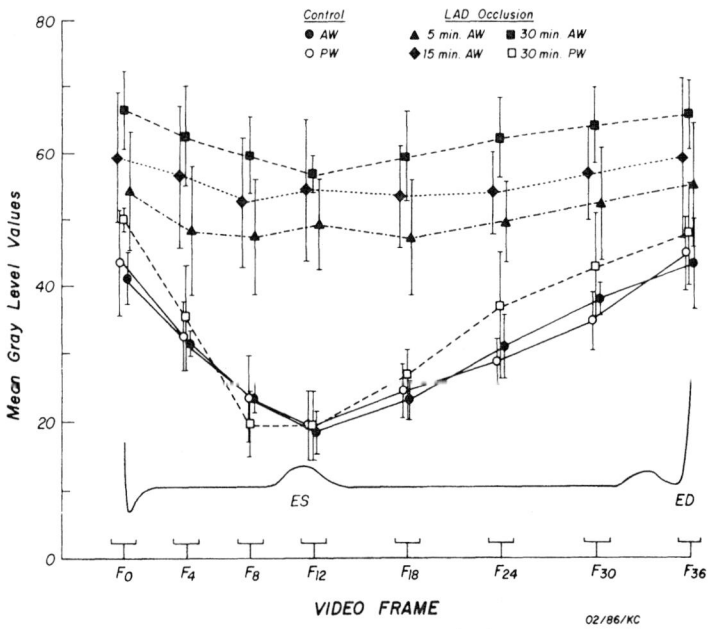

Fig. 4. MGL values (mean ± SD) in the anterior wall (Aw) and posterolateral wall (Pw) measured from the sequential video images representing a complete cardiac cycle for the last six animals. In the control state, MGL decreases during systole and increases during diastole, in both walls. During LAD ligation, at any given time the MGL measured from the anterior wall is significantly increased compared with the control state and there is blunting of the cyclic variation. (Reproduced with permission from [51].)

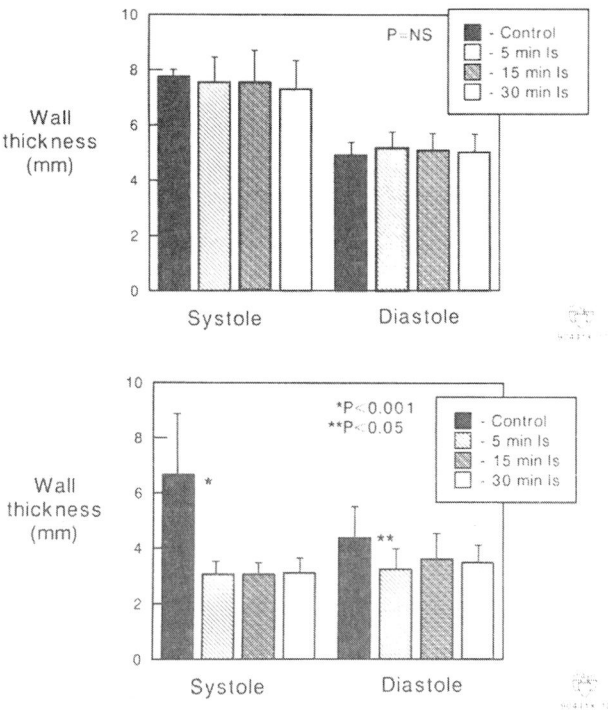

Fig. 5. Changes in the thickness (mm) of the anterior wall (above) and posterolateral wall (below) in the control state and at 5, 15, and 30 min following LAD ligation. Note there is a significant decrease in the thickness of the anterior wall during ischemia, both during systole and diastole.

demonstrated significant decrease in wall thickness (Fig. 5). The results of our study indicate that the echo texture changes associated with acute myocardial ischemia can be recognized as early as five minutes after the onset of ischemia. These changes in the echo texture can be appreciated by epicardial ultrasound examination and potentially could be utilized intraoperatively.

Evaluating the changes in the echo texture of the myocardium using high-frequency echo images [51] we feel offers a potential solution for diagnosing intraoperative myocardial ischemia. In the ultrasound literature it has been well documented both in *in vitro* experiments as well as *in vivo* experiments, that the backscatter (i.e., reflected ultrasound signal) is increased from ischemic myocardium [52–54]. The intensity of the backscatter and its spatial distribution give rise to the texture of the structure imaged. The changes in echo texture on high-frequency epicardial echo images following ischemia (Fig. 2) are similar to those seen on *in vitro* experimental myocardial ischemia (Fig. 6) [53]. Thus, texture changes together with wall motion changes may provide a reliable combination of measures for assessing myocardial ischemia intraoperatively. Although our study demonstrates a prom-

374

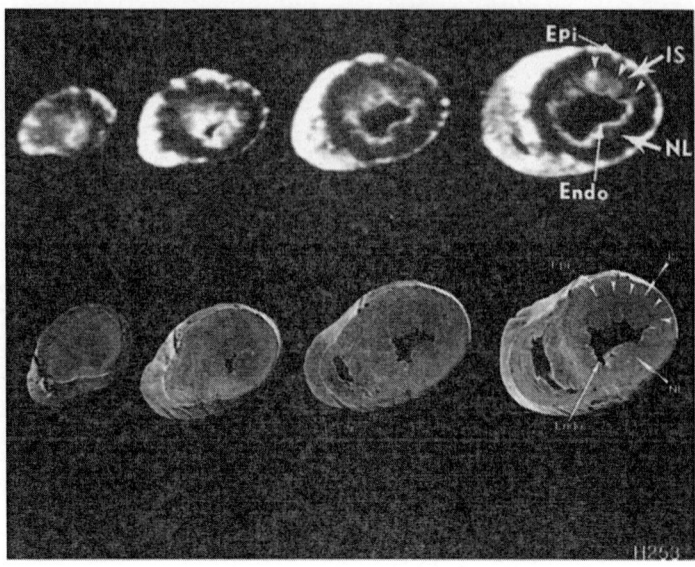

Fig. 6. Four anatomical sections (lower panel) and the corresponding compound echo images (upper panel) taken from a canine heart excised after 30 min of LAD ligation. The normally perfused myocardium apperas a lighter shade of red while the region perfused by occluded LAD artery appears a darkers shade of red. The corresponding compound echo images reveal altered texture and increased brightness in the regions associated with increased redness. Is = ischemia, NL = Normal, Endo = Endocardium, Epi = Epicardium. (Reproduced with permission from [53].)

ising role, there are limitations present which need to be addressed:

1. Currently, the transducer probe is not suitable to image the posterior wall of the left ventricle.
2. The short focus of the transducer (< 2 cm) offers some difficulty to interpret the echo texture in the subendocardial region during end systole.
3. We do not know the echo texture of chronically ischemic myocardium commonly prevalent in human population.

Doppler estimation of coronary blood flow

Intraoperative Doppler evaluation of coronary artery blood flow in the resting state and following hyperemic response can indicate the degree of myocardial perfusion, normal or decreased. Although Doppler can estimate coronary blood flow accurately [55], many conditions other than coronary stenosis can markedly alter coronary reactive hyperemic response [56–58].

Therefore, it is not an ideal technique to identify underperfused ischemic myocardium.

In summary, detection of myocardial ischemia intraoperatively is a difficult problem. However, assessment of changes in wall motion along with echo texture using epicardial high frequency echocardiography or transesophageal echocardiography may aid in early recognition of intraoperative myocardial ischemia.

References

1. Marx, GF, Mateo CV and Orkin LR: Computer analysis of post anesthetic deaths. Anesthesiology 39: 54, 1973.
2. Lunn JN and Mushin WW: Mortality associated with anaesthesia. London, Nuffield Provincial Hospitals Trust, 1982.
3. Val PG, Pelletier LC, Hernandez MG, Jais JM, Chaitman BR, Dupras G and Solymoss BC: Diagnostic criteria and prognosis of perioperative myocardial infarction following coronary bypass. J Thorac Cardiovasc Surg 86: 878, 1983.
4. Morton BC, McLaughlin PR, Trimble AS, and Morch JE: Myocardial infarction in coronary artery surgery. Circulation 52 (Supplement 1): 198, 1975.
5. Chaitman BR, Alderman EL, Sheffield, LT, Tong T, Fisher L, Mock MB, Weins RD Kaiser GC and Roitman D, et al.: Use of survival analysis to determine the clinical significance of new Q waves after coronary bypass surgery. Circulation 67: 302, 1983.
6. Espinoza J, Lipski J, Litwak R, Donoso E and Dack S: New Q wave after coronary artery bypass surgery for angina pectoris. Am J Cardiol 33: 221, 1974.
7. Rose MR, Glassman E, Isom OW and Spencer FC: Electrocardiographic and serum enzyme changes of myocardial infarction after coronary artery bypass surgery. Am J Cardiol 33: 215, 1974.
8. Kotrly KJ, Kotter GS, Mortara D and Kampine JP: Intraoperative detection of myocardial ischemia with an ST segment trend monitoring system. Anesth Analg 63: 343, 1984.
9. Graeber GM: Creatine kinase (CK): Its use in the evaluation of perioperative myocardial infarction. Surg Clin North Am 65 (3): 539, 1985.
10. Ellis AK, Little T, Masud ARZ and Klocke FJ: Patterns of myoglobin release after reperfusion of injured myocardium. Circulation 72: 639, 1985.
11. Seguin JR, Saussine M, Ferriere M and Chaptal PA: Myoglobin to predict myocardial infarction during heart surgery. The Lancet January 25: 220, 1986.
12. Senyk J, Malm A and Bornmyr S: Intraoperative cardiothermography. Eur Surg Res 3: 1, 1971.
13. Robicsek F, Masters TN, Svenson RH, Daniel WG, Daugherty HK, Cook JW and Selle JG: The application of thermography in the study of coronary blood flow. Surgery 84 (6): 858–864, 1978.
14. Mills SA, Jobsis FF and Seaber AV: A fluorometric study of oxidative metabolism in the *in vivo* canine heart during acute ischemia and hypoxia. Ann Surg 186 (2): 193, 1977.
15. Kaplan JA and Wells PH: Early diagnosis of myocardial ischemia using the pulmonary arterial catheter. Anesth Analg 60: 789, 1981.
16. Likoff M, Reichek N, St. John Sutton M, et al.: Epicardial mapping of segmental myocardial function: A echocardiographic method applicable in man. Circulation 66: 1050, 1982.

17. Smith, JS, Cahalan MK, Benefiel DJ, Byrd BF et al.: Intraoperative detection of myocardial ischemia in high risk patients: Electrocardiography versus two-dimensional transesophageal echocardiography. Circulation 72: 1015, 1985.

18. Topol EJ, Weiss JL, Guzman PA, Dorsey-Lima A, and Blank TJJ: Immediate improvement of dysfunctional myocardial segments after coronary revascularization: Detection by intraoperative transesophageal echocardiography. J Am Coll Cardiol 4: 1123, 1984.

19. Ross J Jr.: Electrocardiographic ST segment analysis in the characterization of myocardial ischemia and infarction. Circulation 53 (Supplement I): 73, 1976.

20. Borer JS, Brensike JF, Redwood DR et al.: Limitations of the electrocardiographic response to exercise in predicting coronary artery disease. N Eng J Med 293: 367, 1975.

21. Epstein, SE: Value and limitations of the electrocardiographic response to exercise in the assessment of patients with coronary artery disease. Am J Cardiol 43: 667, 1978.

22. Froelicher VF, Thompson AJ, Longo MR, et al.: Value of exercise testing for screening asymptomatic men for latent coronary artery disease. Prog Cardiovas Dis 18: 265, 1976.

23. Barnard RJ, Buckberg GD and Duncan HW: Limitations of the standard transthoracic electrocardiogram in detecting subendocardial ischemia. Am Heart J 99: 476, 1980.

24. Chaitman BR, Bourassa MG, Wagniart P, Corbara F and Ferguson RJ: Improved efficacy of treadmill exercise testing multiple lead ECG system and basic hemodynamic response. Circulation 57: 71, 1978.

25. Reitan JA: Noninvasive monitoring. In: Saidman LJ, Smith NT (eds.): *Monitoring in Anesthesia*. John Wiley and Sons, New York, 1978, p. 85.

26. Kaplan JA: The present status of the electrocardiogram in the operating room. In: Gravenstein JS, Newbower RS, Ream AK and Smith NT (eds.): Essential Noninvasive Monitoring in Anesthesia. Grune and Stratton, New York, 1980, p. 89.

27. Arbeit SR, Rubin IL and Gross H: Dangers in interpretating the electrocardiogram from the oscilloscope monitor. JAMA 211: 453, 1970.

28. Roy WL, Edelist G and Gilbert B: Myocardial ischemia during noncardiac surgical procedures in patients with coronary artery disease. Anesthesiology 51: 393, 1979.

29. Battler A, Froelicher VF, Gallagher KP, Kemper WS, and Ross J Jr.: Dissociation between regional myocardial dysfunction and ECG changes during ischemia in the conscious dog. Circulation 62: 735, 1980.

30. Roberts R and Sobel BE: Elevated plasma MB creatine phosphokinase activity: A specific marker for myocardial infarction in perioperative patients. Arch Intern Med 136: 421, 1976.

31. Graeber, GM, Cafferty PJ, Wolfe RE, et al.: Concentrations of creatine kinase and lactic dehydrogenase in the muscles encountered during median sternotomy and in the walls of the cardiac chambers. Surg Forum 34: 337, 1983.

32. Graeber GM, Snyder RJ, Zajtchuk R et al.: A comparison of serum isoenzyme levels of creatine phospho kinase and lactic dehydrogenase in patients undergoing thoracic operations and patients admitted to a coronary care unit. Ann Thoracic Surg 30: 364, 1980.

33. Kettunen, P: CK isoenzymes and transaminases after coronary arteriography, cardiac surgery and noncardiac thoracotomy. Clin Chem Acta 127: 97, 1983.

34. Block MI, Said JW, Siegel RJ and Fishbein MC: Myocardial myoglobin following coronary artery occlusion: An immunohistochemical study. Am J Pathol 111: 374, 1983.

35. Nishikai, M and Reichlin M: Radioimmunoassay of serum myoglobin in polymyositis and other conditions. Arthritis Rheum 20: 1514, 1977.

36. Roth EF, Barfeld PA, Goldsmith SJ et al.: Sickle cell crisis as evaluated from measurements of hydroxybutyrate, dehydrogenase and myoglobin in plasma. Clin Chem 27: 314, 1981.

37. Reynolds EW and Yu PN: Transmyocardial temperature gradient in dog and man. Circ Res 15: 11, 1964.
38. Barlow CH and Chance B: Ischemic areas in perfused rat hearts: Measurement by NADH fluorescence photography. Science 193: 909, 1976.
39. Barlow CH, Harken AH and Chance B: Evaluation of cardiac ischemia by NADH fluorescence photography. Ann Surg 186: 737, 1977.
40. Tennant R and Wiggers CJ: The effect of coronary occlusion on myocardial contraction. Am J Physiol 112: 351, 1935.
41. Forrestor JS, Wyatt HL, Protasio L and Tyberg JV et al.: Functional significance of regional ischemic contraction abnormalities. Circulation 54: 64, 1976.
42. Gallagher KP, Kumada T, Koziol JA et al.: Significance of regional wall thickening abnormalities relative to transmural myocardial perfusion in anesthetized dogs. Circulation 62: 1266, 1980.
43. Kerber RE, Marcus ML, Ehrhardt J, et al.: Correlation between echocardiographically demonstrated segmental dyskinesis and regional myocardial perfusion. Circulation 52: 1097, 1975.
44. Ross J Jr. and Franklin D: Analysis of regional myocardial function, dimensions and wall thickness in the characterization of myocardial ischemia and infarction. Circulation 53 (Supplement I): 188, 1976.
45. Tomoike H, Franklin D, McKown D et al.: Regional myocardial dysfunction and hemodynamic abnormalities during strenuous exercise in dogs with limited coronary flow. Circ Res 46: 487, 1978.
46. Pandian NG and Kerber RE: Two dimensional echocardiography in experimental coronary stenosis. 1. Sensitivity and specificity in detecting transient myocardial dyskinesis: Comparison with sonomicrometers. Circulation 66: 597, 1982.
47. Asinger R, Elsperger J, Helseth P, et al.: Coronary artery manipulation for canine myocardial ischemia or reperfusion models alters baseline wall thickening. Circulation 74 (Supplement II): 18, 1986.
48. Homans DC, Asinger R, et al.: Regional function and perfusion at the lateral border of ischemic myocardium. Circulation 71: 1038, 1985.
49. Lima JAC, Becker LC, Melin JA, et al.: Impaired thickening of nonischemic myocardium during acute regional ischemia in the dog. Circulation 71: 1048, 1985.
50. McPherson DD, Armstrong M, Rose E. et al.: High-frequency epicardial echocardiography for coronary artery evaluation. In vitro and in vivo validation of arterial lumen and wall thickness measurements. J Am Coll Cardiol 8: 600, 1986.
51. Chandrasekaran K, Greenleaf JF, Kim KH, Edwards WD, Seward JB and Tajik AJ: Epicardial echocardiography in tissue characterization of ischemic myocardium in a canine model. Am J Cardiac Imaging (In Press).
52. Miller JG, Perez JE, and Sobel BE: Ultrasonic characterization of myocardium. Prog Cardiovas Dis XXVII: 85, 1985.
53. Chandrasekaran K, Greenleaf JF, Robinson BS, Edwards WD, Seward JB and Tajik AJ: Echocardiographic visualization of acute myocardial ischemia – in vitro study. Ultrasound Med Biol 12 (10): 785–793, 1986.
54. Rasmussen S, Lovelace DE, Knoebel SB, Ransburg R and Corya BC: Echocardiographic detection of ischemic and infarcted myocardium. J Am Coll Cardiol 3: 733, 1984.
55. Marcus ML, Wright C, Doty D et al.: Measurements of coronary velocity and reactive hyperemia in the coronary circulation of humans. Circ Res 49: 877–891, 1981.
56. Marcus ML, Doty DB, Hiratika LF, Wright CB et al.: Decreased coronary reserve: A mechanism for angina pectoris in patients with aortic stenosis and normal coronary arteries. New Engl J Med 307: 1362–1366, 1982.

57. Olinger GN, Mulder DG, Malony JV et al.: Phasic coronary flow: Intraoperative evaluation of flow distribution, myocardial function, and reactive hyperemic response. Ann Thorac Surg 21: 397–404, 1976.
58. Von Restorff W, Hofling B, Holtz J et al.: Effect of increased blood fluidity through hemodilution on coronary circulation at rest and during exercise in dogs. Pflugers Arch 357: 15–24, 1975.

PART 6: Doppler Echocardiography in Interventions

6.1. Intraoperative color flow Doppler imaging in valvular heart disease

RYOZO OMOTO, SHINICHI TAKAMOTO, SHUNEI KYO,
MAKOTO MATSUMURA & YUJI YOKOTE

Introduction

In the short time since its introduction to the cardiovascular field [1–3], real-time two-dimensional Doppler echocardiography, or color flow Doppler imaging, has convincingly demonstrated and proved its practical value and diagnostic effectiveness in acquired valvular disease, congenital heart disease and aortic aneurysms. The use of intraoperative color flow Doppler imaging in the cardiovascular field is a new application of the technique. There have already been reports from several cardiac centers on the usefulness of this application [4–7] and we can expect substantial development in this field in the future. The color flow Doppler technique has been employed during cardiac surgery at the author's institute since 1984. There are two approaches to its use in surgery. One is to place the probe in direct contact with the surgical field and to take echograms from the surface of the heart (epicardial approach). The other approach uses a transesophageal probe (transesophageal approach [8], transesophageal echocardiography; TEE). Both methods are necessary, but transesophageal echocardiography is likely to develop into the slightly more effective method because color flow mapping by the transesophageal route has made study of intracardiac and intra-aortic flow continuously accessible without the inconvenience of a probe in the operative field or the risk of infection.

This chapter will discuss the three-year experience of intraoperative color flow Doppler imaging in valvular disease at Saitama Medical School. Detailed and technical descriptions of color flow mapping itself are reported in the literature [9].

Methods

Patients

Between April of 1984 and February of 1987, we performed intraoperative color Doppler examinations on 45 patients with valvular heart disease at

I. Cikes (ed.), *Echocardiography in Cardiac Interventions*, 381–394, 1989.
© 1989 *Kluwer Academic Publishers.*

Table 1. Operations for valvular heart disease in 45 patients.

Operation		No.
Aortic valve replacement		18
St. Jude Medical valve	(17)	
Carpentier-Edwards valve	(1)	
Mitral valve replacement		24
St. Jude Medical valve	(20)	
Hancock valve	(2)	
Carpentier-Edwards valve	(2)	
Open mitral commissurotomy		11
Tricuspid annuloplasty		8
Kay's method	(5)	
DeVega's method	(3)	
Mitral annuloplasty		2
Aortic valvuloplasty*		4

* Combined with DeBakey type 1 dissecting aortic aneurysm.

Saitama. Table 1 lists the surgical procedures carried out for valvular lesions in these patients. Intraoperative color flow mapping was performed by the epicardial approach in 22 patients, by the transesophageal approach in 22 patients, and by both in one patient. In Fourty-five patients with valvular heart disease, prosthetic valves, valves repaired by valvuloplasty and valves managed conservatively without a surgical procedure were evaluated by intraoperative color flow mapping.

Instrumentation

The color flow mapping systems in use were the Aloka SSD-880 and SSD-860 with 3.5 and 5 MHz transducers. These 2-D Doppler systems display color flow maps simultaneously with two-dimensional echocardiograms. Flow toward the transducer is displayed in red and flow away from the transducer in blue. The velocity of the flow is in direct proportion to the brightness of the color in seven gradations. Turbulence is encoded in green and is added proportionately to each color in 16 gradations. Actual turbulent flow is usually displayed in a mosaic pattern. Color flow frame rates were from 15 to a maximum of 30 frames per second. With the epicardial approach, the standard transducers for percutaneous examination were gas-sterilized with ethylene oxide for 24 hours prior to intraoperative use. A transesophageal

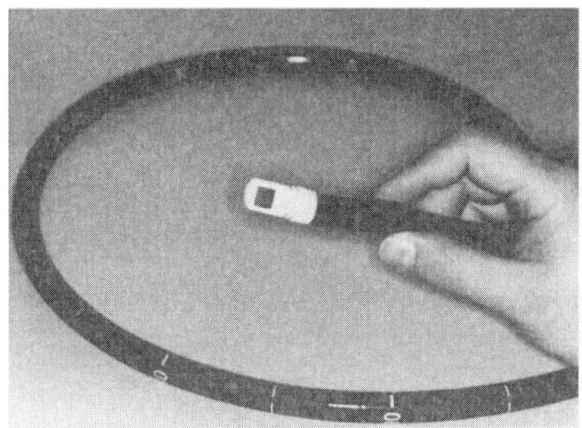

Fig. 1. A transesophageal probe with 5 Mhz phased array transducer (100 cm in length and 11 mm in diameter).

probe with 5 or 3.5 MHz phased-array transducer was connected to each of the color Doppler systems. The transducer was mounted on a modified gastroscope of 100 cm in length and 11 mm in diameter with antero-posterior flexibility (Fig. 1).

The color flow mapping images were recorded on a Sony videotape recorder (VO-5800), and photographed on 35 mm and/or instant color photo film.

Intraoperative scanning

Operative scanning by color flow mapping was performed before and after the cardiac procedures. In the case of valvuloplasty, the competency of the valve was examined preoperatively, intraoperatively (pre- and post-proce-dure), and postoperatively by color flow mapping. For epicardial scanning, the pericardial cavity was filled in some cases with warm saline during scanning for better ultrasound windows. During surgery, valvular regurgita-tion was evaluated semi-quantitatively by the same criteria as was used for the percutaneous color flow mapping described previously [9,10]. The criteria for assessing the severity of regurgitation were based primarily on the extent of the regurgitant jet images in the long-axis and four-chamber views (Fig. 2).

With these criteria, an acceptable correlation has been found between percutaneous color flow mapping and angiographic Sellers' grading [3, 4] or operative findings. Grades were assigned in each case according to the following criteria. In aortic regurgitation, Grade 1 regurgitant jet flow images

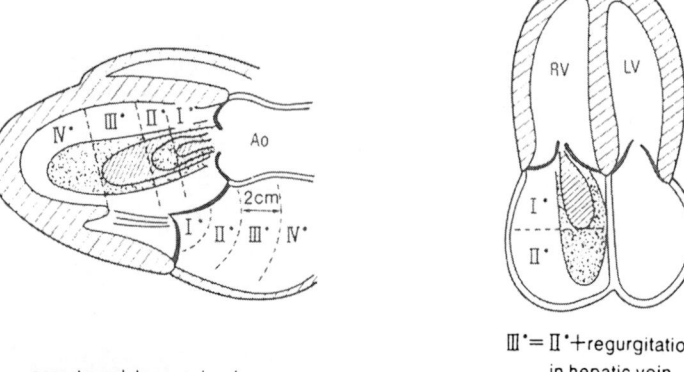

III'= II'+regurgitation
in hepatic vein
Apical four-chamber view

parasternal long-axis view

Fig. 2. Diagram demonstrating how color flow mapping findings can be used to quantitate the severity of valvular regurgitation on a four-grade scale. Severity of valvular regurgitation by color flow mapping is mainly determined from the farthest distance reached by the regurgitant jet.

reach halfway to the tip of the anterior mitral leaflet from the aortic ring in the conventional long-axis view; Grade 2 regurgitant flow images, to the tip of anterior mitral leaflet (AML); Grade 3 flows, to the level of the papillary muscle; and Grade 4, beyond the level of the papillary muscle deeper toward the apex. In mitral regurgitation, Grade 1 regurgitant jet flow images are localized immediately posterior to the mitral valve in the left atrium, not overshooting the midpoint level between the mitral orifice and the valve ring in the conventional long-axis view; Grade 2 regurgitant flows reach almost to the level of the mitral valve ring; Grade 3 flows are present deep to the level of the miral valve ring but within 2 cm from it; Grade 4 flows are present over 2 cm deep to the level of the mitral valve ring and are often visualized diffusely in the enitre left atrium. In tricuspid regurgitation, Grade 1 regurgigant jet flow images are present within the half of the right atrium that is above the tricuspid valve in the conventional apical four-chamber view; Grade 2, present diffusely within the enitre right atrium; and Grade 3, present in the entire right atrium with significant regurgitation in the hepatic vein.

Results

Mitral annuloplasty

According to intraoperative color flow mapping in two non-rheumatic patients with Grade 1 and 2 mitral regurgitation, there was no change in the grade of regurgitation over the period of the procedure (Table 2).

Table 2. Assessment of mitral annuloplasty by color flow mapping: Change of grading of mitral regurgitation.

Patient	Preop.	Intraop.	Postop.
1	2	2 → 2	2
2	1	1 → 1	0

Open mitral commissurotomy

In the 11 patients who underwent open mitral commissurotomy, the grade of mitral regurgitation was assessed intraoperatively by color flow mapping (Fig. 3). Two cases in whom mitral regurgitation had not previously been detected showed Grade 1 mitral regurgitation after the procedure. In three patients, mitral regurgitation was increased during the procedure from Grade 1 to Grade 2. In six patients, the grade of mitral regurgitation was unchanged after mitral commissurotomy. The postoperative evaluation of the grade of mitral regurgitation showed that the severity of mitral regurgitation was almost unchanged (3 patients) or was improved (10 patients), although the grade of one patient increased from Grade 2 to Grade 3 (Table 3).

Table 3. Assessment of open mitral commisurotomy by color flow mapping: Change of grading of mitral regurgitation.

Patient	Preop.	Intraop.	Postop.
1	0	1 → 1	0
2	2	2 → 2	1
3	1	1 → 2	0
4	0	0 → 1	0
5	2	1 → 2	3
6	1	1 → 1	0
7	1	1 → 2	1
8	0	0 → 0	0
9	0	0 → 1	0
10	0	1 → 1	1
11	0	0 → 0	0

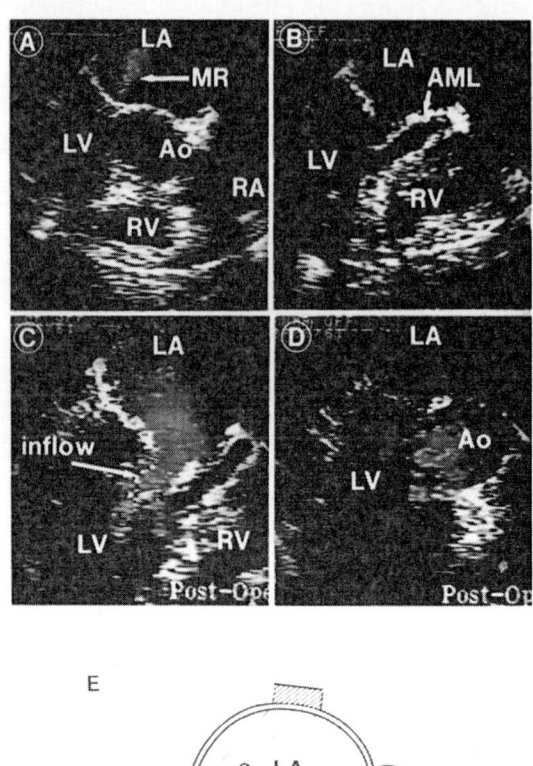

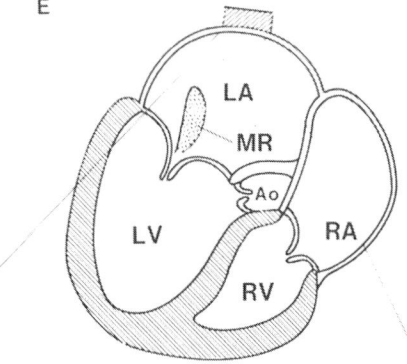

Fig. 3. Intraoperative transesophageal color flow mapping images in a patient with mitral stenosis; 55-year-old male. (A) Color flow mapping in systole. Grade 1 mitral regurgitation (MR) is noted (arrow). (B) B-mode in diastole. Mitral commissurotomy was performed and mitral opening was improved. (C) Color flow mapping in diastole. Inflow blood through the mitral orifice was increased and less turbulent. (D) Color flow mapping in systole. Mitral regurgitant is not seen. (E) Diagram of (A). AML: anterior mitral leaflet. Inflow: inflow blood.

Tricuspid annuloplasty

In eight patients, tricuspid annuloplasty was performed with Kay's or DeVega's procedure (Fig. 4). In all patients with Grade 1, 2, or 3 tricuspid regurgitation, the grade of the regurgitation was decreased to Grade 1 or 2 (Table 4).

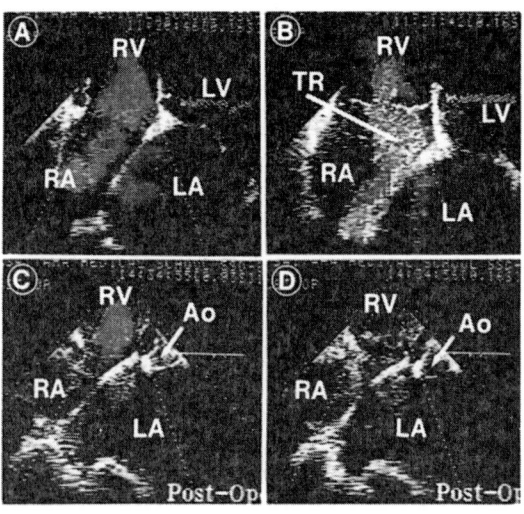

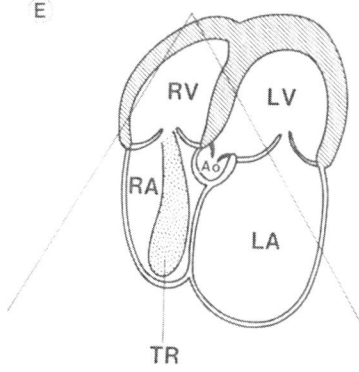

Fig. 4. Intraoperative epicardial color flow maping in a patient with tricuspid regurgitation associated with mitral stenosis and regurgitation; 72-year-old male. (A) Color flow mapping in diastole. Inflow blood through the tricuspid valve is increased before tricuspid annuloplasty. (B) Color flow mapping in systole. Remarkable tricuspid regurgitation (TR) is seen in mosaic pattern (arrow). (C) Color flow mapping in diastole. Inflow blood is decreased. (D) Color flow mapping in systole. Tricuspid regurgitation is not seen after tricuspid annuloplasty with Kay's procedure. (E) Diagram of (B).

388

Table 4. Assessment of tricuspid annuloplasty by color flow mapping: Change of grading of tricuspid regurgitation.

Patient	Preop.	Intraop.	Postop.
1	2	2 → 1	1
2	2	2 → 1	0
3	2	2 → 1	1
4	1	1 → 0	0
5	2	2 → 1	2
6	2	2 → 0	1
7	3	3 → 0	1
8	3	3 → 0	0

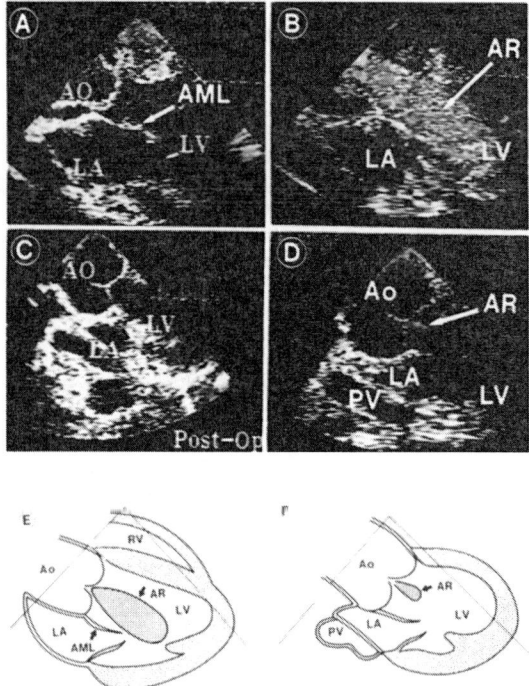

Fig. 5. Intraoperative epicardial color flow mapping in a patient with Grade 3 aortic regurgitation associated with DeBakey type 1 dissecting aortic aneurysm; 32-year-old male. (A) B-mode in diastole. An intimal flap is prolapsing into the left ventricular outflow tract. (B) Color flow mapping in diastole. Grade 3 aortic regurgitation (AR) is imaged (arrow). (C) B-mode in systole after aortic valvuloplasty. (D) Color flow mapping in systole demonstrating effect of aortic valvuloplasty. Aortic regurgitation was decreased to minimum (arrow). (E) Diagram of (B). (F) Diagram of (D).

Aortic annuloplasty

Aortic regurgitation was repaired in four patients with DeBakey type 1 dissecting aortic aneurysm (Fig. 5). The grade of the regurgitation present in three patients was reduced from Grade 3 to Grade 1 in two cases, and to Grade 2 in one. In the other patient, there was an improvement from Grade 2 to Grade 1 (Table 5).

Table 5. Assessment of aortic valvuloplasty by color flow mapping: Change of grading of aortic regurgitation.

Patient	Preop.	Intraop.	Postop.
1	3	3 → 2	1
2	2	2 → 1	0
3	3	3 → 1	0
4	3	3 → 1	1

Untouched valve

The principal valvular lesions alone were operated, but the concomitant mild valvular disorders were left untreated. The flow patterns in those valves in

Table 6. Assessment of untouched valve by color flow mapping: Change of grading of regurgitation.

Lesion	Grading preop.	No.	Grading intraop.	No.
Aortic regurgitation	2	3	2 → 2	2
			2 → 1	1
	1	5	1 → 1	5
Mitral regurgitation	2	3	2 → 2	2
			2 → 1	1
	1	4	1 → 1	1
			1 → 0	3
Tricuspid regurgitation	3	2	3 → 2	1
			3 → 1	1
	2	4	2 → 2	1
			2 → 1	1
			2 → 0	2
	1	12	1 → 2	1
			1 → 1	5
			1 → 0	6

which nothing was done about the regurgitation were examined intraoperatively by color flow mapping. Aortic regurgitation of Grades 1 and 2 was seen in eight cases and mitral regurgitation was found in six. After surgical treatment of the principally affected valve, in all but one of the thirteen patients with tricuspid valve regurgitation, the regurgitation in the untouched valves showed either no change or a remission. The exception among these thirteen had a Grade 1 regurgitation which was uniquely aggravated to Grade 2 (Table 6).

Prosthetic valve

The inherent leaks in the St. Jude Medical valve were also studied by means of color flow mapping, employing both the epicardial and the transesophageal approaches. With the former approach, the inherent leaks were depicted in 3 (38%) out of 8 cases that underwent mitral valve replacement (MVR), and in 3 (27%) of 11 cases treated with aortic valve replacement (AVR). With the transesophageal approach, images of the inherent leaks were obtained in all 12 MVR cases and in 3 (50%) of the 6 AVR cases

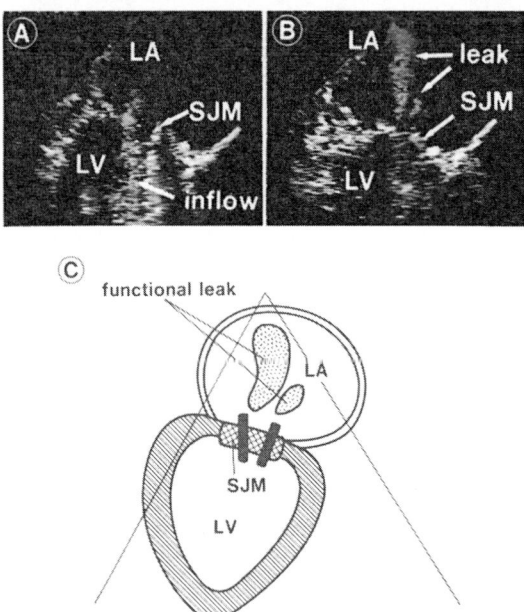

Fig. 6. Intraoperative transesophageal color flow mapping in a mitral valve replacement; 66-year-old female. (A) Color flow mapping in diastole. Inflow blood through St. Jude Medical valve (SJM) is seen. (B) Color flow mapping in systole. Inherent transvalvular leaks through St. Jude Medical valve in mitral position are seen. (C) Diagram of (B).

Table 7. Assessment of St. Jude valve by intraoperative color flow maping.

Approach	Valve Replacement		Detection of Inherent Leak
Epicardial	Mitral	8	3 (38%)
Epicardial	Aortic	11	3 (27%)
Transesophageal	Mitral	12	12 (100%)
Transesophageal	Aortic	6	3 (50%)

(Table 7). These functional leaks appeared as between 2 and 5 narrow regurgitant jets (Fig. 6).

In one patient who was given a porcine valve in MVR surgery, paravalvular leaks were detected intraoperatively by the transesophageal approach. These leaks had appeared around the external border of the suture ring of the porcine valve, whereas the inherent leaks in the St. Jude Medical valve mentioned above were transvalvular leaks, passing through the valve orifice and around the hinges of the prosthetic valve (Fig. 7).

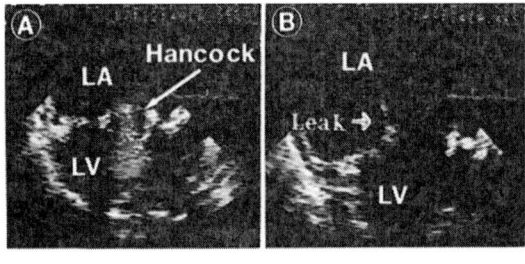

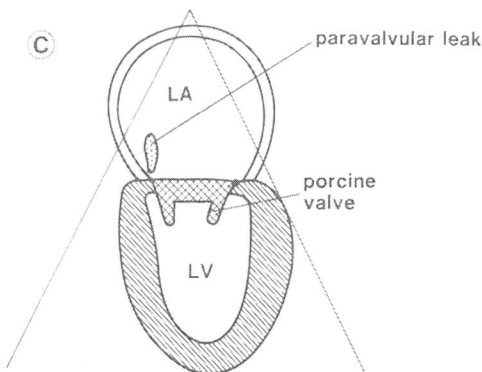

Fig. 7. Intraoperative transesophageal color flow mapping in a mitral position; 58-year-old female. (A) Color flow mapping in diastole. Inflow blood through porcine valve in mital position (Hancock) is seen. (B) Slight paravalvular leak from the edge of the ring of the Hancock valve is demonstrated. (C) Diagram of (B).

Discussion

Echocardiography was already being employed in a variety of ways for the intraoperative evaluation of cardiac surgery well before the development of color flow mapping, and its usefulness is well known. Numerous reports presenting the details of such uses have appeared elsewhere.

Since color flow mapping makes possible the visualization of blood flow, it is naturally to be expected that its intraoperative application will be of very great value; and in the author's three years of experience with intraoperative color flow mapping at Saitama Medical School, it has become clear that this technique is both safe and easy to perform, and is an extremely useful aid to the cardiac surgeon. Fourty-five cases of valvular disease have now been treated with the help of intraoperative color flow mapping at this medical school. After valvuloplasty has been carried out, it is essential for the surgeon to confirm the competency of the valve, because, should a marked valvular regurgitation appear after the completion of the surgical procedure, replacement of the valve must be undertaken without delay. Accordingly, if reliance cannot be placed in the method of evaluation of competency used during valvuloplasty, the surgeon may well prefer to replace the valve instead.

The introduction of color flow mapping into the area of valvular surgery is likely to motivate cardiac surgeons to undertake valvuloplasty with more willingness than hitherto. If the valve can be salvaged by means of valvuloplasty instead of being resected, the patient is very fortunate. It is of similar importance to be able to judge reliably during an operation whether a mild degree of valvular regurgitation may safely be left untouched or not.

Among the fourty-five cases in which intraoperative color flow mapping was employed, there were none in which it was decided to replace a valve after an attempt at valvuloplasty. Also, there were no cases in which regurgitant flow increased significantly after the valve was left untouched. However, there was no doubt of the great usefulness of intraoperative color flow mapping to the surgeon in this series of cases.

A number of problems remain in relation to the use of the same criteria for intraoperative grading – assessment of degree - of valvular regurgitation using the present technique as when percutaneous color flow mapping is performed. It is probably necessary to establish proper criteria for intraoperative assessments. Within this series of fourty-five cases, however, the assessments made by percutaneous color flow mapping before and after surgery were on the whole found to be in agreement with those made intraoperatively, and so it may be considered that it was permissible from a practical standpoint to follow these same criteria.

Intraoperative color flow mapping revealed inherent leaks in a high proportion of St. Jude Medical valves. In particular, when the transesophageal approach was used, the technique clearly indicated inherent leaks in all of these valves in MVR cases. A paravalvular leak was detected intra-operatively in one case, but it was very slight in degree, and so was left untouched. Three days after the operation this leak disappeared of its own accord. It is highly significant that a minor paravalvular leak of this type should have been observed to correct itself soon after surgery.

It should be possible to distinguish between inherent leaks and para-valvular leaks by their location. Inherent leaks are transvalvular leaks, and generally appear at the orifice of a prosthetic valve, whereas paravalvular leaks are usually seen around the border of the suture ring of such a valve.

The number of cases performed at Saitama Medical School is still small, but the author considers that this series has demonstrated the importance and usefulness of intraoperative color flow mapping in the examination of patients with valvular disorders.

This new modality, which facilitates immediate evaluation of the cardio-vascular procedure just completed, whether it is applied routinely or selectively, cannot but produce more insight and better results at a very small price in terms of effort and risk. Intraoperative color flow mapping in cardio-vascular surgery has permitted precise diagnosis, quick assessment of the degree of surgery necessary, and timely evaluation of the effects of surgery prior to chest closure. In conclusion, intraoperative color flow mapping has the potential to ensure improved results in cardiovascular surgery.

References

1. Omoto R, Yokote Y, Takamoto S, Tamura F, Asano H, Namekawa K, Kasai C, Tsukamoto M and Koyano, A: Clinical significance of newly developed real-time intracardiac two-dimensional blood flow imaging system (2-D Doppler). Jpn Circ J 47: 191, 1983.
2. Bommer WJ: Basic principles of flow imaging. Echocardiography 2: 501–509, 1985.
3. Sahn DJ: Real-time two-dimensional Doppler echocardiography flow mapping. Circulation 71: 849–853, 1985.
4. Takamoto S, Kyo S, Adachi H, Matsumura M, Yokote Y and Omoto R: Intraoperative color flow mapping by real-time two-dimensional Doppler echocardiography for evaluation of valvular and congenital heart disease and vascular disease. J Thorac Cardiovasc Surg, 90: 802–812, 1985.
5. Maurer G, Czer L, DeRobertis M, et al.: Intraoperative Doppler color flow mapping in valvular and congenital heart disease. Circulation 72: (Suppl. III), 206, 1985. Abstract.
6. Czer L, Maure G, DeRobertis M, Kass R, Lee M, Chaux A, and Matloff J: Utility of intra-operative color Doppler flow imaging after surgical correction of valvular regurgitation. Am Coll Cardiol 7: 160, 1986. Abstract.
7. Czer LSC, Maurer G, DeRobertis M, Bolger AF, Kass RM, Lee ME, Blanche C, Chaux A and Matloff JM: Intraoperative evaluation of mitral regurgitation: Superiority of Doppler color flow mapping. Circulation 74: (Suppl. II), 394, 1986. Abstract.
8. Goldman ME, Thys, D, Ritter S, Hillel, Z and Kaplan J: Transesophageal realtime

Doppler flow imaging: A new method for intraoperative cardiac evaluation. J Am Coll Cardiol 7: 1, 1986. Abstract.

9. Omoto, R (Ed.): Color atlas of real-time two-dimensional Doppler echocardiography (2nd ed.). Shindan-To-Chiryosha Co., Tokyo, 1987 (distributed by Lea & Febiger, Philadelphia).

10. Omoto R, Yokote Y, Takamoto S, Kyo S, Ueda K, Asano H, Namekawa K, Kasai C, Kondo Y and Koyano A: The development of real-time two-dimensional Doppler echocardiography and its clinical significance in acquired valvular disease with special reference to the evaluation of valvular regurgitation. Jpn Heart J 25: 325–340, 1984.

6.2. Doppler for guiding and flow measurement in coronary artery surgery

H. ENGEDAL, K. MATRE & L. SEGADAL

Introduction

The main steps in coronary arterial revascularization procedures, based upon preoperative coronary cinearteriograms, are the following:

1. Identify the diseased arteries in the operative field.
2. Select the optimal site for graftanastomosis.
3. Perform the surgical revascularization which usually involves bypass grafting.
4. Check the functional result by measuring blood flow in established grafts.

For step (1) and (2) the surgeon usually has to rely on anatomical knowledge and operative experience, while electromagnetic flowmeters are used as a routine for step (4) at many cardiac centres. The Doppler technology provides means to ease these 3 tasks challenging the surgeon.

Identification of coronary arteries and grafts

The need for special detection techniques exists when the arteries are not directly visible on the surface of the exposed heart. This may be due to intra-myocardial course, epicardial fat coverage, epi- and pericardial adhesions after pericarditis, radiation treatment and earlier operative interventions. The last group represents an increasing number of coronary artery surgery cases per year, demanding more surgical skill than primary operations. Dissection based on experience and guesswork is at best timeconsuming, with the risk of unnecessary traumatization of tissue, and in worst case damaging to native vessels and open grafts. To guide the dissection, different invasive techniques have been developed: introduction of angioscopes, catheters and probes through the coronary ostia from aorta, and retrograde probing of arteries through a peripheral incision. Opposed to these methods Doppler guiding is completely non-traumatic.

I. Cikes (ed.), *Echocardiography in Cardiac Interventions*, 395–405, 1989.
© 1989 *Kluwer Academic Publishers.*

Technical considerations

Although Doppler transducers designed for coronary mapping and flow measurement have not been commercially available until recently, several surgical groups have used the method by adapting and modifying existent equipment [1–4]. Non-directional and directional, continuous-wave Doppler (CWD) and pulsed-wave Doppler (PWD) have all been successfully applied. The range of ultrasonic frequencies has been from 8 to 20 MHz to optimize signals due to the short distance, usually less than 10 mm, between ultrasound transducer crystal and target blood flow. Our experience relates to 7 years use of 10 MHz PWD with different pencil-like probes (Fig. 1). Pulsed Doppler is preferable to CWD as it gives depth resolution reducing unwanted signals from superficial tissue structures and neighbouring vessels. Slimmer probes are made with the single crystal needed in PWD. Coronary blood flow velocities are within the range of pulse repetition rate (PRF) capacity of the equipment, avoiding the problem of aliasing. As the main goal is accurate precision in localizing the arteries, the success of mapping depends on the slim design of an easy held probe convenient to use all over the cardiac surface. Although flexible transducerhandles of different length and varying approach angles may be advantageous, normally a single probe with axial ultrasound beam of 1–3 mm width and a short, rigid handle may satisfy all demands for tracing. Transducers must be sterilized either by gas or autoclaving, tested for current leakage, and connected to the Doppler by an isolation transformer for optimal patient safety.

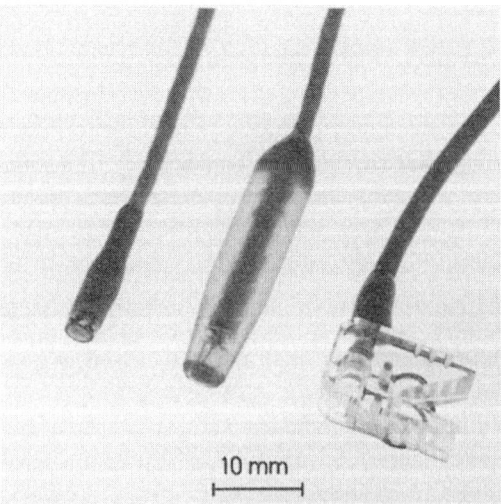

10 mm

Fig. 1. From left to right: Two pen-probes for coronary mapping, and one 4 mm clip-on probe for graft flow measurement.

Clinical application

At reoperations Doppler mapping may start once the sternotomy is completed when preservation of open grafts is wanted. Moving the probe over the scarred surface of the beating heart in CWD or PWD mode allows the surgeon to register the audible velocity signal from graft flow through a loudspeaker, and guide the early dissection to free the necessary part for cannulation. The normal moisture in the operative field provides sufficient contact for ultrasound transmission, excluding the need for coupling gel. Both at primary procedures and reoperations Doppler guiding may be useful for quick identification of the internal mammary artery (IMA), which is not always easily seen. By tracing its course the dissection of a pedicle with electrocautery may be fastened and made more safe. At this mapping stage IMA flow velocity may be recorded in-situ with the pen-probe, and in this way provide early information concerning the suitability as a bypass graft (Fig. 2). Low, zero and reversed velocity precludes the antegrade use of IMA. The potential for retrograde grafting may also be evaluated by directional Doppler registration after proximal inflow occlusion of IMA.

Mapping of the native arteries is difficult on a beating heart, and better

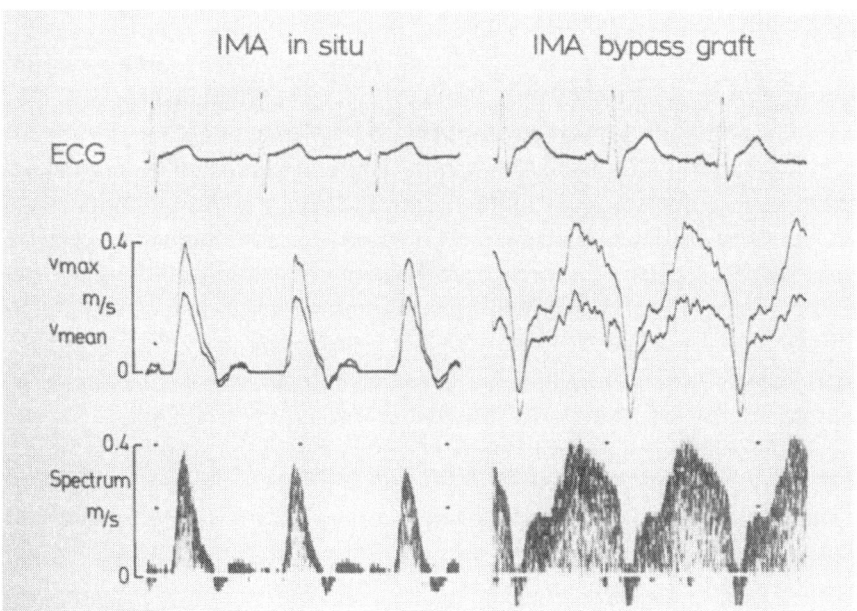

Fig. 2. Maximum velocity (v max), mean velocity (v mean) and velocity spectrum in internal mammary artery (IMA) before dissection (left panel) and as a bypass graft to LAD (right panel). Note increase in diastolic flow.

398

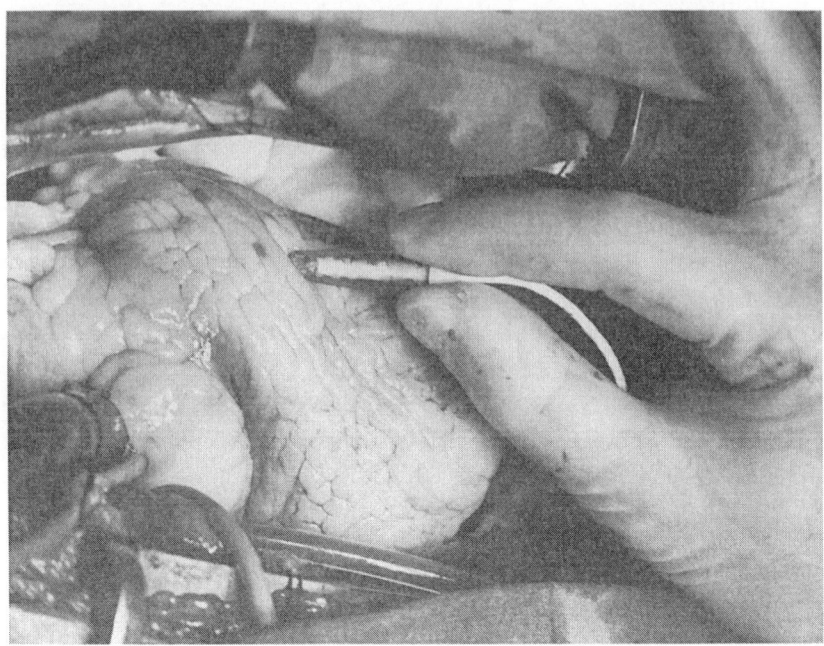

Fig. 3. Mapping of LAD on a fibrillating heart.

postponed until the patient is on cardiopulmonary bypass. During systemic cooling the heart rate slows, and this reduced movement makes accurate identification easier. Even easier is the mapping on a fibrillating heart, and we prefer this condition for examination (Fig. 3). A directional Doppler transducer will have no problem in separating between arterial and venous blood flow, using a combination of audible signal and velocity display. Identification is made more distinct with pulsatile flow on the cardiopulmonary bypass, causing higher pulsesynchronous peak velocity in the arteries. Mapping has by this method been possible with perfusion pressure as low as 20 mm Hg. Normally one can expect to hear Doppler signal from a vessel that is visualized by coronary arteriography. The option of pulsatile flow has made it possible to localize segments not filled with contrast at angiography.

In addition to the need for tracing of deeply situated left anterior descending artery (LAD), there is often a question about the correct numbering of diagonal branches from LAD and marginal branches from the circumflex artery (CFX). One or more of these have in 15–20% of cases a partial or complete intramyocardial course. Systematic counting of Doppler detections along LAD and CFX in a distal direction enables the surgeon to find the correct branches for grafting in accordance with the arteriograms.

Cardiac surgeons using crystalloid cardioplegia must finish their Doppler identification procedure before aortic crossclamping. Infusion of blood cardioplegia provides enough moving red cells for ultrasound reflection and Doppler shift registration. Intermittent or continuous blood cardioplegia thereby makes Doppler mapping obtainable during the crossclamp period.

Selection of site for graftanastomosis

Once the vessel in need of grafting has been identified the question of optimal site for anastomosis has to be answered. For hemodynamic reasons this should be just distal to the stenotic part, providing maximum antegrade flow in the run off area, with grafting at the widest possible vessel diameter. The usual practice is to compromise with this principle, and rather choose the site where the artery is exposed without dissection. This is often quite peripheral to the significant stenosis, at a segment with less diameter. The result is establishment of blood supply partly retrograde in the ischemic area, with longer grafts than desirable and necessary. Doppler mapping makes accurate identification of the stenosis possible by registering the highest velocity signal along the vessel (Fig. 4). Occluded coronary arteries are difficult to trace distal to angiographically documented stop in contrast filling, and vessel

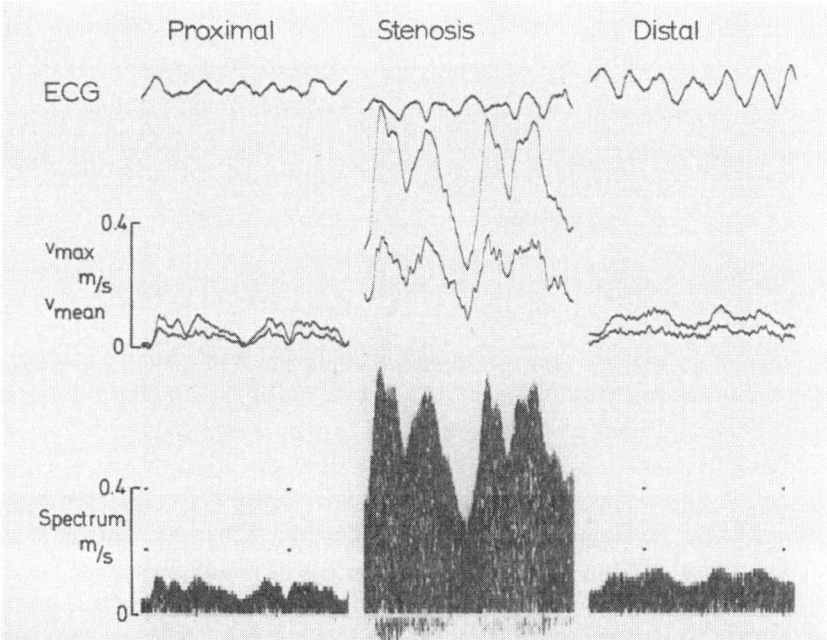

Fig. 4. Localization of stenosis in LAD by recording of sevenfold increase in velocity at the stenosis (middle panel) compared to proximal (left panel) and distal segment (right panel).

identification may be limited to the central flow conducting part. Accompanying veins are often detectable, and then give an indirect lead to the artery one is looking for.

Having localized the stenosis it remains to identify the optimal anastomosis site if this is deeply situated. Pulsed Doppler is also a tool for depth measurement, of special value when parts of LAD are intraseptal or intracavitary, and other branches deep intramyocardially. Changing the depth of the small sample volume makes it possible to measure the accurate distance from the epicardial surface to the intravascular blood stream along the ultrasound beam. This information allows the surgeon to avoid traumatic dissection where the artery is most inaccessible and rather attack it a more superficial segment.

Coronary arteries as a rule have more normal vessel walls with less atheromatosis in their intramyocardial segments. Selecting these hidden parts more suitable for anastomosis is an additional reason for using Doppler guidance in coronary bypass grafting.

Flow measurement

Theoretical considerations

Electromagnetic flow probes has been the only commercially available equipment for graft flow measurement, and therefore been used routinely for intraoperative evaluation of coronary bypass procedures. Methodological weaknesses like manufacturers calibration errors in the range of 9–50% [5], the need for intermittent mechanical zero calibration, good probe- vessel contact and dependency of hematocrit [4] have made many cardiac centres abandon the practice. This has been done in spite of the obvious value for immediate assessment of operative result [6, 7], while some aspects of prognostic value has been questioned [8].

Calculation of blood flow by Doppler technique is based on the equation:

$$Q = v \cdot A$$

Where Q = flow, v = average blood velocity over the cross-section, A = cross-sectional area. The Doppler shift equation (Chapter 6.5) means that the angle between the ultrasound beam and the direction of blood flow must be accurately determined before v can be calculated. Velocity profile necessary for v recording may be (a) measured by a multirangegated PWD unit, (b) averaged by a sample volume including the whole trans-sectional flow area, or (c) assumed to be known. The different methods have been shown to work in vitro with good accuracy, that is systemic errors of 6% or less [9]. In vivo non-invasive measurements are liable to considerable errors in the range of 10-14% standard errors. These are caused mainly by failing measurement of cross-sectional area and angle of approach, pitfalls that may be avoided or reduced with invasive application of specially designed probes.

Methods

Internal vessel diameter may be measured by ultrasound, using either A-, M- or 2D-mode. We have found the wall thickness of human saphenous veins in the calf to be fairly constant (0,37 mm ± 0,02 mm) measured by caliper. Using this as a standard subtraction factor with cylindrical probes with fixed internal diameter slightly less than the external vein graft diameter, we have shown Doppler to be superior to electromagnetic flow for in vitro measurement, resulting in a correlation coefficient of 0,98 and a slope of regression line 0,97, compared to true flow [4]. These probes will also eliminate the other factors affecting area measurement accuracy; time varying diameter and non-circular cross-section. The angle problem is solved by designing the clip-on probes with a fixed, known angle between the crystal and cylindrical axis. Feeding internal diameter and angle into a flow calculator using 10 MHz PWD results in a rapid digital readout of flow in ml/min (VINGMED SD-100, VINGMED SOUND A/S, Horten, Norway). Beam width of 3 mm is used, while sampling depth is varied to encompass the complete flow area. Time-varying estimates of maximum and mean velocities within the sample volume are displayed as curves. A velocity spectrum analyzer enables the operator to improve the depth adjustment to optimize the signal. Using cylindrical probes the wall motion filter of the Doppler may be reduced, thus including low velocity components in the mean velocity estimate.

Clinical application

Graft flow measurement is normally done after weaning from cardiopulmonary bypass, in a stable hemodynamic situation. Clip-on probes with 4 mm internal diameter, slightly compressing the vein grafts, has been applicable in most cases (Fig. 5). With access to 3 and 5 mm probes the demand is satisfied concerning vein grafts. Even smaller probes may be desirable for accurate measurement in IMA-grafts. Stripping of its pedicle in a short segment of IMA is required for accurate flow calculation, but useful evaluation of its function may be obtained by recording flow velocity in m/sec with a pen transducer or clip-on probe at a suitable part of the pedicle. A striking

402

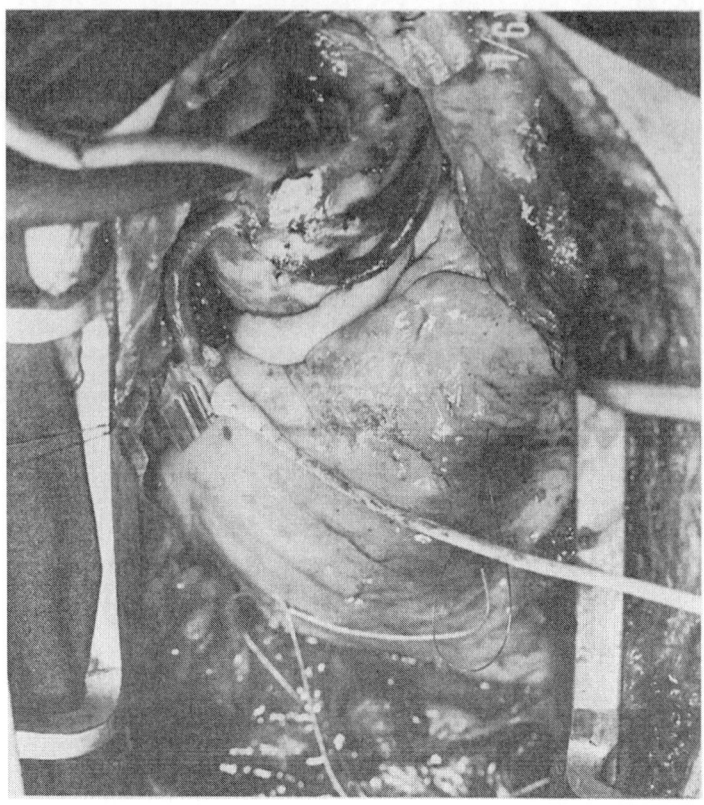

Fig. 5. Flow measurement in vein graft to right coronary artery with 4 mm clip-on probe.

change in flow pattern and increase in flow values has been documented when comparing in-situ pregraft with established bypassfunction of IMA (Fig. 2). Difficulties in weaning from cardiopulmonary bypass is an indication for graft flow measurement at this stage, being the only method to decide if the graft is functioning, and to what extent. If no flow is recorded one has to look for technical faults. Twisted, kinked or stretched grafts are unveiled by inspection, while anastomoses are checked by thin Fogarty catheters introduced through graft incision or side branch, and withdrawn after balloon inflation. Flow values less than 50 ml/min predict an increased risk for graft occlusion [6]. To assess the capacity of the run-off area injection of 3–12 mg papaverine in the graft is better than hyperemic response to graft occlusion. The latter depends on the severity of native coronary stenosis in contrast to the papaverine test, which normally yields doubling, and in some cases triple increase of basic flow (Figs. 6 and 7). Recordings exceeding 50 ml/min has no relation to graft patency rate, and need not be supplemented by papaverine injections. Registration of graft flow enables the surgeon to document not

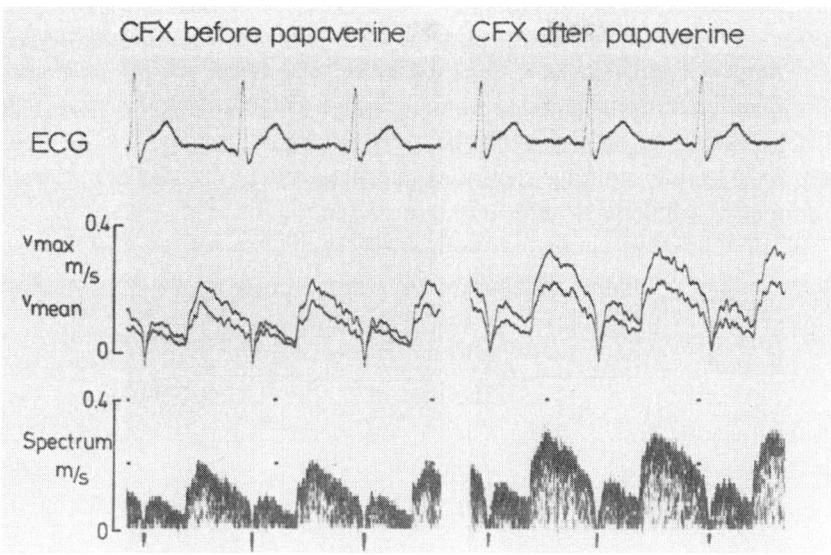

Fig. 6. Maximum and mean velocity in a vein graft to circumflex artery (CFX) before (left panel) and after 3 mg papaverine (right panel). Calculated flow increased from 55 to 90 ml/min, mostly due to velocity increase in diastole.

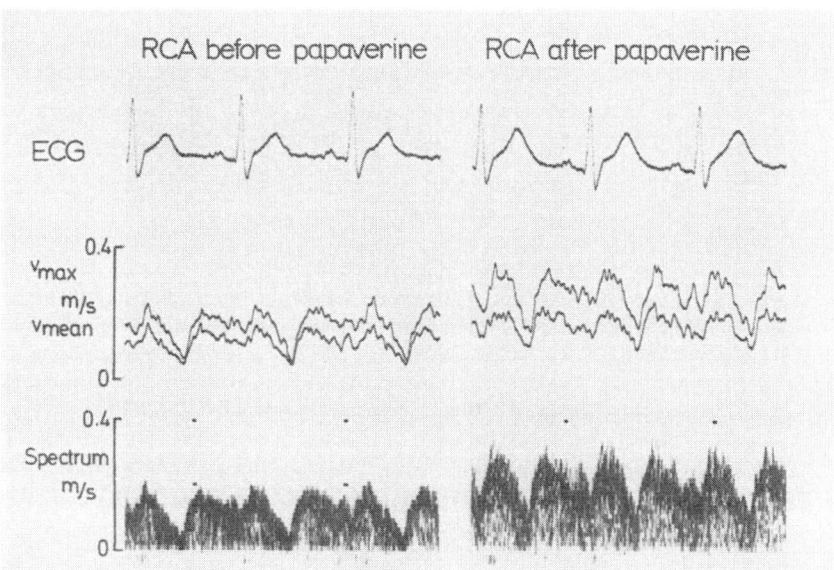

Fig. 7. Maximum and mean velocity in vein graft to right coronary artery (RCA) before (left panel) and after 3 mg papaverine (right panel). Calculated flow increased from 60 to 110 ml/min, due both to systolic and diastolic velocities increase.

404

only that anatomical corrections have been made, but more informative that a certain functional result has been achieved. Filing these flow measurements in the surgical report has been most useful in those cases where patients are referred with recurrent symptoms and occluded grafts. Low flow values, with small increase after papaverine in the initial procedure, will weaken the argument for a second grafting attempt of the same vessel. Satisfactory primary recordings strengthens the indication for reoperation.

The qualitative phasic flow velocity curves may represent additional information for graft patency prediction [10], and therefore be useful in surgical decisionmaking, but further studies are needed.

Conclusions

Available Doppler equipment provides the cardiac surgeon with a guiding tool for:
1. Easier and more safe identification of hidden coronary arteries and grafts in primary procedures and specially reoperations.
2. Better selection of grafting site.
   Doppler is preferable to electromagnetic technique in coronary bypass flow measurement, which is:
3. Necessary to unveil technical errors.
4. Recommended for documentation of functional result.
5. Useful for prediction of prognosis.
6. Important for decisionmaking concerning reoperative revascularization.

References

1. Moulder PV, Teague MJ, Manuele VJ, Brunswick RA, Daicoff GR: Intraoperative Doppler coronary artery finder. Ann Thor Surg 24: 430–432, 1977.
2. FitzGerald DE, Fortescue-Webb CM, Ekeström S, Liljeqvist L, Nordhus O: Monitoring coronary artery blood flow by Doppler shift ultrasound. Scand J Thor Cardiovasc Surg 11: 119–123, 1977.
3. Wright CB, Doty DB, Eastham CL, Marcus ML: Measurements of coronary reactive hyperemia with a Doppler probe. J Thor Cardiovasc Surg 80: 888–897, 1980.
4. Segadal L, Matre K, Engedal H, Resch F, Grip A: Estimation of flow in aortocoronary grafts with a pulsed ultrasound Doppler meter. Thorac cardiovasc Surgeon 30: 265–268, 1982.
5. Moran JM, Burke DW, Loeb JM, Roberts AJ, Sanders Jr JH, Michaelis LL: Accuracy in coronary graft flow measurement. Ann Thorac Surg 32: 506–509, 1981.
6. Grondin PR: How valuable is perioperative flow measurement in aortocoronary bypass grafts? Ann Thorac Surg 31: 398–399, 1981.
7. Segadal L: Assessment of flow in aortocoronary grafts. Seminars in Ultrasound, CT, and MR, 6: 68–72, 1985.

8. de Rijbel RJ, Schipperheyn JJ: The use of electromagnetic flow measurements for detection of early stenosis in aortocoronary bypass grafts. Ann Thorac Surg 31: 402–408, 1981.
9. Gill RW: Measurement of blood flow by ultrasound: Accuracy and sources of error. Ultrasound in Med & Biol 11: 625–641, 1985.
10. Balderman SC, Moran JM, Scanlon PJ, Pifarrè R: Predictors of late aorta-coronary graft patency. J Thorac Cardiovasc Surg 79: 724–728, 1980.

6.3. Color flow evaluation of coronary anastomosis

SHUNEI KYO, RYOZO OMOTO, SHINICHI TAKAMOTO &
MAKOTO MATSUMURA

Introduction

Surgical intraoperative assessment of the technical adequacy of coronary artery bypass graft anastomoses has been difficult due to a lack of appropriate tools and technology [1]. Several clinical attempts have been reported using intraoperative epicardial ultrasonic techniques to assess the anatomical structure [2], the color blood flow image [3], and the blood flow velocity profile [4] of the native coronary artery and/or of the aorto-coronary bypass graft. In the surgeon's point of view, the color flow mapping real-time two-dimensional Doppler echocardiography (2-D Doppler) is considered to the most appropriate technology to assess the coronary artery intraoperatively among current ultrasonic equipments, because this technology can provide the information about the anatomical structure and blood flow dynamics of the coronary artery simultaneously, which can minimize the interruption of the surgery for the evaluation of the technical adequacy of the results of aorto-coronary bypass surgery [5].

The purpose of this study is to demonstrate the clinical feasibility of 2-D Doppler echocardiography for intraoperative assessment of coronary bypass graft anastomoses.

Material and methods

Intraoperative 2-D Doppler examination of aoro-coronary bypass graft was performed on eleven patients undergoing elective aorto-coronary bypass surgery (Table 1). All patients were male aged 47 to 68 years old. 21 saphenous vein grafts and 6 internal mammary artery grafts were bypassed with a standard median-sternotomy and cardiopulmonary bypass on these patients. The average number of bypass grafts was 2.5, and complete revascularization was performed in all patients. After completion of coronary bypass grafts, and just after weaning from cardiopulmonary bypass, the bypassed grafts and their anastomoses were examined by epicardial 2-D Doppler with a high resolution transducer. The 2-D Doppler system used was the XA-340 pro-

I. Cikes (ed.), *Echocardiography in Cardiac Interventions*, 407–414, 1989.
© 1989 *Kluwer Academic Publishers.*

408

Table 1. Study group.

Elective aorto-coronary bypass surgery		11 patients
Age: 47–68 (Average 56.2 ± 6.0) years old		
Sex: Male : Female = 11 : 0		
Coronary lesion:	LMT disease	2 patients
	2 vessels disease	3 patients
	3 vessels disease	6 patients
Location of bypass graft:	LIMAG – LAD	6 grafts
	SVG – RCA	4 grafts
	SVG – LAD	8 grafts
	SVG – CX	9 grafts

duced by Aloka Co., Tokyo, Japan. The XA-340 system has a proto-type of linear-array scanner with a linear type transducer of 7.5 MHz frequency; the pulse repetition frequencies of this system are 2 and 4 KHz. To avoid the perpendicular direction of the Doppler echo beam to the blood flow through the vessels we used a special triangular stand-off between the probe and the vessels to be imaged (Fig. 1). Compression of the vessels was avoided by filling the pericardial cradle with warm saline as necessary. The lowest velocity displayed in color was around 2 cm/sec on the XA-340 system. Before intraoperative use the transducer is gas sterilized with ethylene oxide for at least 24 hours. Simultaneously the coronary blood flow volume was measured with an electromagnetic flow meter (MFV 1100, FG flow probe: 3, 4, 5 mm, produced by Nihonkoden Co., Tokyo, Japan). Informed consent was ob-

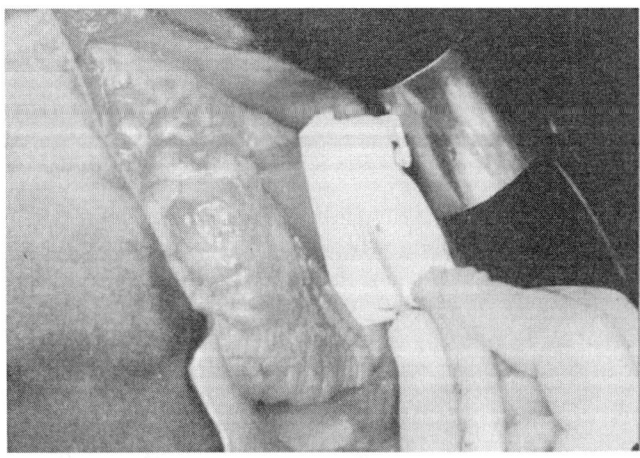

Fig. 1. Intraoperative epicardial 2-D Doppler technique for visualization of coronary artery using 7.5 MHz linear array transducer.

tained before the operation. No arrhythmia or other complications related to intraoperative 2-D Doppler were noted.

Results

Figure 2 shows representative color blood flow images in the proximal right coronary artery and left anterior descending coronary artery. While it is usually not easy to visualize the distal portion of the native coronary artery with this system, the visualization of the coronary bypass grafts was relatively good. The color blood flow image in the bypassed graft was visualized in 19 of 21 (90%) studied saphenous vein grafts. By electromagnetic flow meter, the average of graft flow was measured as 68.9 ± 28.1 ml/min (15 − 140 ml/min). The 2-D Doppler failed to detect the flow image when the graft flow was less than 20 ml/min measured by electromagnetic flow meter (Fig. 3).

In the case of internal mammary artery grafts, the 2-D Doppler failed to visualize the flow image in 2 of 6 grafts and electromagnetic flow meter failed to measure the flow volume in 4 of 6 grafts in which electromagnetic flow probe could not be fitted on two grafts. Figure 4 shows representative 2-D Doppler images of the saphenous vein grafts and the internal mammary artery graft in a 66-year-old male. All three grafts were confirmed to be patent with a good graft flow by intraoperative 2-D Doppler examination.

One minor abnormality in a proximal anastomosis of saphenous vein graft

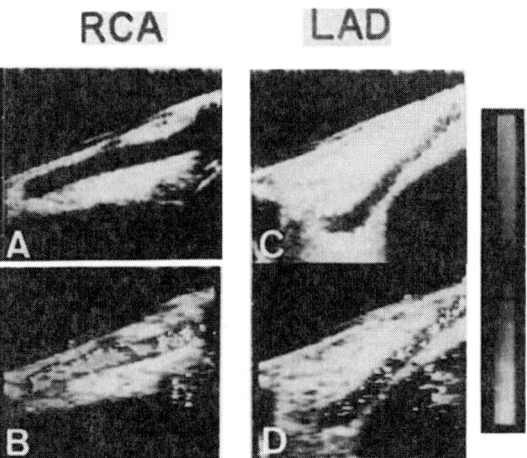

RCA   LAD

Fig. 2. 2-D Doppler images of proximal right coronary artery (RCA) and left anterior descending coronary artery (LAD) using 7.5 MHz linear-array transducer by means of intra-operative epicardial approach.

410

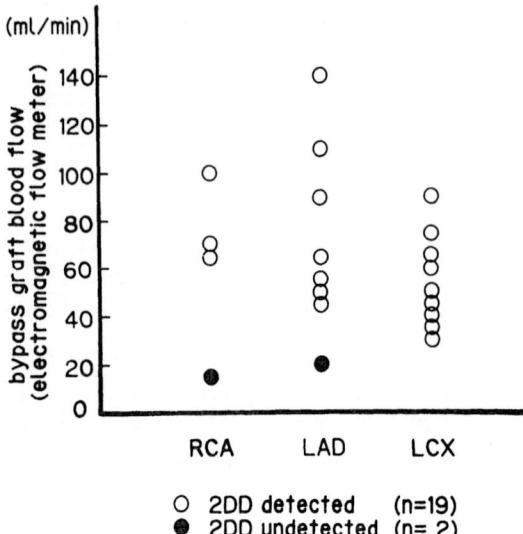

Fig. 3. 2-D Doppler detection of saphenous vein graft flow by means of intraoperative epicardial approach. 2-D Doppler fails to visualize the blood flow image when the graft flow volume is less than 20 ml/min (solid circle).

was noted (Fig. 5). A surplus small part of the saphenous vein graft protruded into the aortic lumen at the proximal anastomosis, but the flow through the anastomosis was not disturbed so much in the 2-D Doppler echocardiogram. A representative 2-D Doppler image of the distal anastomosis of the internal mammalian graft is shown in Fig. 6. T-bar shape of the

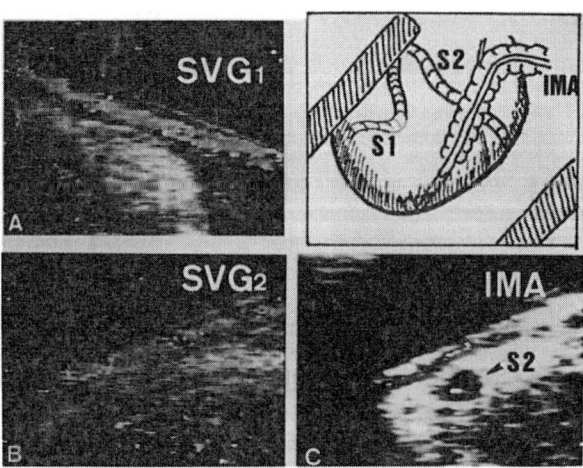

Fig. 4. Intraoperative epicardial 2-D Doppler evaluation of aorto-coronary bypass grafts. Satisfactory graft flows are demonstrated in both saphenous vein grafts and internal mammary artery graft. SVG = saphenous vein graft; IMA = internal mammary artery graft. C: The cross-section of the saphenous vein graft (S2) is also seen.

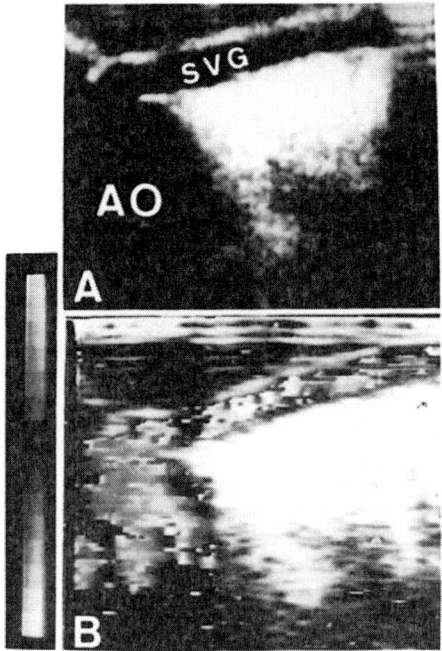

Fig. 5. 2-D Doppler image in proximal anastomosis of saphenous vein graft. A surplus small segment of saphenous vein graft protrudes into the aortic lumen at the proximal anastomosis, but the color blood flow image in the graft is not disturbed much. AO = ascending aorta; SVG = saphenous vein graft.

flow through the anastomosis can be clearly seen, but the 2-D echo image of the anatomical structure in the small anastomosis of internal mammalian arterial graft was not so clearly visualized by the 7.5 MHz transducer in our system.

Discussion

Several attempts have been made to achieve non-invasive imaging of the coronary artery by ultrasound [6, 7, 8, 9]. Sahn [2] first reported the use of 2-D echocardiography for intraoperative evaluation of native coronary artery and saphenous vein graft using a 9 MHz scanner. Hiratzka [1] also reported the intraoperative evaluation of coronary artery bypass graft anastomosis using a 12 MHz scanner. The current commercially available model of phased-array color flow mapping Doppler echo system carries transducer with only 2.5, 3.5, and 5.0 MHz frequencies which may not be sensitive enough to visualize the anatomical structure of the native coronary artery. In this study we used a proto-type of the linear 2-D Doppler system (XA-340)

412

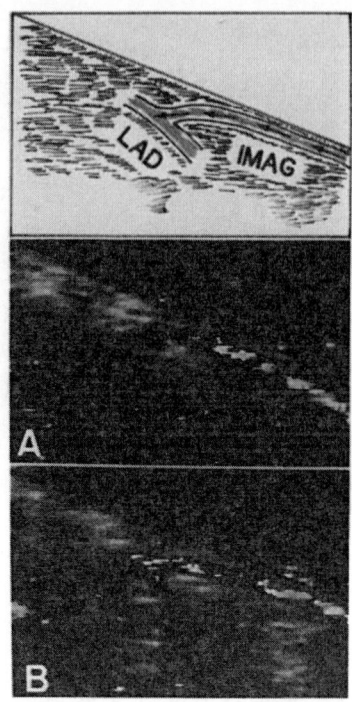

Fig. 6. 2-D Doppler images in distal anastomosis of internal mammary artery graft (IMAG). The blood flow through T-bar shape of anastomosis of IMAG to left anterior descending coronary artery (LAD) is clearly seen.

designed for the examination of peripheral vessels which carries a 5.0 and 7.5 MHz scanner. With 7.5 MHz, probe color blood flow images of the proximal coronary artery and the saphenous vein graft were clearly visualized by an intraoperative epicardial approach, but the color flow visualization of the distal coronary artery and the internal mammary artery graft was success-ful in only a limited number of the studied case. In order to improve the visualization of these small arteries, a special 2-D Doppler scanner should be designed for intraoperative epicardial use which carries a transducer probe with a frequency higher than 9 MHz. Utilizing the recent technological improvement in 2-D Doppler system and transducer, although it is possible in only a limited number of patients and in the limited area of the bypass graft, it has been possible to visualize the graft blood flow of the saphenous vein and the internal mammalian artery by even the transthoracic approach. Figure 7 presents a 2-D Doppler blood flow image of a saphenous vein graft from the precordial window using a newly developed commercially available linear-array 2-D Doppler system (SSD-350, produced by Aloka Co., Tokyo, Japan). The potential for imaging coronary anatomy and flow at the

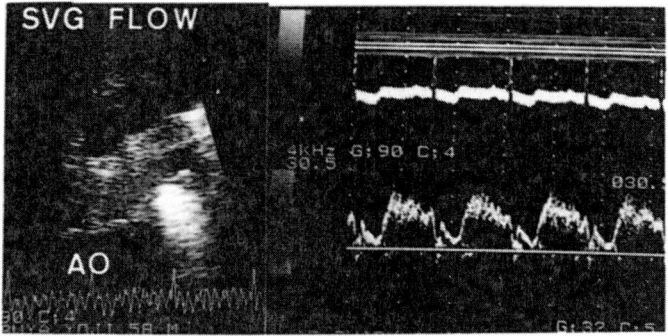

Fig. 7. 2-D Doppler image of saphenous vein graft flow from precordial window (transthoracic approach) using a convex type transducer of 5 MHz frequency of the newly developed linear-array 2-D Doppler system (Aloka, SSD-350). The velocity wave form of the graft flow is recorded simultaneously by FFT (fast-Fourier transform method) pulsed Doppler spectral analysis. AO = ascending aorta; SVG = saphenous vein graft.

operating table may permit the surgern to confirm the optimal position to place the coronary bypass graft and the technical adequacy of coronary artery bypass graft immediately after anastomosis. Also the potential for imaging the anatomy and flow of the coronary bypass graft in the outpatient echo laboratory may permit the surgeon and cardiologist to confirm the good graft patency and the good postoperative condition of the patients after aorta-coronary bypass graft surgery without having to repeat coronary angiography. Improvements in the color flow mapping Doppler echo system in the future should make available to the cardiologist and the surgeon a comprehensive ultrasonic method for evaluation of coronary anatomy and flow dynamics both in the outpatient clinic and operating room without angiography.

References

1. Hiratzka LF, McPherson DD, Lamberth WC, Jr., Brandt B. III, Armstong ML, Schroder E, Hunt M, Kieso R, Megan MD, Tompkins PK, Marcus ML, Kerber RE: Intraoperative evaluation of coronary artery bypass graft anastomoses with high-frequency epicardial echocardiography: experimental validation and initial patient studies. Circulation 73: 1199–1205, 1986.
2. Sahn DJ, Barratt-Boyes BG, Graham K, Kerr A, Roche A, Hill D, Brandt PWT, Copeland JG, Mammana R, Temkin LP, Glenn W: Ultrasonic imaging of the coronary arteries in open-chest humans: Evaluation of coronary atherosclerotic lesions during cardiac surgery. Circulation 66: 1034–1044, 1982.
3. Takamoto S, Kyo S, Adachi H, Matsumura M, Yokote Y, Omoto R: Intraoperative color flow mapping real-time two-dimensional Doppler echocardiography for evaluation of

414

valvular and congenital heart disease and vascular disease. J Thorac Cardiovasc Surg 90: 802–812, 1985.

4. Kajiya F, Ogasawara Y, Tsujioka K, Nakai M, Goto M, Wada Y, Tadaoka S, Matsuoka S, Mito K, Fujiwara T: Evaluation of human coronary blood flow with an 80 channel 20 MHz pulsed Doppler velocimeter and zero-cross and Fourier transform methods during cardiac surgery. Circulation 74 (Suppl III): 53–60, 1986.

5. Kyo S, Adachi H, Takamoto S, Matsumura M, Yokote Y, Omoto R: Intraoperative evaluation of the effects of coronary revascularization by color flow mapping 2-D Doppler echocardiography and thermocardiography. JACC 7: 150A, 1986. (Abstr.)

6. Weyman WE, Feigenbaum H, Dillon JC, Johnston KW, Eggleton RC: Noninvasive visualization of the left main coronary artery by cross-sectional echocardiography. Circulation 54: 169–174, 1976.

7. Hiraishi S, Yashiro K, Kusano S: Noninvasive visualization of coronary arterial aneurysm in infants and young children with mucocutaneous lymph node syndrome with two-dimensional echocardiography. Am J Cardiol 43: 1225–1233, 1979.

8. Yoshikawa J, Katao H, Yanagihara K, Takagi Y, Okumachi F, Yoshida K, Tomita Y, Fukaya T, Baba K: Noninvasive visualization of the dilated main coronary arteries in coronary artery fistulas by cross-sectional echocardiography. Circulation 65: 600–603, 1982.

9. Kyo S, Takamoto S, Matsumura M, Yokote Y, Omoto R: Transesophageal 2-dimensional echo-Doppler visualization of left main coronary arterial anatomy and flow. J Am Coll Cardiol 9: 179A, 1987. (Abstr.)

6.4. Intraoperative Doppler color flow mapping in dissecting aneurysm of the aorta

SHINICHI TAKAMOTO & RYOZO OMOTO

Dissecting aneurysm of the aorta (DAA) is a severe disease, frequently involving a broad area of the thoracic and abdominal aorta, the mortality of which is still high even in intensive medical or surgical treatment due to the complicated pathophysiology of the dissection of the aorta [1, 2]. Preoperative assessments of DAA by 2-D echography [3, 4], CT scanning [5], RI angiography [6] and cine-aortography [7] have their own limitations.

A real-time two-dimensional Doppler echocardiography (2-D Doppler) system [8] can afford to perform color flow mapping on a real-time echogram simultaneously. By this 2-D Doppler color flow mapping great progress is being made in the diagnosis and evaluation of cardiovascular diseases [9]. The authors have first reported application of 2-D Doppler to the dissecting aortic aneurysm [10]. However, 2-D Doppler has its own limitations consistent wih echography also, that is, the echo does not penetrate into bone or the lung. While transcutaneous 2-D Doppler can only display parts of the aorta due to the narrowness of the beam windows on the chest wall, intraoperative use of 2-D Doppler has no obstacle before the aorta and total imaging of the dissecting aorta in the operative field can be obtained with information of blood flow dynamics [11]. Clinical significance of intraoperative color flow mapping in the dissecting aneurysm of the aorta is discussed in this chapter.

Methods

The 2-D Doppler system used was the Aloka SSD-880 utilizing a phased-array transducer with 3.5 MHz of frequency. Flow toward the transducer is displayed in red and flow away from it in blue. Velocity of the flow is in direct proportion to the brightness of the color. Variance of velocity is displayed by a mixture of green color. 2-D Doppler images were stored on a Sony video-cassette recorder (VO 5800) and photographed on a 35 mm color film. A transducer was gas-sterilized for at least 24 hours with ethylene-oxide. Before and after the vascular procedure during the operation of DAA, direct scanning by 2-D Doppler along the aorta was performed both in short and long axis views.

I. Cikes (ed.), *Echocardiography in Cardiac Interventions*, 415–422, 1989.
© 1989 *Kluwer Academic Publishers*.

416

Case presentations

Typical cases are presented

Case 1. T.M. 39 year-old male, DeBakey type I + aortic regurgitation.
Before a vascular procedure 2-D Doppler displayed grade 3 of aortic regurgitation along the mitral valve with a mosaic flow pattern of yellow and blue dots which indicated a very fast turbulent flow. Intimal flap was visualized to extend to the aortic ring proximally and to the distal end of the aortic arch distally. Large entry was displayed with blood flow image from a true lumen to a false lumen just above the aortic ring in the dilated aortic root (Fig. 1). Good amounts of blood flow existed in both true and false lumens which indicated existence of a large re-entry.

After replacement of the aortic valve and the ascending aorta, no aortic regurgitation was displayed in the left ventricle. Smooth flow from the aortic

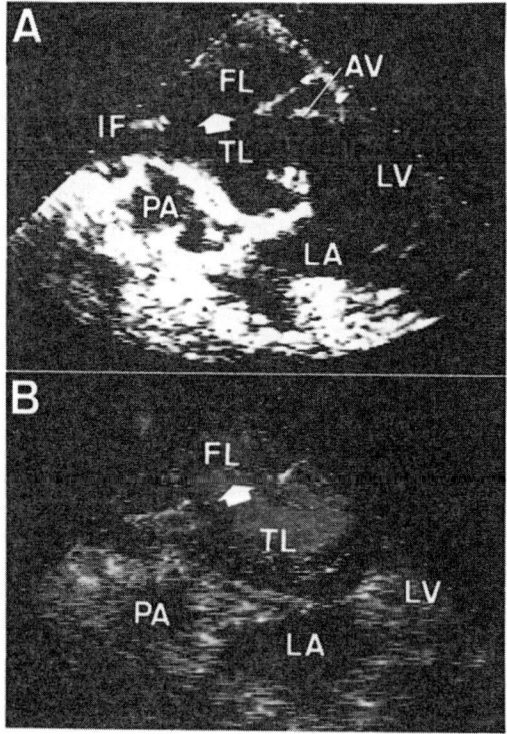

Fig. 1. (A) Intra-operative 2-D echogram images of Case 1 in long axis views of the aortic root. Entry is shown with arrow. LV = left ventricle, LA = left atrium, PA = pulmonary artery, IF = intimal flap, AV = aortic valve, TL = true lumen, FL = false lumen. (B) Intraoperative 2-D Doppler images of Case 1 in a long axis view of the aortic root. An intimal flap and blood flow through the large entry to the false lumen at the dilated aortic root are shown.

root through the graft to the true lumen in the aortic arch was displayed. Significant blood flow was not displayed in the false lumen in the aortic arch, which implied that the entry no longer existed.

Case 2. T.O. 23 year-old male, DeBakey type III.
2-D Doppler revealed the aortic dissection from the distal origin of the left subclavian artery to the abdominal aorta. The proximal end of the large false lumen was filled with thrombus and a small jet flow from the small true lumen to the false lumen through the dissected edge of the intercostal artery

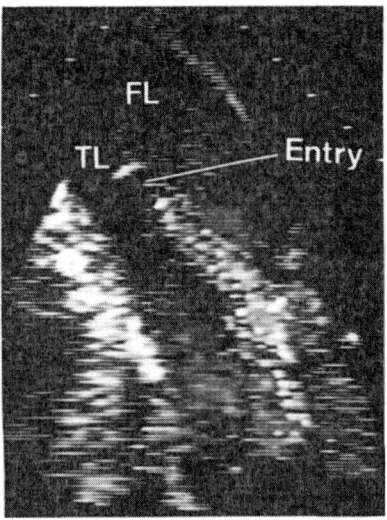

Fig. 2. Intraoperative 2-D Doppler image of Case 2 in a long axis view of the descending aorta. Before the vascular procedure a jet flow of a mosaic pattern is shown to eject from the entry. Site and size of the entry is clearly displayed by intraoperative color flow mapping.

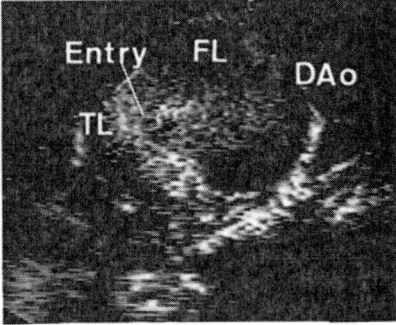

Fig. 3. Intraoperative 2-D Doppler images of Case 2 in a short axis view of the descending aorta (DAo). Before the vascular procedure, form the dissected edge of the intercostal artery a small jet flow to the false lumen is shown. Mural thrombus in the false lumen is also displayed. Such a small flow through the tiny entry is clearly shown in intraoperative color flow mapping.

418

(Fig. 3) was shown clearly. The main entry was displayed in the middle of the descending aorta with a jet flow of a mosaic pattern of a turbulent flow (Fig. 2) and both lumens in the proximal abdominal aorta were perfused with a vivid blue flow pattern away from the transducer.

After graft replacement of the descending aorta smooth flow was shown from the aortic arch through the graft to the two lumens in the abdominal aorta. However, small leakage from the proximal anastomosis of the graft to the cavity wrapped by the remaining aneurysmal wall and its precise site were detected (Fig. 4).

Case 3. M.A. 65 year-old male. DeBakey type III + AAA (Fig. 5).
From the abdominal approach through a median laparatomy the distal descending aorta was shown to be dissected and blood flow with fast velocity in the small true lumen and very slow flow in the false lumen were displayed. The celiac axis was displayed to be perfused from the false lumen (Fig. 5-A). The superior mesenteric artery was perfused from the true lumen through the narrow channel which was produced by circumferential dissection around the origin of the superior mesenteric artery, which we named 'bridge formation' (Fig. 5-B). Both renal arteries were perfused by the true lumen but at the left renal artery, 'bridge formation' was alsof shown (Fig. 5-C). The abdominal aorta was dilated above the bifurcation and blood flow pattern was shown only in the true lumen in the abdominal aortic aneurysm without

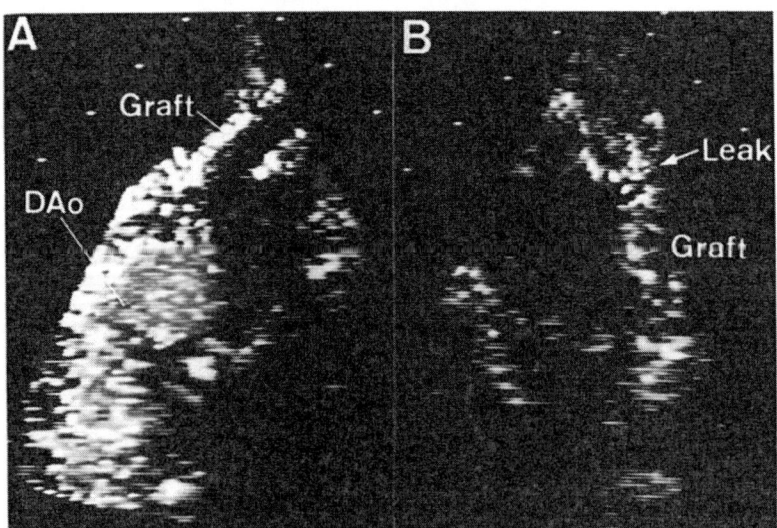

Fig. 4. Intraoperative 2-D Doppler images of graft anastomosis in the descending aorta (DAo) in Case 2. (A) Long axis view of the descending aorta. (B) Short axis view of the descending aorta at the level of the anastomosis. Small leakage is shown in the upper right site of the anastomosis.

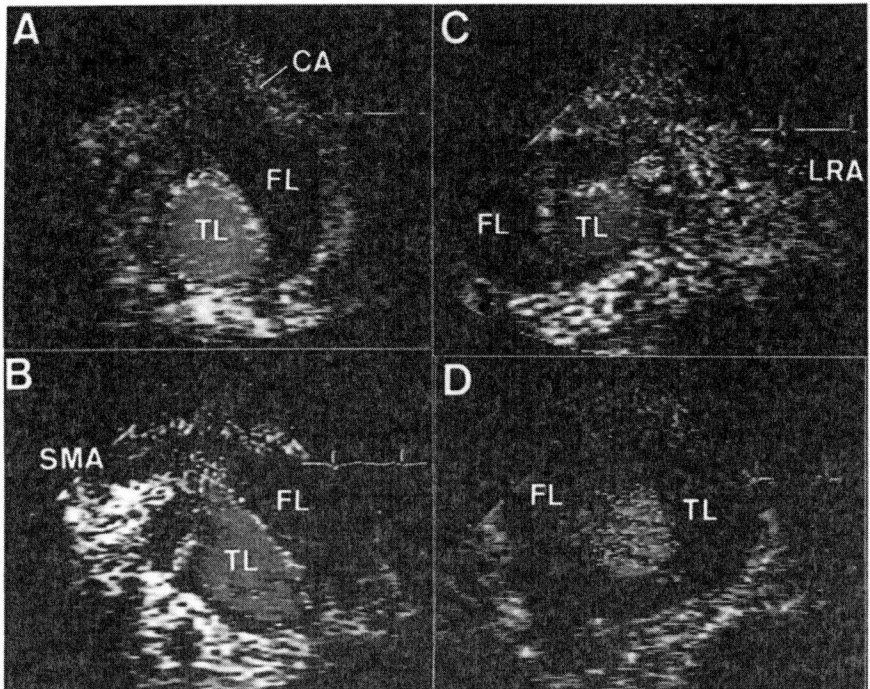

Fig. 5. Intraoperative 2-D Doppler images of Case 3 in serial short axis views of the abdominal aorta. Before surgery, (A) The celiac axis (CA) is perfused from the false lumen. (B) At the root of the superior mesenteric artery (SMA) circumferential dissection occurs and produces a narrow channel from the true lumen, which we named 'bridge formation'. (C) At the left renal artery 'bridge formation' is also seen. (D) At the abdominal aortic aneurysm blood flow exists only in the true lumen without a re-entry.

a re-entry (Fig. 5-D). This information confirmed that the operation of abdominal aortic aneurysmectomy and the graft replacement with fenestration was appropriate. After the vascular procedure it was confirmed that flow in the false lumen increased and the blood supply to the major branches were maintained.

Discussion

Color flow mapping by 2-D Doppler has brought great progress to non-invasive diagnosis in cardiovascular diseases. If the aorta is dilated and in contact with the chest wall without the lung in between, transcutaneous 2-D Doppler can obtain clear color flow mapping in the aneurysmal cavity. However, with the transcutaneous 2-D Doppler it has usually been difficult to obtain images of the entire thoracic aorta due to the poor penetration of the echo in the thorax.

The intraoperative 2-D Doppler easily gave the image of the thoracic aorta in the operative field without obstacle by direct scanning of the aorta. In addition to direct scanning of the thoracic aorta, abdominal aorta could be imaged by transcutaneous scanning of 2-D Doppler during the operation as well, although the clarity of its image is less than with direct scanning. If this information is inhibited by air in the gastrointetinal tract, direct scanning of the abdominal aorta through the minilaparatomy is also feasible. These scannings of operative 2-D Doppler can offer images of the whole aorta from the ascending to the abdominal aorta in a short time and without contrast medium. Moreover, intraoperative 2-D Doppler can supply 3-D information of the structure and flow dynamics in the dissected aorta by obtaining serial 2-D imaging in both short and long axis views. Cine-aortography offers 2-D images of limited views with a limited volume of contrast medium, yet can hardly supply complete 3-D information. Furthermore, this information is confined to the intra-vascular cavity. Dynamic CT with contrast medium injection displays rough information of blood flow but not precise instantaneous flow dynamics. RI angiography is a simple noninvasive method but precise information of dissection cannot be obtained.

By this total imaging of DAA, site and size of entry and reentry: extension of dissection; thrombus formation; relationship to the neighboring organ; blood flow dynamics in the true and false lumens, in the entry and re-entry, and in the major branches of the aorta and the heart could all be obtained by the 2-D Doppler. With this information the precise and most appropriate operative procedure can be determined. The site of the aortic incision, site of the aortic clamp, range of the graft replacement, graft replacement or simple closure of the entry, closure of the entry or opening of re-entry, anastomosis with a true lumen or with double lumens, need for additional arterial reconstruction to the branches of the aorta or not are all determinable by use of the 2-D Doppler system intraoperatively. Although the operative procedure and approach are roughly determined by preoperative cine-aortography, recently by transesophageal 2-D Doppler [12], final determination of the precise procedure is confirmed by intra-operative 2-D Doppler. In Case 3 blood flow status of the celiac axis was not clearly demonstrated pre-operatively even by cine-aortography. 2-D Doppler guaranteed appropriateness of the operative procedure which was a key to operative success, and this was evidenced by an uneventful post-operative course.

After vascular procedure, 2-D Doppler reveals information about intimal tear caused by the vascular clamp, closure of entry or opening of re-entry, blood flow dynamics in the true lumen and the remaining false lumen, and in graft anastomosis and the major branches of the aorta. At the anastomosis site even small leakage can be shown and the precise site of leakage can be identified as in Case 2. Thus, intraoperative 2-D Doppler can check the operative effect and evaluate the post-operative state. Especially, confirmation of good perfusion in the major branches of the aorta by 2-D Doppler is particularly important in order to obtain successful effect of the operation as Case 3.

Since the operation for DAA is mainly aimed at closure of an entry or opening of a re-entry and replacement of the dilated aorta, and not necessarily replacement of the whole dissected aorta, it leaves large parts of the dissected aorta in situ frequently. We sometimes encountered cases in which the operations were done successfully but post-operative courses were exaggerated due to loss of perfusion to the branches of the aorta. Unconsciousness due to brain ischemic damage, liver and kidney dysfunction, intestinal ischemia and necrosis are causes of post-operative complications and mortality [1]. It is very difficult to carry out invasive angiography in such a critical condition with large parts of the dissection left post-operatively. Post-operative 2-D Doppler also may not provide sufficient information due to air in the paralytic bowel.

Therefore, the keys to success in the operation for DAA are appropriate selection of the operative procedure, good anastomosis and adequate perfusion in the major branches of the aorta. In order to check these operative effects during the operation, there have not been any effective examinations previously. If intraoperative 2-D Doppler revealed some defects in a graft anastomosis or in perfusion of the major branches of the aorta, repair of the anastomosis or additional arterial reconstruction could be carried out soon before the patient fell into a critical condition.

The operation of DAA has the high mortality of 30-50% in the acute stage and around 20% in the chronic stage [1, 2]. Post-operative complications relating to the stenotic and obstructive lesions in DAA have often been reported [1, 13]. However, proper selection of the procedure and judging the operative results by utilizing intra-operative 2-D Doppler might lead to a reduction of the high operative mortality.

References

1. DeBakey ME, McCollum CH, Crawford ES, Morris GC, Howell J, Noon GP, Lawrie G: Dissection and dissecting aneurysms of the aorta, Twenty-year follow-up of five hundred twenty-seven patients treated surgically. Surgery 92: 1118–1134, 1982.
2. Wheat MW Jr: Acute dissecting aneurysms of the aorta, diagnosis and treatment – 1979. Am Heart J 99: 373–387, 1980.
3. DeMaria AN, Bommer .W, Neumann A, Weinert L, Borgen H, Mason DT: Identification

and localization of aneurysms of the ascending aorta by cross-sectional echocardiography. Circulation 59: 755–761, 1979.

4. Kasper W, Meinertz T, Kersting F, Lang K, Just H: Diagnosis of dissecting aortic aneurysm with suprasternal echocardiography. Am J Cardiol 42: 291–294, 1978.

5. Godwin JD, Herfkens RL, Skioldebrand CG, Federle MP, Lipton MJ: Evaluation of dissections and aneurysms of the thoracic aorta by conventional and dynamic CT scanning. Radiology 136: 125–133, 1980.

6. Kusakabe K, Watanabe N, Saito R, Maki M, Yamazaki T, Shigeta A: Diagnosis of aortic aneurysm with radionuclide angiography. Nippon Acta Radiologica 40: 866–877, 1980.

7. Hayashi K, Meaney TF, Zelch JV, Tarar R: Aortographic analysis of aortic dissection. Am J Roentgenol 122: 769–782, 1974.

8. Namekawa K, Kasai C, Tsukamoto M, Koyano A. Imaging of blood flow using autocorrelation. Ultrasound in Medicine & Biology 8: 138, 1982.

9. Omoto R (ed.): Color atlas of real-time two-dimensional Doppler echocardiography. Shindan-To-Chiryo Co. Tokyo, 1984.

10. Takamoto S: Aortic disease, In color atlas of real-time two-dimensional Doppler echocardiography. 1st Ed. Edited by R. Omoto. Shindan-to Chiryo Co., Tokyo, 1984.

11. Takamoto S, Kyo S, Adachi H, Matsumura M, Yokote Y, Omoto R: Intraoperative color flow mapping by real-time two-dimensional Doppler echocardiography for evaluation of valvular and congenital heart disease and vascular disease. J Thorac Cardiovasc Surg. 90: 802, 1985.

12. Takamoto S, Kyo S, Matsumura M, Hojo H, Yokote Y and Omoto R: Total visualization of thoracic dissecting aortic aneurysm by trans-esophageal Doppler color flow mapping. Circulation 74: Suppl. II: 132, 1986.

13. Shumacker HB Jr, Isch JH, Jolly WW: Stenotic and obstructive lesions in acute dissecting thoracic aortic aneurysms. Ann Surg 181, 662–669, 1975.

6.5. Doppler monitoring of cardiac output using an implantable aortic transducer

LEIDULF SEGADAL, KNUT MATRE & HOGNE ENGEDAL

Continuous hemodynamic monitoring after cardiac surgery is mandatory. Knowledge of the performance of the heart, and in particular display of trends is necessary to take appropriate action in due time. Equipment for continuous measurements of blood pressure in heart chambers and great vessles has been available for some time, and pressure trends are of great help in the postoperative care. Unfortunately, even the combined observation of pre- and after-load is not always sufficient for the evaluation of the performance of a heart chamber. Knowledge of stroke volume and flow makes it possible to quantify peripheral vascular resistance and heart work, necessary for the right measures to be taken before organ failure is manifest.

Many methods have been devised to measure cardiac output, invasively or noninvasively. The single widely used method in postoperative care is the thermo-dilution technique. By this method a central catheter is needed, preferably in the pulmonary artery, useful also for measurement of pulmonary artery and wedge pressure. The estimation of flow, however, can only be made intermittently, by injections of cold saline, and the central catheter is not without harmful effects.

Electromagnetic flow measurement can be made continuously, but the need for zero-flow calibration and the encircling probe around the vessel makes this method impractical except for experimental purposes.

A step further in the development of a continuous method for post-operative cardiac output measurement was taken by Keagy and collaborators, when in 1983 they described a technique, tested in dogs, for measuring aortic flow by a removable, extraluminal ultrasound Doppler probe, with transmitting frequency of 20 MHz [1]. They fixed the small probe to the ascending aorta by suturing a Gore-tex graft in the shape of a pocket to the vessel wall. Excellent individual correlation with electromagnetic flow measurements were achieved in five dogs.

Independently we had been working with a very similar method for several years, and the first clinical study (Matre et al. 1985) [2] showed that this method was possible to applicate in clinical practice without complications. Our fixation method was simple: A small pocket was dissected on the anterior wall of the ascending aorta between the epicardium and the

I. Cikes (ed.), *Echocardiography in Cardiac Interventions*, 423–429, 1989.

424

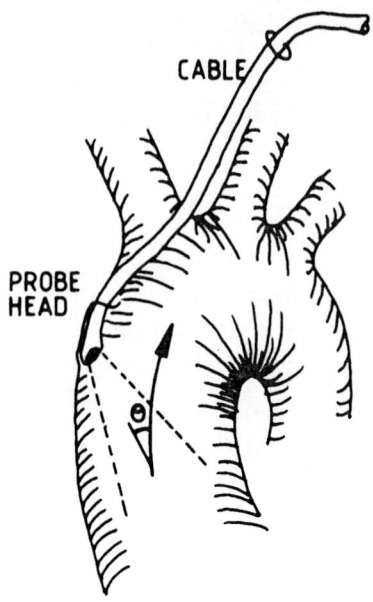

Fig. 1. Placement of invasive extractable Doppler probe on the ascending aorta. (From: Matre et al., 1985 [2] Courtesy Butterworth & Co).

adventitia (Fig. 1). The pocket was narrowed at its entrance after the placement of the probe by one or to sutures of prolene 7–0. The probe itself, transmitting 10 MHz pulsed ultrasound, was shaped almost like one half of a longitudinally divided pear, with the flat side against the aortic lumen. The adult probe measured 6 mm at the largest cross-sectional diameter (Fig. 2). The cable was led cranially behind sternum and through a small incision in

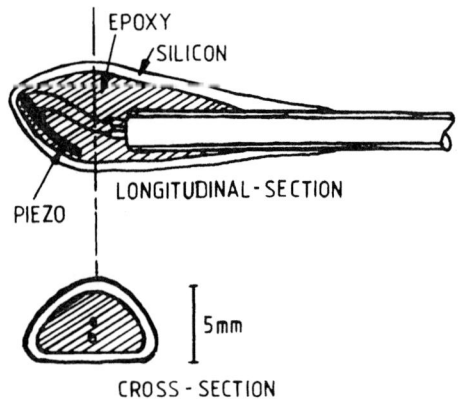

Fig. 2. Implantable Doppler probe. The piezo-electric crystal is backed by epoxy for stability. Probe and cable covered with silicone rubber. (From: Matre et al., 1985 [2] Courtesy Butterworth & Co.)

jugulum. It was easily removed the first or second day after the operation by gentle traction in the cable without any harm to the patient or the probe. Unfortunately, the correlation to the reference method, thermodilution, was relatively poor (r = 0.77).

Keagy et al. later reported application of this method in children using a 20 MHz probe attached to aorta by thin metal tines [3].

In 1986 another norwegian group presented clinical experience with a different type of extraluminal, extractable Doppler probe for aortic flow measurement [4]. In order to cover a larger portion of the cross-sectional area they used 2 MHz and a fairly large crystal of 4×8 mm. The chest drain sized probe and cable were fixed to the aortic wall by a double suture, kept tight in a long tourniquet, and led through the skin in the epigastrium. Recordings from 8 patients with this technique also gave a correlation co-efficient of 0.77, when compared with thermodilution measurements.

Method

Blood velocity measurement by the ultrasound Doppler technique is based on the frequency shift of reflected ultrasound. The velocity is connected to the shift of frequency (f_1), the transmitted frequency (f_0) and the sound velocity in blood (c) by the Doppler equation: [5]

$$v = \frac{f_1 \cdot c}{2 \cdot f_0 \cdot \cos \theta}$$

where θ is the angle between direction of the blood flow and the direction of the ultrasound beam. If the mean cross-sectional velocity (v) is known blood flow in aorta is:

$$Q = \pi \cdot r^2 \cdot v$$

Cardiac output is 5–8% larger when the aortic blood flow is measured distal to the coronary arteries [5]. The difficulties by application of this well known principle to the invasive postoperative measurement of aortic flow is mainly:

1. Probe-size. In order to have a non-traumatic system, particularly in children, the width of the probe should not exceed 5–6 mm. As the size of the crystal has to be even smaller the frequency should be 5 MHz or higher, because the diameter of the crystal should exceed 5 times the wave-length in order to achieve a homogeneous ultrasound field. As the sound attenuation is larger by higher frequencies, the opposite part of the aorta can hardly be reached when the frequency is 10 mHz or higher. The width of the sample

volume, using flat crystals, will be of the same size as the crystal, making it difficult to get Doppler shift recordings from more than a very limited part of the aortic cross-section.

2. Probe-fixation. Very small movements of the probe may critically alter the direction of the narrow ultrasound beam and therefore a very stable fixation is needed.

3. Angle-estimation. Even if the acustic angle of the transmitted beam in relation to the contrast surface of the probe is known, the varying curvature of the aorta from one patient to another makes it difficult to estimate the angle between ultrasound beam and blood stream. Furthermore, the angel will vary from the outer to the inner part of the sample volume, particularly when long sampling volumes are used, as the beam enters the curved vessel obliquely.

4. Estimation of diameter. Both mechanical measurement of wall thickness and outer diameter as well as echographic measurement has been used, both methods probably with an error less than 5% [2, 4]. The variations of diameter due to alterations in blood pressure is less known. Experimental studies indicate that the use of a fixed systolic diameter introduces only small errors when the blood-pressure is within physiological limits. In severe hypotension or hypertension, however, a larger error may be introduced [6].

5. Sample volume. Ideally a uniform sampling over one complete cross-section of aorta should take place. From what is already mentioned it is obvious that some compromize must be chosen. The available equipment limits the effective sampling volume to a width of 4 to 8 mm and a length of 8 to 30 mm, and the sampling becomes more heterogeneous by augmenting length [7]. Probe-technology and electronical compensations, will probably reduce these limitations in the near future. Presently, the technique relies on a representative position of a limited sample volume.

6. Flow profile. If the mean velocity profile of the aorta is flat, as it probably is in smaller animals and children, central measurement of flow with a small sampling volume will implicate only minor errors [6, 8, 9]. In most adult patients however, the mean profile is skewed and irregular, according to recent studies [10, 11, 12]. Therefore, when a small sample volume is taken as representative, substantial over- or underestimation of cardiac output may occur in some of the patients. Concerning flow profile, the most serious limitation is the possible alterations of the profile due to changing cardiac output and aortic pressure.

Practical considerations

Despite all theoretical limitations, the method is, even at this stage of development, a very useful technique and in some patients the measurements are in excellent agreement with other methods (Figs. 3, 4 and 5). High quality Doppler technology and dedicated probes are necessary [2]. The technique of probe fixation is essential, and whichever method used, must be performed with skill and concern. The longitudinal alignment is particularly important. The sample volume should initially be placed at a depth of about 1/3 of the aortic diameter and, with a short length, moved to and from in different depths, to test the variations in mean velocity. Small variations indicate a flattened profile an give reason to expect reliable measurements. The sample volume should then be lengthened to between 12 and 16 mm, the highpass filtration set to a minimum, and the sensitivity and gain controls adjusted regularly. Trend display of the time average velocity seems to be more useful than the displayed absolute value of cardiac output. In some patients correct cardiac output is achieved over a broad range, when compared to thermodilution measurements. In order to cope with the possible errors, one has to distinguish between sources of error being constant for one patient and those rising from changes in the hemodynamic condition. The constant errors may be reduced by calibration by another reliable method, for instance by thermo- or dye-dilution technique or by electromagnetic calibration. In one of our series this procedure improved the

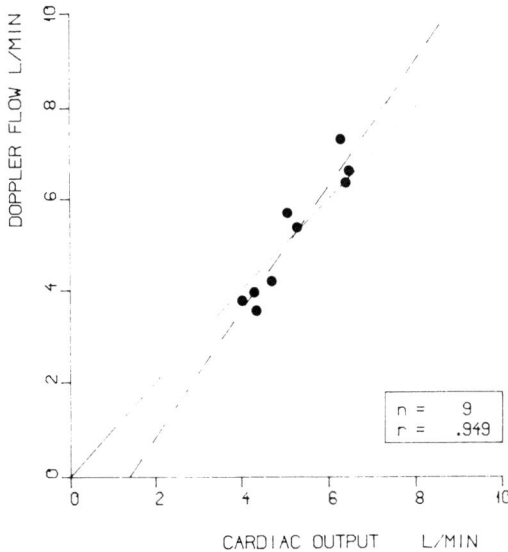

Fig. 3. Correlation between Doppler cardiac output measurements (y-axis) and average of three simultaneous thermodilution measurements (x-axis) in one patient. Line of identity and regression line (dashed) is drawn.

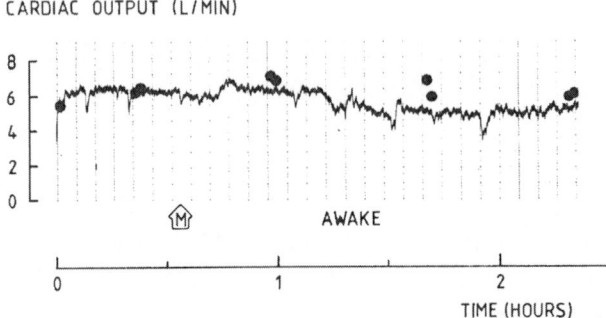

CARDIAC OUTPUT (L/MIN)

Fig. 4. Cardiac output variations in a postoperative stable situation. Doppler measurement = continous curve. Thermodilution = dots. M = morphine administration. (From: Matre et al. 1985. [2] Courtesy Butterworth & Co.)

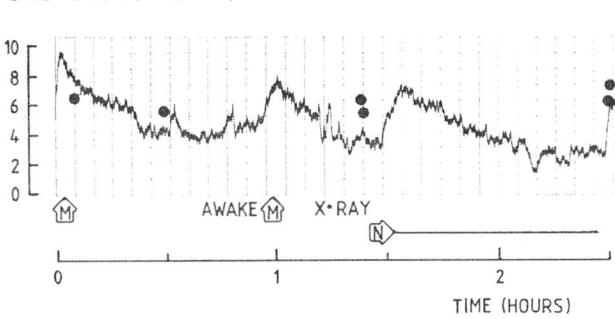

CARDIAC OUTPUT (L/MIN)

Fig. 5. Cardiac output variations immediately after the operation in an unstable patient. N = nitroprusside infusion. Other symbols as in Fig. 4. (From: Matre et al. 1985 [2] Courtesy Butterworth & Co.)

correlation of later measurements from r = .53 to r = .74 [13]. The dynamic errors are more difficult to adjust for. In our series there is a tendency for Doppler measurements to overestimate changes in flow, even if the mean of all recordings correlates well with the mean of the thermodilution measurements (Fig. 3). This tendency is also found in other studies [2, 4].

Present state

The continous cardiac output monitoring by the extractable Doppler probe has given us a new dynamic parameter which, used with care, provides a very promising tool in the postoperative care of selected cardiac patients. Probably most reliable results are achieved in patients with small aortas and normal aortic valves. The greatest value is the possibility of immediate detection of changes in cardiac output. Care must be taken when the method is used in patients with prosthetic or abnormal valves, and when flow rate or pressure is beyond normal physiological limits. It is preferable when the use of a thermo-dilution catheter is impractical or contraindicated, but still close observation of the cardiac performance is desired [4].

Better knowledge of the variations of the flow profile, improved probe technology and sophisticated on-line compensating computations will probably make this method a relatively cheap, safe and reliable technique for monitoring operated hearts at risk. Combined with pressure monitorings, trend curves of cardiac output, heart work and peripheral as well as pulmonary vascular resistance may be produced on-line, giving critically ill patients a better postoperative care and chance of survival.

References

1. Keagy BA, Lucas CL, Hsiao HH, Wilcox BR: A removable extraluminal Doppler probe for continuous monitoring of changes in cardiac output. J Ultrasound Med 2: 357, 1983.
2. Matre K, Segadal L, Engedal H: Continuous measurement of aortic blood velocity, after cardiac surgery, by means of an extractable Doppler ultrasound probe. J Biomed Eng 7: 84, 1985.
3. Keagy BA, Wilcox BR, Lucas CL, Henry GW, Boudino M: A removable, extraluminal ultrasound probe for monitoring postoperative cardiac output in the pediatric open heart patient. Circulation, Abstracts 72: III: 148, 1985.
4. Svennevig JL, Grip A, Lindberg H, Geiran O, Hall KV: Continuous monitoring of cardiac output postoperatively using an implantable Doppler probe. Scand J Thor Cardiovasc Surg 20: 145, 1986.
5. Brubakk AO, Gisvold SE: Measurement of instantaneous blood-flow velocity in the human aorta using pulsed Doppler ultrasound. Cardiovasc res. 16: 26, 1982.
6. Matre K, Segadal L: Evaluation of an extractable Doppler ultra sound probe for continous cardiac output monitoring, by simultaneous measurement of velocity, diameter, flow and pressure in cats. Cardiovasc Res 22: 855, 1988.
7. Hatle L, Angelsen BAJ: Doppler ultrasound in cardiology. Philadelphia, 1982, Lea and Febiger, Philadelphia 1982.
8. Paulsen PK, Hasenkam JM: Three-dimensional visualization of velocity profiles in the ascending aorta in dogs, measured with a hot-film anemometer. J Biomech 16: 201, 1983.
9. Lucas CL, Keagy BA, Hsiao HS, Johnston TA, Henry GW, Wilcox BR: The velocity profile in the canine ascending aorta and its effects on the accuracy of pulsed Doppler determinations of mean blood velocity. Cardiovasc Res 18: 282, 1984.
10. Segadal L, Matre K: Blood velocity distribution in the human ascending aorta. Circulation 76: 90, 1987.
11. Vieli A, Jenni R, Anliker M: Spatial velocity distributions in the ascending aorta of healthy humans and cardiac patients. IEEE Trans BME 33: 28, 1986.
12. Jenni R, Vieli A, Ruffmann K, Krayenbuehl HP, Anliker M: A comparison between single gate and multigate ultrasonic Doppler measurements for the assessment of the velocity pattern in the human ascending aorta. Eur Heart J 5: 948, 1984.
13. Segadal L, Matre K: Continuous postoperative cardiac output measurement. Clinical evaluation of invasive Doppler method. To be published.

6.6. Doppler echocardiography and cardiac pacing

GILBERT J. PERRY & NAVIN C. NANDA

I. Introduction

The ability of Doppler echocardiography to evaluate changes in flow non-invasively on a beat to beat basis has made it quite valuable as a means of evaluating pacemaker physiology. Combined Doppler echocardiographic studies of the left atrium and mitral inflow have been used to evaluate left atrial size and function [1, 2] while Doppler echocardiographic studies of aortic flow velocity have been used to evaluate the effect of different pacing modes or different AV intervals on resting stroke volume [1, 3–10]. These studies are useful in evaluating patients for ventricular versus dual chamber pacemakers, and for optimizing the AV interval in patients who have received dual chamber pacemakers. Doppler echocardiographic studies can also be used to document atrial capture [11] to exclude pacemaker induced valvular regurgitation [3] and to investigate the hemodynamic alterations in patients with the pacemaker syndrome. This chapter will review the role that combined Doppler echocardiographic studies have played in improving our understanding of pacemaker physiology, and the clinical applications of these techniques.

II. Use of Doppler echocardiography in choosing the pacing mode

A. Combined Doppler-echocardiographic evaluation of atrial function

A variety of mechanisms contribute to the fall in cardiac output observed during ventricular pacing, including loss of AV synchrony, an abnormal sequence of ventricular activation, induction of atrioventricular regurgitation, and loss of the normal heart rate response to exercise [3, 12–13]. The most important of these at rest is probably loss of the normal atrial contribution to ventricular filling [12]. The importance of synchronous atrial contraction for maintenance of stroke volume varies widely from patient to patient, depending on factors such as left atrial size and contractility [1], the presence of mitral stenosis, heart rate, and ventricular compliance [14]. All of these para-

I. Cikes (ed.), *Echocardiography in Cardiac Interventions*, 431–447, 1989.
© 1989 *Kluwer Academic Publishers*.

432

meters are readily evaluated during a Doppler echocardiographic examination.

A simple, indirect assessment of atrial function can be attained by measuring left atrial size by 2-D guided M-mode echocardiography from the standard parasternal long axis window. In a study of 26 patients with multi-programmable pacemakers by Labovitz et al. [1] left atrial size was found to be an important predictor of the decrease in stroke volume following loss of AV synchrony. Changes in stroke volume in this study were determined by measuring changes in the Doppler time-velocity integral in the ascending aorta. Patients with normal left atrial size had on average a $32 \pm 11\%$ fall in stroke volume when their pacemakers were reprogrammed from AV synchronous pacing (DVI) to asynchronous ventricular pacing (VVI), compared to an $11 \pm 13\%$ fall in patients with enlarged left atria (> 2.2 cm/m^2). These investigators concluded that this difference reflected the inability of large, compliant left atria to contract vigorously enough to significantly contribute to ventricular filling. Atrial contractility can be assessed by 2-D echocardiography by examining the left atrium from the suprasternal window, but this approach has not yet been explored as a means of predicting stroke volume dependence on AV synchrony.

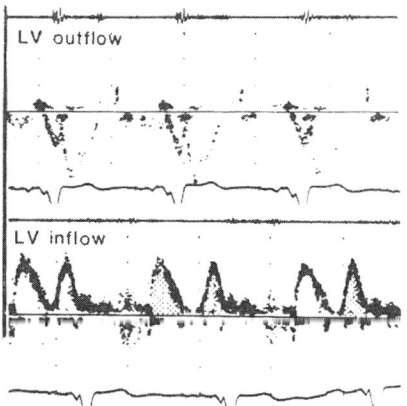

Fig. 1. Determination of the atrial contribution to ventricular filling by Doppler evaluation of left ventricular inflow. Using an apical window, the Doppler cursor is placed in the left ventricle just beneath the mitral valve to record mitral inflow. The second beat shows measurement of the time-velocity integral of total left ventricular inflow. The third beat measures that portion of inflow due to atrial contraction. The ratio of atrial to total inflow was found to correlate with the fall in stroke volume during asynchronous pacing in this study. Stroke volume in this study was determined from the time-velocity integral of total left ventricular inflow.
(Reproduced with permission from Iwase M, Sobota I, Yokota M et al: Evaluation by pulsed Doppler echocardiography of the atrial contribution to left ventricular filling in patients with DDD pacemakers. Am J Cardiol 58: 104–9, 1986.)

Doppler echocardiography allows more direct assessment of atrial function. In this approach, the pulsed Doppler sample volume is aligned parallel to mitral inflow at the center of the mitral annulus. The ratio of the Doppler time-velocity integral of the atrial component of ventricular filling ('A'-wave) to the time velocity integral of total ventricular filling reflects the relative proportion of ventricular filling resulting from properly timed atrial systole, and should be closely related to the fall in stroke volume with loss of AV synchrony (Figs. 1 and 2). Iwase et al. [2] studied 26 patients in this manner and found a significant correlation (r = .62, p. 005) between the ratio of atrial to total left ventricular inflow and the percent increase in ventricular inflow which occurred when the dual chamber pacemakers in these patients were reprogrammed from asynchronous to synchronous mode. These investigators and others have noted an increase in the ratio of atrial to total left ventricular filling with age [2, 14] and in patients with decreased left ventricular compliance, suggesting that such patients may be particularly good candidates for sequential pacing.

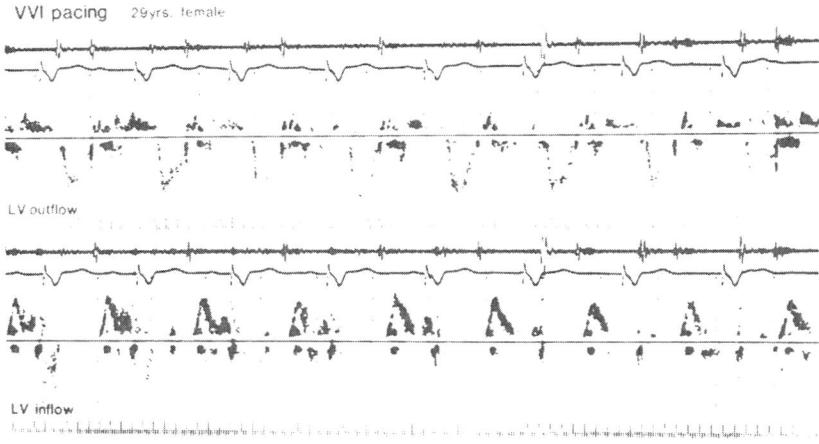

Fig. 2. Left ventricular outflow and inflow velocity during VVI pacing. An 'A' wave in the mitral Doppler tracing due to left atrial contraction is observed immediately after a P wave appearing in diastole (bottom tracing, 3rd–5th beats), but the left ventricular outflow and inflow time-velocity integrals remain almost unchanged, irrespective of the presence of a preceding P wave, because the left atrial contribution to left ventricular filling is small. Atriogenic diastolic reflux is also seen in a long PR interval (first and second beats).

(Reproduced with permission from Iwase M, Sotobata I, Yokota M et al: Evaluation by pulsed Doppler echocardiography of the atrial contribution to left ventricular filling in patients with DDD pacemakers. Am J Cardiol 58: 104–9, 1986.)

B. Doppler echocardiographic evaluation of the effect of AV synchrony on stroke volume

Doppler echocardiographic techniques allow direct measurement of the effect of altering pacing parameters on stroke volume. Stroke volume is typically determined by Doppler echocardiography by multiplying the mean flow velocity through a valve or blood vessel by the cross-sectional area of that conduit [16–20] (Figs. 3 and 4). The most widely utilized and documented method has been to determine flow and cross-sectional area in some portion of the ascending aorta or high left ventricular outflow tract. The major source

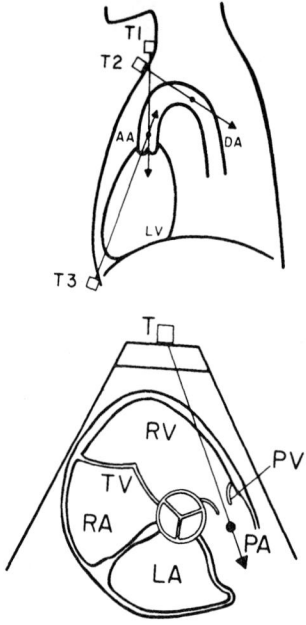

Fig. 3. Doppler techniques for measurement of cardiac output. Top: The transducer is placed in the suprasternal notch and angled inferiorly to pass the ultrasonic beam through the ascending aorta (T1) or the descending aorta (T2). The transducer may also be placed over the cardiac apex and angled superiorly to obtain Doppler shifts from the proximal ascending aorta (T3). Note that the ultrasonic beam is kept nearly parallel to the walls of the aorta in all three transducer positions to obtain maximum Doppler shifts. AA = ascending aorta; DA = descending aorta; LV = left ventricle. Bottom: An alternate technique for measuring cardiac output is to pass the ultrasonic beam parallel to the long axis of the pulmonary artery (PA), which is imaged by two-dimensional echocardiography in the standard parasternal short-axis plane. The Doppler sample volume (black dot) is placed beyond the pulmonary valve (PV) in the midlumen of the pulmonary artery (PA). LA = left atrium; RA = right atrium; TV = tricuspid valve; T = transducer; RV = right ventricle.
(Reproduced with permission from Schuster AH, Nanda NC: Doppler echocardiography – Part I: Doppler cardiac output measurements: Perspective and comparison with other methods of cardiac output determination. Echocardiography 1: 46, 1984.)

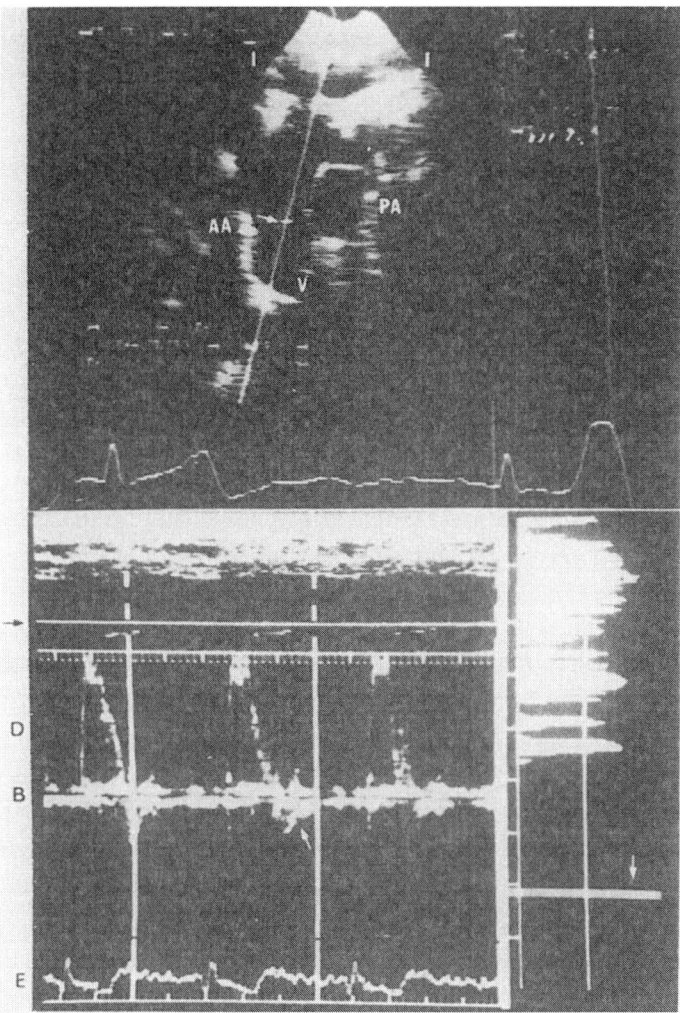

Fig. 4. Doppler estimation of left ventricular output. Top: The examination was begun by placing the Doppler cursor line parallel to the walls of the ascending aorta (AA), imaged from the suprasternal transducer position. The Doppler sample volume (arrow) was placed well above the level of the aortic valve (V) to avoid interference from valve noises. The position of the transducer was then adjusted to record the maximum Doppler frequency shift signal. This was done because, in some patients, including the patient shown here, the maximum Doppler frequency shift signal is obtained when the Doppler cursor line is nearly but not absolutely parallel to the vessel walls. The maximal systolic aortic diameter (d = 2.5 cm, r = 1.25 cm) was measured at the level of the Doppler sample volume and the aortic cross-sectional area C calculated as r^2 = 4.9 cm^2. PA = pulmonary artery; I = innominate vein. Bottom: Because the systolic aortic Doppler (D) flows s/waveform is roughly triangular in shape, the area under the velocity curve A was obtained by multiplying the maximum velocity (125 cm/sec) with the duration of flow (0.24 sec), and dividing by 2. This equals 15 cm sec/sec. Stroke volume was then obtained by multiplying the area under the velocity curve A with the cross-sectional area

of the vessel C, and was calculated as 73.5 ml. Multiplying the stroke volume with the heart rate (approximately 60 beats per minute) gave a cardiac output of 4.4. liter/min in this patient. Doppler sample volume position is denoted by a black arrow on the M-mode and a white arrow on the A-mode. The small vertical time markers at the bottom are spaced 0.04 = sec apart. B = Doppler baseline; E = electrocardiogram.

(Reproduced with permission from Main J, Nanda NC, Saini VD: Clinically useful Doppler calculations and illustrative case examples. In: Nanda NC, (Ed), Doppler Echocardiography. Igaku-Shoin. p. 511, 1985.)

of error in Doppler calculation of absolute stroke volume by this method appears to be determination of aortic diameter [16–18, 21]. Difficulties include the changing size of the aorta throughout the cardiac cycle, the necessity to be perpendicular to the walls of the aorta in order to avoid overestimating aortic diameter, the need for a high quality study in order to confidently identify inner aortic borders, and uncertainty as to the optimal site for measurement of aortic diameter [16]. Aortic flow velocity, on the other hand, can be measured accurately and reproducibly, with an intraobserver variability of $3.2 \pm 2.9\%$ and an interobserver variability of $5.4 \pm 3.4\%$ [20]. As a result of this and the fact that mean aortic diameter does not change significantly with alterations in cardiac output, it is possible to measure changes in stroke volume quite accurately by Doppler techniques by measuring the change in the Doppler time-velocity integral of aortic flow (Fig. 5). Changes in the Doppler time velocity integral have been shown to correlate well with changes in stroke volume determined by thermodilution [17, 22]. Flow velocity can be measured in the ascending aorta from the suprasternal window or the right parasternal window, or in the high left ventricular outflow tract from the apical window. We favor the latter approach (Fig. 6), which has the advantages of being available in almost all patients, and of being well away from the operative site in patients undergoing studies at the time of pacemaker implantation.

Our laboratory has been interested in using Doppler techniques to study the change in resting stroke volume which occurs when switching from AV synchronous to asynchronous pacing. In one study of seven patients with programmable dual chamber pacemakers, investigators from our laboratory found a mean 18% fall in aortic time-velocity integral when these pacemakers were reprogrammed from DVI mode to VVI mode [4]. Other investigators have reported similar results, with the increase in Doppler aortic velocity when switching from asynchronous ventricular pacing to sequential AV pacing at a fixed heart rate ranging from 16–35% (Table 1). It is clear from the results of these various studies that synchronous atrial contraction contributes importantly to resting cardiac output, and that this can be measured using Doppler techniques.

Table 1. Improvement in stroke volume as determined by aortic flow velocity upon switching from VVI to atrial synchronous pacing.

Author	N	# Pts who increased stroke volume	% Increase in stroke volume	Predictors of increased stroke volume
Nanda [4]	6	5/6	18%	
Zugibe [3]	10	10/10	20%	
Stewart [5]	29		16%	Pacemaker syndrome, intact Va conduction
Labowitz [1]	26	21/26	27%	Left atrial size
Faerestrand [7]	13	11/13	21%	
Forfang [6]	8		35%	LV disease (see text)

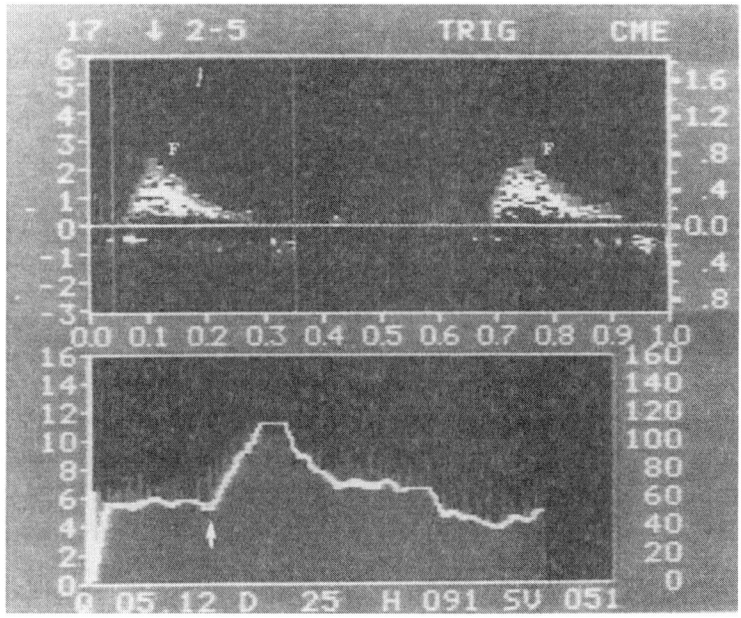

Fig. 5. Doppler estimation of cardiac output. Top panel: Free-standing, commercially available continuous-wave Doppler equipment (Carolina Medical Electronics) was utilized in a volunteer to obtain ascending aortic flow (F) from the suprasternal approach. The peak aortic flow velocity is about 0.8 meter/sec (numbers on the right). The numbers on the left represent Doppler frequency shifts in kHz. Bottom panel: On-line measurements of cardiac output were obtained nearly continuously. The initial cardiac output, which was in the range of 5.5 to 6 liter/min, rose to 12 liter/min following inhalation of amyl nitrite (arrow) and then fell to 5.12 liter/min when the effects of the drug wore off. An aortic diameter (D) valve of 25 mm, obtained from two-dimensional echocardiographic examination, was used in the calculation of Doppler cardiac outputs. The numbers on the left denote cardiac output in liters per minute, and those on the right stroke volume in milliliters. Values at end of examination: Q = cardiac output, 5.12 liter/min; H = heart rate, 91 beats per min; SV = stroke volume, 51 ml.
(Reproduced with permission from Schuster AH, Nanda NC, et al.: Doppler evaluation of cardiac output. In: Nanda NC, (Ed), Doppler Echocardiography. Igaku-Shoin, p. 165, 1985.)

438

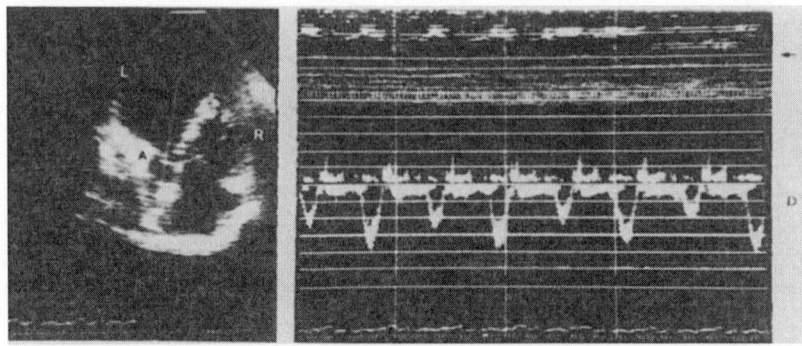

Fig. 6. Left panel: Two-dimensional echocardiogram, recorded from the left ventricular apex, in a patient with pulsus alternans due to cardiomyopathy. The bright dot on the cursor line marks the position of the Doppler sample volume in the left ventricular outflow tract near the aortic valve. A = aortic valve; L = left ventricle; R = right ventricle. Right panel: Pulsed Doppler (D) recording demonstrating alternation of blood flow velocity in the left ventricular outflow tract. The Doppler tracing is inverted, indication that the direction of systolic flow is away from the ultrasonic transducer and toward the aorta.
(Reproduced with permission from Schuster AH, Nanda NC: Doppler echocardiographic features of mechanical alternans. Am Heart J 107: 580–583, 1984.)

It has been suggested in the past that patients with poor left ventricular function may be particularly sensitive to loss of AV synchrony. However, in both the study of Labovitz et al. [1] and in another Doppler study of 29 patients by Stewart et al. [5] left ventricular function was found not to be a predictor of the importance of preserved AV synchrony. Forfang et al. [6] in a relatively small study, reported that 4 patients with left ventricular 'disease' suffered a 47% decrease in stroke volume as measured by Doppler time-velocity integral, compared to only a 23% fall in 4 patients with isolated conduction defects and normal left ventricles. Three of four patients with left ventricular 'disease' in this study had previously undergone aortic valve replacement for aortic stenosis and were thus clearly a group of patients who would be expected to have relatively non-compliant ventricles and therefore a marked dependence on preserved atrial synchrony [14].

A similar approach can be used to evaluate candidates for dual chamber pacemakers. Most patients, of course, will not have temporary programmable dual chamber pacemakers in place prior to permanent pacemaker implantation. However, many candidates for dual chamber pacing will already have a temporary or permanent ventricular pacemaker, and most of these patients will have AV dissociation during ventricular pacing due to retrograde AV block. When the atria and ventricles are disassociated as a result of VVI pacing, the stroke volume can be observed to vary on a beat-to-beat basis depending on the relationship of atrial and ventricular contraction

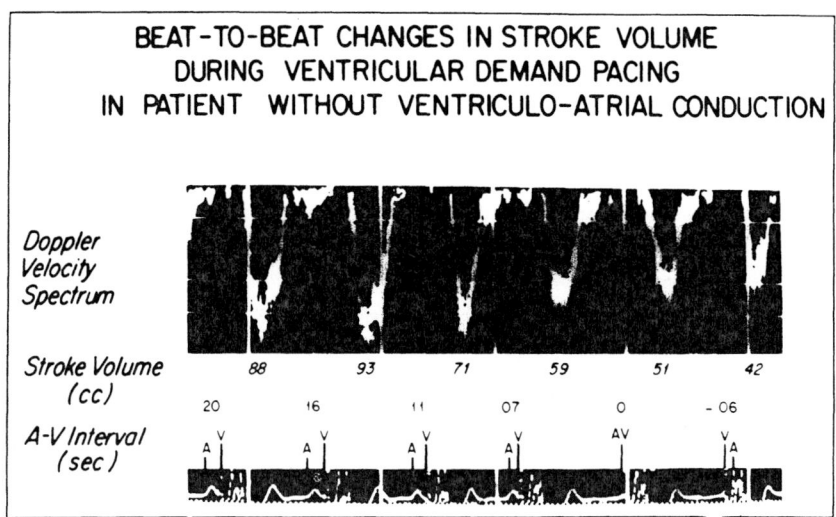

Fig. 7. Beat to beat changes in stroke volume during VVI pacing in a patient with atrioventricular dissociation. When atrial systole fortuitously precedes ventricular systole by a physiologic interval (first three QRS complexes), the stroke volume is much higher than when atrial systole coincides with ventricular systole.
(Reproduced with permission from Stewart WJ, et al.: Doppler ultrasound measurement of cardiac output in patients with physiologic pacemakers. Effects of left ventricular function and retrograde ventriculoatrial conduction. Am J Cardiol 54: 308, 1984.)

during any given cardiac cycle (Fig. 7). Comparison of the Doppler time-velocity integral when atrial precedes ventricular contraction by a relatively physiologic interval compared to the time-velocity integral when atrial and ventricular systole are poorly related yields a direct estimate of the importance of synchronous AV contraction for maintenance of stroke volume. A preliminary study by Halperin et al. [8] measured the variation in beat-to-beat Doppler mean aortic velocity during AV disassociated ventricular pacing to derive a variance index. They found that a high variance index in this setting is predictive of the magnitude of the benefit derived from AV sequential compared to ventricular pacing. Similar results have been reported by other investigators using changes in pulse pressure measured with a blood pressure cuff to approximate alterations in stroke volume [23]. In patients in sinus rhythm, the ventricular pacing rate can be increased slightly above the sinus rate, and the fall in the Doppler time-velocity integral recorded to yield an estimate of the importance of AV synchrony. With the latter approach, other factors which may contribute to a fall in stroke volume with ventricular pacing, such as disordered ventricular contraction or induction of valvular regurgitation, must also be considered. Patients who do not have AV disassociation during ventricular pacing due to intact retrograde conduction are almost always candidates for dual-chamber pacemakers without further evaluation, due to the high prevalence of the 'pacemaker syndrome' in these patients if they receive ventricular pacemakers [12].

The physiologic benefit from DDD pacemakers relative to VVI pacemakers derives not only from preservation of atrial synchrony but also from the ability of these pacemakers to increase heart rate in response to increased atrial activity [24]. Thus, in patients with relatively well preseved sinus function and AV block, DDD pacemakers may provide a significant advantage even if there is relatively little difference in stroke volume between VVI and DVI pacing modes, as a result of the ability to increase heart rate normally with exercise. This has limited the clinical relevance of evaluation of atrial function in choosing pacing modes in the past. There are significant disadvantages associated with dual chamber pacemakers, however, including longer implantation time, higher cost, shorter pacemaker lifetime, pacemaker 'endless loop' tachycardia, and the inability to use these pacemakers in patients in atrial fibrillation or flutter. For these reasons there has been considerable interest in developing a physiologic pacemaker which will increase its firing rate in response to some physiologic indicator of exercise or increased demand other than artrial rate. Various ventricular pacemakers now undergoing clinical testing are capable of increasing heart rate in response to respiratory rate [25], QT interval [26], or body motion [27], thereby allowing an increase in heart rate in response to exercise without resorting to dual chamber pacing. If these rate-responsive single chamber pacemakers are successful and become more widely available, the contribution of atrial synchrony to rest and exercise stroke volume will become a much more important criterion for choosing between dual chamber and single chamber rate sensitive pacemakers. Doppler echocardiographic determination of left atrial size, left atrial function (size of the 'A' wave), and the change in aortic flow velocity during atrial synchronous vs asynchronous rhythms allows noninvasive assessment of the contribution of AV synchrony to stroke volume and should gain more widespread clinical use and acceptance as these newer pacemakers become available.

III. Optimization of AV pacing intervals by Doppler echocardiography

Dual chamber pacemakers allow individualization of a number of pacing parameters, one of which is the AV interval. Many studies have demonstrated that the AV interval can influence cardiac output [2, 3, 6, 7, 9–11, 28]. The optimal AV interval is influenced by such factors as the presence of mitral valve disease, left ventricular compliance [6], atrial contractility, heart rate [9], whether the rhythm is paced or endogenous, and the pacing mode [28].

Doppler echocardiography provides a means of optimizing the AV interval in a given patient under varying physiologic conditions.

Several Doppler studies have documented that altering AV intervals causes a measurable difference in resting stroke volume determined from the aortic or mitral time-velocity integral. Zugibe et al [11] studied 7 patients in DVI mode at rest at a fixed heart rate of 70–72 beates per minute, and found that aortic flow volocity was maximal in most patients at an AV interval between 150–200 msec. The optimal AV interval varied from patients to patients, however, and in some patients, changes within the relatively physiologic range of 100–200 msec caused significant changes in stroke volume (Fig. 8). Faerestrand et al [7] measured peak aortic velocity from the apical view in 13 patients in DDD mode, and found that the optimal AV interval varied from 100–250 msec in different patients. Iwase et al [2] have reported

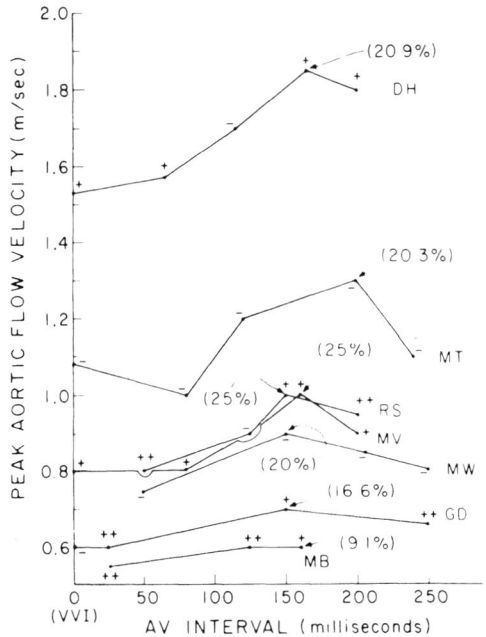

Fig. 8. Peak aortic flow velocity at different AV intervals (7 patients). + = mitral regurgitation present; ++ = increased mitral regurgitation; - = mitral regurgitation not evaluated by Doppler. The number in parenthesis indicates the maximum increase in peak aortic flow velocity obtained in a given patient relative to the VVI value, or the shortest AV interval (in patients in whom VVI values were not available). The optimal AV interval occurred between 150 to 200 msec. Note that the optimal AV interval varied from patient to patient, and that in some patients small changes in AV delay within the physiologic range caused significant changes in stroke volume.

(Reproduced with permission from Zugibe FT Jr, Nanda NC, Barold SS, Akiyama T. Usefulness of Doppler echocardiography in cardiac pacing: Assessment of mitral regurgitation, peak aortic flow velocity, and atrial capture. PACE 6: 1350, 1983.)

similar results, using the transmitral time-velocity integral as an estimate of stroke volume in 20 patients with DDD pacemakers reprogrammed to DVI mode at a pacing rate of 70. Considering all AV intervals between 50 and 250 msec in 50 msec increments, they found a mean 46% difference in transmitral time-velocity integral between the best and the worst AV interval, and a mean difference of 18% between the best and worst AV interval within the relatively physiologic range of 100–200 msec. On the other hand, only 5 of 20 patients had an improvement of more than 5% at any AV interval compared to a 'standard' AV interval of 150 msec. Thus, the three published Doppler studies concerning the effect of AV interval on stroke volume in DVI mode have all concluded that while in most patients the optimal AV interval is in the 150–200 msec range, there is significant variability in the individual patient. Improvements in resting stroke volume on the order of 5–15% appear to be possible in some patients in DVI mode by individualizing their AV interval rather than using an arbitrary 'normal' value, but the number of patients who would be benefited by such an approach remains uncertain.

An important consideration when using Doppler or other methods to optimize the AV interval is the fact that the optimal AV interval differs significantly from DVI to VDD mode [28]. Forfang et al [6] investigated the optimal AV interval in 8 patients with VDD pacemakers using aortic flow velocities from the suprasternal window. The optimal AV interval varied widely in this study; in several instances, very short AV intervals (< 100 msec) maximized stroke volume. Patients with aortic valve disease were particularly sensitive to changes in AV intervals, likely due to decreased ventricular compliance causing increased dependence on optimal AV synchrony. In one such patient, the optimal AV interval of 75 msec resulted in a relative stroke volume 25% higher than the stroke volume at a 'physiologic' AV interval of 150 msec. Wish et al [28] have reported data that suggest that the lower optimal AV interval demonstrated in studies of VDD pacing modes [6, 29] are a result of more prolonged left atrial to ventricular activation times for a given programmed AV interval when atrial sensing (VDD mode) as opposed to atrial pacing (DVI mode) occurs. Patients with DDD pacemakers optimized in DVI mode suffered a mean 21% fall in thermodilution cardiac output when in VDD mode at the same rate, due to a mean 75 msec prolongation of left atrial to ventricular activation time. It is thus important when adjusting the AV interval of DDD pacemakers to consider which pacing mode is likely to be controlling the patient's rhythm the majority of the time, and to optimize the AV interval to that mode. Using Doppler techniques to determine aortic flow velocity at several AV intervals may also allow an AV delay to be found which results in a reasonably good stroke volume in both pacing modes. Some newer pacemakers allow programming of different AV delays depending on whether the atrial event is sensing of endogenous atrial activity or pacing, in which case Doppler flow velocities can be used to optimize each AV interval independently.

Doppler echocardiography has also been used to study the relationship of the optimal AV interval to the heart rate. Halpering et al [6] found that the optimal AV interval in DVI mode was shorter at a paced rate of 90 than at a paced rate of 70 in four of five patients studied. This same study found that the improvement in aortic flow velocity at the optimal AV interval relative to a non-physiologic AV interval was much greater at a heart rate of 70 than at a rate of 90. These findings suggest that AV synchrony is most important for maintenance of cardiac output at slower heart rates, while at more rapid rates, for example during exercise, an appropriate increase in heart rate may be more important for maintenance of cardiac output then preservation of AV synchrony. Further studies are necessary to determine whether the AV interval which optimizes resting stroke volume is different from that which maximizes exercise capacity, and if so, which parameter ought to be maximized.

In conclusion, Doppler aortic flow velocity appears to be a relatively simple and accurate means of studying the relation of AV interval to stroke volume. This approach has been invaluable in improving our understanding of pacemaker physiology, but the clinical utility of routinely using Doppler to adjust AV intervals remains uncertain, since the percentage of patients who can be significantly benefited by using individually optimized AV intervals rather than 'standard' intervals is unknown. A study investigating the number of patients benefited and the magnitude of the improvement which occurs in resting stroke volume and exercise capacity when patients previously paced at 'standard' AV intervals are reprogrammed to 'optimal' AV intervals using Doppler flow velocities needs to be performed to validate the clinical utility of this technique. Patients who are very dependent on preservation of atrial synchrony, for example patients with decreased ventricular compliance, will likely be most sensitive to changes in AV interval, and may be good candidates for Doppler studies to optimize the AV interval. When using Doppler flow velocities to adjust the AV interval, the physician needs to keep in mind that subsequent alteration in heart rate or pacing mode may alter the optimal AV interval in a given patient, and that the AV interval which maximizes resting stroke volume may not be the optimal AV interval to maximize exercise capacity.

444

IV. Evaluation of pacemaker induced valvular regurgitation by Doppler echocardiography

Ventricular pacing may cause deterioration in stroke volume by mechanisms other than loss of AV synchrony, including induction of valvular regurgitation, and alteration of the normal ventricular activation sequence [3, 12–13]. In an experimental model, contrast echocardiographic techniques with agitated saline has been used to investigate the influence of the pacing site on the amount of regurgitation induced [13]. In this study, significant differences

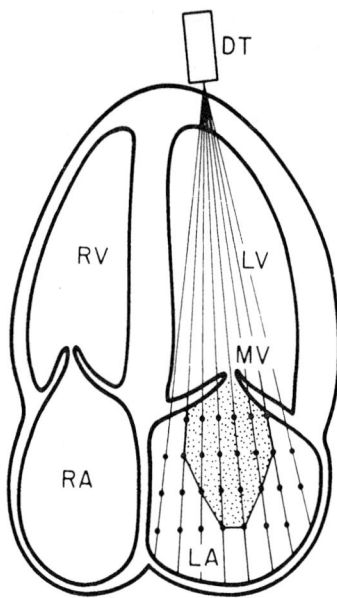

Fig. 9. Principles of 2-dimensional color Doppler flow mapping. Conventional pulse Doppler evaluates the frequency shift of an emitted ultrasound pulse, and thereby blood flow velocity, from one point in a two dimensional plane. Color Doppler machines measure Doppler shifts at multiple points in a 2-dimensional plane. The frequency shifts are analyzed for direction, magnitude and variance, and the resulting flow information is color coded and superimposed on a standard two-dimensional echocardiographic display. Flow towards the transducer is traditionally represented by shades of red, and flow away from the transducer by shades of blue, with brighter shades of red or blue corresponding to higher blood flow velocities. The variance of the Doppler shift between adjacent pixels, which reflects disturbance of flow, is coded by shades of green. Mitral regurgitation is readily identified by the abnormally directed, frequently turbulent flow extending from the mitral valve into the left atrium during ventricular systole. The percentage of the left atrium occupied by the regurgitant flow has been shown by us to correlate with the severity of regurgitation [33].
(Reproduced with permission from Adhar GC, Abbasi AS, Nanda NC: Doppler echocardiography in the assessment of mitral regurgitation and mitral valve prolapse. In: Nanda NC, (Ed), Doppler Echocardiography. Igaku-Shoin. p. 201, 1985.)

in the severity of mitral regurgitation were noted at different ventricular pacing sites, with regurgitation occurring with right ventricular apical pacing, and only mild regurgitation with left ventricular basal pacing. Induction of significant mitral regurgitation with ventricular pacing has also been reported in man [3, 30], although its incidence remains unknown. It is now possible to directly visualize and semiquantitate regurgitant lesions without resorting to contrast injection by using color Doppler flow mapping (Fig. 9) [31–33]. We have observed a patient who had marked worsening of mitral regurgitation by color Doppler when his dual chamber pacemaker was reprogrammed from an AV interval of 150 msec to 100 msec [11]. Thus, color Doppler can be used to document and semiquantitate pacemaker induced regurgitation, and in the cause of AV sequential pacemakers, it may be possible to re-program the AV interval to minimize the amount of regurgitation.

V. Evaluation of atrial capture by Doppler echocardiography

Echocardiographic analysis of mitral valve motion and Doppler analysis of mitral inflow patterns can be used to document atrial capture [3, 34–35]. This may be useful in patients with AV sequential pacemakers, in whom it is often difficult from the surface electrocardiogram to separate atrial activity from the electrical artifact of the atrial pacemaker. The presence of a normal 'A' wave in the M-mode mitral valve trace or the Doppler mitral inflow trace confirms normal synchronous atrial activity. In the case of AV dissociation, the 'A' wave of the Doppler inflow trace may be seen to wander throughout the cardial cycle (Fig. 2). Unfortunately, VA conduction, which is very important clinically because of its proclivity to result in the pacemaker syndrome in the case of ventricular pacemakers, or endless loop tachycardias in the case of dual chamber pacemakers, is less easy to diagnose from analysis of mitral valve motion or inflow. Although no 'A' wave is seen either in the M-mode mitral trace or the Doppler mitral trace during VA conduction due to concurrence of atrial and ventricular systole, other conditions, such as atrial fibrillation or a very rapid heart rate, may cause absence of the 'A' wave. Color Doppler evaluation of right sided flows may be of use in the diagnosis of VA conduction. We have observed retrograde systolic flow in the superior vena cava as a result of VA conduction, analogous to the cannon 'A' waves seen on physical examination. Thus, combined Doppler and echocardiographic examination may be a useful noninvasive means of evaluating the presence of atrial systole and its relation to ventricular systole in those patients in whom this is not clear from the surface electrocardiogram.

References

1. Labovitz AJ, Williams GA, Redd RM, Kennedy HL: Noninvasive assessment of pacemaker hemodynamics by Doppler echocardiography: importance of left atrial size. J Am Coll Cardiol, 6: 196–200, 1985.
2. Iwase M, Sotobata I, Yokota M, et al: Evaluation by pulsed Doppler echocardiography of the atrial contribution to left ventricular filling in patients with DDD pacemakers. Am J Cardiol, 58: 104–9, 1986.
3. Zugibe F, Nanda NC, Barold SS, Akiyama T: Usefulness of Doppler echocardiography in cardiac pacing: assessment of mitral regurgitation, peak aortic flow velocity and atrial capture. PACE, 6: 1350–7, 1983.
4. Nanda NC, Bhandari A, Barold SS, Falkoff M: Doppler echocardiographic studies in sequential atrioventricular pacing. PACE, 6: 811–4, 1983.
5. Stewart WJ, Dicola VC, Harthorne JW, et al: Doppler ultrasound measurement of cardiac output in patients with physiologic pacemakers. Am J Cardiol, 54: 308–12, 1984.
6. Forfang K, Otterstad JE, Ihlen H: Optimal atrioventricular delay in physiologic pacing determined by Doppler echocardiography. PACE, 9: 17–20, 1985.
7. Faerestrand S, Ohm OJ: A time-related study of the hemodynamic benefit of atrioventricular synchronous pacing evaluated by Doppler echocardiography. PACE, 8: 838–48, 1985.
8. Halperin JL, Teichholz LE, Steinmetz MY, et al: Selection of patients for dual-chamber pacing by noninvasive means: the VVI-variance index. Circulation, 70: II-409, 1984. (Abstract).
9. Halperin JL, Rothlauf EB, Stern EH, et al: Pulsed-Doppler echocardiographic assessment of hemodynamic function during dual-chamber cardiac pacing. Circulation, 68: III-379, 1983. (Abstract).
10. Kafka W, Holdebrandt U, Delius W: Hemodynamic advantage of AV-sequential pacing with respect to the AV-delay. PACE, 8: A–38, 1985. (Abstract).
11. Switzer DF, Nanda NC: Doppler-echocardiographic assessment of cardiac pacemakers. Cardiol Clin, 3: 631–53, 1985.
11. Tscheliessnigg KH, Stenzl W, Dacar D: Hemodynamic importance of a constant AV delay. PACE, 8: A–38, 1985. (Abstract).
12. Ausubel K, Furman S: The pacemaker syndrome. Annals Int Med, 103: 420–9, 1985.
13. Maurer G, Torres MAR, Corday E, et al: Two-dimensional echocardiographic contrast assessment of pacing-induced mitral regurgitation: relation to altered regional left ventricular function. J Am Coll Cardiol, 3: 986–91, 1984.
14. Judy WV, Hall JH: Non-invasive analysis of pacemaker induced cardiodynamics. Circulation, 70: II-408, 1984. (Abstract).
15. Miyatake K, Okamoto M, Kinoshita N, et al: Augmentation of atrial contribution to left ventricular inflow with aging as assessed by intracardiac Doppler flowmeter. Am J Cardiol, 53: 586–89, 1984.
16. Gardin JM, Tobis JM, Dabestani A, et al: Superiority of two-dimensional measurement of aortic vessel diameter in Doppler echocardiographic estimates of left ventricular stroke volume. J Am Coll Cardiol, 6: 66–74, 1985.
17. Huntsman LL, Stewart DK, Barnes SR, et al: Noninvasive Doppler determination of cardiac output in man. Circulation, 67: 593–601, 1983.
18. Schuster AH, Nanda NC: Doppler echocardiography: Part I: Doppler cardiac output measurements: Perspective and comparison with other methods of cardiac output determination. Echocardiography: A Review of Cardiovascular Ultrasound, 1: 45–54, 1984.

19. Lewis JF, Kuo LL, Nelson JG, et al: Pulsed Doppler echocardiographic determination of stroke volume and cardiac output: Clinical validation of two new methods using the apical window. Circulation, 70: 425–431, 1984.

20. Gardin JM, Dabestini A, Natin K, et al: Reproducibility of Doppler aortic blood flow velocity measurements: studies on intra-observer, inter-observer and day-to-day variability in normal subjects. Am J Cardiol, 54: 1092–8, 1984.

21. Schuster AH, Nanda NC: Doppler echocardiographic measurement of cardiac output: comparison with a non-golden standard. (ed) Am J Cardiol, 53: 257–9, 1984.

22. Elkayam U, Gardin JM, Berkley R, et al: The use of Doppler flow velocity measurement to assess the hemodynamic response to vasodilators in patients with heart failure. Circulation, 67: 377, 1983.

23. Reiter MJ, Hindman MC: Hemodynamic effects of acute atrioventricular sequential pacing in patients with left ventricular dysfunction. Am J Cardiol, 49: 687–92, 1982.

24. Eisenhauer AC, McElroy PA, Weber KT: Chronotropic dysfunction and exercise. Physiologic Principles and Clinical Applications. Weber KT & Janicki JS (eds). Philadelphia: WB Saunders, 1986.

25. Ionescu VL: An 'on demand pacemaker' responsive to respiratory rate. PACE 3: 375, 1980 (Abstract).

26. Rickards AF, Norman J: Relation between QT interval and heart rate. New design of physiologically adaptive cardiac pacemaker. Br Heart J 45: 56–61, 1981.

27. Anderson K, Humen D, Klein GJ, Brumwell D, Huntley S: A rate variable pacemaker which automatically adjusts for physical activity. PACE 6: A12, 1983 (Abstract).

28. Wish M, Fletcher RD, Gottdiener JS, et al: Optimal left atrioventricular sequence in dual chamber pacing-limitations of programmed A-V interval. J Am Coll Cardiol, 3: 507A, 1984 (Abstract).

29. Von Bibra H, Busch U, Wirtzfeld A: The beneficial effect of short AV-intervals in VDD patients. J Am Coll Cardiol 5: 394, 1985.

30. Haas J, Strait G: Pacemaker-induced cardiovascular failure: hemodynamic and angiographic observations. Am J Cardiol 33: 295–299, 1974.

31. Miyatake K, Izumi S, Okamoto M, et al: Semiquantitative grading of severity of mitral regurgitation by real-time two-dimensional Doppler flow imaging technique. J Am Coll Cardiol, 7: 82–8, 1986.

32. Perry GJ and Nanda NC: Diagnosis and quantitation of valvular regurgitation by color Doppler flow mapping. Echocardiography: A Review of Cardiovascular Ultrasound 3: 493–503, 1986.

33. Helmcke F, Nanda NC, Hsiung MC, Soto B, Adey C, Goyal RG, Gatewood R: Color Doppler assessment of mitral regurgitation using orthogonal planes. Circulation 75: 175–183, 1987.

34. Ambrose JA, Meller J, Herman MV, et al: The ventricular A wave and a new echocardiographic index of late diastolic filling of the left ventricle. Am Heart J, 96: 615, 1978.

35. Naito M, Dreifus LS, Mardelli TJ, et al: Echocardiographic features of atrioventricular and ventricule-atrial conduction. Am J Cardiol, 46: 625, 1980.

6.7. Duplex scanning in arterial and venous disease

DAVID C. TAYLOR, GREGORY L. MONETA &
D. EUGENE STRANDNESS

Introduction

A duplex ultrasonic system involves combining B-mode imaging and a pulsed Doppler in a single instrument. Since development of the first clinically useful system in the mid 1970's [1], duplex scanning has rapidly become the most useful and widely applied method for the evalution of arterial and venous disease. It is now the most frequently used noninvasive diagnostic modality in the assessment of extracranial cerebral vascular disease [2].

The major advantage of the duplex system is that it may be used for both screening and serial assessment of the anatomic and hemodynamic abnormalities associated with the development of arterial and venous disease. For example, some soft atherosclerotic plaques and thrombi may have acoustic properties similar to flowing blood, and therefore will be missed by imaging alone. However, these lesions can still be detected by documentation of the increase in flow velocity that occurs through the narrowed segment. While the B-mode image is used to identify echogenic plaques, it also permits accurate placement of the pulsed Doppler sample volume at any point in the vessel within the scan plane. The B-mode image also insures that the vessel is insonated at a known Doppler angle. Unless the system permits automatic correction for the Doppler angle in presenting frequency or velocity data, it is important to make all velocity determinations at a constant Doppler angle. We have found an angle of 60 degrees easy to utilize from site to site and study to study. The only area where the image becomes the primary method of diagnosis is in the assessment of acute deep venous thrombosis. But even here the Doppler is useful in making the diagnosis of a nonocclusive thrombus. In this chapter we will present an overview of current and future applications of duplex scanning in the evaluation of selected surgically important arterial and venous abnormalities.

Carotid disease

Stroke not only causes significant neurological impairment in many patients but it remains the third leading cause of death in North America [3]. Athero-

I. Cikes (ed.), *Echocardiography in Cardiac Interventions*, 449–462, 1989.
© 1989 *Kluwer Academic Publishers*.

450

sclerosis of the cerebral arteries accounts for approximately two thirds of all strokes and it seems to have a particular predilection for the extracranial cerebral arteries, especially the carotid bifurcation [4]. As these vessels are superficial they can easily be examined using duplex ultrasound.

Because it is safe, accurate, and easily repeated, duplex ultrasound has become the preferred noninvasive method for studying the extracranial cerebral circulation. Its accuracy in the diagnosis of carotid artery stenosis and occlusion rivals that of angiography. Using analysis of spectral velocity waveforms obtained from selected locations in the carotid artery, we have shown an 82% overall agreement of duplex ultrasound with contrast angiography [5,6]. This is as good as the inter and intraobsever variability in the interpretation of carotid angiograms [7].

For lesions which narrow the diameter of the artery by less than 50%, the diagnostic information of importance is found in those spectral features that reflect blood flow turbulence. This is seen as spectral broadening (Fig. 1). Classification of disease that produces a greater than 50% diameter reduction depends mainly on the quantification of the peak systolic and end diastolic velocity changes characteristic of high grade lesions (Table 1 and Fig. 1).

Examination of the vertebral arteries, while more difficult and less accurate than assessment of the carotid arteries, can detect flow reversal in cases of subclavian steal syndrome and is able to localize areas of stenosis, especially near its origin from the subclavian artery [8].

In patients who present with transient ischemic attacks or strokes, a

Table 1. Duplex classifaction of internal carotid stenosis.*

(A) Normal: An internal carotid spectrum with a peak frequency below 4 KHz and minimal spectral broadening. (A frequency of 4 KHz corresponds to a peak velocity of 120 cm/sec.) Boundary layer separation within the carotid bulb is almost invariably present.

(B) 1–15% Diameter Reduction: An internal carotid peak spectral frequency below 4 KHz and slight spectral broadening during the deceleration phase of systole. No boundary layer separation is present.

(C) 16–49% Diameter Reduction: The peak spectral frequency is below 4 KHz. Spectral broadening fills the whole systolic window.

(D) 50–75% Diameter Reduction: An internal carotid peak spectral frequency in excess of 4 KHz and marked spectral broadening.

(D+) 80–99% Diameter Reduction: An internal carotid with a peak frequency exceeding 4 KHz, marked spectral broadening and an end diastolic frequency greater than 4.5 KHz (135 cm/sec).

(E) Occlusion: No flow signal in an adequately visualized internal carotid with characteristic low or reversed flow in the common carotid.

* a 5 MHz probe with a Doppler angle of 60 degrees.

duplex study can be important for several aspects of the patient's diagnosis and therapy. When the noninvasive study documents a high grade carotid bifurcation stenosis, appropriate for both the symptoms and the cerebral distribution of the event, it provides strong evidence to suggest the etiology of the problem. Such patients then proceed to carotid angiography and are generally treated by carotid endarterectomy. While it has been suggested that a duplex study can be used as the sole investigation prior to carotid endarterectomy [9], we do not as yet recommend this approach. Pending further studies demonstrating the safety of this approach, we proceed with endarterectomy based on duplex alone only when there is a contraindication to angiography or where angiography is not possible.

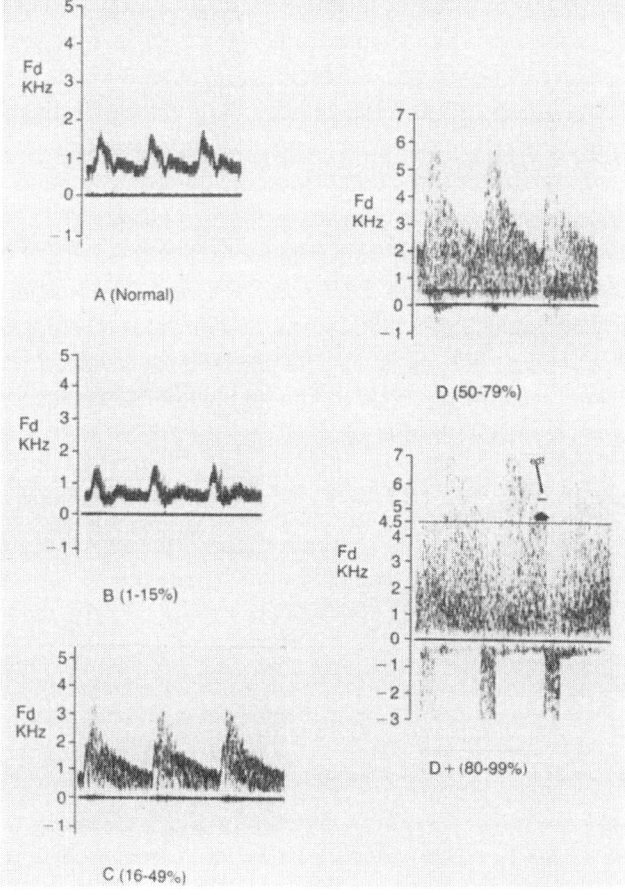

Fig. 1. Typical spectral waveforms seen with increasing degrees of carotid stenosis. With stenosis of less than 50% the major changes in the waveform are manifest as spectral broadening while with stenosis of greater than 50% increases in systolic and diastolic velocities occur (see Table 1).

Duplex scanning is also commonly used in the assessment of asymptomatic patients with cervical bruits. While the management of this group of patients is controversial, there is evidence to suggest that patients with high grade carotid bifurcation lesions may benefit from carotid endarterectomy [10]. We have recently shown that patients with a carotid artery stenosis of greater than 80% diameter reduction are at a particularly high risk to develop ipsilateral TIA's, stroke or carotid occlusions [11]. We currently screen all patients with asymptomatic bruits using duplex ultrasound. If they are found to have high grade stenosis, and are otherwise good surgical candidates, we recommend that they undergo carotid endarterectomy.

Duplex scanning can be used to follow the course of the endarterectomized carotid artery. The incidence of early carotid restenosis following endarterectomy has recently been shown to be in the range of 10–19% [12]. These early lesions are smooth and rarely the cause of symptoms. It is now possible to serially follow these patients and document the natural history of this myointimal lesion and its relationship to long-term outcome. In addition, interventional strategies, such as various drug therapies designed to reduce the incidence of restenosis, could potentially be evaluated by duplex scanning. Unoperated carotid arteries and those contralateral to the operated vessel can also be followed using this method [13].

High resolution imaging has been used to assess the morphology of the atherosclerotic plaque and its relationship to clinical events. It has been suggested that complex, heterogenous plaques with an irregular surface may have a poorer clinical prognosis than the homogenous, fibrous lesions with a smooth intimal surface [14] (Fig. 2).

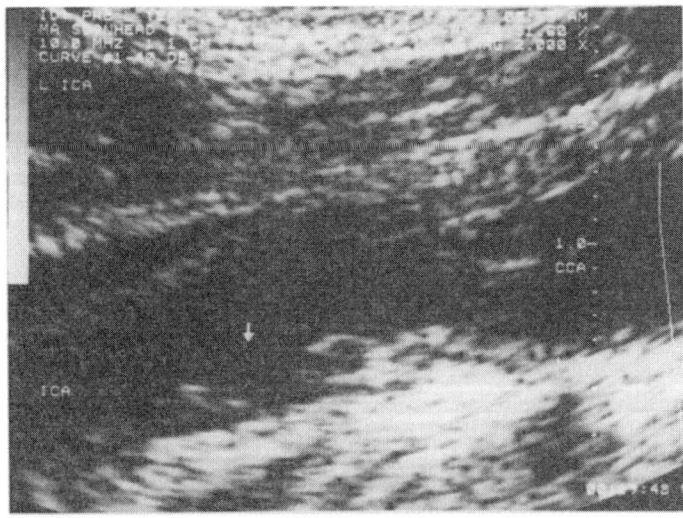

Fig. 2. This B-mode image shows what appears to be a complex ulcerated carotid plaque.

Renal and visceral arteries

One of the more recent applications of duplex ultrasound is in the assessment of intraabdominal vessels. These vessels can be difficult to image due to their distance from the skin surface. However, with careful technique and attention to detail, including the use of lower frequency scanheads (usually 3 MHz), useful information can be obtained.

Renovascular disease is the most common cause of curable hypertension, especially in patients with more severe hypertension [15]. Screening methods to identify these patients have included intravenous pyelography, nuclear renal scans and split renal function tests. These have been disappointing [16] and the only definitive test continues to be angiography.

Duplex ultrasound can be used to scan the renal arteries from their orgin to the renal parenchyma (Fig. 3). Because of their depth, image resolution is often poor. The diagnosis of renal artery narrowing is therefore nearly completely dependent on the detection of a velocity increase in the renal artery. By comparing peak renal artery velocities with those recorded from the aorta it is possible to identify renal artery stenosis that exceeds 60% of the lumen diameter with a sensitivity of 91% and a specificity of 95% [17].

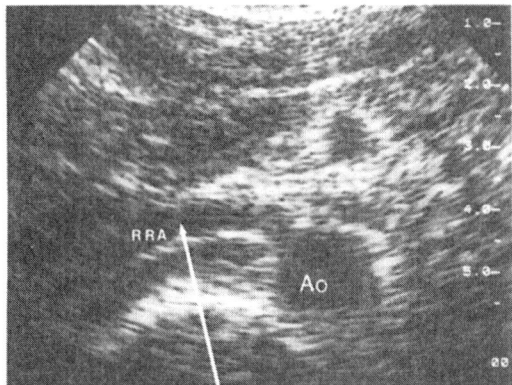

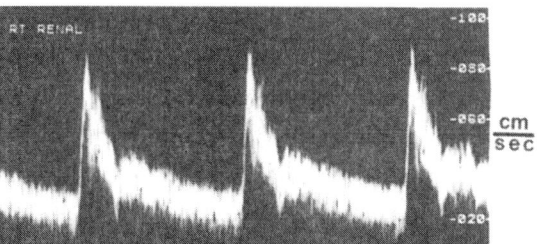

Fig. 3. B-mode image obtained in transverse section showing the right renal artery with the corresponding normal spectral waveform. RRA (right renal artery), AO (aorta).

The use of duplex ultrasound in this fashion to screen selected patients with hypertension for renovascular disease could improve the identification of this patient group for definitive therapy while decreasing the need for angiography. Renal artery duplex scanning is also useful in the followup of patients with either arterial reconstructions or transluminal angioplasty of the renal artery. In these instances duplex ultrasound is employed to detect restenosis and monitor graft patency.

Duplex scanning can also be employed in the assessment of the transplanted kidney. Renal artery stenosis may be a factor in the development of either hypertension or renal failure in the transplant patient [18]. Duplex ultrasound can be used to detect renal artery stenosis in these patients [19]. There is also some preliminary evidence that rejection of the transplant kidney is associated with an increase in renal parenchymal resistance which is reflected in a fall of the end diastolic velocity of the renal artery waveform [20]. This may not only aid in the diagnosis of rejection, but also be useful in monitoring the effects of drugs that are used to halt or reverse the rejection process.

Duplex ultrasound can be used to study blood flow in the celiac and superior mesenteric arteries and has been applied to the study of patients with suspected intestinal angina. In normal subjects there is a maximum increase in superior mesenteric blood flow 30–45 minutes following feeding but virtually no change in celiac artery flow. The shape of the superior mesenteric artery spectral waveform also changes from a high to a low resistance configuration following feeding [21] (Fig. 4). Patients with superior mesenteric artery stenosis have localized velocity increases within the stenosis which are easily detected. In addition, they have a waveform configuration which, even in the fasting state, has a low resistance configuration ie. a marked increase in end diastolic velocity [22]. When there is a high grade stenosis found in both the celiac and superior mesenteric arteries, these findings, in conjunction with an appropriate clinical presentation, are sufficient to make the diagnosis of chronic mesenteric ischemia.

Flow in the portal circulation can be studied by duplex ultrasound. Portal vein patency, direction of portal flow, patency of portosystemic shunts and estimates of portal vein volume flow have all been measured by duplex ultrasound [23].

Peripheral arteries

Dissatisfaction with other noninvasive methods for localizing and estimating the hemodynamic significance of a peripheral arterial lesion [24–26] has led to application of duplex scanning in the evaluation of patients with lower

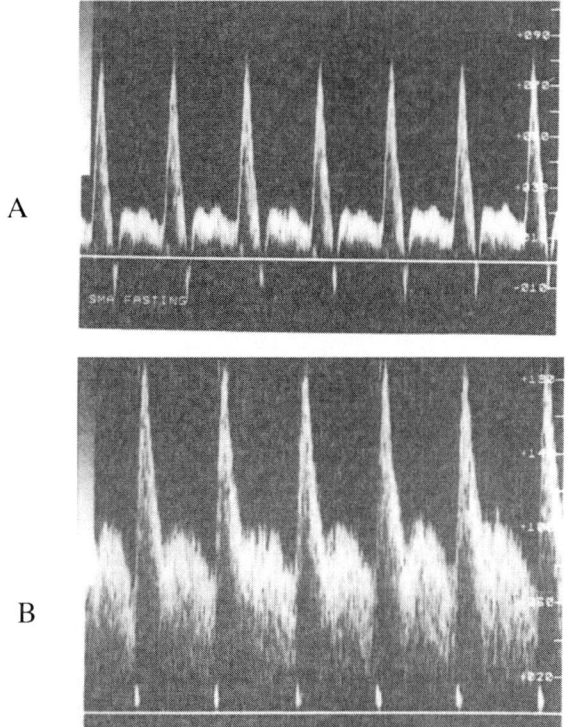

Fig. 4. The spectral waveform from the superior mesenteric artery in the fasting state (A) shows low diastolic flow with evidence of flow reversal during diastole, features characteristic of high end organ resistance. In contrast the spectral waveform from the same artery after a meal (B) shows increased diastolic flow and absence of flow reversal which is associated with low end organ resistance.

extremity atherosclerotic occlusive disease. In these patients the complexity and eccentricity of atherosclerotic lesions, coupled with a propensity for multilevel involvement, often precludes an accurate estimation of hemodynamic significance of an individual stenosis based on angiographic criteria alone. This is particularly true with regard to the iliac artery and the orgin of the deep femoral artery [27, 28]. Direct pressure measurements at the time of angiography, although accurate [29], are not commonly used for either screening or follow-up studies.

Duplex examination of the lower extremity arteries is technically demanding and time consuming. Two to three hours may be required to study both lower extremities. It does, however, provide detailed information about the hemodynamic, and thus clinical, significance of individual arterial lesions. A complete examination includes the distal aorta, the common and external iliac arteries, common femoral arteries, origin of the profunda femoris,

Table 2. Duplex derived arterial velocities in 55 volunteers without evidence of arterial occlusive disease [30]*.

Arterial segment	Peak systolic velocity + SD (cm/sec)
External iliac	119.3 + 5.4
Common femoral	114.1 + 2.4
Proximal superficial femoral	90.8 + 1.5
Distal superficial femoral	93.6 + 1.3
Popliteal	68.8 + 1.8

* a: 25 women, 30 men, average age 51.9 + 14.3 years.

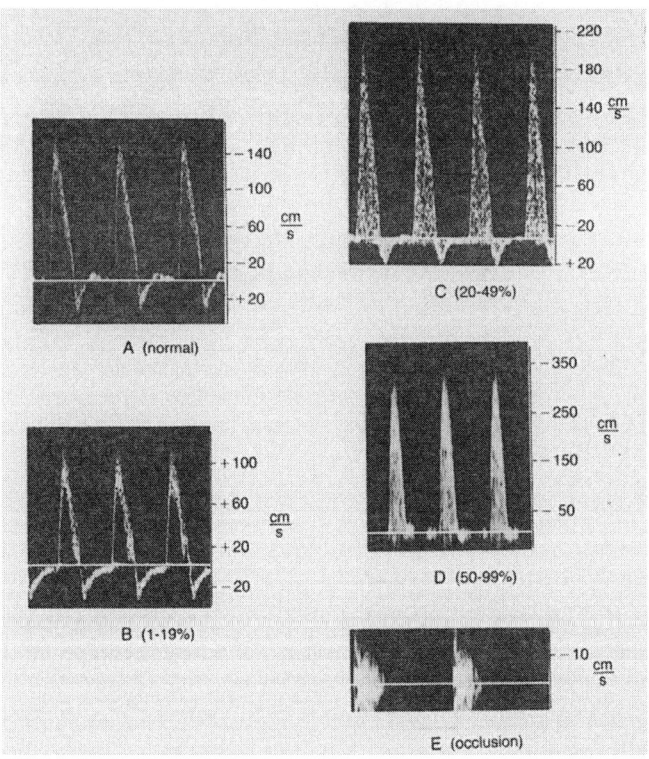

Fig. 5. Examples of spectral waveforms used to classify peripheral arterial stenosis. A: (Normal) A triphasic waveform with systolic forward flow followed by reverse flow in diastole. No significant spectral broadening. B: (1–19% stenosis) Spectral broadening is present in a normal waveform with normal velocities. C: (20–49% stenosis) At least a 30% increase in peak systolic velocity compared to the proximal recording site is combined with marked spectral broadening. D: (50–99% stenosis): There is a greater than 100% increase in peak systolic velocity combined with extensive spectral broadening. Loss of reverse flow results in a monophasic signal. E: (Occulusion): No flow can be demonstrated in an adequately visualized artery.

proximal, mid and distal superficial femoral arteries and the popliteal arteries.

Based on angiographic comparisons of duplex examinations in normal and atherosclerotic limbs, waveform and velocity criteria have been developed to predict the degree of stenosis in lower extremity arteries (Table 2 and Fig. 5). Prospective application of these criteria to the arterial segments noted above yielded, when compared with angiography, an overall 77% sensitivity, 98% specificity and a postive predictive value of 94% in determining the presence of a greater or less than 50% stenosis [30]. These results are similar to those reported for intraobserver varibility in estimating peripheral arterial stenosis from conventional angiograms [31, 32]. Analysis of the end diastolic velocity may eventually permit even more precise quantitation of the degree of stenosis [33].

Peripheral arterial duplex scanning is applicable both in operated and non-operated patients. In non-operated patients it can be used to follow the progression of an individual stenosis in patients and in research studies. It is a valuable adjunct to angiography in the assessment of the iliac artery and can be used as the sole diagnostic procedure prior to transluminal angioplasty [34]. Finally, in operated patients with multilevel disease, where other non-invasive tests cannot specifically examine the treated arterial segment, duplex scanning can be used for serial follow-up of operative reconstructions [35] and individual sites of transluminal angioplasty (Fig. 6).

Venous system

The major deep veins may be examined by either B-mode imaging alone or with the duplex system [36, 37]. Most of the work to date has been with an imaging system that did not permit evaluation of the iliac veins or inferior vena cava. In this circumstance, the patency of the iliac veins has to be estimated by venous outflow studies using plethysmographic methods. However, more recent duplex systems using lower frequency transducers and a pulsed Doppler have permitted evaluation of the iliac veins as well.

Both the Doppler and B-mode image, especially the later, are important in the venous examination below the inguinal ligament. The Doppler is used to study flow characteristics (spontaneity, phasicity and response to distal and proximal compression) while the B-mode may visualize intraluminal thrombus (Fig. 7). Failure of the vein walls to co-apt with gentle probe pressure is used to detect the presence of an intraluminal thrombus [38]. For iliac vein occlusion, it is not possible to utilize co-aptation of the vessel as an index of patency so it is necessary to depend upon the presence or absence of flow. In

458

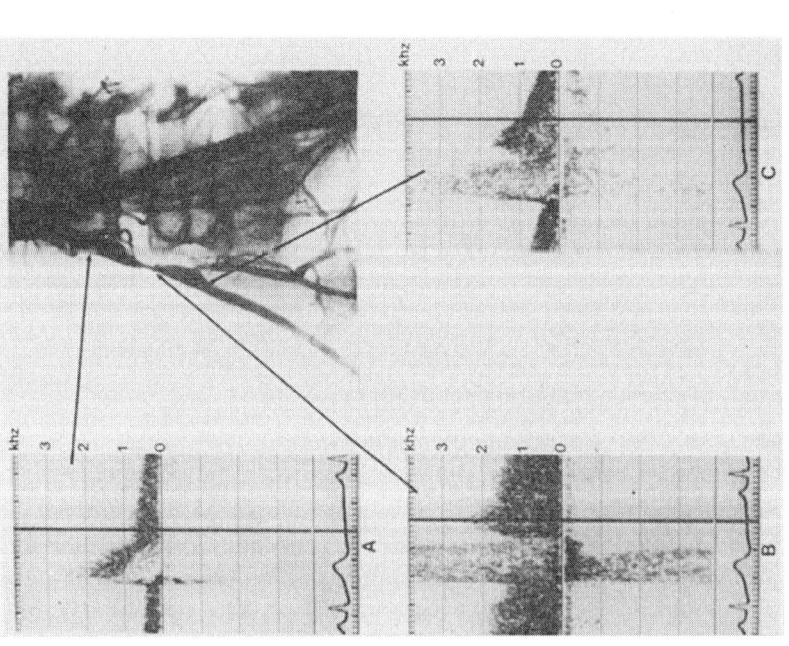

Fig. 6. Iliac artery velocity spectra before (A) and after (B) transluminal angioplasty.

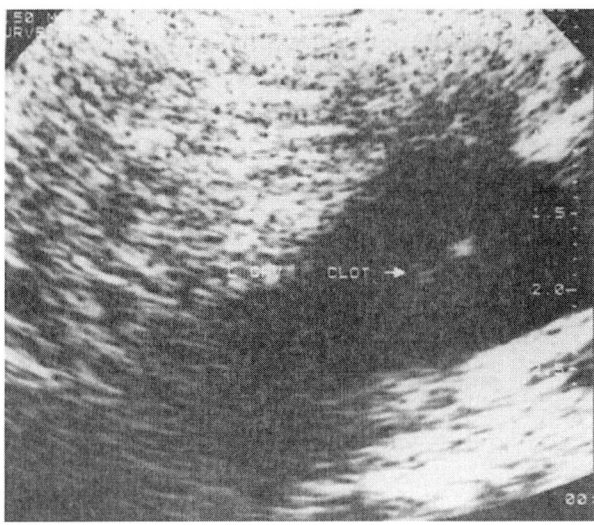

Fig. 7. The arrow points to the tip of a common femoral vein (CFV) thrombus.

addition, Duplex scanning may be used to document extrinsic venous compression as the etiology of impaired venous outflow (Fig. 8).

Duplex scanning can also be applied to other aspects of venous disease as well. In selected patients the B-mode may allow the study of venous valvular motion [39]. In patients with chronic venous incompetence, when compared

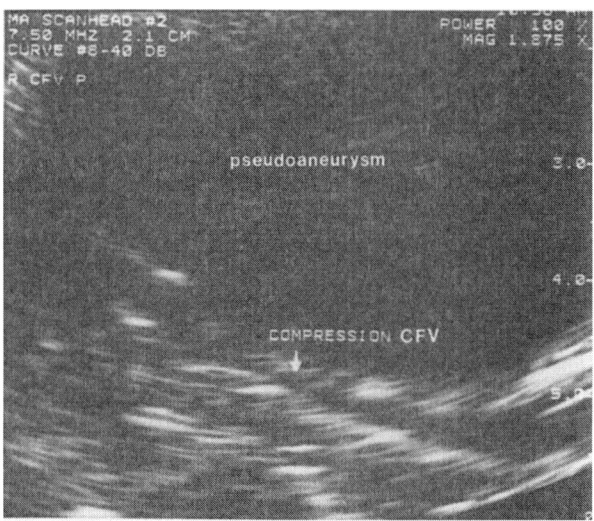

Fig. 8. In this patient a large common femoral artery pseudoaneurysm compressing the common femoral vein (CFV) produced a clinical picture similar to that of deep venous thrombosis.

460

to ambulatory venous pressures, it appears to have both a sensitivity and specificity in excess of 80% in the detection of venous reflux [40]. It is now being used by some investigators to assess serially the course of a deep venous thrombus in response to heparin or fibrinolytic therapy [41]. In addition, the technique appears promising for the study of the natural history of deep venous thrombosis and its relationship to the development of the postthrombotic syndrome.

Conclusions

Duplex scanning combines B-mode ultrasonic imaging with a pulsed Doppler for detection of blood flow velocities. The technique allows serial, accurate, noninvasive assessment of both anatomic and hemodynamic abnormalities. It should be considered the procedure of choice in the non-invasive evaluation of extracranial carotid artery disease. In addition, exciting new areas of application include renovascular hypertension, visceral and peripheral arterial ischemia, and acute and chronic venous disease. Although the equipment is expensive and considerable technical skill is required for many of the examinations, the versatility and accuracy of Duplex scanning promises to make it the mainstay of the noninvasive vascular laboratory.

References

1. Barber FE, Baker DW, Nation WC, et al.: Ultrasonic duplex echo-Doppler scanner. IEEE Trans Biomed Eng 21: 109–113, 1974.
2. Baker JD: How vascular surgeons use noninvasive testing. J Vasc Surg 4: 272–276, 1986.
3. Bernstein EF: The clinical spectrum of ischemic cerebrovascular disease, in Bernstein EF (ed.): Noninvasive Diagnostic Techniques in Vascular Disease. St. Louis, CV Mosby Co, pp. 301–315, 1985.
4. Hass WK, Fields WS, North RR, et al.. Joint study of extracranial arterial occlusion. II. Arteriography, Techniques, Sites and Complications. JAMA 203: 961–968, 1968.
5. Roederer GO, Langlois YE, Chan AW, et al.: Ultrasonic duplex scanning of extracranial carotid arteries: Improved accuracy using new features from the common carotid artery. J Cardiovasc Ultrasonics 1: 373–380, 1982.
6. Roederer GO, Langlois YE, Jager KA, et al.: A simple spectral parameter for accurate classification of severe carotid disease. Bruit 8: 174–178, 1984.
7. Chikos PM, Fisher LD, Hirsh JH, et al.: Observer variability in evaluating extracranial carotid artery stenosis. Stroke 14: 885–892, 1983.
8. Bendick PJ, Jackson VP: Evaluation of the vertebral arteries with duplex sonography. J Vasc Surg 3: 523–530, 1986.
9. Flanigan DP, Schuler JJ, Vogel M, et al.: The role of duplex scanning in surgical decision making. J Vasc Surg 2: 15–25, 1985.

10. Roederer GO, Langlois YE, Lusiani L, et al.: Natural history of carotid artery disease on the side contralateral to endarterectomy. J Vasc Surg 1: 62–72, 1984.

11. Roederer GO, Langlois YE, Jager KA, et al.: The natural history of carotid artery disease in asymptomatic patients with cervical bruits. Stroke 15: 605–613, 1984.

12. Zierler RE, Bandyk DF, Thiele BL, Strandness DE Jr: Carotid artery stenosis following endarterectomy. Arch Surg 117: 1408–1415, 1982.

13. Reilly LM, Lusby RJ, Hughes L, et al.: Carotid plaque histology using real-time ultrasonography: Clinical and therapeutic implications. Am J Surg 146: 188–193, 1983.

14. Gifford RW Jr.: Epidemiology and clinical manifestations of renovascular hypertension, in Stanley JC, Ernst CB, Fry WJ (eds.): Renovascular Hypertension. Philadelphia, WB Saunders Co, 1984, pp. 77–99.

15. Williams GH, Braunwald E: Hypertensive vascular disease, in Braunwald E, Isselbacher KJ, Petersdorf RG, et al. (eds.): Harrison's Principles of Internal Medicine (11th Ed). New York, McGraw-Hill Co, p. 1024, 1987.

16. Treadway KK, Slater EE: Renovascular hypertension. Ann Rev Med 35: 665–693, 1984.

17. Kohler TR, Zierler RE, Martin RL, et al.: Noninvasive diagnosis of renal artery stenosis by ultrasonic duplex scanning. J Vasc Surg 4: 450–456, 1986.

18. Lacombe M: Arterial stenosis complicating renal allotransplantation in man: A study of 38 cases. Ann Surg 181: 283–288, 1975.

19. Reintz ER, Goldman MH, Sais J, et al.: Evaluation of transplant renal artery blood flow by Doppler sound-spectrum analysis. Arch Surg 118: 415–419, 1983.

20. Rigsby CM, Taylor KJW, Weltin G, et al.: Renal allografts in acute rejection: Evaluation using duplex sonography. Radiology 158: 375–378, 1986.

21. Jager K, Bollinger A, Valli C, et al.: Measurement of mesenteric blood flow by duplex scanning. J Vasc Surg 3: 462–469, 1986.

22. Nicholls SC, Kohler TR, Martin RL, et al.: Use of hemodynamic parameters in the diagnosis of mesenteric insufficiency. J Vasc Surg 3: 507–510, 1986.

23. Ackroyd N, Gill R, Griffiths K, et al.: Duplex scanning of the portal vein and portasystemic shunts. Surgery 99: 591–597, 1986.

24. Flanigan DP, Collins JT, Goodreau JJ, et al.: Femoral pulsatility index in the evaluation of aortoiliac occlusive disease. J Surg Res 31: 392–399, 1981.

25. Flanigan DP, Gray B, Schuler JJ, et al.: Correlation of Doppler-derived high thigh pressure and intra-arterial pressure in the assessment of aorto-iliac occlusive disease. Br J Surg 68: 423–425, 1981.

26. Barrie WE, Evans DH, Bell PRF: The relationship between pulsatility index and proximal arterial stenosis. Br J Surg 66: 366, 1979.

27. Moore WS, Hall AD: Unrecognized aortoiliac stenosis. Arch Surg 103: 663–638, 1971.

28. Clifford PC, Cole SEA, Rhys Davies E, et al.: Detection of arterial stenosis: increased accuracy using biplanar angiography and Doppler signal analysis. J Cardiovasc Surg 26: 554–557, 1985.

29. Brener BJ, Raines JK, Darling RC, et al.: Measurement of systolic femoral arterial pressure during reactive hyperemia: an estimate of aortoiliac disease. Circulation 49–50: H259–267, 1974.

30. Jager KA, Phillips DJ, Martin RL, et al.: Noninvasive mapping of lower limb arterial lesions. Ultrasound Med Biol 11: 515–521, 1985.

31. Slot HB, Strijbosch L, Greep JM: Intraobserver variability in single plane aortography. Surgery 90: 497–503, 1981.

32. Thiele BL, Strandness DE Jr.: Accuracy of angiographic quantification of peripheral atherosclerosis. Progress Cardiovasc Diseases 26: 223–236, 1983.

462

33. Nicholls SC, Kohler TR, Martin RL, et al.: Diastolic flow as a predictor of arterial stenosis. J Vasc Surg 3: 498–501, 1986.
34. Jager K, Johl H, Seifert H, et al.: Perkutane transluminale Angioplastie (PTA) ohne vorausgehende diagnostische Arteriographie. VASA Suppl. 15: 24, 1986.
35. Bandyk DF: Postoperative surveillance of femorodistal grafts: the application of Echo-Doppler (Duplex) ultrasonic scanning, in Bergan JJ, Yao JST (eds.): Reoperative Arterial Surgery. Orlando, Grune & Stratton, 1986, pp. 59–80.
36. Sullivan ED, Peter DJ, Cranley JJ: Real-time B-mode venous ultrasound. J Vasc Surg 1: 465–471, 1984.
37. Hannan LJ, Stedje KJ, Skorez MJ, et al.: Venous imaging of the extremities: our first twenty-five hundred cases. Bruit 10: 29-32, 1986.
38. Raghavendra BN, Horii SC, Hilton S, et al.: Deep venous thrombosis: detection by probe compression of veins. J Ultrasound Med 5: 89–95, 1986.
39. Brownlow RL, McKinney WM: Ultrasonic evaluation of jugular venous valve competence. J Ultrasound Med 4: 169–172, 1985.
40. Szendro G, Nicolaides AN, Zukowski AJ, et al.: Duplex scanning in the assessment of deep venous incompetence. J Vasc Surg 4: 237–242, 1986.
41. Stedje KG, Hannan LJ, Karkow WS, et al.: Assessing the results of heparin and streptokinase therapy of deep venous thrombosis using sequential real-time B-mode ultrasound scans. Bruit 9: 197–200, 1985.

6.8. Doppler techniques for intraoperative arterial assessment

R. EUGENE ZIERLER

The results of arterial reconstructive surgery are determined by patient selection and operative technique. Although technical errors are uncommon, they are often responsible for perioperative complications such as occlusion of bypass grafts and stroke after carotid endarterectomy [1–3]. Avoiding these problems requires that the technical result be assessed at the conclusion of the procedure. Simple observation and palpation of the vessels are not adequate, since defects within the lumen rarely affect the external surface and a transmitted pulse may be present in an occluded artery. Therefore, objective methods must be used to assess the surgical result and facilitate immediate correction of technical errors.

Methods for intraoperative assessment are based on either anatomic imaging or flow detection and include contrast arteriography, B-mode ultrasound scanning, the electromagnetic flowmeter, and Doppler ultrasound [4]. While arteriography is generally regarded as the standard assessment technique, it involves arterial puncture, contrast injection, and is relatively time consuming. B-mode scanning is noninvasive but requires complex equipment and provides only anatomic information. The electromagnetic flowmeter is of limited value for intraoperative assessment because many technical errors produce only minimal changes in the volume of flow. Doppler ultrasound provides a simple and rapid technique for evaluating blood flow without puncture or manipulation of vessels. The Doppler assessment not only confirms the presence of flow in the reconstructed arterial segment, but also detects the localized flow disturbances that are associated with minor technical errors.

Doppler methods

Instrumentation

The frequency shift that occurs when ultrasound is reflected by moving blood cells is an example of the Doppler effect. This frequency shift is proportional to blood velocity, transmitted ultrasound frequency, the speed of sound in

I. Cikes (ed.), *Echocardiography in Cardiac Interventions*, 463–471, 1989.
© 1989 *Kluwer Academic Publishers.*

tissue, and the cosine of the angle between the ultrasound beam and the direction of flow. In clinical use, all of these parameters except blood velocity can be kept constant, and the Doppler frequency shift is directly proportional to blood cell velocity. Most Doppler instruments have transmitting frequencies in the range of 3 to 10 MHz, but a 20 MHz Doppler is also available for intraoperative use [5]. Although the depth of tissue penetration by ultrasound is inversely proportional to transmitting frequency, the distances required for intraoperative assessment are short, and the transmitting frequency is not an important consideration.

Doppler instruments operate in either a continuous wave or pulsed mode. A continuous wave system insonates all structures in the path of the ultrasound beam, so the reflected Doppler signal represents the entire flow profile of all vessels present. Pulsed Doppler systems detect flow at a particular depth in tissue by transmitting short bursts of ultrasound, a technique called range-gating [6]. The region where blood flow is detected is referred to as the sample volume, and this can be positioned at any point along the axis of the ultrasound beam. Continuous wave Doppler instruments are generally less expensive and easier to use than the pulsed systems, and they provide a qualitative evaluation of flow patterns [7]. Since a pulsed Doppler detects flow at discrete sites in tissue, it permits evaluation of flow patterns at specific locations within a vessel. This approach is best suited for sophisticated signal processing methods such as spectral analysis [8].

Doppler signal analysis

Listening to the amplified audio output of the instrument is the simplest approach to Doppler signal analysis. The frequency or pitch of the sound is directly proportional to blood velocity, and turbulent flow is characterized by a harsh or grating sound quality. Signals obtained at the site of a severe stenosis are characterized by a localized area of increased frequency and a zone of turbulence distal to the stenotic segment. Less severe lesions may produce only a small zone of turbulence. Thus, an experienced examiner can learn to distinguish between normal and abnormal flow patterns. However, this audible interpretation is purely subjective, and the more subtle flow disturbances associated with some minor lesions or technical errors may not be detected.

A more objective method is the use of a zero crossing frequency meter to generate analog waveforms from the Doppler signal. The analog waveform presents changes in Doppler shift frequency over time with forward and reverse velocity components indicated by positive or negative deflections relative to a zero baseline. As illustrated in Fig. 1, a normal peripheral artery waveform is triphasic with a prominent forward flow phase in systole followed by a brief phase of flow reversal in early diastole and a final smaller forward flow phase. This normal pattern can be altered by arterial disease. A localized increase in the peak systolic frequency is caused by the high velocity jet in a severe stenosis; distal to a stenosis the waveform becomes monophasic with a rounded contour, lower systolic peak, and loss of the reverse flow component (Fig. 1). Although analog waveforms are subject to a variety of errors and artifacts, they are easily obtained with inexpensive equipment and can provide clinically useful information [9].

Spectral analysis is a method for processing Doppler signals that overcomes the limitations of analog waveforms [8]. While the analog waveform represents the Doppler signal as a single line, a spectrum analyzer displays the entire frequency and amplitude content of the signal. The amplitude of the signal is proportional to the number of blood cells passing through the ultrasound beam. Spectral waveforms are generally presented with frequency on the vertical axis, time on the horizontal axis, and amplitude indicated by a gray-scale (Fig. 2).

It is now recognized that various arterial lesions give rise to characteristic spectral waveforms. The center stream flow pattern in a normal artery is laminar with all the blood cells having nearly the same speed and direction. Figure 2 illustrates the center stream spectral waveform from a normal internal carotid artery. In this example, the band of frequencies is narrow, particularly during systole. The relatively low hemodynamic resistance of the cerebral circulation results in forward flow throughout systole and diastole. Resistance in the normal lower extremity arterial circulation is higher, and a phase of flow reversal is present (Fig. 1). Stenoses and arterial wall defects disrupt this normal laminar flow pattern, and the blood cell motion becomes random. These disturbed flow patterns produce spectral waveforms that are characterized by a widening of the frequency band referred to as spectral broadening. Severe stenoses are associated with high velocity jets and turbulence, and the corresponding spectral features are increased peak systolic frequency and spectral broadening. Minor defects such as intimal flaps or wall irregularities cause localized flow disturbances that may be evident only as a relative increase in spectral width.

Examination technique

Sterilized Doppler probes can be applied directly to the external surfaces of the exposed vessels and acoustically coupled with a small amount of blood or saline. Since the Doppler frequency shift is proportional to the incident angle of the ultrasound beam, a constant angle should be maintained during the

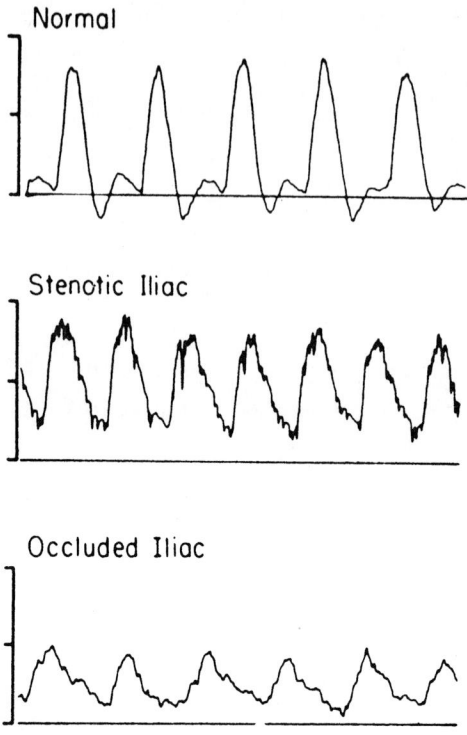

Fig. 1. Analog waveforms taken from the common femoral artery with a continuous wave Doppler. The normal waveform is triphasic with a small reverse flow component (below baseline). Progressive iliac artery disease results in a monophasic waveform without reverse flow.

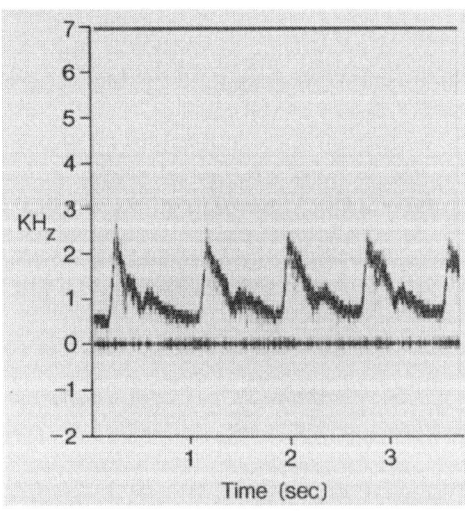

Fig. 2. Spectral waveform taken with a pulsed Doppler from the center stream of a normal internal carotid artery. Flow is forward (positive) throughout the cardiac cycle. The frequency band is narrow with a clear area under each systolic peak, indicating a laminar flow pattern.

examination. Doppler instruments with transmitting frequencies in the range of 8 to 10 MHz are generally used for intraoperative assessment. Continuous wave Doppler signals are most suitable for audible interpretation and generating analog waveforms; more detailed information on flow patterns can be obtained with spectral analysis of pulsed Doppler signals.

After an arterial reconstruction is completed, each vessel in the operative field should be evaluated with a Doppler probe. With experience, the sounds of normal arterial flow in the lower extremity and carotid circulations can be easily recognized. The absence of a flow signal or an abrupt 'water hammer' pulse indicates arterial occlusion. A harsh, high pitched signal is associated with a significant stenosis. Distal to a stenotic lesion, the flow pattern is monophasic and low pitched. By systematically evaluating the exposed vessels, the flow patterns can be determined in the proximal arteries, the reconstructed segment, and the distal branches. The flow contributions of various arteries can be assessed by temporary compression and release of the vessels under evaluation. Anastomotic sites and endarterectomy endpoints should be examined carefully for localized flow disturbances that may indicate a technical error. Detection of minor flow disturbances is greatly facilitated by the use of a pulsed Doppler and spectrum analyzer.

Clinical results

A study on the value of intraoperative Doppler assessment in aortic reconstructive surgery was reported by Keitzer et al. [10]. The results of 35 elective operations that included a qualitative continous wave Doppler evaluation were compared with 22 procedures in which the Doppler was not used. The former group required nine reoperations to manage vascular complications, while 15 reoperations were necessary in the latter group. Overall operative mortality and reoperation rate were significantly lower in the group with intraoperative Doppler assessment. A similar study was carried out on patients having femoropopliteal bypass procedures, and a significant difference was again found in favor of intraoperative Doppler assessment [10].

Both continuous wave Doppler and pulsed Doppler with spectral analysis have been used for intraoperative assessment of in situ saphenous vein bypass grafts [11, 12]. By detecting intact valve cusps and arteriovenous fistulas, these techniques can reduce the need for operative arteriography and shorten operating time. When a 20 MHz pulsed Doppler was used to evaluate 50 consecutive in situ grafts, 6% of anastomoses were considered technically unsatisfactory and competent valve cusps were found at 5% of valve incision sites [12].

Bandyk et al. used a 20 MHz pulsed Doppler and spectrum analyzer to assess the technical results of 20 femoropopliteal and ten femorotibial bypass grafts [13]. Interpretation of center stream spectral waveforms was based on localized increases in peak systolic frequency and spectral width. Operative arteriography was performed in all cases, and lesions considered significant were intimal flaps larger than 2 mm, stenoses of greater than 30% diameter reduction, and intraluminal defects consistent with thrombus. A normal arteriogram and pulsed Doppler spectral waveforms are shown in Fig. 3. Abnormal spectral waveforms were observed in five of the 30 bypass grafts. Operative arteriography identified defects that required correction in three of these five cases (1 graft kink, 2 greater than 30% stenoses); the remaining two grafts had minor defects (1 spasm, 1 20% stenosis). No other significant defects were found by arteriography, and none of the grafts occluded within one month after surgery. If operative arteriography is regarded as the standard test for detecting significant technical errors, pulsed Doppler with spectral analysis had a sensitivity of 100% and a specificity of 93%. The false-positive assessments can be attributed to the ability of the pulsed Doppler method to detect flow disturbances produced by minor arterial lesions.

In a related study, the 20 MHz pulsed Doppler was used to measure blood flow velocity in 24 femoropopliteal and 42 femorotibial bypass grafts [14]. Peak systolic flow velocity was greater in femoropopliteal grafts (90 ± 22 cm/sec) than in femorotibial grafts (68 ± 19 cm/sec). All successful grafts had continuous forward flow in diastole at operation, indicating a hyperemic flow state with decreased peripheral vascular resistance. This diastolic forward flow persisted during the immediate postoperative period, but decreased thereafter. Early graft occlusion was associated with a peak systolic flow velocity less than 40 cm/sec and absence of forward flow in diastole. These intraoperative findings should prompt a search for technical problems or alternate procedures that could increase graft flow velocity.

In carotid endarterectomy, technical errors can be associated with perioperative neurologic complications [2, 3]. Studies based on the use of routine operative arteriography have shown that the incidence of significant technical problems after carotid surgery is between 5 and 10 percent [5]. The qualitative interpretation of continuous wave Doppler signals has been used to identify carotid artery defects requiring immediate correction [7, 15]. In the hands of an experienced examiner, this approach can be extremely valuable.

Zierler et al. assessed the technical results of 50 carotid endarterectomies with both operative arteriography and spectral analysis of 20 MHz pulsed Doppler signals [5]. Flow disturbances consistent with technical errors were observed in seven internal carotid arteries, and in two of these cases operative arteriography showed defects that required correction. No other technical problems were found and no perioperative neurologic complications

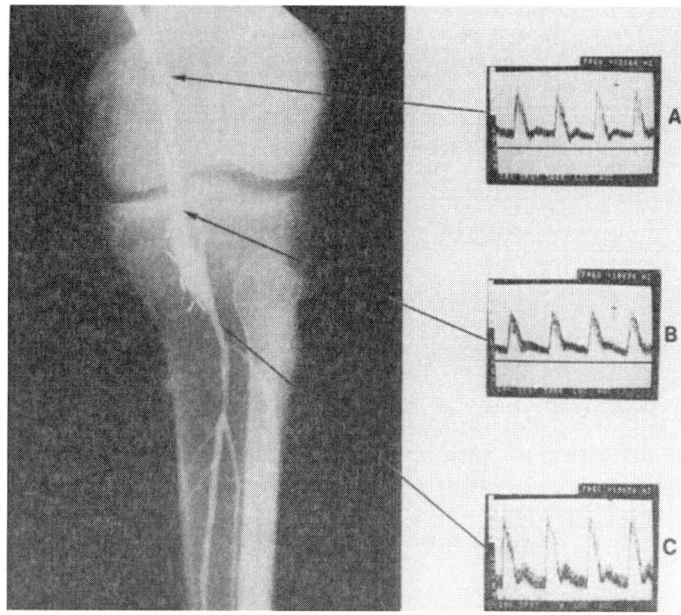

Fig. 3. Normal operative arteriogram and corresponding 20 MHz pulsed Doppler spectral waveforms from a femoropopliteal bypass graft. The vein graft to artery anastomosis is technically satisfactory. No significant flow disturbances are present in the distal graft (A), proximal to the anastomosis (B), or distal to the anastomosis (C).

occurred. Figure 4 shows the intraoperative spectral waveforms from a case in which a significant defect was identified and corrected. The results of Doppler assessment during carotid endarterectomy are similar to those reported for bypass grafts in the leg. This method is very sensitive to relatively minor flow disturbances, so although false-positive assessments do occur, false-negatives are exceedingly uncommon and the negative predictive value is high.

Conclusions

The Doppler methods for intraoperative assessment of arterial surgery are rapid, safe, reliable, and relatively inexpensive. Although they require some skill and experience, the techniques are easily learned. The main disadvantage of the Doppler methods is that they provide no direct anatomic information on the arterial defects identified. An imaging technique such as contrast arteriography or B-mode scanning may be needed to completely characterize a particular defect. The qualitative continuous wave Doppler assessment is the simplest approach and is satisfactory for most routine applications.

470

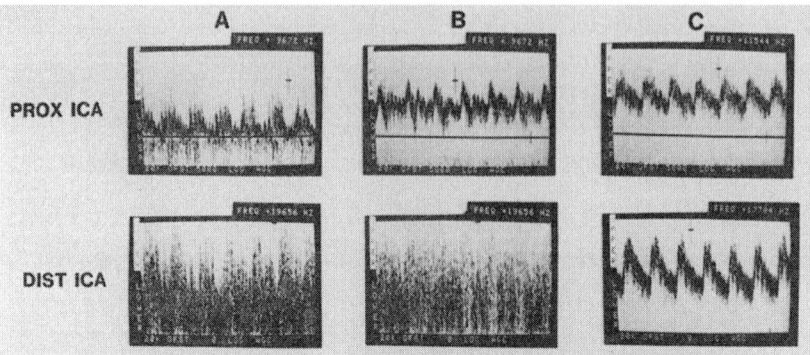

Fig. 4. 20 MHz pulsed Doppler spectral waveforms from intraoperative assessment of a carotid endarterectomy. Prior to endarterectomy (A) the proximal and distal internal carotid waveforms are markedly abnormal. After endarterectomy (B) the proximal waveform is improved, but the distal site remains disturbed. Correction of a distal stenosis results in a normal flow pattern (C).

Pulsed Doppler with spectral analysis provides more detailed information on flow patterns, especially those minor disturbances associated with small arterial defects.

Because of their high negative predictive value, the Doppler assessment methods can be used to select patients for operative arteriography. If this is done, only a small proportion of patients will be subjected to the invasive procedure, and the chances of overlooking a significant defect are extremely low.

Summary

When arterial reconstructive surgery is performed, objective methods are required to identify technical errors that could lead to perioperative complications. Doppler ultrasound provides a simple and rapid approach to intraoperative assessment that gives physiologic information on flow patterns in the reconstructed arteries. The examination is performed by placing a sterile Doppler probe directly on the external surface of the exposed vessels. Continuous wave Doppler signals are best suited for qualitative interpretation by audible analysis or analog waveforms. The characteristic sounds associated with major arterial lesions are easily recognized by an experienced examiner. Detecting the subtle flow disturbances produced by some minor lesions and technical errors requires the use of pulsed Doppler and spectral analysis. Experience with intraoperative Doppler assessment has confirmed its value in aortic reconstructive surgery, bypass grafts in the leg, and carotid endarterectomy. In addition to identifying technical errors such as intimal flaps, residual plaques, and stenoses, Doppler derived velocity measurements can be used to predict long-term patency of bypass grafts. The main disadvantage of the Doppler methods is the lack of direct anatomic information on the arterial defects identified, and other studies are usually required to completely characterize a lesion. Because Doppler methods have a high negative predictive value, they could be used to select patients for operative arteriography.

References

1. LiCalzi LK, Stansel HC: Failure of autogenous reversed saphenous vein femoropopliteal grafing – Pathophysiology and prevention. Surgery 91: 352–358, 1982.
2. Collins GJ, Rich NM, Anderson CA, et al.: Stroke associated with carotid endarterectomy. Am J Surg 135: 221–225, 1978.
3. Towne JB, Bernhard VM: Neurologic deficit following carotid endarterectomy. Surg Gynecol Obstet 154: 849–852, 1982.
4. Zierler RE: Intraoperative Doppler techniques for arterial evaluation. Seminars in Ultrasound 6: 73–84, 1985.
5. Zierler RE, Bandyk DF, Thiele BL: Intraoperative assessment of carotid endarterectomy. J Vasc Surg 1: 73–83, 1984.
6. Baker DW: Pulsed ultrasonic Doppler blood flow sensing. IEEE Trans Sonics Ultrasonics 17: 170–173, 1970.
7. Barnes RW, Garrett WV: Intraoperative assessment of arterial reconstruction by Doppler ultrasound. Surg Gynecol Obstet 146: 896–900, 1978.
8. Zierler RE, Roederer GO, Strandness DE: The use of frequency spectral analysis in carotid artery surgery. In Bergan JJ, Yao JST (eds.): Cerebrovascular Insufficiency. Orlando, Grune and Stratton, Inc., pp. 137–163, 1983.
9. Johnston KW, Marozzo BC, Cobbold RSC: Errors and artifacts of Doppler flowmeters and their solution. Arch Surg 112: 1335–1342, 1977.
10. Keitzer WF, Lichti EL, Brossart FA, et al.: Use of the Doppler ultrasonic flowmeter during arterial vascular surgery. Arch Surg 105: 308–312, 1972.
11. Spencer TD, Goldman MH, Hyslop JW et al.: Intraoperative assessment of in situ saphenous vein bypass grafts with continuous-wave Doppler probe. Surgery 96: 874–876, 1984.
12. Bandyk DF, Jorgensen RA, Town JB: Intraoperative assessment of in situ saphenous vein arterial grafts using pulsed Doppler spectral analysis. Arch Surg 121: 292–299, 1986.
13. Bandyk DF, Zierler RE, Thiele BL: Detection of technical error during arterial surgery by pulsed Doppler spectral analysis. Arch Surg 119: 421–428, 1984.
14. Bandyk DF, Cato RF, Towne JB: A low flow velocity predicts failure of femoropopliteal and femorotibial bypass grafts.f Surgery 98: 799–809, 1985.
15. Seifert KB, Blackshear WM: Continuous-wave Doppler in the intraoperative assessment of carotid endarterectomy. J Vasc Surg 2: 817–820, 1985.

6.9. Doppler guiding of venous and arterial puncture

TIMOTHY SHINE & MICHAEL NUGENT

Doppler techniques can be used to confirm the location of a blood vessel, and this knowledge facilitates venous and arterial puncture. Legler and Nugent [1] have shown that the Doppler reduces the number of needle probes required for internal jugular vein cannulation. Fewer needle probes should reduce the number of complications associated with this procedure. Petzoldt [2] has described a Doppler technique for subclavian vein cannulation. The Doppler has also been used to locate veins and arteries in patients in shock or with severe burns [3], as an aid to percutaneous radial artery cannulation in infants and small children [4], and as a technique for monitoring arterial patency in limbs distal to the site of arterial catheterization. The Doppler also has been used as a noninvasive technique for assessing brachial, radial, and ulnar arterial patency and forearm arterial blood pressure in patients who have undergone cardiac catheterization via the brachial artery [5]. Barnes [6] has shown the Doppler to be a sensitive index of asymptomatic arterial obstruction following cardiac catheterization via the femoral and branchial arterial routes.

Internal jugular vein cannulation

The internal jugular vein collects blood from the brain and superficial parts of the face and neck. Its origin is at the base of the skull as a continuation of the sigmoid sinus. The vein runs in the carotid sheath into the subclavian vein. Facial, lingual, pharyngeal, superior and middle thyroid veins are tributaries of the internal jugular vein. It runs under the sternocleidomastoid muscle and the deep cervical fascia. The internal jugular vein is in the triangle between the two inferior heads of the sternocleido-mastoid muscle. The vein runs close to the carotid vessels, sympathetic chain, stellate ganglion, vagus nerves and phrenic nerves, and the thoracic duct on the left. A direct, almost straight line to the right atrium is formed by the right internal jugular vein, the innominate vein and the subclavian vein.

Using anatomic landmarks, Defalque [9] has described three approaches to cannulation of the internal jugular vein which are defined in relation to the

I. Cikes (ed.), *Echocardiography in Cardiac Interventions*, 473–479, 1989.
© 1989 *Kluwer Academic Publishers*.

474

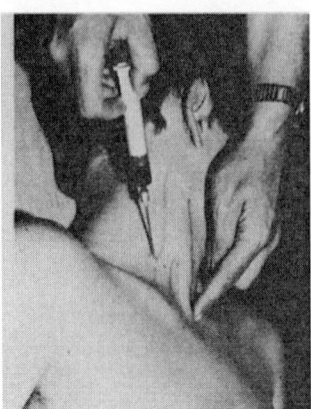

Fig. 1. Posterior approach for cannulation of internal jugular vein: The needle is introduced under the sternocleidomastoid muscle near the junction of the middle and lower third of its lateral border, and aimed at the suprasternal notch. (Used with permission[7]).

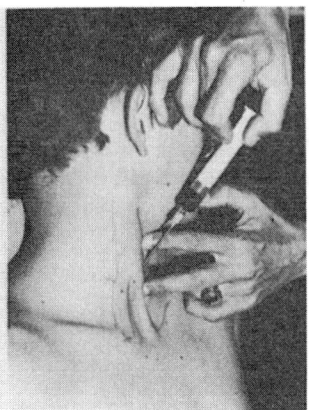

Fig. 2. Anterior approach for cannulation of internal jugular vein: The needle is inserted at the midpoint of the anterior border of the sternocleidomastoid muscle and directed toward the ipsilateral nipple, forming 30 to 15 degree angle with the skin. (Used with permission[7]).

sternocleidomastoid muscle. These are the anterior, central, and posterior approaches (Figs. 1–3). The technique for internal jugular cannulation using the Doppler was first described by Ullman and Stoelting [8] and modified by Nugent and Legler [1]. The internal jugular vein is located using a Parks model 811 Doppler* probe in the central region of the sternocleidomastoid muscle. With the patient in the head-down position and the head turned to the left, the probe is held at 45° to the surface of the skin above the clavicle over the medial border of the lateral (clavicular) head of the sternocleido-

* Parks Medical Electronics, Inc., P.O. Box BB, Beaverton, Oregon 97075.

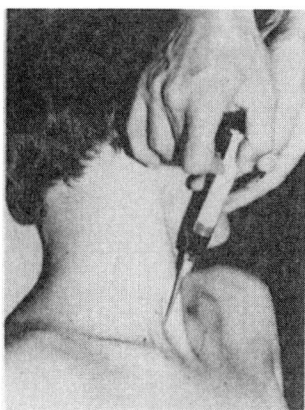

Fig. 3. Central approach for cannulation of internal jugular vein: The needle is inserted in the triangle formed by the two heads of the sternocleidomastoid muscle along the medial border of the lateral (clavicular) head, forming a 30-degree angle with the plane of skin, and directed caudally and slightly lateral to the sagittal plane. The central approach is used when the Doppler is employed to confirm the location of the internal juglar vein (Used with permission[7]).

mastoid muscle (Fig. 4). The probe is moved superiorly and laterally above the clavicle as required until the carotid arterial sound is heard. Arterial sounds have been described as being similar to a pistol shot. More lateral to the carotid is the characteristic venous hum of the internal jugular vein. This low frequency sound is often described as sounding like a windstorm. The location of the vein is marked with an indelible ink marker (Fig. 5). The vein is marked on dry skin just above the probe while the probe is being moved superiorly along the vein. The site is cleansed and sterilely draped prior to catheterization. Legler and Nugent [1] recorded the number of patients that required a single needle pass to correctly place a guide wire in the internal jugular vein using the Seldinger [9] technique. The success rate for single pass internal jugular cannulation increased to 78% using the Doppler from 28% without the Doppler as seen from Table 1.

Table 1. Patients having internal jugular cannulation.

	Single pass of needle	Multiple passes of needle	Total no. of patients	Single pass success rate
With Doppler	17	5	22	77.3% (54.6–92.2)*
Without Doppler	6	15	21	28.6% (11.3–52.2)

$\chi^2 = 10.24$, P = 0.0014. χ^2 (corrected) = 8.38; P < 0.005.
* 95% confidence intervals.

476

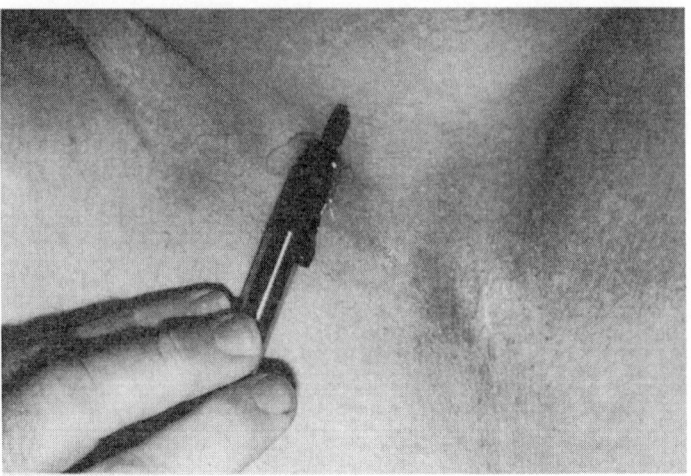

Fig. 4. Echocardiographic gel is placed above the clavicle over the medial border of the lateral (clavicular) head of the sternocleidomastoid muscle.

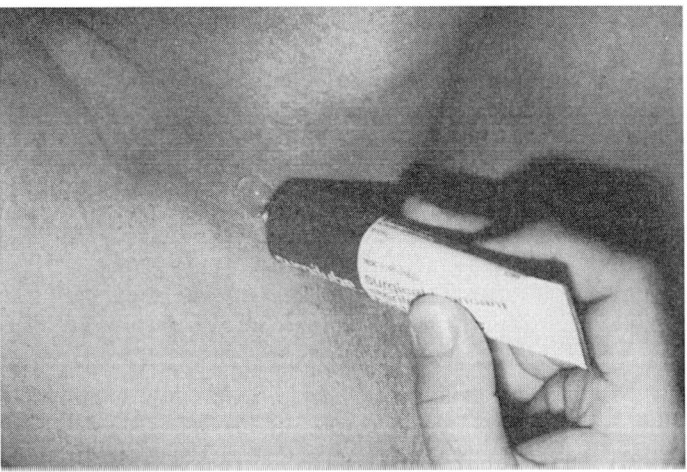

Fig. 5. The probe is held at a 45 degree angle to the surface of the skin and moved superiorly and laterally as required until the carotid arterial sound is heard. Lateral to the carotid sound is the characteristic venous hum of the internal jugular vein. The area above the gel is marked with an indelible ink marker delineating the direction of the internal jugular vein.

Less than three minutes were required in Legler's and Nugent's[1] studies for internal jugular cannulation.

Defalque [7] has described complications associated with the anatomic approaches to internal jugular cannulation. Included are pleural puncture, nerve damage, thoracic duct injury, and hematoma. Internal jugular cannulation is usually a benign procedure, however, fatal hemothorax and fatal hemorrhage have been reported [10]. The 28.6% of patients cannulated with a single pass in Nugent's control group compares favorably with the 43.3% noted in the report by Goldfarb and Lebrec [11] based on their experience with 1,000 patients. Goldfarb and Lebrec [11] also found that 42.7% of patients required three or more passes to cannulate the internal jugular vein using anatomic landmarks. The value of accurate localization of the internal jugular vein using the Doppler is apparent because minimizing the amount of needle exploration should result in a decreased complication rate.

Bazaral and Harlan's [12] ultrasonographic study of the neck has demonstrated other advantages of the Doppler technique. Bazaral [12] showed palpation of the right carotid just firmly enough to clearly feel the carotid pulse, significantly decreased the average size of the jugular and that rotation of the head brought the sternocleidomastoid anterior or medial to the internal jugular vein so that both palpation of the carotid and extreme rotation of the head produces anatomical changes that seem to make cannulation of the jugular difficult. Using the Doppler technique, palpation of the carotid during cannulation is not required.

Subclavian vein cannulation

The technique for Doppler-assisted subclavian vein puncture is that described by Petzoldt et al [2]. The patient lies flat on his back with the head turned to the left for right-sided cannulation. The Doppler probe is applied to the patient's skin below the clavicle and the beam is directed towards the area beneath and beyond the clavicle. The arterial sound is heard first and the probe is moved medially until the continuous low frequency respiratory dependant noise of the subclavian vein is heard. The maximum intensity of the Doppler signal occurs when the ultrasonic beam impinges fully on the blood vessel. This is the most convenient site and direction for venous puncture. Petzoldt [2] used an ultrasound directed puncture employed a needle guide mounted on the ultrasound receptor. He successfully performed 48 subclavian punctures in 50 patients.

Percutaneous radial artery cannulation

Chinyanga [4] used a modified Doppler probe as an aid to percutaneous radial artery cannulation in infants and small children. The modification narrowed the transmitted beam to a width approximating the vessel diameter allowing for a more accurate determination of vessel location. Chinyanga dorsiflexed the hand 30 to 40 degrees and moved the Doppler probe from lateral to medial over the radial artery until the arterial sound was heard clearly. The point of maximum intensity of the Doppler sound was established and a small skin incision was made 5 mm distal to the area where the arterial sound was localized. The angiocath was then introduced at an 15–20° angle. When the tip of the angiocath passes onto the Doppler prism, intensity of the Doppler sound is reduced and may become inaudible. Chinyanga and Smith had an 86.9% success rate in children for radial artery cannulation. Fifty-two percent of the cannulations were successful at the first attempt and 82.6% after a maximum of two attempts.

Table 2. Cannulation of the radial artery in infants and small children with the aid of the Doppler ultrasound device.

Number of patients	23
Age	2 months–4 years (mean 2.20 ± 1.36)
Weight	4.3–20 kg (mean 11.9 ± 4.41)
Total successes	20 (86.9 percent)
Success on 1 attempt	12 (52.1 percent)
Success on 1 and 2 attempts	19 (82.6 percent)

Jelenko and McKinley [3] used the Doppler to locate blood vessels in patients with shock or severe burn. They described using the Doppler for vessel location in patients whose vessels are difficult to find due to surrounding tissue edema. Jenklo and Chinyanga used the Doppler to cannulate brachial and axillary arteries as well as saphenous and brachial veins.

Monitoring complications of arterial catheterization

The Doppler has also been used to assess complications of brachial artery catheterization and other signs of arterial cannulation. Barnes [6] evaluated arterial injury in 100 patients who underwent cardiac catheterization. He found that brachial artery obstruction occurred in 18 patients using the criteria of diminished arterial sounds and decreased arterial blood pressure in the forearm. Two-thirds of the patients who demonstrated Doppler signs of brachial artery obstruction had either no symptoms or only transient symptoms of ischemia. The Doppler proved to be an effective guide to physiologic assessment of complications of arterial catheterization. The reports of brachial artery occlusion as a result of catheterization vary from 0.3% [13] to 65% [14]. Barnes states that 'many of the reported rates of brachial artery occlusion may be underestimated because of the collateral circulation around the elbow which may result in an asymptomatic extremity or even detectable distal pulses coexistant with brachial artery occlusion [6]. Long et al [15] described the use of the Doppler for continuous monitoring of arterial patency during cardiac catheterization. This technique requires positioning of the Doppler probe over a distal branch of the artery to be catheterized. The probe is positioned so that the pulse is continuously audible. The angiographer then has continuous information about the patency of blood flow in the vessel distal to the cannulation sight as well as an indication of the patient's heart rate and cardiac rhythm. Having this audible information available, the angiographer need not take his eye away from the patient.

In summary, the Doppler is useful in cannulating the internal jugular and subclavian veins; and in locating arteries and veins in infants, small children, patients with severe burns, and those in shock. It is also useful as a monitor of patency of arteries distal to sites of arterial catheterization.

References

1. Legler DW, Nugent M: Doppler localization of the internal jugular vein facilitates central venous cannulation. Anesthesiology 60: 481–482, 1984.
2. Petzoldt R, Lutz H, Ehler R, Kresse H, Kohl W: Puncture of veins and arteries assisted by ultrasound. Ultrasound Med Biol 2: 331–333, 1976.
3. Jelenko C, McKinley JC: The elusive artery: Found by sound. JACEP 5: 194, 1976.
4. Chinyanga HM, Smith JM: A modified Doppler flow detector probe – an aid to percutaneous radial arterial cannulation in infants and small children. Anesthesiology 50: 256–258, 1979.
5. Barnes RW, Foster EJ, Janssen A, Boutros AR: Safety of brachial arterial catheters as monitors in the intensive care unit – prospective evaluation with the Doppler ultrasonic velocity detector. Anesthesiology 44: 260–264, 1976.
6. Barnes RW, Petersen JL, Krugmire RB, Strandness DE: Complications of brachial artery catheterization: prospective evaluation with the Doppler ultrasonic velocity detector. Chest 66: 363–367, 1974.
7. Defalque RJ: Percutaneous catheterization of the internal jugular vein. Anesth Analg 53: 116–120, 1974.
8. Ullman JI, Stoelting RK: Internal jugular vein location with the ultrasound Doppler blood flow detector. Anesth Analg 57: 118, 1978.
9. Seldinger SI: Catheter replacement of the needle in percutaneous arteriorgraphy. Acta Radiol 39: 368–376, 1953.
10. McEnany MT, Austen WG: Life-threatening hemorrhage from inadvertent cervical arteriotomy. Ann Thorac Surg 24: 233–236, 1977.
11. Goldfarb G, Lebrec D: Percutaneous cannulation of the internal jugular vein in patients with coagulopathies: An experience based on 1,000 attempts. Anesthesiology 56: 321–323, 1982.
12. Bazaral M, Harlan S: Ultrasonographic anatomy of the internal jugular vein relevant to percutaneous cannulation. Crit Care Med 9: 307–310, 1981.
13. Braunwald E, Swan HJC: Cooperative study on cardiac catheterization. Circulation 37: 1–113, 1968.
14. Kottke BA, Fairbourn FJ II, Davis GD: Complication of aortography. Circulation 30: 843–847, 1964.
15. Long JA, Dunnick NR, Doppman JL: Doppler monitoring of arterial punctures. Radiology 134: 245, 1980.

PART 7: Stress Echocardiography

7.1. Exercise echocardiography

WILLIAM F. ARMSTRONG

Introduction

Coronary artery disease is a leading cause of morbidity and mortality in industrialized nations. A primary goal of modern cardiology is the detection of latent coronary artery disease before any of the permanent sequelae such as myocardial infarction become established. The primary method for large population screening and for evaluation of patients with chest pain syndromes is electrocardiographic monitoring during exercise. Using such a test myocardial ischemia is diagnosed if reproduction of chest pain with co-incident abnormalities of the electrocardiogram occur. Because of the sub-optimal accuracy of routine electrocardiographic monitoring, supplemental imaging is frequently employed in an effort to improve both the diagnostic yield and to obtain prognostic information. This imaging usually has taken form of either thallium perfusion imaging or radionuclide ventriculography [1–5]. More recently echocardiographic imaging has been performed at the time of exercise testing in an effort to obtain analagous information [6–23]. In this chapter we will briefly review the advantages and disadvantages of this technique, its validation with catherization and other imaging modalities, its accuracy in specific subsets of patients, and finally additional prognostic information in patients following acute myocardial infarction which can be obtained from exercise echocardiography.

Types of exercise echocardiography

The term 'stress echocardiography' refers to echocardiographic imaging in conjunction with some stimulus designed to provoke myocardial ischemia. The stress can be a form of exercise such as bicycle ergometry [6–8, 13, 14, 18, 19, 21] or treadmill exercise [9–12, 15, 16, 20, 22, 23], an increase in heart rate with atrial transesophageal pacing [24, 25], a pharmacologic manipulation such as dipyridamole infusion [26] or cold pressor stimulation [27]. This chapter will deal only with echocardiographic imaging in conjunction with exercise. The basic assumption underlying stress echocardiography

I. Cikes (ed.), *Echocardiography in Cardiac Interventions*, 483–494, 1989.

is that myocardial ischemia will result in abnormal ventricular wall motion, or abnormal global ventricular function, which can be detected and quantified using echocardiographic imaging.

Echocardiography has several advantages when compared to other imaging modalities. Perhaps its greatest advantage is its tremendous versatility, as not only ventricular wall motion and overall function, but also valvular structures, wall thickness, pericardial abnormalities, and all complications of coronary disease, such as aneurysm formation with or without thrombus, and papillary muscle dysfunction can be simultaneously assessed. Echocardiography is also portable, and, in comparison with other imaging techniques, relatively inexpensive. The test can be repeated at short intervals and has no known adverse effects. Qualitative results are available immediately and the equipment for quantitative assessment of global and segmental wall motion is becoming widely available at moderate cost. The major disadvantage of echocardiography is the presumed limited success of the examination, especially when dealing with patients at the time of exercise when excessive heart rate and respiratory rate may interfere with imaging. A second disadvantage is that echocardiography relies on the end-effect of ischemia and does not detect early metabolic abnormalities. Early reports of exercise echocardiography noted success rates of only 70–80% [6, 7]. More recent larger studies using modern scanning equipment consistently achieve success rates of 90% or greater in unselected patients [9, 11, 15, 20, 23].

Methodology

Exact protocols for performance of exercise echocardiograms vary with the laboratory in question. The protocol at Indiana University has been developed over a period of three years and involves the following procedure [9, 20]. The patient undergoes routine supine two-dimensional echocardiography in parasternal long and short axis views and in apical two and four chamber views. The optimal transducer positions are marked on the patient's chest. The patient is prepared for treadmill exercise including placement of electrocardiographic leads. Treadmill exercise is performed using a Modified Balke protocol [28] at which time heart rate, blood pressure, cardiac rhythm and electrocardiographic ST-segment and T-wave morphologies are continuously monitored. Exercise intensity is increased at three minute intervals. Exercise is terminated for any one of multiple end-points, including attainment of > 85% maximum age predicted heart rate, reproduction of the patient's usual symptoms, reduction in systolic blood pressure > 20mmHg, significant arrhythmias or development of dyspnea or non-cardiac symptoms precluding further exercise. At termination of the exercise the patient immediately steps off the treadmill, reassumes a supine left lateral position on a bed adjacent to the treadmill apparatus and the two-dimensional echocardiogram is repeated. Because of the proximity of the echocardiographic equipment to the treadmill apparatus, no more than 20 seconds is lost in transferring the patient for the post-exercise echocardiographic examination. The technician rapidly scans both the parasternal and apical windows using previously marked transducer positions.

Our analysis is dependent upon computer generated, digital continuous loop images of the heart [20]. This requires only one high quality cardiac cycle for analysis. As such, post exercise scanning time can be made as abbreviated as possible. The images are processed into a quad screen format whereby a continuous loop of each view at rest is displayed side-by-side with its immediate post-exercise counterpart for either qualitative or quantitative analysis.

Methods of analysis

Exercise echocardiograms can be analyzed by a variety of methods. The simplest involves a qualitative description of regional wall motion in predefined segments of the left ventricle as either being normal, hypokinetic, akinetic or dyskinetic. This assessment, in comparison with the resting view, gives information regarding deterioration of segmental ventricular wall motion with exercise. An abnormal response is defined as development of a new wall motion abnormality. In addition to the qualitative assessment, quantitative parameters of both global and regional wall motion can be determined. The simplest parameters include determination of fractional shortening at the base of the heart or cavity area change [10]. Using a variety of algorithms, including Simpson's rule, left ventricular ejection fraction can be calculated at rest and with exercise [15, 19, 21, 22]. Physiologic information can be added to these measurements and end-systolic pressure volume relationships determined [18]. By constructing multiple chords from a ventricular centroid, regional wall motion along any number of predefined radians can be determined and compared at rest and exercise.

Validation of the technique

Exercise echocardiography has been validated using a number of standards including radionuclide imaging and cardiac catheterization. Heng and coworkers have compared two-dimensional echocardiography and thallium redistribution and found good correlation between the presence of reversible

Table 1. Comparison of exercise echocardiography and thallium scintigraphy (n = 96).

	Sensitivity	Specificity	Overall accuracy	Positive predictive value
Exercise Echo	85%	71%	82%	91%
Thallium	84%	62%	79%	89%

left ventricular wall motion abnormalities and reversible thallium defects. Additionally there was a correlation between reduced exercise ejection fraction by echocardiography and reversible thallium defects [12]. We have previously compared the results of continuous loop exercise echocardiograms to thallium scintigraphy in a cohort of 96 patients who subsequently underwent coronary arteriography [11]. Echocardiograms were reviewed by blinded experienced echocardiographers and graded qualitatively for wall motion abnormalities which developed with exercise. Results of this study, which represents our earliest experience with post exercise echocardiography imaging are presented in Table 1. Overall accuracy of the two tests was virtually identical, and the additive value of either exercise echocardiography or thallium scintigraphy to the electrocardiogram with respect to improved diagnostic accuracy was identical. This cohort included patients with single and multivessel disease. As will be subsequently seen, accuracy is dependent on the extent of disease [17].

While thallium assesses myocardial perfusion abnormalities, radionuclide ventriculography analyzes left ventricular wall motion. This technique has also been compared to exercise echocardiography by a number of investigators. Visser, et al. compared radionuclide ejection fraction and wall motion analysis to similar data derived from exercise echocardiograms [13]. They concluded that the sensitivity of radionuclide ejection fraction and wall motion analysis was greater than that for two-dimensional echocardiography. The specificity of two-dimensional echocardiography was 92% in their study. In contrast to this, Limacher and colleagues from Houston compared exercise radionuclide ventriculography and exercise echocardiography in 41 patients evaluated as part of a larger study [15] (see below). The sensitivity for exercise two-dimensional echocardiography was 92% compared with only 71% for radionuclide ventriculography. These sensitivities are for the entire patient cohort. For patients with single, double and multivessel disease, exercise echocardiography was also more sensitive. The specificity of exercise echocardiography was 88% compared to 82% for radionuclide ventriculography.

The Limacher study comprised a total of 73 patients, all of whom underwent exercise echocardiography and coronary arteriography. Fifty-six of the 73 patients had coronary artery disease at cardiac catheterization. Their ejection fraction at rest was $56 \pm 13\%$ and fell to $53 \pm 16\%$ after exercise ($p < .01$). The combination of an abnormal ejection fraction response and/or development of wall motion abnormalities post-exercise yielded a sensitivity of 91% for exercise echocardiography with a specificity of 88%. Sensitivity was highest for those with three vessel disease (100%) and lowest for those with single vessel disease (64%). Patients with two vesselss disease had intermediate sensitivity (95%). These sensitivity and specificity calculations were based on the combination of ejection fraction response and wall motion analysis. Analysis of wall motion abnormalities alone reduced the accuracy of the test only minimally.

We have also examined the relationship of the accuracy of exercise echocardiography to the presence of single and multivessel coronary artery disease [17]. This study was performed in a cohort of 94 patients, 35 of whom had prior myocardial infarction. The sensitivity for detection of coronary disease in patients with multivessel disease was 96% in those with prior myocardial infarction and 89% in those without prior myocardial infarction. The sensitivities for detecting patients with single vessel disease were 100% and 76% for those with and without prior infarction respectively. Although the vast majority of patients with multivessel disease were identified as having coronary disease, exercise echocardiography specifically identified them as having multivessel disease in only 50% of cases (22/45). This phenomenon which has also been noted with radionuclide technique [1], probably arises because only the most jeopardized segment of myocardium is detected as abnormal when end-points such as chest pain or ischemic electrocardiographic changes are used. As with the study of Limacher, et al. [15] the greatest source of a false negative exercise echocardiogram was single vessel disease.

Clinical utility of exercise echocardiography

We have recently completed a detailed evaluation of the practical additive value of exercise echocardiography to routine treadmill exercise testing in a cohort of 95 patients subsequently studied with coronary arteriography [20]. In this study the exercise echocardiograms were compared to routine analysis of the treadmill electrocardiogram (Fig. 1). The latter were classified as being either normal, when a patient developed no chest pain or electrocardiographic changes; ischemic, when there was a combination of chest pain and ST-segment depression; or ambiguous, when asymptomatic ST-segment depression was seen, when ST-segments were uninterpretable because of baseline abnormalities, or when chest pain or atypical symptoms developed in the absence of electrocardiographic changes. Because this study was performed

488

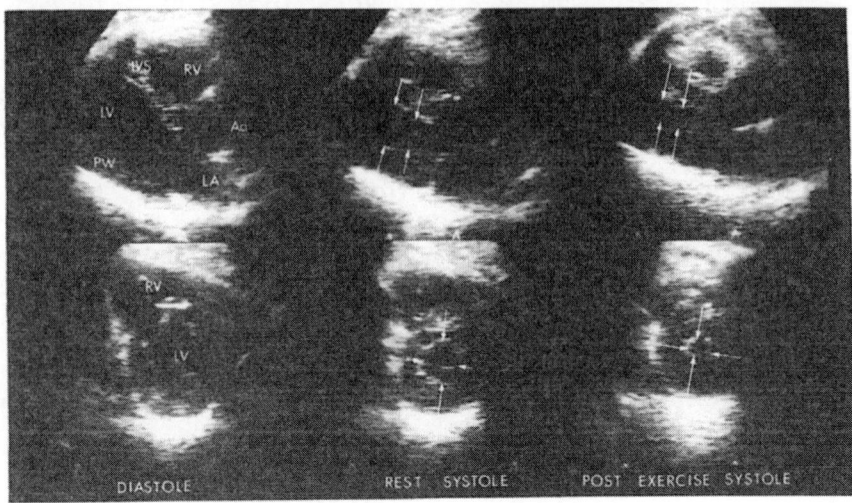

Fig. 1. Example of an exercise echocardiogram in a patient without coronary disease. The patient was a 54 year old hypertensive man with recent onset of exertional chest pain. He walked for 8 minutes on the treadmill before developing his usual chest pain associated with 3 mm of ST-segment depression. Echocardiograms in the long and short axis parasternal views are presented. There is normal systolic wall motion at rest (middle panel) and hyperdynamic wall motion (arrows) post exercise. The coronary arteries were normal at catheterization. (LV = left ventricle, LA = left atrium, RV = right ventricle, RA = right atrium, Ao = aorta, IVS = intraventricular septum, PW = posterior wall.)

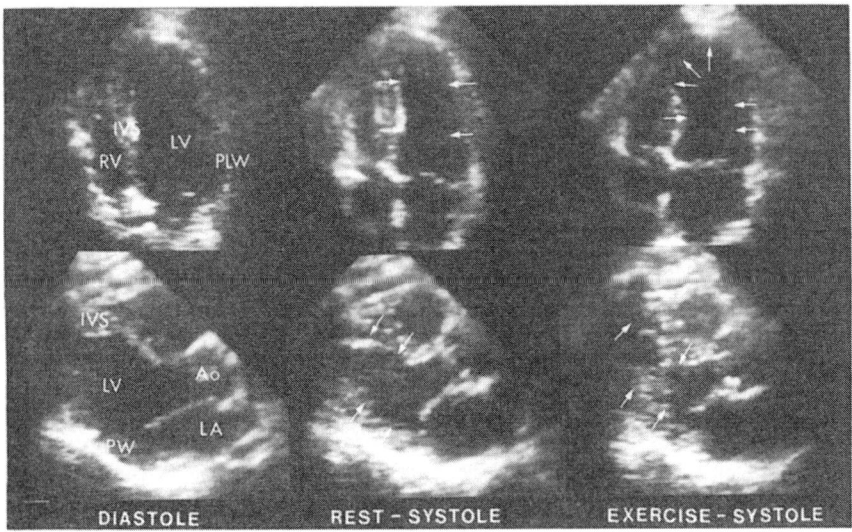

Fig. 2. Rest and post-exercise echocardiograms recorded in a patient without prior myocardial infarction. The parasternal long axis and apical four chamber views are presented. At rest wall motion is normal. Post-exercise the apex and distal anterior septum are akinetic. At catheterization a 95% lesion of the proximal left anterior descending coronary artery and a 60% lesion of the circumflex were found. Orientation and abbreviations are as in Fig. 1.

in a referral center, over a third of patients fell into this category of an ambiguous electrocardiographic response to treadmill exercise. The subset of 59 patients without clinical or electrocardiographic evidence of prior myocardial infarction is of particular interest in this subgroup (Fig. 2). In was in the subset of patients, with an ambiguous electrocardiographic response to treadmill exercise and without prior myocardial infarction, in whom exercise echocardiography was of greatest value. The exercise echocardiogram correctly classified 14/18 patients otherwise considered as non-diagnostic on the basis of routine treadmill exercise testing. Of the 20 patients with an ischemic treadmill response, 19 had coronary disease on angiography, 18 of whom had an abnormal exercise echocardiogram. Twenty-one patients had a normal symptomatic and electrocardiographic response to treadmill exercise, 13 of whom had coronary disease at subsequent angiography. Exercise echocardiography correctly identified nine of these patients as having myocardial ischemia as the basis of their presenting complaints.

In a comparison of the concordance of the two studies it was found that exercise echocardiography provided the correct diagnosis with regards to presence or absence of coronary disease in 48 patients. In this subgroup treadmill exercise provided the correct diagnosis in only 24, an incorrect diagnosis in 10 and was nondiagnostic in 14 patients. Exercise echocardiography provided incorrect information in 11 patients, only three of whom were correctly identified by analysis of the electrocardiogram at the time of treadmill exercise testing. It thus appeared that exercise echocardiography was superior to routine analysis of the exercise electrocardiogram for the diagnosis or exclusion of coronary disease.

False negative studies occurred most often in patients with single vessel disease. False positive exercise echocardiograms occurred in two patients with cardiomyopathy and resting segmental wall motion abnormalities which were also noted on contrast ventriculography. We have further evaluated the specificity of resting versus exercise induced wall motion abnormalities and found that the specificity of the latter for coronary disease is 100% for posterior wall and 97% for anterior wall motion abnormalities [16]. When mild resting abnormalities are considered as abnormal specificity decreases to 92% [16].

Prognostic information available from exercise echocardiogram

As noted above exercise echocardiography can be used for the detection of coronary disease. Additionally it may play a role for assessing its severity with regards to single versus multivessel disease. Obviously this latter observation when present bears some relation to patient prognosis, as those patients with preserved ventricular function and single vessel disease will have a better short and long term prognosis than those with multivessel lesions and poor left ventricular function [29, 30]. The specific ability of exercise echocardiography to determine prognosis following myocardial infarction has been investigated by three different groups [21–23]. Starling and his colleagues from San Antonio evaluated the role of left ventricular ejection fraction determined with echocardiography at the time of limited treadmill exercise in the convalescent period following myocardial infarction [21]. Detailed wall motion analysis was not undertaken in their study. They found by multivariant analysis that left ventricular ejection fraction < 40% at rest correlated with a higher likelihood of cardiac death over a one year followup. The combination of a reduced ejection fraction and an ischemic ST-segment response furthermore identified a smaller subgroup of specially high likelihood of early cardiac death.

A more detailed analysis has been undertaken by Jaarsma et al. from the Netherlands [22]. This group evaluated the role of limited exercise testing combined with two-dimensional echocardiographic imaging in 49 patients studied within three weeks of an index myocardial infarction. Because of preexisting myocardial infarction, wall motion abnormalities were present at rest in all patients. Remote transient wall motion abnormalities were present in 18 of the 49 patients following exercise. Within this subgroup, 17 had multivessel coronary disease. Only five of the remaining 25 without remote exercise induced wall motion abnormalities had multivessel disease. Sixteen patients experienced a new ischemic event on follow-up ranging from 8–12 weeks after discharge. A new exercise induced wall motion abnormality was present in 12 of the 16 patients (75%). These authors concluded that exercise echocardiography was of value in identifying patients with multivessel disease in the convalescent phase following myocardial infarction, or who were of high likelihood to suffer recurrent myocardial infarction or develop unstable angina. Ejection fractions were calculated in these patients as well but were of limited value in assessing patient prognosis.

We have recently completed a study of 40 patients also studied with immediate post exercise treadmill echocardiography in the convalescent phase following myocardial infarction [23]. Thirty patients had Q-wave infarctions and the remainder had non-Q-wave infarctions. The electrocardiogram in the monitored leads revealed abnormalities of the ST-segment or T-wave at rest in 37 of 40 patients (92.5%). The echocardiographic portion of the study included assessment of qualitative wall motion abnormalities at rest and following exercise as well as comparison of rest and post exercise ejection fraction. Followup at the time of data analysis ranged from 6–10 months with a mean 7.4 months. A positive exercise echocardiogram in this setting was defined as development of a new remote wall motion abnor-

491

mality post-exercise or worsening of multiple preexisting wall motion abnormalities (Fig. 3). A 'good' clinical outcome was seen in 20 patients, 19 of whom had a negative post-exercise echocardiogram defined by the above criteria. Twenty patients had a poor clinical outcome, prospectively defined as development of unstable angina, recurrent myocardial infarction, documentation of multiple vessel coronary disease at cardiac catheterization or cardiac death. The exercise echocardiogram was positive for remote or worsening wall motion abnormalities in 16 of these 20 patients (80% sensitivity for detection of adverse outcome). Exercise echocardiography was superior to routine analysis of a treadmill electrocardiogram in this patient population. Neither the resting nor post-exercise ejection fraction, or the change in ejection fraction, was of value in identifying patients likely to experience an adverse outcome in this series. There was disagreement between the treadmill electrocardiogram and echocardiographic results in 15 patients; the correct clinical outcome was predicted by results of echocardiography in 13 (87%) of these patients in which there was a discrepancy. In distinction to the low specificity for multivessel coronary disease in our stable patient population (noted previously) [17], exercise echocardiography correctly predicted the presence of multivessel disease in 14 of 15 post infarct patients (93%) subsequently studied with angiography. This study as well as that by Jaarsma et al. helps establish a role for exercise echocardiography in assessing prognosis following myocardial infarction.

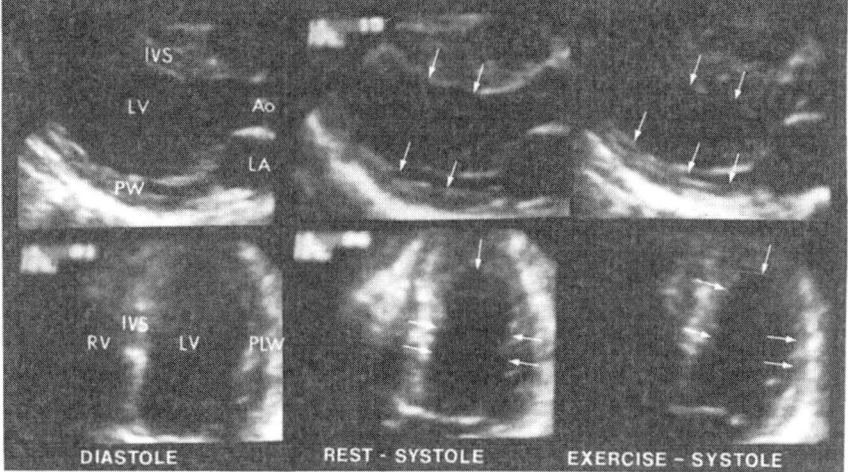

Fig. 3. Rest and post-exercise echocardiograms in a patient studied following an inferior myocardial infarction. The parasternal long axis and apical 4 chamber views are presented. At rest (middle pannel) the infero-posterior wall is akinetic and the posterolateral wall (4 chamber view) is hypokinetic. Post exercise the posterolateral wall becomes dyskinetic consistent with additional exercise induced ischemia.

492

Summary

Exercise echocardiography is an exciting new technique which is readily applicable in the majority of patients with known or suspected coronary artery disease. Its accuracy appears equivalent to that of routine planar thallium imaging and to radionuclide ventriculography. As with other imaging techniques its accuracy is highest in those patients with multivessel disease and lowest in those with single vessel disease. In experienced hands it adds valuable information to the analysis of the electrocardiogram at the time of treadmill exercise testing and may provide vital information in patients in the convalescent phase following myocardial infarction.

References

1. Rigo P, Bailey IK, Griffith LSC, et al.: Value and limitations of segmental analysis of stress thallium myocardial imaging for localization of coronary artery disease. Circulation 61: 973–981, 1980.
2. Kennedy JW: The detection of coronary artery disease with radionuclide techniques: a comparison of rest-exercise thallium imaging and ejection fraction response. Circulation 61: 610–619, 1980.
3. Osbakken MD, Okada RD, Boucher CA, Strauss HW, Pohost GM: Comparison of exercise perfusion and ventricular function imaging; an analysis of factors affecting the diagnostic accuracy of each technique. J Am Coll Cardiol 3: 272–283, 1984.
4. Port SC, Oshima M, Ray G, McNamee P, Schmidt DH: Assessment of single vessel coronary artery disease: results of exercise electrocardiography, thallium-201 myocardial perfusion imaging and radionuclide angiography. J Am Coll Cardiol 6: 75–83, 1985.
5. Maddahi J, Abdulla A, Garcia EV, Swan HJC, Bernman DS: Noninvasive identification of the left main and triple vessel coronary artery disease: improved accuracy using quantitative analysis of regional myocardial stress distribution and washout of thallium-201. J Am Coll Cardiol 7: 53–60, 1986.
6. Wann LS, Faris JV, Childress RH, Dillon JC, Weyman AE, Feigenbaum H: Exercise cross-sectional echocardiography in ischemic heart disease. Circulation 60: 1300–1308, 1979.
7. Morganroth J, Chen CC, David D, et al.: Exercise cross-sectional echocardiographic diagnosis of coronary artery disease. Am J Cardiol 47: 20–26, 1981.
8. Mason SJ, Weiss JL, Weisfeldt ML, Garrison JB, Fortuin NJ: Exercise echocardiography: detection of wall motion abnormalities during ischemia. Circulation 59: 50–59, 1979.
9. Robertson WS, Feigenbaum H, Armstrong WF, Dillon JC, O'Donnell J, McHenry PW: Exercise echocardiography: a clinically practical addition in the evaluation of coronary artery disease. J Am Coll Cardiol 2: 1085–1091, 1983.
10. Berberich SN, Zager JR, Plotnick GD, Fisher ML: A practical approach to exercise echocardiography: immediate postexercise echocardiography. J Am Coll Cardiol 3: 284–290, 1984.
11. West SR, Vasey CG, Armstrong WF et al.: Comparison of continuous loop exercise echocardiography and thallium scintigraphy for detection of coronary artery disease. Circulation 72 (Suppl III) 58, (abstract), 1985.

12. Heng MK, Simard M, Lake R, Udhoji VH: Exercise two-dimensional echocardiography for diagnosis of coronary artery disease. Am J Cardiol 54: 502–507, 1984.
13. Visser CA, VanderWieken RL, Kan G et al.: Comparison of two-dimensional echocardiography with radionuclide angiography during dynamic exercise for the detection of coronary artery disease. Am Heart J 106: 528–534, 1983.
14. Ginzton LE, Conant R, Brizendine M, Lee F, Mena I, Laks MM: Exercise subcostal two-dimensional echocardiography a new method of segmental wall motion analysis. Am J Cardiol 53: 805–811, 1984.
15. Limacher MC, Quinones MA, Poliner LR, Nelson JG, Winters WL, Waggoner AD: Detection of coronary artery disease with exercise two-dimensional echocardiography. Circulation 67: 1211–1218, 1983.
16. Vasey CG, Armstrong WF, Ryan T, McHenry PL, Feigenbaum H: Prediciton of the presence and location of coronary artery disease by digital exercise echocardiography. J Am Coll Cardiol 7: 15A (abstract), 1986.
17. Armstrong WF, O'Donnell J, Feigenbaum H: Exercise echocardiography: effect of prior myocardial infarction and extent of coronary disease on accuracy. J Am Coll Cardiol 10: 531–538, 1987.
18. Ginzton LE, Laks MM, Brizendine M, Conant R, Mena I: Noninvasive measurement of the rest and exercise peak systolic pressured/end systolic volume ratio; sensitive two-dimensional echocardiographic indicator of left ventricular function. J Am Coll Cardiol 4: 509–516, 1984.
19. Crawford MH, Amon KW, Vance WS: Exercise 2-dimensional echocardiography. Am J Cardiol 51: 1–6, 1983.
20. Armstrong WF, O'Donnell J, Dillon JC, McHenry PL, Morris SN, Feigenbaum H: Complimentary value of two-dimensional exercise echocardiography to routine treadmill exercise testing. Ann Intern Med. In press, 1986.
21. Starling MR, Crawford MH, Henry RL, Lembo NJ, Kennedy GT, O'Rourke RA: Prognostic value of electrocardiographic exercise testing and noninvasive assessment of left ventricular ejection fraction soon after acute myocardial infarction. Am J Cardiol 57: 532–537, 1986.
22. Jaarsma W, Visser CA, FunkeKupper AJ, Res JCJ, Van Eenige J, Roos JP: Am J Cardiol 57: 86–90, 1986.
23. Ryan T, Armstrong WF, O'Donnell JO, Feigenbaum H: Risk stratification following myocardial infarction using exercise echocardiography. Am Heart J 114: 1305–1316, 1987.
24. Chapman PD, Doyle TP, Troup PJ, Gross CM, Wann LS: Stress echocardiography with transesophageal atrial pacing: preliminary report of a new method of detection of ischemic wall motion abnormalities. Circulation 70: 445–450, 1984.
25. Iliceto S, D'Ambrosio G, Sorinio M, et al.: Comparison of postexercise and transesophageal atrial pacing two-dimensional echocardiography for detection of coronary artery disease. Am J Cardiol 57: 547–553, 1986.
26. Picano E, Distante A, Masini M, Morales MA, Lattanxi F, L'Abbate A: Dipyridamole-echocardiography test in effort angina pectors. Am J Cardiol 56: 452–456, 1985.
27. Gondi B, Nanda BC: Cold pressor test during two-dimensional echocardiography: usefulness in detection of patients with coronary disease. Am Heart J 107: 278–285, 1984.
28. McHenry PL, Phillips JS, Knoebel SB: Correlation of computer quantitated treadmill exercise electrocardiogram with arteriographic location of coronary artery disease. Am J Cardiol 30: 747–752, 1972.
28. McHenry PL, Phillips JS, Knoebel SB: Correlation of computer quantitated treadmill exercise electrocardiogram with arteriographic location of coronary artery disease. Am J Cardiol 30: 747–752, 1972.

29. Proudfit WJ, Bruschke AVG, MacMillan JP, Williams GW, Sones FM: Fifteen year survival of patients with obstructive coronary artery disease. Circulation 68: 986–997, 1983.
30. Cass Principal Investigators and their associates: Coronary artery surgery (CASS); a radomized trial of coronary artery bypass surgery. Circulation 68: 939–950, 1983.

7.2. Stress echocardiography with transesophageal atrial pacing

SABINO ILICETO & PAOLO RIZZON

Wall motion abnormalities (WMA) are a very sensitive and early marker of myocardial ischemia; they may be present at rest but are particularly evident during exercise. Therefore, various cardiac imaging techniques have recently been used to study left ventricular (LV) WMA induced either by spontaneous or stress-induced ischemia.

Two-dimensional echocardiography (2D Echo) is by far the most widely used form of cardiac imaging as compared to other methods. Its advantages include: 1) a relative low cost; 2) ease of execution and exam repeatibility; 3) the possibility, unique to this method, of displaying, in real time, sections of the heart in various tomographic planes.

Despite all this, while it is doubtlessly an ideal tool for studying LV kinetics in resting conditions, 2D Echo is less useful during physical exercise due to some technical drawbacks which make the exam difficult to carry out and interpret. Indeed, during physical exercise (in either the supine or upright position) using a bicycle ergometer or a treadmill, chest movements and, above all, hyperpnea limit the attainment of good quality standard tomographic planes for a sufficient number of consecutive cardiac cycles. In fact, due to frequent interposition of lung tissue, only a few consecutive cycles can be recorded making the interpretation of the images and the segmentary evaluation of the wall motion extremely hard. Moreover, not all patients can always reach adequate levels of physical exercise and at times there may even be contraindications. For these reasons several attempts have been made at replacing it with other sorts of stress which could both induce ischemia under various clinical conditions and be used in conjunction with 2D Echo [1–5].

Drug tests (ergonovine and dipyridamole), handgrip, and cold pressor test have all given satisfactory results in certain instances but, despite this, physical exercise has proven irreplaceable as a routine practice. Recently, the attention of some research groups has been directed towards atrial pacing. This technique was introduced in 1967 by Sowton [6] as a stress test to assess the presence and severity of coronary artery disease (CAD). Subsequently, several Authors proposed atrial pacing as a valid alternative to exercise [7–13]. Unlike this latter, during atrial pacing cardiac volumes decrease and blood pressure does not change significantly; therefore, in some cases, this

I. Cikes (ed.), *Echocardiography in Cardiac Interventions*, 495–508, 1989.
© 1989 *Kluwer Academic Publishers*.

496

stress does not allow one to obtain a rate-pressure product as high as that reached with physical exercise [14]. Despite these drawbacks, this stress has shown, especially if used in conjunction with cardiac imaging techniques [15–19], a diagnostic accuracy, in the detection of significant CAD, which is as good as that obtained during physical exercise.

Furthermore, atrial pacing is a very low risk stress test: it can even be used on patients unable to carry out adequate physical exercise or with contra-indications to it [12] because of the gradual and controlled increase in heart rate and myocardial oxygen demand and the immediate return to baseline haemodynamic conditions when stimulation ceases.

Despite these interesting aspects atrial pacing was not widely used in the past because of its invasive nature. Recently, transesophageal, non-invasive stable stimulation of the atria has been developed. Chapman [20] and our group [21–27] have suggested using transesophageal atrial pacing (TAP) together with two-dimensional echocardiography (TAP-2D Echo) as a stress test for studying ischemia-induced localized WMAs.

Transesophageal atrial pacing

Transesophageal atrial stimulation was proposed for the first time more than 30 years ago [28] exclusively for the diagnosis and treatment of arrhythmias. In subsequent years its routine utilization [29–32] was limited by lack of consistent atrial capture and patient discomfort resulting from high current requirements. Routine use of the transesophageal approach has recently become possible thanks to improvements in this technique [33–34].

Recent studies have, in fact, demonstrated that it is possible to minimize the intensity of the current needed to capture the atria and, consequently, patient discomfort by: 1) using a bipolar catheter with electrodes spaced approximately 30 mm apart; 2) finding the best positioning for the catheter (near the left atrium); 3) using long-lasting pulses of 10 msec. In our laboratory the catheters we use have 2 electrodes spaced 29 mm apart (Fig. 1). The catheter is introduced through the nares into the distal oeso-phagus (Fig. 2), then the proximal electrode is connected to the V1 lead of a standard electrocardiograph to find the best position, corresponding to the largest amplitude and most rapid deflection of the atrial electrogram. After sticking the proximal end of the catheter to the nose with a plaster, the electrodes are connected to the pacer with the cathode connected to the proximal electrode. We use either a commercially available instrument for transesophageal electrophysiologic studies or a simpler one, expressly built for the purpose, which can emit square wave pulses lasting up to 20 msec, amplitude up to 30 mA, at an increasing rate of up to 200 beats/min.

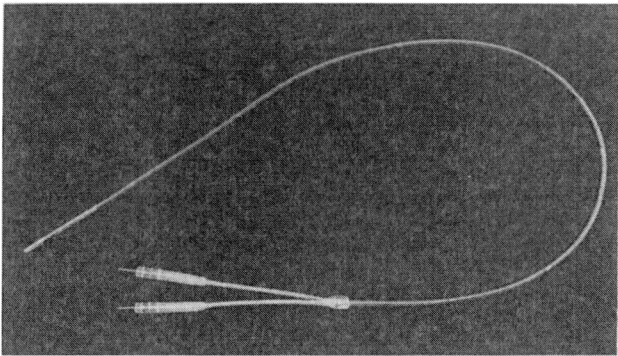

Fig. 1. Transesophageal bipolar catheter for atrial stimulation. The electrodes are spaced 29 mm apart.

A slow pacing rate is used at the beginning so as to be sure that the ventricle is not paced and to find the minimum current intensity which enables stable capture of the atria. Then the rate is gradually increased up to 150 b/min to identify those patients requiring atropine-sulfate (0.02 mg/kg i.v.) premedication because of low Wenckebach point. Then the pacing protocol is followed, starting at 110 b/min and slowly increasing the rate.

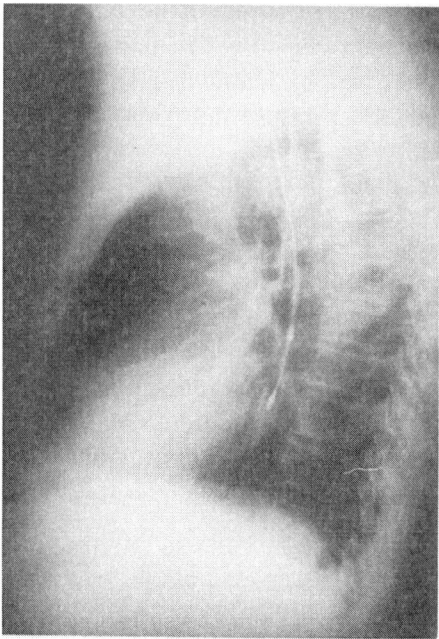

Fig. 2. Lateral chest X-ray in a patient in whom the transesophageal catheter has been inserted through the nares into the distal oesophagus.

Pacing is stopped if chest pain occurs or when the maximum heart rate of 150 b/min is reached. At high rates the Wenckebach phenomenon frequently appears and, in any case, the duration of the cycle shortens so much as to make an analysis of the wall motion very difficult with echocardiographic methods. We prefer to carry out the pacing in a continuous manner rather than stop it at each step because, in this way, more easily reproducible hemo-dynamic alterations are obtained [35], even if it becomes difficult to monitor any ST-segment change, because of artifacts induced by the stimulation.

Patients usually tolerate the whole procedure very well as long as they have been carefully told in advance to help by swallowing the transducer and as long as the aims and manner of the pacing have been adequately ex-plained. Only in some cases premedication with oral diazepam is necessary. Local anesthetics are not necessary to introduce the transducer. In a series of over 300 consecutive patients transesophageal stimulation was not obtained in 18% of cases. In some cases it was not possible to introduce the catheter because of abnormalities in the first part of the respiratory apparatus; in other cases stable atrial capture could not be obtained or the pacing was interrupted because of the appearance of a burning sensation in the epi-gastric or low retrosternal site. These disorders, when present, are generally slight, do not lead to interruption of the exam, and are easily distinguished from the chest pain often suffered by patients. We have never come across major complications during TAP except in the case of one patient with severe multivascular CAD who developed ventricular arrhythmias during the test, which quickly returned to normality without needing any drugs after stopping pacing. Homeral pressure does not change significantly during pacing or recovery.

2D Echo during TAP

Exam recording

After inserting and positioning the transducer and after evaluating the pacing efficiency and deciding whether or not atropine premedication is advisable, a standard echocardiogram is done in basal conditions. Pacing is then begun, monitoring the ECG and humeral arterial pressure and recording the apical 4-chambers, 2-chambers and long axis views at the end of each step. By means of these views, it is possible to obtain images of sufficiently good quality in most patients.

Two-dimensional echocardiographic exams are in no way affected by TAP. The patient lies preferably in the left lateral decubitus. In this way he does not hyperventilate and is ready for all the time needed to record an adequate number of cardiac cycles in all the tomographic planes at each pacing step. In our experience, in no case was image quality worse during the execution of the test than during rest conditions. The whole procedure, from the introduction of the transducer to the end of pacing and recording, usually takes no longer than 20 minutes. Only one doctor assisted by a nurse is needed.

Reading the exam

In a large proportion of coronary patients, during atrial pacing new WMAs appear. The main information that the test supplies concerns the site, severity and extent of these abnormalities. Since wall motion evaluations are both subjective and qualitative, we have evaluated the influence of inter- and intra-observer variability in interpreting the test [21]. We have found that even when interpreting images obtained at the maximum pacing rate there is a good degree of agreement both between two observers and among evaluations made by the same observer. In particular, we have never come across a disagreement greater than one index of the semiquantitative evaluation scale we use (diskinesia, akinesia, hypokinesia, normokinesia).

Sensitivity and specificity

Using the presence of WMAs during pacing as the criterion for a positive test, we found a sensitivity of 78% and specificity of 85% in a series of more than 200 consecutive patients without prior myocardial necrosis.

Sensitivity decreases to 60% in patients with single vessel disease and to 75% in coronary patients with normal ventricular wall motion during basal conditions. In these patients, who are the most difficult to diagnose because of less severe CAD and normal LV function at rest, diagnostic sensitivity is still acceptable.

The diagnostic accuracy of TAP-2D Echo proved to be greater than that of the exercise ECG (Fig. 3) and comparable to that of post-exercise 2D Echo [23] (Fig. 4).

Our findings therefore support Heller's [15] and McKay's [19] data which show that both ECG changes and perfusion defects induced by atrial pacing compare favourably with those produced by exercise testing.

500

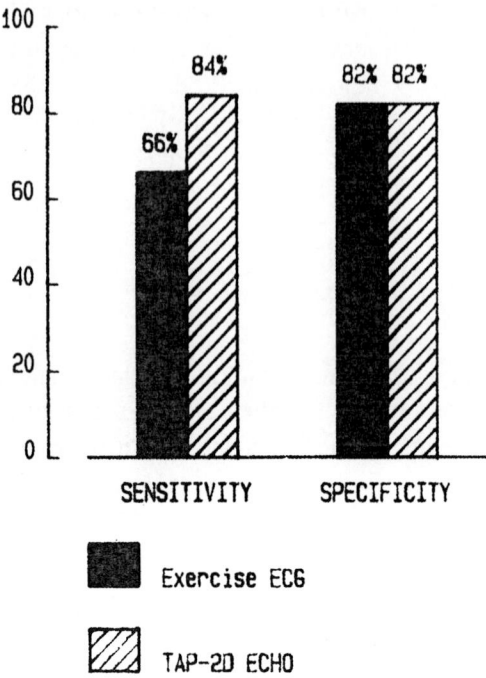

Fig. 3. Sensitivity and specificity of transesophageal atrial pacing (TAP) – two-dimensional echocardiography (2D-Echo) and exercise electrocardiography (ECG) in the detection of coronary artery disease (CAD) in 117 patients without previous myocardial infarction.

Severity and extent of WMAs

Various studies have shown that the severity of ischemia-induced LV functional deterioration is greater in patients with multivessel CAD than in those with single-vessel disease [36–37]. Moreover, it has been shown that, even in patients with single-vessel disease both the site and severity of the stenoses affect the type of ventricular response to stress [38–39]. The severity and extent of WMAs induced by pacing are also correlated with the severity and extent of CAD [25]. We have been able to check this by quantifying both the severity of CAD by a coronary score [36], and the severity of LV WMAs by a wall motion score. This was done by dividing the LV into 9 segments and giving each of them a score corresponding to a semiquantitative judgment of wall motion [21].

We have found a significant correlation between wall motion score during pacing and coronary score, supporting the empirical observation that the most serious and extensive wall motion alterations during pacing are usually detected in patients with more severe CAD.

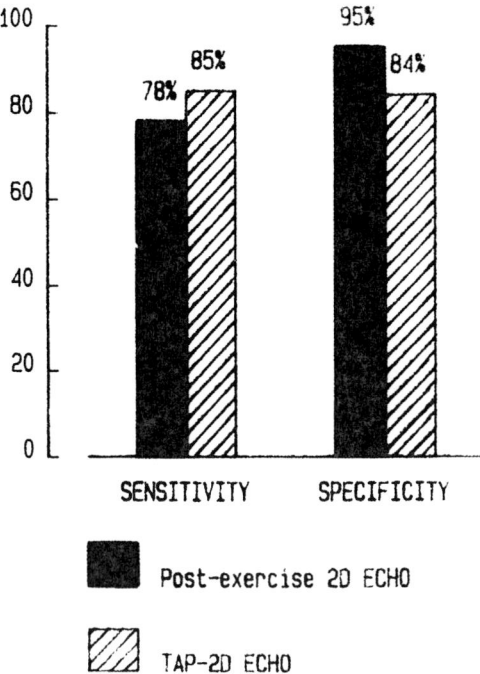

Fig. 4. Sensitivity and specificity of transesophageal atrial pacing (TAP) – two-dimensional echocardiography (2D`Echo) and post-exercise echocardiography in the detection of coronary artery disease (CAD) in 78 patients [23].

Onset of WMAs

2D Echo is the only cardiac imaging technique commonly used in clinical practice which enables a real and correct monitoring of ventricular wall motion throughout the entire length of a stress-inducing test. We have thus been able to verify that the WMAs observed at the maximum pacing rate often appear at lower rates and worsen over the course of the test.

Figure 5 summarizes the observations on a group of 33 patients with CAD and normal ventricular wall motion at rest (unpublished data). As one can see, the patients with multivessel disease develop WMAs which are more severe and which start at lower pacing levels. In particular, 24 out of 33 patients develop WMAs at rates of less than 110 or 120 b/min. Of these, 19 had multivessel disease and 5 had single-vessel disease (4 out of these 5 had critical proximal stenoses of the left anterior descending artery).

502

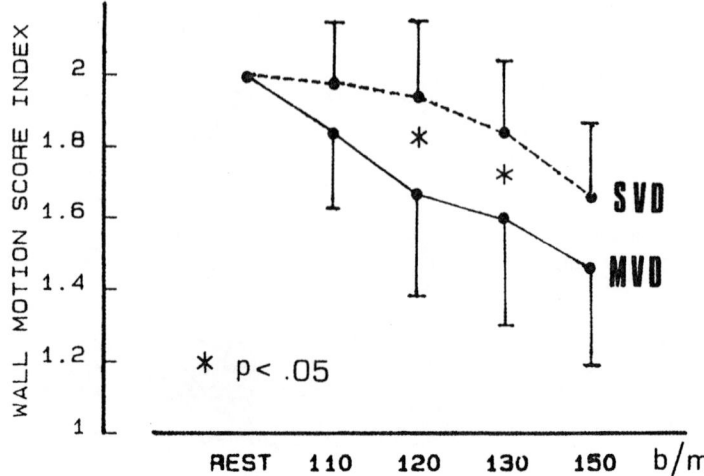

Fig. 5. Wall motion score index (WMSI) at rest and at four steps of atrial pacing in patients with single-vessel disease (SVD) and 22 patients with multivessel disease (MVD).

Correlation between WMA site and CAD distribution

An analysis of the distribution of WMAs gives some indications as to the area of the heart affected by CAD. We have analyzed the segmentary motility in 119 consecutive patients without previous myocardial infarction. These patients were subjected to diagnostic 2D Echo during TAP and selective coronary angiography (unpublished data). The LV was divided into 9 segments arbitrarily grouped into 2 vascular territories: anterior, tributary of the left anterior descending artery (including anterior wall, septum and apex) and posterior, depending on the circumflex and the right coronary (including diaphragmatic and lateral wall). For each segment we calculated: 'sensitivity' taken as percentage of pathological segments in patients with critical coronary stenosis in the corresponding vascular territory and 'specificity' taken as percentage of normokinetic segments in patients without critical coronary stenosis in the corresponding territories.

In the presence of coronary stenosis on the left anterior descending artery, the segments most frequently affected by WMAs are those of the interventricular septum. When right coronary and/or circumflex lesions are present the most affected segments are those of the diaphragmatic wall. The lateral wall is only rarely the site of WMAs. Furthermore, there is a low specificity of abnormalities appearing in the posterobasal segment: this is very probably due to a relatively greater difficulty in interpreting the wall motion of this segment, especially in the case of hypokinesis.

Clinical applications of TAP-2D Echo

The large amount of information supplied by TAP-2D Echo on ischemic LV contractility can be used in clinical practice for the routine evaluation of patients with CAD. We have been using this test for 3 years and, in our experience, it has been particularly useful for the detection [22–23] and evaluation [25] of CAD, for the postoperative evaluation of patients after bypass surgery [26] and in the prognostic evaluation of patients with acute myocardial infarction [24].

Detection of CAD

TAP 2-D Echo presents a good diagnostic accuracy [27], greater than that of exercise ECG and comparable to that of exercise echocardiography. However, it does not replace the abovesaid methods in clinical practice.

Atrial pacing is, in fact, an artificial stress that does not reproduce the alterations of real life and which, even if done transesophageally, still does have a minimum degree of invasivity. Therefore, for CAD diagnosis, pacing must be seen as an alternative stress to be used when exercise tests cannot be carried out or interpreted. TAP-2D Echo is particularly useful: 1) in patients unable to reach an adequate level of physical exercise for muscular-skeletal or cardiovascular reasons; 2) in patients whose exercise ECG is not interpretable because of the presence of non-specific ST-changes; 3) in patients whose echocardiographic images obtained during or after exercise are not of a sufficiently good quality to enable one to correctly evaluate the ventricular wall motion.

Evaluation of the effect of coronary artery bypass surgery

Several studies have demonstrated that coronary artery bypass surgery improves overall and regional left ventricular function during exercise [40–43]. This beneficial effect is particularly evident in those patients in whom a greater impairment of left ventricular function occurs during exercise [42]. Therefore, preoperative evaluation of LV function during exercise is useful not only for the assessment of the effect of surgical revascularization, but also for the identification of those patients who have a good LV function at rest but present a viable myocardium at jeopardy and are, therefore, more likely to benefit from coronary artery bypass surgery.

However, preoperative exercise evaluation is not always obtainable because in some patients it is contraindicated, inadequate or not perform-

504

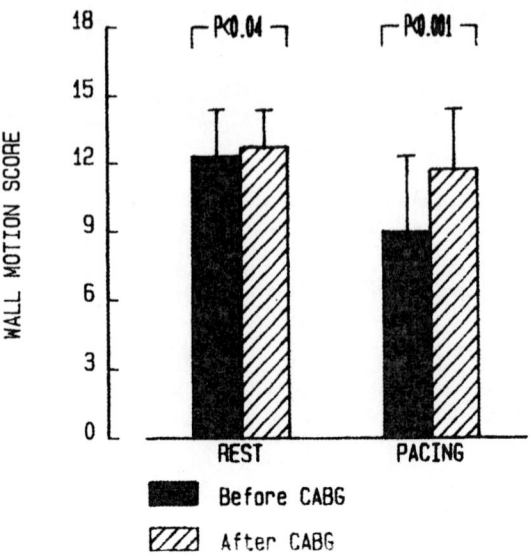

Fig. 6. Wall motion score at rest and during pacing, before and after coronary artery bypass grafting (CABG).

able. In these cases an alternative stress such as pacing can be very useful.

Moreover, atrial pacing has the advantage over physical exercise that it produces an easily-reproducible stress level since it is independent of the patient's general physical conditions and his/her tolerance to exercise. This aspect is particularly important in comparative studies for evaluating the effects of drug or surgical interventions. Our experience is currently based on 35 patients who underwent TAP-2D Echo before and one month after surgery [26].

Figure 6 shows LV wall motion score (WMS) before and after surgery, at rest and during pacing. One can see how there have been no significant variations in resting wall motion while there is a considerable improvement in ventricular contractility during pacing.

Moreover, the behaviour of the WMS during pacing correlated with clinical and electrocardiographic data. All 27 patients in whom the atrial pacing WMS improved or remained normal after surgery had neither chest nor ischemic electrocardiographic changes during exercise testing, although 13 of them had angina and 19 ST depression in preoperative studies; conversely, 5 of the 8 patients with a decreased or unchanged atrial pacing WMS had either angina or ST depression during physical exercise.

Identification of patients with myocardial infarction and multi-vessel disease

Most complications of myocardial infarction occur in the first year after the acute event. Clinical and laboratory data obtainable from survivors on their hospital discharge have been utilized to identify high risk patients who might be usefully submitted to agressive diagnostic procedures and therapeutic interventions. The presence and extent of additional myocardium at risk is a good indicator of future cardiac events and can be detected by means of exercise electrocardiography and myocardial scintigraphy [44–52].

However, in myocardial infarction survivors, exercise testing is not always performable [51–52] because of physical limitations or contraindications such as early post-infarction angina and congestive heart failure. Because of such limitations approximately 20–30% of all patients surviving a myocardial infarction cannot be appropriately evaluated although these patients are the most likely to have future cardiac events. In these patients atrial pacing can be safely performed and provides accurate prognostic information [12].

In patients without contraindications to early exercise testing, atrial pacing is at least as accurate, for diagnostic purposes, as physical exercise [11].

We submitted a series of 62 patients with first myocardial infarction to TAP-2D Echo, before coronary angiography.

Asinergy in regions 'remote' from infarcted myocardium was observed in 75% of patients with multi-vessel disease but also in 52% of patients with single-vessel disease. This diagnostic accuracy is not excellent, but similar to that reported by Morris [48] who used exercise nuclear ventriculography. If the test is used for diagnostic purposes, however, the low specificity must not be considered an important limit since, as Gibson [47] has recently demonstrated, coronary angiographic results are less predictive of future cardiac events than the evaluation of the extent of stress-induced ischemic myocardium. Therefore, it is not unlikely that information obtained with TAP 2D-Echo can also be satisfactorily utilized for prognostic stratification, independently of coronary angiographic data.

References

1. Mitamura H, Ogawa S, Hori S, Yamazaki H, Handa S, Nakaruma Y: Two-dimensional echocardiographic analysis of wall motion abnormalities during handgrip exercise in patients with coronary artery disease. Am J Cardiol 48: 711–719, 1981.
2. Kurtz RG, Lemire MS, Chene R, Stacewicz M, Pitt B: Cold pressor test echocardiography. (Abstr.) Am J Cardiol 47: 453, 1981.
3. Gondi B, Nanda N: Cold pressor test during two-dimensional echocardiography: usefulness in detection of patients with coronary disease. Am Heart J 107: 278–285, 1984.
4. Bernstein RF, Grossman RG, Child JS, Krivokapich J, Thessonboom S: Isoproterenol

506

stress echocardiography: a new method for detecting coronary artery disease. (Abstr.) Circulation 70: II-184, 1984.

5. Picano E, Distante A, Masini M, Morales MA, Lattanzi F, L'Abbate A: Dipyridamole-Echocardiography test in effort angina pectoris. Am J Cardiol 56: 452–456, 1985.

6. Sowton GE, Balcon R, Gross G, Frick MH. Measurement of the angina threshold using atrial pacing. Cardiovasc Res 1: 301–7, 1967.

7. Hecht HS, Chew CY, Burnam M, Schnugg SJ, Hopkins JM, Singh BN: Radionuclide ejection fraction and regional wall motion during atrial pacing in stable angina pectoris: comparison with metabolic and hemodynamic parameters. Am Heart J 101: 726–33, 1981.

8. Tzivoni D, Benhorin J, Keren A, Gottlieb S, Stern S: Comparison of right atrial pacing soon after myocardial infarction with treadmill testing 6 months later. Am J Cardiol 49; 1594–99, 1982.

9. Markham RV Jr, Winniford MD, Firth BG, Nicod P, Dehmer GJ, Lewis SE, Hillis LD: Symptomatic, electrodcardiographic, metabolic, and hemodynamic alterations during pacing induced myocardial ischemia. Am J Cardiol 51: 1589–94, 1983.

10. Arbogast R, Bourassa MG: Myocardial function during atrial pacing in patients with angina pectoris and normal coronary arteriograms. Am J Cardiol 32: 257–63, 1973.

11. Tzivoni D, Gottlieb S, Keren A, Benhorin J, Chenzbraun A, Waksman R, Stern S: Early right atrial pacing after myocardial infarction. I. Comparison with early treadmill testing. Am J Cardiol 53: 414–7, 1984.

12. Tzivoni D, Gottlieb S, Keren A, Benhorin J, Chenzbraun A, Klein J, Stern S: Early right atrial pacing after myocardial infarction. II. Results in 77 patients with predischarge angina pectoris, congestive heart failure, or age older than 70 years. Am J Cardiol 53: 418–20, 1984.

13. Tzivoni D, Keren A, Gottlieb S, Granot C, Benhorin J, Gazala E, Golhman J, Stern S: Right atrial pacing soon after myocardial infarction. Circulation 65: 330–5, 1982.

14. Slutsky R, Watkins J, Peterson K, Karliner J: The response of left ventricular function and size to atrial pacing, volume loading and afterload stress in patients with coronary artery disease. Circulation 63: 864, 1981.

15. Heller GV, Aroesty JM, McKay RG, Silverman KJ, Come PC, Kolodny GM, Grossman W. The pacing stress test: thallium-201 myocardial imaging after atrial pacing. Diagnostic value in detecting coronary artery disease compared with exercise testing. JACC 3: 1197–205, 1984.

16. Tobis J, Nalcioglu O, Johnston WD, Seibert A, Iseri LT, Roeck W, Henry WL: Digital angiography in assessment of ventricular function and wall motion during pacing in patients with coronary artery disease. Am J Cardiol 51: 668–75, 1983.

17. Johnson RA, Wasserman AG, Leiboff RH, Katz RJ, Bren GB, Varghese PJ, Ross AM: Intravenous digital left ventriculography at rest and with atrial pacing as a screening procedure for coronary artery disease. JACC 2: 905–10, 1983.

18. Mancini GBJ, Petersonf KL, Gregoratos G, Higgins CB: Effects of atrial pacing on global and regional left ventricular function in coronary heart disease assessed by digital intravenous ventriculography. Am J Cardiol 53: 456–61, 1984.

19. McKay RG, Aroesty JM, Heller GV, Silverman KJ, Parker JA, Als AV, Come P, Kolodny GM, Grossman W: The pacing stress test reexamined: correlation of pacing-induced hemodynamic changes with the amount of myocardium at risk. JACC 3: 1469–81, 1984.

20. Chapman PD, Doyle TP, Troup PJ, Gross CM, Wann SL: Stress echocardiography with transesophageal atrial pacing: preliminary report of a new method for detection of ischemic wall motion abnormalities. Circulation 70: 445, 1984.

21. Iliceto S, Sorino M, D'Ambrosio G, Papa A, Favale S, Rizzon P: Detection of coronary

artery disease by 2-dimensional echocardiography during transesophageal atrial pacing: sensitivity and specificity. (abstr.) Circulation 70 (Suppl. II): 185, 1984.

22. Iliceto S, Sorino M, D'Ambrosio G, Papa A, Favale S, Biasco G, Rizzon P: Detection of coronary artery disease by two-dimensional echocardiography and transesophageal atrial pacing. J Am Coll Cardiol 5: 1188–97, 1985.

23. Iliceto S, D'Ambrosio G, Sorino M, Papa A, Amico A, Ricci A, Rizzon P: Comparison of post exercise and transesophageal atrial pacing two-dimensional echocardiography for detection of coronary artery disease. Feasibility, specificity and sensitivity. Am J Cardiol 57: 547–553, 1986.

24. Iliceto S, Sorino M, D'Ambrosio G, Lopriore V, Ricci A, Papa A, Amico A, Chiddo A, Rizzon P: Atrial pacing in the detection and evaluation of coronary artery disease. Eur Heart Journal 7 (suppl C): 59–67, 1986.

25. Papa A, Iliceto S, D'Ambrosio G, Sorino M, Graziadei R, Rizzon P: Value of wall motion abnormalities during atrial pacing in the prediction of the extent of coronary artery disease (abstr.). Eur Heart Journal 6: 14, 1985.

26. Iliceto S, Ricci A, Lopriore V, Papa A, Bortone S, Antonelli A, Chiddo A, Rizzon P: Atrial pacing-induced wall motion abnormalities. Improvement after coronary artery by-pass graft surgery. (abstr.) Circulation 72: III-354, 1985.

27. Iliceto, S, Sorino M, D'Ambrosio G, Papa A, Amico A, Rizzon P: Wall motion abnormalities induced by atrial pacing in patients with suspected coronary artery disease. Analysis of 176 cases studied by 2D Echo during transesophageal atrial pacing (abstr.) Eur Heart Journal 6: 124, 1985.

28. Zoll PM: Resuscitation of the heart in ventricular standstill by external electrical stimulation. JAMA 247; 768–71, 1952.

29. Burack B, Furman S: Transesophageal cardiac pacing. Am J Cardiol 23: 469–72, 1969.

30. Rowe GG, Terry W, Neblett I: Cardiac pacing with an esophagal electrode. Am J Cardiol 24: 548–50.

31. Lubell DL: Cardiac pacing from the esophagus. Am J Cardiol 27: 641–44, 1971.

32. Gallagher JJ, Smith WM, Kasell J, Smith WM, Grant AO, Benson DW: The use of the esophageal lead in the diagnosis of mechanisms of reciprocating supraventricular tachycardia. Pace 3: 440–444, 1980.

33. Gallagher JJ, Smith WM, Kerr CR, Kasell J, Cook L, Reiter M, Sterba R, Harte M: Esophageal pacing: a diagnostic and therapeutic tool. Circulation 65: 336–41, 1982.

34. Benson DW, Sanford M, Dunnigan A, Benditt D: Transesophageal atrial pacing threshold: role of interelectrode spacing, pulse width and catheter insertion depth. Am J Cardiol 53: 63–7, 1984.

35. Thadani U, Lewis JR, Mathew TM, West RO, Parker JO. Reproducibility of clinical and hemodynamic parameters during pacing stress testing in patients with angina pectoris. Circulation 60: 1036–44, 1974.

36. De Pace NL, Iskandrian AS, Hakki A, Kane SA, Segal BL: Value of left ventricular ejection fraction during exercise in predicting the extent of coronary artery disease. J Am Coll Cardiol 1: 1002–1010, 1983.

37. Johnson LL, McCarthy DM, Sciacca RR, Cannon PJ: Right ventricular ejection fraction during exercise in patients with coronary artery disease. Circulation 60; 1284, 1979.

38. Leong K, Jones RH: Influence of the location of left anterior descending coronary artery stenosis in left ventricular function during exercise. Circulation 65: 109–114, 1982.

39. De Pace NL, Iskandrian AS, Nadell R, Colby J, Hakky A: Variation in the size of jeopardized moycardium in patients with isolated left anterior descending coronary artery disease. Circulation 67: 988, 1983.

508

40. Huikuri HV, Korhonen UR, Linnaluoto MK, Takkunen JT. Effect of coronary artery bypass grafting on left ventricular response to isometric exercise. Am J Cardiol 54: 514–8, 1984.

41. Rahimtoola SH. Postoperative exercise response in the evaluation of the physiologic status after coronary bypass surgery. Circulation 65 (suppl. II): 106–14, 1982.

42. Barry WH, Pfeifer JF, Lipton MJ, Tilkian AG, Hultgren HN. Effects of coronary artery bypass grafting on resting and exercise hemodynamics in patients with stable angina pectoris: a prospective, randomized study. Am J Cardiol 37: 823–30, 1976.

43. Freeman MR, Gray RJ, Berman DS, Maddahi J, Raymond MJ, Forrester JS, Matloff JM: Improvement in global and segmental left ventricular function after coronary bypass surgery. Circulation 64 (suppl. II): 34–9, 1981.

44. Markiewicz H, Houston N, DeBusk RF. Exercise testing soon after myocardial infarction. Am J Cardiol 56: 26-31, 1977.

45. Theroux P, Waters DD, Halphen O, Debaisieux JC, Mizgala HT. Prognostic value of exercise testing soon after myocardial infarction. N Engl J Med 301: 341–5, 1979.

46. Gibson RS, Watson DD, Craddock GB, Crampton RS, Kaiser DL, Denny MJ, Beller GA: Prediction of cardiac events after uncomplicated myocardial infarction: a prospective study comparing predischarge exercise thallium-201 scintigraphy and coronary angiography. Circulation 68: 321–36, 1983.

47. Gibson RS, Taylor GJ, Watson DD, Stebbins PT, Martin RP, Crampton RS, Beller GA. Predicting the extent and location of coronary artery disease during the early post-infarction period by quantitative thallium201 scintigraphy. Am J Cardiol 47: 1010–8, 1981.

48. Morris DD, Rozanski A, Berman DS, Diamond GA, Swan HJC: Non invasive prediction of the angiographic extent of coronary artery disease after myocardial infarction: comparison of clinical, bicycle exercise electrocardiographic, and ventriculographic parameters. Circulation 70; 192–201, 1984.

49. Nicod P, Corbett JR, Firth BG, Lewis SE, Rude RE, Huxley R, Willerson JT. Prognostic value of resting and submaximal exercise radionuclide ventriculography after acute myocardial infarction in high-risk patients with single and multivessel disease. Am J Cardiol 52: 30–6, 1983.

50. Turner JD, Schwartz KM, Logic JR, Sheffield LT, Kansal S, Rortman PI, Mantle JA, Russel RO, Rackley CE, Rogers WJ: Detection of residual jeopardized myocaridum 3 weeks after myocardial infarction by exercise testing with tallium-201 myocardial scintigraphy. Circulation 61: 729–35, 1980.

51. Fioretti P, Brower RW, Simoons ML, Bos RJ, Baardman T, Beelen A, Hugenholtz PG: Prediction of mortality during the first year after acute myocardial infarction from clinical variables and stress test hospital discharge. Am J Cardiol 55: 1313–8, 1985.

52. Krone RJ, Gillespie JA, Weld FM, Miller PJ, Moss AJ: Multicenter Postinfarction Research Group. Low-level exercise testing after myocardial infarction: usefulness in enhancing clinical risk stratification. Circulation 71: 80–9, 1985.

7.3. Stress Doppler echocardiography

STEVE M. TEAGUE & JAMES A. HEINSIMER

Introduction

Perhaps the most serious intervention a cardiologist can recommend to
patients under his care is cardiac surgery. Doppler ultrasound has proven
merit in identifying patients with critical mitral and aortic stenosis, as well as
severe aortic regurgitation who may warrant such intervention [1, 2, 3].
However, the most common complaint that patients bring to a clinical cardiologist is that of chest pain, mandating that the presence and severity of
coronary artery disease be established. It is the purpose of this chapter to
introduce the emerging role of Doppler ultrasound in the identification and
classification of patients with coronary artery disease by stress testing. The
merit of Doppler examination during stress testing lies in the ability to quantitate ventricular function by noninvasive measurement of velocity, acceleration, and volume of blood leaving the left ventricle during systolic ejection.

Velocity and acceleration as indices of ventricular function

Electrokymographic studies by Ring and colleagues in the early 1950's were
among the first to suggest that the rate of ejection of blood into the aorta
could detect abnormal cardiac function. Rudewald used a direct technique to
measure the instantaneous acceleration of blood in the human aorta, showing
a decrease in the instantaneous acceleration of blood with increasing age [4].
Rushmer was first to report ventricular performance correlates of ascending
aortic flow acceleration and peak velocity in coronary models. Utilizing
canines instrumented with electromagnetic blood flow cuffs surrounding the
ascending aorta, Rushmer observed dramatic and immediate decrements in
ascending aorta ejection velocity and acceleration following the ligation of
coronary arteries [5]. Similarly, Kezdi and co-workers examined ventricular
ejection during myocardial infarction in an animal model and found that
aortic flow velocity and mean acceleration decreased by 16% and 23%
respectively as a result of myocardial infarction [6]. Other canine studies
showed increases in peak acceleration and velocity of ejection following

I. Cikes (ed.), *Echocardiography in Cardiac Interventions*, 509–520, 1989.

calcium gluconate, ouabain, or isoproterinol infusion [7, 8]. Increases in maximal acceleration and velocity correlated with a rise in left ventricular maximal dp/dt as well as the maximal velocity of circumferential left ventricular fiber shortening.

Early studies in man investigated peak acceleration and velocity in patients with coronary disease during cardiac catheterization. Miniaturized electromagnetic blood flow meters were attached to the tips of cardiac catheters and positioned in the ascending aorta for such measurements. In patients with chronic coronary disease, the magnitude of resting ejection velocity and acceleration related to the severity of angiographic coronary disease [9]. Both velocity and acceleration showed positive correlation with angiographic ejection fractions ($R = 0.88$) in twelve such patients. A study of 40 patients undergoing catheterization correlated peak velocity and acceleration with stroke volume, but neither velocity or acceleration stratified patients ranked by left ventricular end diastolic pressure, cardiac index, or ejection fraction [10]. During atrial pacing, it was shown that ejection velocity and acceleration diminish at the heart rate-related threshold for angina [11]. Pacing studies subsequent to bypass grafting showed that rate-related angina and decrements in ejection dynamics were abolished. Hemodynamic studies have shown a correlative rise in left ventricular end diastolic pressure, and a fall in left ventricular ejection fraction during incremental atrial pacing in coronary patients during catheterization [12].

Recently, noninvasive Doppler studies have been reported in 92 patients suffering acute myocardial infarction. Velocity and acceleration were depressed compared to 73 age-matched controls [13]. Both ejection indices successfully discriminated survivors from nonsurvivors.

Thus, a large body of information utilizing indirect and direct techniques would seem to indicate that a decrase in left ventricular ejection velocity or acceleration is a marker of decreased left ventricular performance, as might occur with myocardial ischemia or myocardial infarction.

Doppler examination of ventricular function

Ultrasonic Doppler techniques make it no longer necessary to utilize invasive methods to assess ejection dynamics in the ascending aorta. As Fig. 1 illustrates, a small, hand-held Doppler probe can be placed in the suprasternal notch, affording an excellent ultrasonic window for the assessment of flow in the ascending aorta. In similar fashion, the apical window allows interrogation of blood leaving the ventricle in the left ventricular outflow tract, but it is often difficult to obtain or maintain this window during a stress testing protocol due to patient motion and increased depth of respiration. On

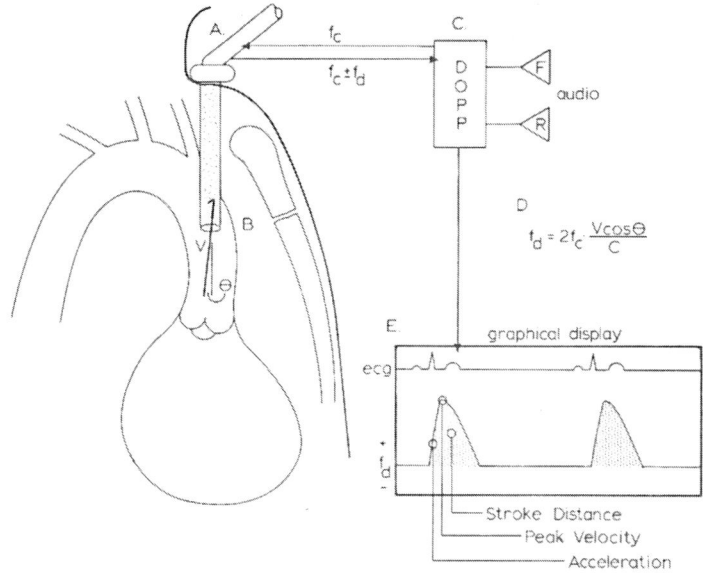

Fig. 1. The suprasternal Doppler examination. (A) Doppler probes with an offset handle are easily positioned in the suprasternal notch affording an ultrasonic view of blood ejected into the ascending aorta (B). The interaction of ultrasound with blood results in the carrier frequency (fc) being increased by a finite amount (fd), governed by the Doppler equation (D). The Doppler shift is proportional to fc, the velocity of blood flowing in the ascending aorta (V), the angle theta between the flow and the Doppler beam, and the speed of propogation, C. Doppler shifts are presented acoustically, and upon a visual display (E). Microprocessors determine the acceleration, the peak velocity and the stroke distance of individual pulses.

the other hand, the suprasternal notch is a stable viewing site for patients exercising upright on the treadmill or supine during bicycle exercise.

From this vantage point a wealth of Doppler information can be obtained. The graphic display in Fig. 1 illustrates typical systolic ejection pulses correlated with the electrocardiogram. Acceleration is determined as the maximal slope of the upstroke portion of the ejection pulse, while peak velocity is the maximal deviation from baseline. The stroke distance is calculated as the integrated area under the Doppler velocity pulse, and represents the distance ejected blood travels during systole. If multiplied by the cross sectional area of the ascending aorta, the stroke distance gives a quantitative approximation of the stroke volume [14]. Modern instrumentation goes beyond the simple graphical display of this pulse, and utilizes microprocessor technology to determine values for acceleration, velocity, and stroke distance or volume on a beat-to-beat basis. Practically, these numerical results can be displayed upon the graphical display or appear as a printout from a chart recorder. Such digital processing may go one step further, and compile a numerical average of all beats recorded during the observation, rejecting beats contaminated by noise or motion artifact [14].

Clinical validation

Suprasternal Doppler examinations have been performed in a wide variety of patients, from resting studies in the catheterization laboratory, to stress studies during treadmill or bicycle exercise.

Studies during cardiac catheterization

It is important that previous findings utilizing velocity sensing catheters in the ascending aorta be duplicated using noninvasive ultrasonic Doppler techniques. Sabbah et al. have reported positive correlations between Doppler ultrasonic peak acceleration in the ascending aorta and angiographic ejection fraction in 36 patients undergoing diagnostic cardiac catheterization [16]. Ejection fraction ranged from 20–90% as illustrated in Fig. 2. Patients with ejection fractions less than 40% invariably had peak accelerations less than 10 m/sec^2, while patients with ejection fractions greater than 60% had peak accelerations greater than 12 m/sec^2. In the intermediate range between 40 and 60%, there was a great deal of overlap in the data, raising some concern that only patients with very low or high ejection fractions can be discriminated from normal patients reliably using the technique.

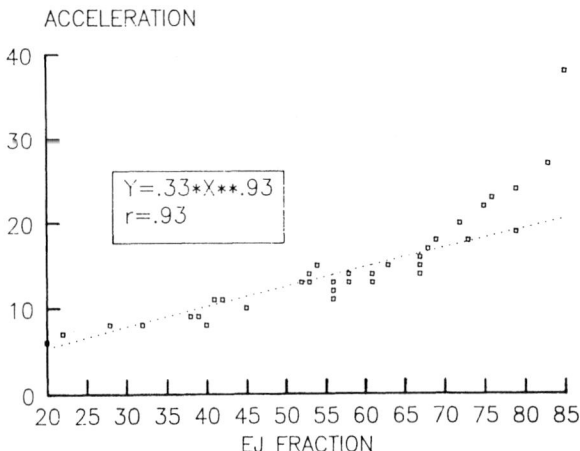

Fig. 2. Catheterization correlates. Correlation between ejection fraction and Doppler maximal acceleration in 36 patients. The insert and the dotted line show a power curve best fit and regression analysis. After Sabbah, et al. [16], with permission.

To investigate the effect of coronary occlusion upon global ventricular function, we studied 25 patients utilizing suprasternal Doppler assessments of ejection velocity and acceleration simultaneous with coronary angioplasty. Similar to Rushmer's results in dogs subjected to coronary ligation, we observed immediate decrements in peak velocity and acceleration coincident with balloon inflations at proximal coronary stenoses. However, significant decrements (−30% in acceleration: −50% in peak velocity) were only observed in patients with demonstrable myocardial ischemia; those with chest pain or ST segment shifts during balloon inflation. In patients without pain or ST change during balloon inflation, no significant change in Doppler ejection was observed. Grouping patients according to the presence or absence of chest pain during balloon inflation, composite coronary tree diagrams showed that patients with decrements in Doppler ejection had significantly more proximal lesions undergoing angioplasty. The typical lesion showing profoundly impaired Doppler ejection during inflation was a left anterior descending stenosis proximal to both the first septal perforator and first diagonal branch. These catheterization studies lend support to the hypotheses that the suprasternal Doppler examinations can estimate elements of resting ventricular function, as well as directional changes in ventricular function during cardiovascular stress. Our angioplasty experience suggests that the degree of change in ascending aortic ejection dynamics grossly correlates with the extent of myocardium under ischemic jeopardy.

Studies during treadmill exercise

One of the earliest descriptions of the use of Doppler echocardiography during exercise testing was reported by Daley and coworkers in 1985 [17], demonstrating that stroke volume, peak flow velocity, and acceleration of flow in the ascending aorta could be reproduceably measured during bicycle and treadmill exercise, showing a rise in acceleration and peak velocity in normal subjects. Gardin and coworkers demonstrated that Doppler aortic flow velocity could be measured successfully during supine bicycle exercise. Aortic peak flow velocity increased by 45% compared to resting measurements in normal subjects [18].

A number of technical points are common to the success of these studies. First, it is important that the transducer be applied in a stable manner in the suprasternal notch. We find this easiest to achieve by holding the probe as if it were a pencil, and resting the palm against the patient's sternum. The sternum forms a stable platform against which the examiner can lightly press, maintaining stable transducer contact as the patient exercises to more and more vigorous work loads. The examiner must develop a keen sense of the acoustic

Doppler signal, and attempt to stay at the same interrogation site throughout the examination, maximizing signal strength and Doppler pitch. Only in this way can confidence be gained that the trends seen in the Doppler parameters during stress represent actual physiologic information and not artifact or poor signal acquisition. Although data obtained at rest and at peak tolerated exercise are of most interest, it is important to obtain Doppler data at intermediate levels to assure that the endpoints of the trend represent a continuium. We routinely obtain a continuous strip of 20 optimal quality beats at one minute intervals throughout exercise. As such studies generate considerable amounts of data, it is important that the Doppler instrument feature calculation of running averages of beat-by-beat measurements, as well as final report generation, disclosing the trend of Doppler ejection dynamics as the exercise progresses. It is the trend of Doppler ejection profiles that indicates impairment of ventricular function during stress.

Clinical treadmill-Doppler studies have focused on three distinct patient groups; patients without evidence of organic heart disease, patients with angiographically proven coronary artery disease without prior infarction, and patients status post myocardial infarction performing limited treadmill exercise to determine the presence of multivessel disease. Bryg compared stress Doppler trends of 17 patients with angiographic evidence of coronary disease to 20 healthy young volunteers during Doppler treadmill exercise [19]. He found that both volunteers and patients with angiographic single vessel disease were capable of augmenting peak ejection velocity from rest to peak exercise by 80%, although the Doppler peak exercise data was recorded immediately post exercise. Patients with multivessel disease did not augment velocity, with a flat trajectory between rest and peak exertion.

Our laboratory first reported Doppler treadmill stress testing in coronary patients in 1984 [20]. To date, 170 patients have been studied prior to coronary angiography. We have excluded patients with prior infarction or abnormal electrocardiographic findings. The angiographic ejection fractions of these patients have all been in the normal range of 50 to 80%. We have studied this restricted group to see if Doppler ejection trends can detect coronary patients in a population who, although normal by resting measurements, may develop evidence of impaired ejection capacity during the stress of exercise as a manifestation of the presence and extent of coronary artery disease. In general, our results are comparable to those of Bryg. We find that patients with normal coronary arteries are able to double ejection velocity between rest and peak exertion. On the other hand, patients with severe and extensive three vessel or left main coronary artery disease often have peak exercise values lower than those measured at rest. These patients also have early positive treadmill tests and, occasionally, a fall in systolic blood pressure between rest and peak exertion. Patients with this constellation of stress intolerance have usually undergone coronary artery bypass grafting. At the other extreme, we observed patients with single vessel disease who are inseparable from normal peers on the basis of the Doppler treadmill examination. Usually, these patients have single vessel coronary artery disease, and often those lesions are located in the mid or distal segments of the involved vessel.

The most common ischemic trend is inability to augment ejection velocity between rest and peak exertion, and this is generally seen in patients with two vessel coronary artery disease. Patients with proximal LAD stenosis or three vessel coronary disease may have this type of response as well, usually when collateral flow from less diseased vessels is present.

In summary, the Doppler ejection trajectory from rest to peak exertion appears to assess the degree of global ventricular impairment, rather than the number of diseased vessels, as Fig. 3 illustrates. The degree of compensation is determined by the slope of the trajectory when the exercise ejection velocity is plotted against the exercise heart rate from rest to peak exertion. Patients with high trajectory slopes are compensated: they may be normal or they may have anatomically limited coronary artery disease. Patients with negative or flat trajectory slopes physiologically appear to decompensate and have significant proximal or multivessel coronary disease.

In patients developing diagnostic ischemic ST segment depression, the Doppler examination does not appear to significantly increase the sensitivity

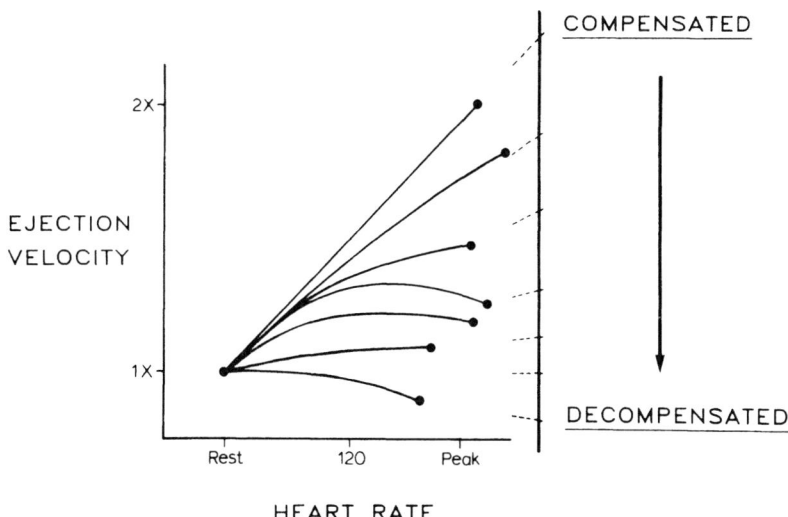

Fig. 3. Doppler treadmill response types. Plotting ejection velocity vs. heart rate from examinations done at rest, peak exertion and intermediate workloads, a variety of Doppler response trajectories are measurable in patients with various manifestations of coronary disease (see text).

or specificity of the treadmill electrocardiographic response in detecting coronary disease. We have found the Doppler stress test to be of chief value in patients unable to achieve target heart rate without ST segment changes [21]. If the patient can achieve a heart rate of at least 120 beats per minute during the treadmill exertion, we found that the slope of the Doppler velocity trajectory (Fig. 3) separates patients with and without coronary disease at the $p = .001$ level. It is in this subgroup that Doppler exercise examination appears to possess the greatest value. In our cohort of 170 patients, 30% had negative, inadequate stress tests.

Data congruent with the trajectory hypothesis have been reported by Metha et al., who studied Doppler responses of 165 patients 3–4 weeks following myocardial infarction undergoing limited treadmill testing [22]. Peak velocity, maximal acceleration, and the systolic velocity integral were all significantly lower at peak exercise in patients with positive stress tests and abnormal systolic blood pressure responses. In the 63 who underwent coronary angiography, treadmill peak velocity and maximal acceleration trajectories were significantly lower in patients with three vessel disease than patients with only one and two vessel disease. Individual values of a maximal acceleration in peak velocity at peak exercise were 65% predictive of three vessel disease, rising to 80% when the Doppler value was combined with the onset time of diagnostic ST depression.

Correlations with radionuclide methods

To further investigated the relationship between the Doppler stress response and the degree of ventricular compensation or decompensation, we studied 72 patients undergoing multigated nuclide radioangiography during graded supine bicycle exercise. All patients were free of prior myocardial infarction, and at subsequent coronary angiography 13 had normal coronary arteries, while 59 had coronary disease. The graph in Fig. 4 compares the change in radionuclear ejection fraction versus the percentage change in Doppler peak ejection velocity from rest to peak exertion. It is apparent that there is only a general positive trend correlating ejection fraction and peak velocity. There is a great deal of scatter around the linear regression through these data, which has a r value of .75. There is some tendency for a fall in ejection fraction to correlate with a fall in velocity, but far more patients have only impaired rise in peak velocity with a fall in ejection fraction. On the other hand, patients who augment ejection fraction greater than 5% augment peak velocity greater than 20% from rest to peak exertion.

Taking a rise in ejection fraction of less than 5% as the diagnostic thres-hold for coronary artery disease, a vertical line was drawn. To establish a

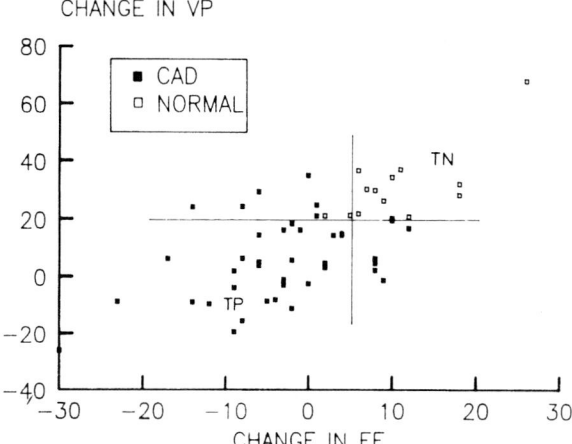

Fig. 4. Nuclear Doppler correlation. The percentage change in peak ejection velocity is plotted against the change in ejection fraction from rest to peak exertion in 72 patients. The legend defines patients with or without coronary artery disease. TP = true positive, TN = true negative (see text).

diagnostic threshold for the Doppler responses, we elected a +20% change in peak velocity (VP), resulting in the horizontal line. The graph is divided into 4 quadrants defined by the intersecting lines. Patients without coronary disease (true normals) by both Doppler and nuclear techniques should lie in the upper right quadrant, while patients truly positive for coronary disease should lie in the lower left quadrant. Nuclear and Doppler studies were concordant for true negative and positive responses in 58 of 73 patients. However, in the lower right and upper left quadrants the noninvasive tests are discordant. In the lower right quadrant coronary patients are nuclear false negatives, while they are Doppler true positives. In the upper left quadrant patients are nuclear true positives, but Doppler false negatives. Although both tests are reasonably accurate in the identification of ischemic responses, there is a subset of patients where the change in ejection fraction and the change in peak ejection velocity is decoupled. Technical errors and measurement scatter could explain some of this disagreement, but the following analysis shows why one should expect only general correlation between ejection velocity and ejection fraction: these indices measure different aspects of ventricular function.

Theoretical considerations

The relationship between the dynamics of ventricular contraction and ejection into the ascending aorta may be modeled mathematically. Refering to

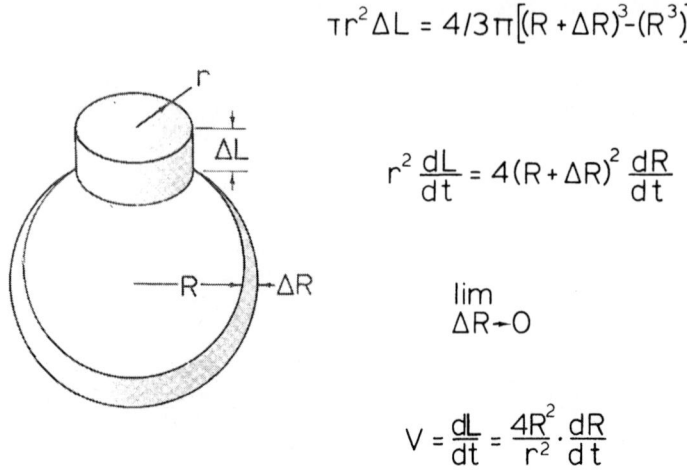

$$\pi r^2 \Delta L = 4/3\pi\left[(R+\Delta R)^3-(R^3)\right]$$

$$r^2\frac{dL}{dt} = 4(R+\Delta R)^2\frac{dR}{dt}$$

$$\lim_{\Delta R\to 0}$$

$$V = \frac{dL}{dt} = \frac{4R^2}{r^2}\cdot\frac{dR}{dt}$$

Fig. 5. Theoretical relationship between ventricular contraction and ascending aortic flow (see text).

Fig. 5, the left ventricle is modeled as a simple sphere characterized by radius R. The aorta is described a cylinder of radius r. During a short portion of total ejection, delta t, the spherical ventricle changes by a small amount, delta R, while the volume of blood displaced from the sphere into the aorta creates a cylinder of radius r and height l. To satisfy conservation of mass, the displacement of blood into the aorta must be equal to the change in the volume of the sphere. If the equation is then cast in differential form, dl/dt and dR/dt, it can be shown that dl/dt (or the velocity of blood flowing into the model aorta) is proportional to the square of the radius of the spherical ventricle and the radius of the cylindrical aorta times the rate of change of R. Thus, the velocity observed in the ascending aorta should most correlate with the velocity of circumferential fiber shortening, dR/dt, scaled by the dimension of the chamber and the dimension of the aorta.

Offsetting effects of chamber diameter and shortening velocity explain why some patients with markedly impaired velocity of circumferential fiber shortening with low ejection fractions but dilated ventricles have normal ejection velocity. If, during a stress test, the velocity of circumferential fiber shortening diminishes due to ischemia or other factors, and the ventricle fails to compensate by dilation, ejection velocity may fall. Correlating this model with observations in canine models cited earlier in this chapter, it appears that Doppler ejection parameters are quite distinct from traditional measurements of ventricular funtion such as dp/dt and ejection fraction, but are correlated in a general sense. Velocity, it appears, relates to the geometry as well as contractile properties of the chamber.

Summary

The velocity and acceleration of blood ejected from the left ventricle are sensitive markers of systolic left ventricular performance. Clinical studies in coronary patients have correlated Doppler ejection dynamics with the irreversible effects of myocardial infarction, and the reversible ischemia induced by exercise stress testing and coronary angioplasty. The magnitude of the Doppler measurement or stress response appears to correlate with the degree of ventricular dysfunction or extent of ischemic jeopardy, helping to identify patients in a high risk category that may deserve serious consideration for surgical or angioplasty intervention. The equipment to perform these studies is technically sophisticated but inexpensive, and examinations can be done by paratechnical personnel after moderate training. Doppler examinations show high potential for improving the cost effectiveness of ventricular performance monitoring during stress testing.

References

1. Hatle L, Brubakk A, Tromsdal A, Angelsen B: Noninvasive assessment of pressure drop in mitral stenosis by Doppler ultrasound. Br Heart J 40: 131, 1978.
2. Stamm BR, Martin RP: Quantification of pressure gradients across stenotic valves by Doppler ultrasound. J Am Coll Cardiol 2: 707, 1984.
3. Teague SM, Heinsimer JA, Andersonf JL, Sublett K, Olson EG, Voyles WF, Thadani U: Quantification of aortic regurgitation utilizing continuous wave Doppler ultrasound. J Am Coll Cardiol 8 (3): 592, 1986.
4. Rudewal B: Hemodynamic of the human ascending aorta as studied by of a differential pressure technique. Acta Physiol Scand 54 (Suppl. 187): 1, 1962.
5. Rushmer RF, Watson N, Harding D, Baker D: Effects of acute coronary occlusion upon the performance of right and left ventricles in intact unanesthetized dogs. Am Heart J 66: 522, 1963.
6. Kezdi P, Stanely EL, Marshall WJ Jr., Kordenat RK: Aortic flow velocity and acceleration as an index of ventricular performance during myocardial infarction. Am J Med Sci 257: 61, 1969.
7. Hof RP, Hof A: Acceleration of blood in the aorta: A parameter useful for evaluating cardiotonic and afterload reducing substances. J Pharmacol Methods 6: 87, 1981.
8. Noble MIM, Trechard D, Guz A: Left ventricular ejection in conscious dogs: Measurement and significance of the maximum acceleration of blood from the left ventricle. Circ Res 19: 139, 1966.
9. Bennett ED, Else W, Miller GAH, Sutton GC, Miller HC, Noble MIM: Maximum acceleration of blood from the left ventricle in patients with ischemic heart disease. Clin Sci Mol Med 46: 49, 1974.
10. Kolettis M, Jenkins BS, Webb-peploe MM: Assessment of left ventricular function by indices derived from aortic flow velocity. Br Heart J: 38: 18, 1976.
11. Jewitt D, Gabe I, Mills C, Maurer B, Thomas M, Shillingford J: Aortic velocity and acceleration measurements in the assessment of coronary heart disease. Eur J Cardiol 1: 299, 1974.

12. Mann T, Brodie B, Grossman W, McLaurin LP: Effects of angina on the left ventricular diastolic pressure-volume relationship. Circulation 55 (5): 761, 1977.

13. Metha N, Bennett DE: Impaired left ventricular function in acute myocardial infarction assessed by Doppler measurement of ascending aortic blood velocity and maximum acceleration. Am J Cardiol 57: 1052, 1986.

14. Teague SM: Measurement of ventricular function using Doppler ultrasound. In: Kisslo JA ed. *Basic Doppler Echocardiography*. New York, Churchill Livingstone Publishers, pp. 65–70, 1985.

15. Stein PD, et al.: Blood velocity and acceleration: Comparison of CW Doppler and electromagnetic flowmetry. Federation Proceedings 44 (5): 1565, 1985.

16. Sabbah HS, Khaja F, Brymer JF, et al.: Noninvasive evaluation of left ventricular performance based on peak aortic blood acceleration measured with a continuous-wave Doppler velocity meter. Circulation 74 (2): 323, 1985.

17. Daley PJ, Sagar KB, Wann LS: Doppler echocardiographic measurement of flow velocity in the ascending aorta during supine and upright exercise. Br Heart J 54: 562, 1985.

18. Gardin JM, Kozlowski J, Dabestani A, Murphy M, Kusnick C, Allfie A, Russell D, Henry WL: Studies of Doppler aortic flow velocity during supine bicycle exercise. Am J Cardiol 57: 327, 1986.

19. Bryg RJ, Labovitz AJ, Mehdirad AA, Williams GA, Chaitman BR: Effect of coronary artery disease on Doppler-derived parameters of aortic flow during upright exercise. Am J Cardiol 58: 14, 1986.

20. Teague SM, Mark DB, Radford M, Robertson J, Albert D, Porter J, Waugh RA: Doppler velocity profiles reveal ischemic exercise responses. Circulation 70 (Supp. II): 185, 1984.

21. Teague SM, Mark DB, Radford M, Robertson J, Albert D, Waugh RA: Doppler ejection dynamics during ischemic exercise responses. Circulation 72 (Supp. III): 448, 1985.

22. Metha N, Bennett G, Mannering D, Dawkins K, Ward DE: Non-invasive Doppler measurement of ascending aortic blood velocity detects impairment of the left ventricular functional response to exercise in post-infarction patients. Am J Cardiol 58: 879, 1986.

PART 8: Cardiovascular Drug Interventions

8.1. Echocardiography in the assessment of cardiovascular drug interventions

BERNARD CLARKE & DEREK GIBSON

Introduction

Echocardiography would seem particularly well adapted to studying the effects of drugs with actions on the heart. Ventricular cavity size has been estimated by cross-sectional echocardiography (CSE), wall and valve motion studied in detail with a repetition rate unsurpassed by any other imaging technique with M-mode, while Doppler allows blood flow velocity and its changes with time to be assessed throughout the heart and great vessels. The present review does not aim to cover the whole literature on the use of these methods for clinical pharmacology. Rather, we attempt to derive more general principles concerning the value and limitations of these methods. Although they have given rise to much useful information over the last 15 years, it might be argued that the overall results have not been wholly commensurate with their apparent potential. Known effects of drugs have been confirmed, but little light has been shed on their basic mechanisms of action or on their therapeutic use in disease.

To document the effects of a drug requires first knowledge of the physical basis and likely performance of the technique of measurement. It is next necessary to differentiate changes related to drug administration from those due to artefact or random variation. Once an effect has been defined, this change must be interpreted in terms of basic mechanisms, bearing in mind particularly loading conditions and possible reflex adjustment. Finally, if such a change can be substantiated beyond reasonable doubt, then its relation to therapeutic action must be defined. The indication for drug administration is usually patient benefit, for example prolongation of life, or improvement in symptoms, so that these ends may bear no clear relation to a change in cardiac function as demonstrated in an acute drug study. When the results of using echocardiography to study drug action are considered, it will be found that difficulties arise at each of these stages.

I. Cikes (ed.), *Echocardiography in Cardiac Interventions*, 523–539, 1989.
© 1989 *Kluwer Academic Publishers*.

Methods

M-mode echocardiography

M-mode echocardiography has been used for more than a decade for studying drugs, and there is thus considerably more experience with it than with cross-sectional echocardiography or Doppler. Though drug effects have usually been monitored in terms of left ventricular transverse dimension and its rate of change, the method can also be used to detect valve motion, and so detect variation in the duration of the isovolumic periods. Changes in the timing of wall motion and in the extent and timing of posterior wall thickness can also be detected. M-mode echo has proved of little value in studying right sided events. For a pharmacological study, records of appreciably higher standard than those acceptable for routine diagnosis are required. The recommendations of the American Society of Echocardiography (ASE) should be followed [1], and a paper speed of at least 75, and preferably 100 mm/s should be used. The value and limitations of M-mode in clinical pharmacology have been reviewed in detail elsewhere [2].

Cross-sectional echocardiography

The particular virtue of cross-sectional echocardiography is the information it gives about wall motion of both left and right ventricles. This should allow more reliable estimates of volume, particularly when wall motion is non-uniform. It is also possible to detect regional abnormalities of function. Cavity volumes have been calculated in a variety of ways, usually from pairs of apical views, using Simpson's rule. An alternative is based on a multiple parasternal views, which has the advantage that range rather than lateral resolution is used. Though all underestimate absolute ventricular volume in comparison with angiography, this need not necessarily be a disadvantage in a pharmacological study when a change is being sought. Analysis of regional function, usually subjective, has been extensively used in patients with coronary artery disease. Methods using cross-sectional echocardiography to document disturbances of timing objectively have not achieved general acceptance, due mainly to their complexity and to problems with localisation of endocardium on single top frames [3, 4].

Doppler

Doppler methods are being used increasingly to study drug effects, by both pulsed and continuous wave (CW) techniques. The former method allows the site at which measurement is being made to be located, while only the latter is applicable when high blood velocities associated with valvular stenoses are being studied. As with M-mode, the repetition rate of these techniques is high, so that blood velocities and accelerations can reliably be measured. In addition, the Doppler method is an absolute one, so that external calibration is not required. It does however also share with M-mode the potential disadvantage that conclusions about overall function are drawn from regional measurements: unless a multigate system is used, it must be assumed that flow profiles are uniform, an assumption that may well be justified when cardiac output is normal or near normal, but which may not apply when it is low. When the appropriate cross-sectional area is known, these simple Doppler methods can be adapted to measure flow. This requires an imaging method, the most suitable non-invasive ones being either M-mode or cross-sectional echo. M-mode allows a diameter to be measured continuously throughout the cardiac cycle, and so is particularly appropriate for the ascending aorta. Though range resolution is of the order of 1–2 mm at 3.5 MHz, even this degree of uncertainty in dimension is equivalent to 5–10% error when cross sectional areas are derived. In addition, the cross sectional area must be shown to be estimated at the level at which peak flow occurs, particularly if CW Doppler is being used. When flow rates are low, aortic cusp opening is incomplete, so that the effective valve area is very significantly less than that of the aortic root. Even for what would seem to be the straightforward problem of estimating aortic area, it may be significant that several different conventions have been recommended [5]. For A–V valve areas, the problem is more complex. They can only be measured by cross-sectional echo, using lateral rather than range resolution, which is of the order of 3–4 mm at 3.5 MHz. In addition, A–V valve areas have long been known to vary throughout the cardiac cycle, so that multiple determinations must be made, making determinations of mitral or tricuspid flow very time consuming. In an attempt to avoid using these area estimates at all, the idea of stroke distance has been introduced as the simple time integral of the flow curve [6]. While the method may have some value in detecting trends in large series of patients, it fails to solve the problem of changes in cross sectional area occurring independent of those in velocity [7]. Whether colour flow mapping will allow some of these problems, particularly those related to inhomogenous flow, to be circumvented remains to be seen.

526

General problems

Reproducibility

Since a clinical pharmacological study is likely to involve measurement before and after drug administration, appropriate allowance must be made for spontaneous variability. Although it is likely that there will be placebo control, the extent of spontaneous variability in echocardiographic measurements must be allowed for in experimental design. Its extent varies with the technique used and has been studied in greatest detail for the M-mode. Here, major determinants include the position of the subject [8], the individuals recording and measuring the record and the position on the chest from which measurements are made [9]. This variability has been documented in a number of studies [10], and amounts to 3–4 mm for dimensions between measurements made within a few minutes of each other, with an overall coefficient of variation of 1 to 8%. Variability increases with the time interval between measurements. Its extent can be reduced by standardising the time in the cardiac cycle at which measurements are made, since LV dimension falls by 2–3 mm and that of the right ventricle increases by a similar amount due to anterior motion of the interventricular septum during inspiration. Although variability might theoretically be reduced by standardising the position within the ventricle from which M-mode records are made by reference to the cross-sectional display, this does not appear to be the case in practice [11]. It is, of course, reduced as the number of replicate determinations is increased. This variability is probably in part methodological, and in part physiological, representing true variation in the cardiovascular system. Nevertheless, its presence represents a major limitation of the technique, since it is of the same order of magnitude of changes produced by drug action. Its effects must therefore be reduced by appropriate experimental design which includes use of replicate samples and measurement by a blinded observer. The reproducibility of cross-sectional echocardiographic estimates of left ventricular cavity volume have been studied only occasionally and reported in a number of ways. Thus Touche et al. [12] found a standard deviation of 23 ml between duplicate determinations, Schiller et al. [13] a correlation coefficient of only 0.80 for the same measurement made by different observers, and Starling et al. of 0.85 [14]. A much higher value (0.98) has been reported by Schnittger in patients studied after cardiac transplantation [15] in whom left ventricular endocardial echoes are of much greater amplitude than normal. Apart from this special case, it appears that failure of reproducibility will constitute a major limitation in using cross-sectional echocardiographic volume estimates since differences between duplicate determinations are large compared with anticipated drug effects. In patients with ischaemic heart disease, considerable variability has been demonstrated between different assessments of regional disturbances of left ventricular wall motion [16]. This has both between and within observer components, and has major implications if the method is used in studying the effects of drugs on regional wall motion.

Estimates of the reproducibility of Doppler estimates of flow velocity have been reported by a number of observers, based on assessments made on a single occasion. Values reported are in the range 6–8% for peak flow [17], 15% for time to peak flow [18], 4% for velocity-time integrals [19] and 6% for stroke volumes [20]. Corresponding values for cross sectional area are 6% for the aortic valve and 14% for the mitral valve [21].

Loading conditions

Observed left ventricular performance is affected by a number of other circulatory variables, not directly related to the heart. These are referred to, generically, as loading conditions. Observed cardiac action can thus be regarded as the resultant of assumed intrinsic capability and the external circumstances in which it is called upon to function. In so far as it affects systolic function, this assumed intrinsic capability is frequently referred to as contractility. Any drug with a cardiac action has the potential of changing loading conditions, either directly or by a reflex mechanism. The possibility of such changes must thus always be allowed for in the experimental design.

(1) *Heart rate.* Changes in heart rate have a major effect on cavity dimensions. Not surprisingly, the mechanism of change in rate is probably more important that the magnitude of the change rate itself. Again, these effects have been studied in greatest detail with respect to the M-mode. When rate is increased by atrial pacing, there is a progressive reduction in end-diastolic (Dd) and end-systolic dimensions (Ds), although fractional shortening remains constant [22]. By contrast, when the same range of heart rate change is brought about by exercise, Dd increases, Ds falls, and fractional shortening increases. Effects of heart rate changes on VCF are harder to interpret due to the additional effect of rate on ejection time. Other possible mechanisms of heart rate change include direct action, sympathetic stimulation, vagal withdrawal, either reflex or atropine induced, those occuring during infancy and childhood when there is a progressive decline, and those associated with an increase in physical fitness [22, 23, 24]. Interaction of these with drug action is complex, so that there can be no unique relation between heart rate changes and cavity dimensions, and therefore no method of 'correction' is possible which does not presuppose the mechanism which it is intended to

correct. Nevertheless, the idea that rate changes can be corrected for is a pervasive one and frequently appears in the literature. It can give rise to major problems. For example, if one uses a regression equation based on spontaneous rate changes in adults, which are probably in part due to changes in sympathetic activity and in part to variation in parasympathetic withdrawal to 'correct' for rate changes caused by a drug that slows heart rate purely by a vagal action, then the possibility of introducing a 'pseudo-inotropic' effect is obvious. Little information is available concerning the effects of rate changes on cross-sectional echocardiographic estimates of LV volume or regional motion. They are potentially important when, for example, a beta blocking drug is being studied. In a Doppler study in normal subjects undergoing exercise testing after administration of β-blockade, no effect was seen on maximal acceleration, peak velocity, or systolic velocity integral measurements made at rest [25]. In contrast, a similar study from the same group in which patients receiving β-blockade following myocardial infarction showed that SVI was increased at rest, comcomitant with the expected decrease in heart rate of following drug administration [26].

(2) *Arterial pressure.* Left ventricular cavity size and end-systolic volume are affected to a major extent by changes in arterial pressure, which behave as alterations in afterload. On M-mode, an increase in arterial pressure by phenylephrine administration is associated with an fall in fractional shortening and VCF [27], and a variable increase in end-diastolic dimension. Again, there is little information available using cross-sectional or Doppler techniques. In view of this relation, therefore, arterial pressure should always be recorded whenever cavity size or its rate of change during systole is being measured.

Changes in peripheral resistance may be associated with compensatory increase in flow so that arterial pressure remains unchanged. This causes large changes in the amplitude of LV wall motion as well as in systolic and probably diastolic measurements. Indeed, changes in left ventricular cavity size and rates of change of dimension during systole have occurred much more frequently and reproducibility with drugs having an action on the peripheral resistance than with those thought to alter inotropic state. For example, amrinone [28] and isoprenaline have both inotropic and vasodilator effects, complicating any echocardiographic assessment of their actions.

(3) *Central blood volume.* Changes in blood volume have a major effect on cavity dimensions. Movement to 80 degree head-up tilt causes a significant reduction in Dd and Ds with no significant change in VCF [27]. Large changes can be brought about by lower body negative pressure [29], or by infusion of dextran [30]. Clearly such changes are closely related to those

occurring with a change in heart rate due to atrial pacing or with the increase in cardiac output due to exercise, demonstrating the way in which these external factors can interact with one another.

Systolic left ventricular function

Ideas on the assessment of systolic left ventricular function are complicated by lack of definition of the term itself. At a mechanistic level, the function of the left ventricle during systole is to generate pressure and flow appropriate to the demands of the circulation. However, the term is used in other senses, including a purely descriptive one of observed cardiac action, or to encompass specific measurements such as fractional shortening or ejection fraction. It is also used at a more fundamental level to imply some quality of the ventricle independent of loading conditions that can be used to quantify its performance, and so to be similar in its meaning to contractility. In addition, it is generally assumed, often implicitly, that systolic ventricular function as described in this last sense is a simple scalar quantity, and that changes in it are qualitatively similar whatever their underlying cause. Depression of function by disease is thus identical in its nature, though not necessarily in its extent to that caused by a drug with a negative inotropic action. It is within this rather loose framework of ideas that the role of echocardiography must be considered.

Blood flow. Left ventricular stroke volume can be estimated using Doppler echocardiography, and this approach has been used, for example, to examine changes brought about by dobutamine [5], hydralazine, isosorbide dinitrate, and sodium nitroprusside [31]. Other characteristics of the flow pattern can also be studied. In his pioneering studies, Light [32] demonstrated the potential value of estimates of peak aortic velocity estimated using a suprasternal approach for documenting drug action in patients in the intensive care unit, and more recently Mehta and Bennett [33] have demonstrated similar changes in patients in the period after acute myocardial infarction. Peak acceleration of aortic blood flow can be determined as the rate of rise of the pressure; flow velocity traces obtained by spectral analysis cannot easily be differentiated, but the calculation can easily be made as V/t where V is peak velocity and t the time to peak velocity. This ratio is not necessarily peak acceleration which can only be derived from continuous differentiation, but is the minimum value capable of explaining the observed velocity. Peak acceleration has been studied in detail in the dog by Noble et al. [34], and, unlike peak velocity, has the interesting property of being independent of arterial pressure and of ventricular filling pressure. It is closely related to the initial ventricular impulse described by Rushmer [35]. Peak acceleration increases with positive inotropic stimuli, and is greatly reduced by incoordinate ventricular contraction, induced, for example, by ventricular disease or abnormal activation. It may thus have potential value in studying drug effects in man, although this does not appear to have been extensively exploited.

Left ventricular volume. Theoretically, stroke volume can also be estimated using M-mode or cross-sectional echocardiography. Volume estimates from the M-mode have had a chequered history. Even if absolute values are unreliable, changes induced by drugs may be reliable directionally in patients with ventricular disease, since discrepancies from predicted values tend to be similar at end-systole and end-diastole. However, these estimates are semi-quantitative at best and should probably be avoided. Cross-sectional echocardiographic estimates should be more reliable, but this has not proved to be the case owing to the poor reproducibility of individual determinations. Stroke volume estimates can be combined with those of arterial pressure to calculate stroke work and thus to construct Starling curves, using end-diastolic volume as a measure of preload [36], dissociating changes in contractility from loading conditions.

Another method of assessing intrinsic left ventricular function (contractility) has been to study end-systolic pressure-volume relations or their derivatives. This approach [37] is based in the experimental observation that end-systolic tension of isolated muscle depends only on end-systolic length and is unaffected by end-diastolic length or mode of contraction, whether isometric or isotonic. In the intact heart the aim is to determine elastance, defined as:

$$E = P/(V - Vo),$$

at end-systole.

Where E is elastance, P pressure, V observed volume, and Vo the volume at which pressure is zero, i.e. the intercept on the pressure axis. E reaches a maximum, Emax, at end-systole. E has proved to be unaffected by arterial pressure or ventricular filling pressure, but is increased with a positive inotropic stimulus. It therefore has the properties of a measure of contractility. In order to calculate it, Vo must be derived. This is performed by infusing a pressor agent such as phenylephrine to generate a series of pressure volume curves as arterial pressure rises. The end-systolic points of these curves are found to lie on a single straight line passing through Vo, which has a slope of Emax.

In order to calculate Emax in this way, pressure and volume must be measured invasively. An alternative approach has been to examine pressure-dimension relations at end-ejection. Cavity dimension is measured by M-mode echocardiography, and end-ejection taken as the timing of A2 on a simultaneous phonocardiogram. Aortic pressure at this time can be assessed from a simultaneous indirect carotid pulse and a sphygmomanometer. The relative height of the dicrotic notch is used to derive the absolute pressure as the corresponding interval between peak systolic and diastolic pressure from the sphygmomanometer determination [38]. The method has been used both to detect left ventricular disease in patients with thalassaemia, to exclude it in those after a 'switch' operation for complete transposition and to document the actions of dobutamine [38, 40, 41, 42]. The results can be considered either in terms of the relations between pressure and dimension, or dimension can be cubed to approximate to volume. This approach is an interesting one. It must be assumed that any reflex effect caused by phenylephrine infusion does not alter left ventricular inotropic state. It has also become apparent that pressure-volume relations at end-ejection are not identical with those at maximum elastance ('end-systole'), with the former being sensitive to afterload [37, 43]. Finally, the definition of end-systole itself may be ambiguous in patients with LV disease [44].

A number of these methods, therefore, including estimation of peak aortic acceleration, construction of Starling curves and measurement of end-systolic pressure-volume relations all allow ventricular performance to be assessed independent of loading conditions. In this they differ from more commonly used quantities such as ejection fraction, shortening fraction, or VCF, which are sensitive to both preload and afterload. In spite of having these characteristics in common, it does not follow that the 'contractility' they measure is a single entity. Peak acceleration has the physical dimensions of $cm/s-2$; an inotropic effect demonstrated from Starling curves, if it has physical dimensions at all, is the slope of stroke work against end-diastolic volume, i.e. it represents a force per unit area, whereas Emax represents elasticity, i.e. the rate of change of pressure with volume. These quantities are of course, all different from one another, as they are from the original definition of contractility in terms of 'Vmax', the maximum velocity of contractile element shortening independent of preload and afterload [45]. Such considerations demonstrate the necessity, as was pointed out by Lord Kelvin a century ago [46], of establishing an unambiguous system of measurement with absolutely definite units before considered interpretation is possible.

Effect of afterload on left ventricular function

The effect of vasodilator administration on cardiac function is due to altered loading conditions and associated reflex adjustments. The success of echocardiography in documenting their use in terms of changes in cardiac action stresses the importance of extracardiac factors in determining observed function. The effects of nitroglycerin have been studied by many authors [16, 27, 31, 47, 48]. Normal subjects and patients with ischaemic heart disease have been studied. Similar effects are seen in both groups. Reduction of arterial pressure occurs, with a fall in Dd by 2 mm and Ds by 3 mm. Isosorbide dinitrate reduced Dd by 5 mm and Ds by 7 mm in a group of dyspnoeic patients, all in NYHA Class III–IV [49]. Increased flow velocity in the left anterior descending artery has been reported using cross-sectional echo-guided measurements after nitroglycerin administration in patients with hypertrophic cardiomyopathy [48]. Cooper et al. [50] described a fall in LV outflow gradient from 39 to 23 mm Hg following intravenous injection of verapamil in a child with hypertrophic cardiomyopathy, using simultaneous CW Doppler and cardiac catheterisation.

Diastolic left ventricular function

Isovolumic relaxation time. Although the exact time of onset of diastole is uncertain, from the practical point of view, it may be taken as starting at end-ejection. This marks the onset of the period of isovolumic relaxation, which ends with the opening of the mitral valve, and the onset of ventricular filling. Isovolumic relaxation time can be measured simply and reliably from an echophonocardiogram as the interval between the onset of A2 and the initial separation of the mitral valve cusps. The timing of A2 can be validated from an aortic echogram and that of the onset of filling from a Doppler record. At first sight, it might appear that changes in isovolumic relaxation time represent changes in relaxation. Unfortunately, this is not the case. Iso-volumic relaxation time is very sensitive to loading conditions, being shortened when aortic pressure is low and left atrial pressure high [51]. In patients with left ventricular disease, nitroglycerin causes striking prolongation, not because of any change in diastolic ventricular properties but simply because left atrial pressure falls [51]. With normal loading conditions, iso-volumic relaxation time is frequently prolonged in patients with ventricular disease, particularly hypertrophy or coronary artery disease. In these circumstances, shortening by drug administration, e.g. verapamil to patients with hypertrophic cardiomyopathy [52] has been taken as evidence of improvement in diastolic function, but such claims cannot be substantiated unless altered loading conditions have been excluded as a cause. The effect of external conditions may vary with the subjects studied; in normal subjects, for example, exercise causes no change in isovolumic relaxation time, whereas in patients with left ventricular hypertrophy, the abnormal prolongation present at rest gives place to abnormal shortening with exercise [53].

Ventricular filling. Abnormalities during ventricular filling can be determined using M-mode or Doppler. On the M-mode, the peak rate of dimension increase and peak rate of thinning of the posterior wall are both reduced. Changes in dimension have been shown angiographically to precede those in filling, so the two entities must not be regarded as identical. On the Doppler, peak early diastolic velocity is reduced as is deceleration of blood flow following this peak. The extent to which these measurements are affected by loading conditions has not been determined in detail, but experimental work suggests a possible interaction [18]. These two approaches have been compared by Spirito et al. [54]; in general they parallel one another though agreement in individual patients is not complete. Their potential use in detecting drug action has been demonstrated in a small number of studies, usually involving patients with left ventricular hypertrophy in which modifications with beta receptor antagonists or slow channel blocking drugs has been demonstrated, usually with a return towards normal values [52, 55]. Intravenous diltiazem had no effect on LV dimensions or fractional shortening in patients with hypertension, but shortened isovolumic relaxation time by 15 msec [56]. Doppler can also be used to study the effects of left atrial systole. Left ventricular diastolic disease is frequently associated with an increase in the contribution of left atrial systole to ventricular filling. This may be apparent as an increase in the percentage of the stroke volume entering at this phase of the cardiac cycle above the normal value of 30–35% to 50% or more. On the Doppler, peak flow rate during atrial systole (A) is increased and may be greater than that during early filling (H), so that the A/H ratio is greater than 1.0. The same phenomenon can also be quantified as a relative increase in the flow velocity-time integral. This method is also potentially available for assessing drug action. An increase in the relative height of the 'a' wave is a feature of early hypertension, and it responds to treatment with antihypertensive agents [57]. The interpretation of events during atrial systole is complex, and many factors are involved. The effects of heart rate do not appear to have been studied in detail, but these are likely to differ from those in systole. As filling time falls, diastasis selectively shortens so that rapid filling and atrial systole become superimposed. The separation and relative heights of the two peaks are thus likely to depend critically on filling time. In patients with disease, the relative height of the left atrial flow pulse is of course, affected by some diastolic abnormality of the left ventricle, but also requires an increase in the force of systolic contraction of the left atrium. The relation between the two depends on the quantitative relation between the extent of LV diastolic disease and that of increased force of left atrial contraction. There is no information on this question in the literature at all.

It is difficult to see how these different effects can be dissociated in intact man using current methods. Many drugs active on left ventricular diastole have negative inotropic effects, such as beta or slow channel blockers; reduction in the contribution of left atrial systole to overall filling they might cause could as well be due to inhibition of atrial systolic contraction than to any change in ventricular diastolic properties. The effects of changes of either atrial, or ventricular loading conditions on atrial systole have still to be defined, both in normal man or in patients with diastolic left ventricular disease. It is quite possible, for example, that the characteristics of atrial systole will þe altered by an increase in atrial pressure, ventricular preload here representing atrial afterload. The extent to which ventricular afterload varies the force of atrial contraction has also not been determined, but again it seems possible that compensatory mechanisms invoked by increased resistance to ventricular ejection might include an augmented contribution of atrial systole independent of any abnormality of diastolic function of the left ventricle.

Incoordinate left ventricular function

In normal subjects, characteristic asynchrony is present, probably facilitating optimum coupling between myocardium and circulation. In disease, these subtle relations are often lost, and incoordination may appear to any stage in the cardiac style. During systole, its presence mimics reduced contractility by reducing the peak rate of pressure rise, and peak aortic acceleration. The effect of drugs with a positive inotropic action has not been established in detail. The effect of thrombolysis on left ventricular wall motion has been analysed using cross-sectional echocardiography and significant improvement noted on the basis of subjective analysis [58]. The extent to which such changes can be documented must be limited by the complex changes in timing as well as amplitude of wall motion documented by more objective methods of analysis.

Abnormal changes in ventricular cavity shape during isovolumic relaxation are common in acute and chronic coronary artery disease. Their amplitude is paradoxically increased by TNT administration and reduced by a pressor stimulus [16], probably reflecting their marked load dependence. The effect of beta blockade depends critically on the pattern of wall motion in the control state even within a homogeneous population of patients with coronary artery disease [59]. Slow ventricular filling in patients with hypertrophic cardiomyopathy and coronary artery disease is again associated with striking

535

asynchrony, and a uniform reduction in the rate of outward wall motion, whose presence again poses considerable problems in analysing drug effects in such patients.

Conclusions

It might be concluded from the foregoing that difficulties attending on the use of echocardiographic imaging and Doppler techniques to study drug action are so substantial as to limit their application. We believe this view to be an oversimplification. Echocardiographic methods, particularly M-mode and Doppler, are excellent means of quantifying many aspects of cardiac action, both systolic and diastolic, and that their overall reproducibility is adequate to allow the effects of drugs to be observed. Indeed, it is their very excellence in this field that has highlighted the conceptual difficulties arising when these simple observations come to be interpreted in the light of basic mechanisms. The effect of loading conditions are substantial, incompletely studied and ill understood, particularly during diastole, and their effects are compounded by reflex adjustments. In systole and isovolumic relaxation their consequences are often greater than any direct effect on myocardial function, and indeed it is here that echocardiographic methods have been particularly successful in documenting the actions of drugs such as vasodilators. Even when loading conditions can be allowed for, conceptual difficulties remain, as for example in assessing contractility, when at least three entities exist fulfilling the appropriate criteria, all with different physical dimensions and therefore representing three independent entities. Yet these are not reasons for abandoning the techniques but rather for peservering with them. It is clear that further understanding of drug action on the heart will depend more on improved ideas than improved techniques. This development is essential if any progress is to be made in the hitherto almost intractable problems of treating patients with ventricular disease.

References

1. Sahn DJ, DeMaria AN, Kisslo J, Weyman A: Recommendations regarding quantitation in M-mode echocardiography. Results of a survey of echocardiographic measurements. Circulation 58: 1072–1083, 1978.
2. Gibson DG: Use of M-mode echocardiography in clinical pharmacology. Brit J Pharmacol 7: 443–449, 1979.
3. Gibson DG, Brown DJ, Logan-Sinclair RB: Analysis of regional left ventricular wall movement by phased array echocardiography. Br Heart J 40: 1334–1338, 1978.
4. Henry WL: Evaluation of ventricular function using two-dimensional echocardiography. Am J Cardiol 49: 1319–1323, 1982.

536

5. Ihlen H, Amlie JP, Dale J et al.: Determination of cardiac output by Doppler echocardiography. Br Heart J 51: 54–60, 1984.

6. Rowles JM, Haites NE: Doppler ultrasound measurement of cardiac output; transcutaneous aortovelography. Br J Hosp Med 31: 292–297, 1984.

7. Gibson DG: Stroke distance – an improved measure of cardiovascular function. Br Heart J 53: 121–122, 1985.

8. Felner, JM, Blumenstein BA, Schlant RC, Carter AD, Alimurung BN, Johnson MJ, Sherman SW, Klicpera MW, Kutner MH, Druker LW: Sources of variability in echocardiographic measurements. Am J Cardiol 45: 995–1004, 1980.

9. Popp RL, Filly K, Brown OR, Harrison DC: Effect of transducer placement on echocardiographic measurements of left ventricular dimension. Am J Cardiol 35: 537–540, 1975.

10. Martin MA: Reproducibility of M-mode echocardiography. Clinical Echocardiography. pp 1–7. Eds Hunter S and Hall R. Castle House Publications Ltd, Kent, United Kingdom, 1986.

11. Pietro DA, Voelkel AG, Ray BJ, Parisi AF: Reproducibility of echocardiography. A study evaluating the variability of serial echocardiographic measurements. Chest 79: 29–32, 1981.

12. Touche T, Prasquier R, Merillon JP, Barthelemy M, Hanoun HC, Vervin P, Gourgon R: Mesure des volumes ventriculaires gauches par echocardiographie bidimensionalle a partir d'une coupe apicale. Arch Mal Coeur 3: 691–700, 1980.

13. Schiller NB, Acquatella H, Ports TA, Drew D, Goeerke J, Ringertz H, Silverman NH, Brundage B, Botvinick EH, Boswell R: Left ventricular volume from paired biplane two-dimensional echocardiography. Circulation 60: 547–555, 1979.

14. Starling MR, Crawford MH, Sorensen SG, Levi B, Richards KL, O'Rourke RA: Comparative accuracy of apical biplane cross-sectional echocardiography and gated radionuclide angiography for estimating left ventricular size and performance. Circulation 63: 1075–1084, 1981.

15. Schnittger I, Fitzgerald PJ, Daughters GT, Ingels NB, Kantrowitz NE, Schwarzkopf A, Mead CW, Popp RL: Limitations of comparing left ventricular volumes by two-dimensional echocardiography, myocardial markers and cineangiography. Am J Cardiol 50: 512–519, 1982.

16. Hall RJC, Doran J, Pusey C, McHaffie D, Gibson DG: The effect of nitroglycerin, beta blockade with acebutalol and isometric stress on incoordinate left ventricular function. Eur Heart J 3: 23–28, 1982.

17. Bennett ED, Barclay SA, Davis AL, Mannering D, Mehta N: Ascending aortic blood velocity and acceleration using Doppler ultrasound in the assessment of left ventricular function. Cardiovasc Res 18: 632–638, 1984.

18. Wallmeyer K, Wann S, Sagar KB, Kalbflesch J, Klopfenstein S: The influence of preload and heart rate in Doppler echocardiographic indexes of left ventricular performance: comparison with invasive indexes in an experimental preparation. Circulation 74: 181–186, 1986.

19. Lewis JF, Kuo LC, Nelson JG, Limacher MC, Quinones MA: Pulsed Doppler echocardiographic determination of stroke volume and cardiac output: clinical validation of two new methods using an apical window. Circulation 70: 425–431, 1984.

20. Nicolosi GL, Pungercic E, Cervesato E, Modena L, Zanuttini D: Analysis of inter-observer and intraobserver variation of interpretation of echocardiographic and Doppler flow determination of cardiac output by the mitral orifice method. Br Heart J 55: 446–448, 1986.

21. Zoghbi, WA, Quinones MA: Determination of cardiac output by Doppler echocardiography: a critical appraisal. Herz. 11: 258–268, 1986.
22. DeMaria AN, Neumann A, Schubart PJ, Lee G, Mason DT: Systematic correlation of cardiac chamber size and ventricular performance determined with echocardiography and alterations in heart rate in normal persons. Am J Cardiol 43: 1–9, 1979.
23. Ehsani AA, Hagberg JM, Hickson RC: Rapid changes in left ventricular dimensions and mass in response to physical conditioning and deconditioning. Am J Cardiol 42: 52–56, 1978.
24. Roeske WR, O'Rourke RA, Klein A, Leopold G, Karliner JS: Noninvasive evaluation of ventricular hypertrophy in professional athletes. Circulation 53: 286–291, 1976.
25. Boyle G, Mehta N, Prindle K, Bennett ED: Ascending aortic blood velocity and acceleration measured by Doppler ultrasound in normal and B-blocked subjects during treadmill exercise. Clin Sci 71: 54, 1986.
26. Mehta N, Bennett D, Mannering D, Dawkins K, Ward DE: Usefulness of noninvasive Doppler measurement of ascending aortic blood velocity and acceleration in detecting impairment of the left ventricular functional response to exercise three weeks after myocardial infarction. Am J Cardiol 58: 879–884, 1986.
27. Redwood DR, Henry WL, Epstein SE: Evaluation of the ability of echocardiography to measure acute alterations in left ventricular volume. Circulation 50: 901–904, 1974.
28. Lejemtel TH, Keung E, Sonnenblick EH, Ribner HS, Matsumoto M, Davis R, Schwartz W, Alousi AA, Davolos D: Amrinone: a new non-glycosidic, non-adrenergic cardiotonic agent effective in the treatment of intractable myocardial failure in man. Circulation 59: 1098–1104, 1979.
29. Nixon JV, Murray RG, Leonard PD, Mitchell JH, Blomqvist G: Effect of large variations in preload on left ventricular performance characteristics in normal subjects. Circulation 65: 698–703, 1982.
30. Quinones MA, Gaasch WH, Cole JS, Alexander JK: Echocardiographic determination of left ventricular stress – velocity relations in man, with reference to the effects of loading and contractility. Circulation 51: 689–700, 1975.
31. Elkayam U, Gardin JM, Berkley R, Hughes CA, Henry WL: Use of Doppler flow velocity measurements to assess the haemodynamic response to vasodilators in patients with heart failure. Circulation 67: 377–383, 1983.
32. Light LH: Non-injurious ultrasonic technique for observing flow in the human aorta. Nature 224: 1119–1121, 1969.
33. Mehta N, Bennett DE: Impaired left ventricular function in acute myocardial infarction assessed by Doppler measurement of ascending aorta blood velocity and maximum acceleration. Am J Cardiol 57: 1052–1058, 1986.
34. Noble MI, Trenchard D, Guz A: Left ventricular ejection in conscious dogs. I. Measurement and significance of the maximum acceleration of blood from the left ventricle. Circ Res. 19: 139–147, 1966.
35. Rushmer RF: Initial ventricular impulse. A potential key to cardiac evaluation. Circulation 29: 268–283, 1964.
36. Bradley RD: Intensive Care. In: Oxford Textbook of Medicine. 2: pp 14. Oxford University Press, Oxford, United Kingdom, 1983.
37. Sagawa K: Editorial: The end-systolic pressure-volume relation of the ventricle: definition, modifications and clinical use. Circulation 63: 1223–1227, 1981.
38. Marsh JD, Green LH, Wynne J, Cohn FF, Grossmann W: Left-ventricular end-systolic pressure-dimension and stress-length relations in normal human subjects. Am J Cardiol 44: 1311–1317, 1979.

538

39. Colan SD, Borow, KM, Gamble WJ, Sanders SP: Effects of enhanced afterload (methoxamine) and contractile state (dobutamine) on left ventricular late-systolic wall stress-dimension ratio. Am J Cardiol 52: 1304–1309, 1983.

40. Borow KM, Arensman FW, Webb C, Radley-Smith R, Yacoub MH: Assessment of left ventricular contractile state after anatomic correction of transposition of the great arteries. Circulation 69: 106–112, 1984.

41. Borow KM, Propper R, Bierman FZ, Grady S, Inati A: The left ventricular end-systolic pressure-dimension relation in patients with thalassemia major. Circulation 66: 980–985, 1982.

42. Mercier JC, DiSessa TG, Jarmanaki JM, Nakanishi T, Hiraishi S, Isabel-Jones J, Friedman WF: Two-dimensional echocardiographic assessment of left ventricular volumes and ejection fraction in children. Circulation 65: 962–969, 1982.

43. Nishioka O, Maruyama Y, Askikawa K, Isoyama S, Satoh S, Suzuki H, Watanabe J, Watanabe H, Shimizu Y, Ino-oka E: Effects of changes in afterload impedance on left ventricular ejection in isolated canine hearts: dissociation of end-ejection from end-systole. Cardiovasc Res. 21: 107–118, 1987.

44. Marier DL, Gibson DG: Limitations of two frame method for displaying regional left ventricular wall motion in man. Br Heart J 44: 555–559, 1980.

45. Braunwald E, Ross Jr. J, Sonnenblick EH: Mechanisms of contraction in the normal and failing heart. N Engl J Med 277: 1012, 1967.

46. Thomson W, Lord, Kelvin: Electrical Units of Measurement. The practical applications of electricity, a series of lectures delivered at the Institute of Civil Engineers. pp 149–175, 1884.

47. Burggraf GW, Parker JO: Left ventricular volume changes after amyl nitrite and nitroglycerine in man, as measured by ultrasound. Circulation 49: 136–143, 1974.

48. Miyatake K, Izumi S, Yamagishi M, Beppu S, Sakakibara H: Analysis of native coronary flow by two – dimensional Doppler echocardiography. Circulation 74: 1863, 1986.

49. Gomes JAC, Carambas CR, Moran HE, Dhatt MS, Calon AH, Caracta AR, Damato AN: The effect of isosorbide dinitrate on left ventricular size wall stress and left ventricular function in chronic refractory heart failure. Am J Med 65: 794–802, 1978.

50. Cooper M, Shaddy R, Silverman R, Enderlein M: Usefulness of Doppler echocardiography for determining haemodynamic improvement with intravenous verapamil in hypertrophic cardiomyopathy. Am J Cardiol 56: 201–202, 1985.

51. Mattheos M, Shapiro E, Oldershaw PJ, Sacchetti R, Gibson DG: Non-invasive assessment of changes in left ventricular relaxation by combined phono-, echo- and mechanography. Br Heart J 47: 253–260, 1982.

52. Hanrath P, Mathey D, Kremer P, Sonntag F, Bleifeld W: Effect of verapamil on left ventricular isovolumic relaxation time and regional left ventricular filling in hypertrophic cardiomyopathy. Am J Cardiol 45: 1258–1264, 1980.

53. Oldershaw PJ, Dawkins KD, Ward DE, Gibson DG: Effect of exercise on left ventricular filling in left ventricular hypertrophy. Br Heart J 49: 568–573, 1983.

54. Spirito P, Maron B, Bonow RO: Noninvasive assessment of left ventricular diastolic function: comparative analysis of Doppler echocardiographic and radionuclide angiographic techniques. J Amer Coll Cardiol 7: 518–526, 1986.

55. Lorrell BH, Paulus WJ, Braunwald E: Improved diastolic function and systolic performance in HCM after nifedipine. N Engl J Med 303: 801–803, 1980.

56. Suwa M, Hiroba Y, Kawamura K: Improvement in left ventricular diastolic function during intravenous and oral diltiazem therapy in patients with hypertrophic cardiomyopathy: an echocardiographic study. Am J Cardiol 54: 1047–1053, 1984.

57. Phillips RA, Coplan NL, Krakoff LR, Yeager K, Ross RS, Gorlin R, Goldman ME:

Doppler echocardiography analysis of left ventricular filling in treated hypertensive patients. J Amer Coll Cardiol 9: 317–322, 1986.

58. Charuzi Y, Beeder C, Marshall LA, Sasaki H, Pack NB, Geft I, Ganz W: Improvement in regional and global left ventricular function after intracoronary thrombolysis: assessment with two-dimensional echocardiography. Am J Cardiol 53: 662–665, 1984.

59. von Bibra H, Gibson DG, Nityanandan K: Effects of propranolol on left ventricular wall movement in patients with ischaemic heart disease. Br Heart J 43: 293–300, 1980.

Index of Subjects

Aortic dissection, 415–421, see also Transesophageal echocardiography intraoperative
Doppler color flow mapping, 415
  entry site, 420
  planing of operative procedure, 420
  reentry site, 420
  type I, 416
  type III, 417, 418
Arterial assessment, see Intraoperative arterial
assessment, Duplex
  scanning
Arterial pacing, see Stress echocardiography
Arterial puncture, see Doppler guiding of
vessels puncture

Balloon atrial septostomy, 41–55
  advantage, 55
  blade atrioseptostomy catheter, 51
  cardiac function changes, 45
  color flow Doppler guiding, 49–55
  contrast echocardiography, 42
  entry phase, 43
  inflation phase, 44
  Miller balloon catheter, 50
  pullback, 44
  results, 45
  technique, 42
  two-dimensional echocardiography, 41

Cardiac output, see Doppler monitoring of
cardiac output
Cardiac catheterization, 77–88, see also Color
Doppler guiding of
  atrial septostomy, Transseptal cardiac
catheterization,
  Transvenous mitral commissurotomy
  ultrasonic guidance of, 77–88
    active localization system, 79
    advantages, 86
    catheter directivity, 81
    catheter transducer, 78
    coronary arteries, 85
    disadvantages, 87

    efficacy testing, 82
    future directions, 87
    localization accuracy, 85
    passive localization system, 79
    transponder localization system, 80
Cardiac masses, see Transesophageal echocardiography
Cardiac pacing, 89–97, 431–445
  Doppler echocardiography in, 431
    choosing the pacing mode, 431
    effect of AV synchrony on stroke
volume, 434
    evaluation of atrial capture, 445
    evaluation of pacemaker physiology,
431
    left atrial size, 432
    optimization of AV pacing intervals,
440
    pacemaker induced valvular
regurgitation, 444
  ultrasonically marked pacing system,
89–97
    flashing marker, 90
    follow-up methods, 94–97
    high frequency vector detection, 95
    implantable pacemaker, 91
    lead impedance measurement, 96
    localization electronic, 89
    marker transducer, 89
    marking in 2-D echocardiographic
image, 94
    marking in M-mode echocar-
diographic image, 94
    passive marking system, 90
    spike-marker differential diagnosis,
96
    temporary pacemaker, 90
    transponder marking system, 90
Color flow Doppler, 41–55, 149, see also
Intraoperative echocardiography
  and contrast echocardiography, 149
  aortic dissection, 415–421
  balloon atrial septostomy, 41–55

guiding of coronary artery anastomosis, 407
transesophageal, 291–295
Congenital heart disease, see Intraoperative echocardiography
Contrast agents, see Contrast echocardiography
Contrast echocardiography, 149–173, 179–186, 191–205, 363–365
  advantages, 166
  clinical application, 156
  color Doppler flow imaging and, 149
  complex congenital heart diseases, 161
  contrast agents, 150, 179, 191
    carbonated water, 185
    carbon dioxide, 150, 180, 191
    Decholin 185
    dextrose, 150, 179, 303
    dimethylsulfoxide, 150, 185
    Echoson, 183
    ether, 185
    fat emulsions, 185
    fluorochemicals, 184
    gelatin, 182, 191, 185
    Hemaccel, 150
    hydrogen peroxide, 181, 191
    indocyanine green, 149, 179, 191
    Iopamidol, 202
    isopropyl alcohol, 185
    liposyn, 150
    milk, 185
    microspheres, 185
    paraldehyde, 150, 185
    perfluorocarbon compounds, 150
    polygelin, 150, 182
    propylene glycol, 150, 185
    Renografin, 185, 191
    saccharide particles, 183
    saline, 150, 179, 303
    sodium bicarbonate – ascorbic acid mixture, 181, 191
    sonicated agents, 185
    sonicated plasma, 185
    Sorbitol, 202
  demonstration of shunts, 156
  left-sided valvular insufficiency, 163
  M-mode echocardiography, 152
  myocardial contrast echocardiography, 171, 191–205, 363–365
  negative contrast effects, 157
  positive contrast effects, 157
  problems related to physic and instrumentation, 155
  problems related to contrast agents, 154
  pulmonary insufficiency, 163
  pulmonary transmission, 150
  qualitative contrast echocardiography, 152
  quantitative contrast echocardiography, 152
  structure identification, 156
  surface tension, 186
  toxicity, 151
  tricuspid insufficiency, 162
  two-dimensional echocardiography, 153
  valvular insufficiency, 162
  videodensitometry, 168, 197
  viscosity, 186
Coronary artery surgery, see Coronary graft flow measurement, Doppler
  guiding of coronary artery surgery, Stress echocardiography
Coronary graft flow measurement, 395, 401
Coronary venous retroperfusion, 117–128
  assessment of global cardiac function, 124
  assessment of the efficacy of retroperfusion, 124
  clinical application, 122
  computation of ventricular function, 125
  echocardiographic assessment, 117
  historical events, 117
  ischemia demonstrated by 2-D echocardiography, 122
  limitations, 127
  measurement of alterations of regional wall motion and thickness, 124
  proposal for improvements, 127
  significance of wall thickening changes, 126
  ultrasonic test for viability, 125

Diastolic left ventricular function, 531
Doppler color flow mapping, see Color flow Doppler guiding of atrial
  septostomy, Intraoperative echocardiography, Transesophageal echocardiography
Doppler monitoring of cardiac output, 423–429
  angle estimation, 426
  estimation of diameter, 426
  flow profile, 426
  implantable Doppler aortic transducer, 423–429
  probe fixation, 426
  probe size, 425
  sample volume, 426
Doppler guiding of vessels puncture, 473–479
  internal jugular vein cannulation, 473

monitoring complication of arterial
    catheterization, 478
  radial artery cannulation, 477
  subclavian vein cannulation, 477
Drug interventions, 523–535
  arterial pressure, 528
  blood flow, 529
  central blood volume, 528
  cross-sectional echocardiography, 524
  diastolic left ventricular function, 531
  Doppler, 525
  echocardiography in, 523
  effect of afterload, 531
  heart rate, 527
  incoordinate left ventricular function,
    534
  isovolumic relaxation time, 532
  left ventricular volume, 530
  loading conditions, 527
  M-mode echocardiography, 524
  reproducibility, 526
  systolic left ventricular function, 529
  ventricular filling, 533
Duplex scaning, 449–460
  advantage, 449
  arterial disease, 449
  atherosclerotic plaque, 452
  carotid disease, 449
  celiac arteries, 454
  intestinal angina, 454
  peripheral arteries, 454
  renal arteries, 453
  stroke, 450
  superior mesenteric arteries, 454
  to follow endarterectomy, 452
  to screen patients with hypertension, 454
  transient ischemic attack, 450
  transplanted kidney, 454
  venous disease, 449
  venous system, 457
  vertebral arteries, 450
  visceral arteries, 453

Endocarditis, see Transesophageal echocardiography
Endomyocardial biopsy, 14, 19–40
  left ventricle, 19–27
    complications, 26
    contraindications for, 20
    echocardiographic monitoring, 21
    indications for, 20
    King's bioptome, 21
    limitations, 25
    location of the biopsy site, 23

methods, 20
  morphological variation, 26
right ventricle, 31–40
  biopsy technique, 33
  Caves-Schults forceps, 31
  echocardiographic technique, 31
  internal jugular approach, 36
Exercise echocardiography, see Stress echocardiography

Hypertrophic cardiomyopathy, see Intraoperative echocardiography

Infective endocarditis, see Transesophageal
  echocardiography
Intracardiac echocardiography, 3–17
  atrial pacing, 11
  contrast injection, 11
  limitations, 16
  LV cavity dimensions, 4
  M-mode, 4, 59
  myocardial biopsy, 14
  pericardial thickness, 14
  rate of dimensions change, 10
  shortening fraction, 10
  trans-septal puncture, 14
  two-dimensional, 4
  wall excursions, 10
  wall thickness, 10
Intraoperative echocardiography, 301–311,
  313–329, 351–361, 367–375, 381–393,
  395–404, 407–413, 463–471
  acute myocardial ischemia, 367–375
  backscatter, 373
  change in the echo texture, 372
  Doppler estimation of coronary blood
    flow, 374
  perioperative myocardial infarction, 367
  color flow Doppler evaluation of
    coronary anastomosis, 407–413
  color flow Doppler imaging, 381–393
    criteria for assessing the severity of
      regurgitation, 383
    epicardial approach, 381
    in aortic annuloplasty, 387
    inherent leaks, 391, 393
    in mitral annuloplasty, 384
    in open mitral commissurotomy, 385
    in prosthetic valve, 390
    in tricuspid annuloplasty, 387
    in untouched valve, 389
    paravalvular leaks, 391, 393
    transesophageal approach, 381
    transvalvular leaks, 391

544

valvular heart disease, 381
in congenital heart disease, 331–341
  arterial level, 339
  assessment of the surgical result, 341
  atrial level, 334
  atrial septal defect, 334
  atrioventricular level, 335
  color-coded Doppler echocardiography, 341
  complete transposition of the great arteries, 334
  dehiscence of ventricular septal defect, 337
  idiopathic hypertrophic subaortic stenosis, 338
  Mustard's procedure, 336
  outflow tract obstruction, 337
  persistent superior left caval vein, 334
  technique, 331
  tetralogy of Fallot, 335, 337
  total anomalous pulmonary venous drainage, 334
  ventriculo-arterial level, 337
  Waterston anastomosis, 340
contrast echocardiogram, 168, 303, 363–365
  cardioplegic perfusion, 363–364
  limitations, 364
  myocardial perfusion, 363
  sonicated albumin, 365
Doppler guiding in coronary artery surgery, 395–404
  flow measurements, 395, 400
  graft flow measurement, 401
  identification of coronary arteries, 395
  identification of coronary grafts, 395
  identification of the internal mammary artery, 397
  in reoperations, 397
  mapping of the native arteries, 397
  selection of site for graft anastomosis, 399
left ventricular performance, 351–361
  effects of coronary artery bypass grafting, 356
  effects of valve surgery, 357
  intraoperative myocardial infarction, 356
  left ventricular function, 355
  limitations, 360
in subvalvular aortic obstruction, 343–350

fibromuscular ridge, 343
hypertrophic cardiomyopathy, 343
membranous type, 343
procedure, 344
results after repair, 347
results before repair, 345
tunnel stenosis, 343
valvular heart disease, 301–311, 313–329
  aortic valve disease, 308
  color flow Doppler, 305
  comparison of contrast vs. color flow echocardiography, 310
  contrast echocardiography, 303
  ejection fraction, 315
  hypertrophic cardiomyopathy, 309
  left ventricular compliance, 321
  left ventricular mass, 317
  left ventricular mechanics, 323
  methodology, 301
  mitral regurgitation, 306
  mitral stenosis, 309
  myocardial function, 309
  myxoma, 309
  tricuspid valve disease, 307
  two-dimensional echocardiography, 301

Laser angioplasty, 99–113
  ablation of AV node, 103
  ablation of His bundle, 103
  ablation of left ventricular thrombi, 105
  ablation of vegetative mass, 105
  argon, 100
  arterial system, 106
  atherosclerotic plaques, 106
  atrial chamber, 103
  atrial septostomy, 103
  cardiac valves, 105
  catheter-directed laser, 99
  clot destruction, 102
  clot dissolution, 106
  CO_2, 100
  complications, 111
  contrast microbubble, 109
  coronary artery obstructions, 107
  direct firing of laser, 99
  electrocatheter system, 112
  elimination of arrhythmogenic foci, 104
  enlarging of coarctation, 106
  excimer, 100
  fluoroscopy, 101
  laser catheter visualization, 107
  laser firing, 108

laser therapy, 99
neodymium, 100
peripheral arteries, 107
ultrasound imaging, 100
valvuloplasty, 105
venous system, 101
ventricular chamber, 103, 233–234
Left ventricular performance, 351–361
Left ventricular compliance, 321

Mitral commissurotomy, see Transvenous mitral
    commissurotomy
Myocardial contrast echocardiography, see
    Contrast echocardiography
Myocardial function in valvular heart disease,
    301
Myocardial ischemia, 367–375, see also
    Transesophageal echocardiography
    back-scatter, 373
    change in the echo texture, 372
    Doppler estimation of coronary blood
        flow, 374
    electrocardiographic monitoring, 367
    following hyperemic response, 374
    in resting state, 374
    intraoperative epicardial echocardio-
        graphy in, 367
    laser fluorometry, 370
    perioperative myocardial infarction, 367
Myocardial perfusion, 191–205, see also
    Contrast echocardiography

Pacing system, see Cardiac pacing
Passive marking system, 79, 90
Perfusion myocardial, see Myocardial perfusion
Pericardiocentesis, 133–144
    blind techniques, 133
    ECG guidance, 133
    echocardiographic guidance, 135
        A- and M-mode guidance, 135
        apical approach, 138
        complications, 143
        contrast method, 136
        direction of the needle, 139
        left parasternal approach, 138
        needle guide attachement, 137, 140
        pericardial biopsy, 142
        pericardial window, 142
        posterior thoracic approach, 138, 141
        remote transducer position, 137
        right parasternal approach, 138
        right-sided approach, 138
        two-dimensional echocardiography,
            137

ultrasonic marking of the needle tip,
    144
xiphocostal approach, 138
fluoroscopic guidance, 133
Prosthetic valve malfunction, see Trans-
    esophageal echocardiography

Retroperfusion, see Coronary venous retro-
    perfusion

Stress echocardiography, 483–492, 495–505,
    509–519
    advantages, 484
    bicycle ergometry, 483
    clinical utility, 487
    cold pressor stimulation, 483, 495
    methods of analysis, 485
    pharmacologic manipulation, 483, 495
    prognostic information, 488
    protocols, 484
    transesophageal pacing, 483, 495–505
    treadmill exercise, 483
    stress Doppler echocardiography,
        50–519
        acceleration, 509
        corelations with radionuclide
            methods, 516
        during cardiac catheterization, 512
        during treadmill exercise, 513
        ejection dynamics, 510
        velocity, 509
    validation of the technique, 485
    with transesophageal atrial pacing,
        495–505
        correlation between WMA and
            CAD, 502
        detection of CAD, 503
        exam recording, 489
        evaluation of effect of coronary
            surgery, 503
        identification of patients with multi-
            vessel disease, 505
        identification of patients with myo-
            cardial infarction, 505
        onset of WMAs, 501
        reading the exam, 499
        severity and extent of WMAs, 500
        sensitivity and specificity, 499
Subvalvular aortic obstruction, see Intraopera-
    tive echocardiography
Systolic left ventricular function, 529

Transesophageal echocardiography, 209–222,
    227–244, 249–258, 261–270, 273–280,

281–289, 291–297
  air embolism, 232
  aortic dissection, 249–258, 294
  artifact in the aorta, 254
    ectasia of the aorta, 254
    false lumen, 250
    intimal flap, 252
    true lumen, 250
    type A, 252
    type B, 252
  cardiac masses, 261–270
    atrial myxomas, 261
    cardiac thrombi, 261
    cardiac tumors, 261
    extracardiac masses, 261, 268
    left atrial appendage thrombi, 262
    left atrial spontaneous echo contrast, 267
  Doppler color flow mapping, 236, 291–297
    aortic aneurysm, 294
    effects of vasoactive drugs on intracardiac shunting, 295
    effects of vasoactive drugs on valvular regurgitation, 295
    iatrogenic atrial septal defect, 294
    intimal flap, 294
    intimal tear, 294
    left atrial myxoma, 293
    mitral regurgitation, 292
  Doppler echocardiography, 220, 235
  early studies, 227
  future directions, 243
  infective endocarditis, 273–280
    endocarditis-associated abscesses, 277
    perivalvular abscesses, 277
    valvular vegetations, 273
  in the intensive care unit, 235
  ischemia and infarction, 237–243
  left ventricular function during anesthesia, 233–234
  mechanical probes, 230
  M-mode transducer, 277
  phased-array probes, 230
  prosthetic valve malfunction, 281–289
    abnormal rocking, 286
    bioprostheses, 281
    early diastolic hump, 286
    endocarditis of prosthetic valve, 281
    mechanical prostheses, 281
    paravalvular leak, 286
    transvalvular regurgitation, 287
    valve degeneration, 283

    valve thrombi, 285
  technique and standard views, 209–222
    aortic valve view, 212
    biatrial view, 217
    left ventricular short axis view, 216
    mitral valve view, 213
    M-mode echocardiography, 209
    non-standardized views, 218
    pulmonary artery view, 217
    two-dimensional echocardiography, 210
Transponder marking system, 80, 90
Transseptal cardiac catheterization, 14, 57–65
  complications, 57
  indications, 57
  intracardiac M-mode echocardiography, 59
  limitations, 64
  M-mode echocardiography, 59
  methods, 57
  needle tip echo transmitter, 65
  pericardial effusion, 59
  results, 62
  two-dimensional echocardiography, 61
Transvenous mitral commissurotomy, 67–75
  balloon catheter, 67
  dilating manipulation, 69
  mitral commissurotomy under direct vision, 72
  results, 75
  two-dimensional echocardiography assessment, 74
  two-dimensional echocardiography guidance, 67

Ultrasonic guidance of
  balloon atrial septostomy, 41–55
  cardiac catheterization, 77–88
  coronary artery surgery, 395–404
  endomyocardial byopsy, 19–40
  laser angioplasty, 99–113
  marked pacing leads, 89–97
  mitral commissurotomy, 67–75
  transseptal cardiac catheterization, 57–65
  vessels puncture, 473–479
Ultrasonically marked pacing system, see Cardiac pacing
Ultrasonically marked cardiac catheters, see Cardiac catheterization

Valvular heart disease, see Contrast echocardiography, Intraoperative echocardiography
Vegetations, 273, 281

Venous disease, see Duplex scanning
Venous puncture, see Doppler guiding of vessels puncture
Venous system and laser, 101
Vessels puncture, see Doppler guiding of vessels puncture

DEVELOPMENTS IN CARDIOVASCULAR MEDICINE

Recent volumes

Perry, H.M., ed.: Lifelong management of hypertension. 1983. ISBN 0-89838-582-2.

Jaffe, E.A., ed.: Biology of endothelial cells. 1984. ISBN 0-89838-587-3.

Surawicz, B., Reddy, C.P., Prystowsky, E.N., eds.: Tachycardias. 1984.
 ISBN 0-89838-588-1.

Spencer, M.P., ed.: Cardiac Doppler diagnosis. 1983. ISBN 0-89838-591-1.

Villarreal, H., Sambhi, M.P., eds.: Topics in pathophysiology of hypertension. 1984.
 ISBN 0-89838-595-4.

Messerli, F.H., ed.: Cardiovascular disease in the elderly. 1984. ISBN 0-89838-596-2.

Simoons, M.L., Reiber, J.H.C., eds.: Nuclear imaging in clinical cardiology. 1984.
 ISBN 0-89838-599-7.

Ter Keurs, H.E.D.J., Schipperheyn, J.J., eds.: Cardiac left ventricular hypertrophy. 1983.
 ISBN 0-89838-612-8.

Sperelakis, N., ed.: Physiology and pathophysiology of the heart. 1984.
 ISBN 0-89838-615-2.

Messerli, F.H., ed.: Kidney in essential hypertension. 1984. ISBN 0-89838-616-0.

Sambhi, M.P., ed.: Fundamental fault in hypertension. 1984. ISBN 0-89838-638-1.

Marchesi, C., ed.: Ambulatory monitoring: Cardiovascular system and allied applications.
 1984. ISBN 0-89838-642-X.

Kupper, W., MacAlpin, R.N., Bleifeld, W., eds.: Coronary tone in ischemic heart disease.
 1984. ISBN 0-89838-646-2.

Sperelakis, N., Caulfield, J.B., eds.: Calcium antagonists: Mechanisms of action on cardiac muscle and vascular smooth muscle. 1984. ISBN 0-89838-655-1.

Godfraind, T., Herman, A.S., Wellens, D., eds.: Calcium entry blockers in cardiovascular
 and cerebral dysfunctions. 1984. ISBN 0-89838-658-6.

Morganroth, J., Moore, E.N., eds.: Interventions in the acute phase of myocardial infarction. 1984. ISBN 0-89838-659-4.

Abel, F.L., Newman, W.H., eds.: Functional aspects of the normal, hypertrophied, and
 failing heart. 1984. ISBN 0-89838-665-9.

Sideman, S., Beyar, R., eds.: Simulation and imaging of the cardiac system. 1985.
 ISBN 0-89838-687-X.

Van der Wall, E., Lie, K.I., eds.: Recent views on hypertrophic cardiomyopathy. 1985.
 ISBN 0-89838-694-2.

Beamish, R.E., Singal, P.K., Dhalla, N.S., eds.: Stress and heart disease. 1985.
 ISBN 0-89838-709-4.

Beamish, R.E., Panagio, V., Dhalla, N.S., eds.: Pathogenesis of stress-induced heart disease. 1985. ISBN 0-89838-710-8.

Morganroth, J., Moore, E.N., eds.: Cardiac arrhythmias. 1985. ISBN 0-89838-716-7.

Mathes, E., ed.: Secondary prevention in coronary artery disease and myocardial infarction. 1985. ISBN 0-89838-736-1.

Lowell Stone, H., Weglicki, W.B., eds.: Pathology of cardiovascular injury. 1985. ISBN 0-89838-743-4.

Meyer, J., Erbel, R., Rupprecht, H.J., eds.: Improvement of myocardial perfusion. 1985. ISBN 0-89838-748-5.

Reiber, J.H.C., Serruys, P.W., Slager, C.J.: Quantitative coronary and left ventricular cineangiography. 1986. ISBN 0-89838-760-4.

Fagard, R.H., Bekaert, I.E., eds.: Sports cardiology. 1986. ISBN 0-89838-782-5.

Reiber, J.H.C., Serruys, P.W., eds.: State of the art in quantitative coronary arteriography. 1986. ISBN 0-89838-804-X.

Roelandt, J., ed.: Color Doppler Flow Imaging. 1986. ISBN 0-89838-806-6.

Van der Wall, E.E., ed.: Noninvasive imaging of cardiac metabolism. 1986. ISBN 0-89838-812-0.

Liebman, J., Plonsey, R., Rudy, Y., eds.: Pediatric and fundamental electrocardiography. 1986. ISBN 0-89838-815-5.

Hilger, H.H., Hombach, V., Rashkind, W.J., eds.: Invasive cardiovascular therapy. 1987. ISBN 0-89838-818-X

Serruys, P.W., Meester, G.T., eds.: Coronary angioplasty: a controlled model for ischemia. 1986. ISBN 0-89838-819-8.

Tooke, J.E., Smaje, L.H.: Clinical investigation of the microcirculation. 1986. ISBN 0-89838-819-8.

Van Dam, R.Th., Van Oosterom, A., eds.: Electrocardiographic body surface mapping. 1986. ISBN 0-89838-834-1.

Spencer, M.P., ed.: Ultrasonic diagnosis of cerebrovascular disease. 1987. ISBN 0-89838-836-8.

Legato, M.J., ed.: The stressed heart. 1987. ISBN 0-89838-849-X.

Safar, M.E., ed.: Arterial and venow systems in essential hypertension. 1987. ISBN 0-89838-857-0.

Roelandt, J., ed.: Digital techniques in echocardiography. 1987. ISBN 0-89838-861-9.

Dhalla, N.S. et al., eds.: Pathophysiology of heart disease. 1987. ISBN 0-89838-864-3.

Dhalla, N.S. et al., eds.: Heart function and metabolism. 1987. ISBN 0-89838-865-1.

Dhalla, N.S. et al., eds.: Myocardial Ischemia. 1987. ISBN 0-89838-866-X.

Beamish, R.E. et al., eds.: Pharmacological aspects of heart disease. 1987. ISBN 0-89838-867-8.

Ter Keurs, H.E.D.J., Tyberg, J.V., eds.: Mechanics of the circulation. 1987. ISBN 0-89838-870-8

Sideman, S., Beyar, R., eds.: Activation, metabolism and perfusion of the heart. 1987. ISBN 0-89838-871-6.

Aliot, E., Lazzara, R., eds.: Ventricular tachycardias. 1987. ISBN 0-89838-881-3.

Schneeweiss, A. et al., eds.: Cardiovascular drug therapy in the elderly. 1987. ISBN 0-89838-883-X.

Chapman, J.V., Sgalambro, A., eds.: Basic concepts in Doppler echocardiography. 1987. ISBN 0-89838-888-0

Chien, S. et al., eds.: Clinical hemocheology. 1987. ISBN 0-89838-807-4.

Morganroth, J., ed.: Congestive heart failure. 1987. ISBN 0-89838-955-0.

Messerli, F.H., ed.: Cardiovascular disease in the elderly. 2nd ed. 1988. ISBN 0-89838-962-3.

Heintzen, P.H., Bürsch, J.H., eds.: Progress in digital angiocardiography. 1988. ISBN 0-89838-965-8.

Scheinman, M.A., ed.: Catheter ablation of cardiac arrhythmias. 1988. ISBN 0-89838-967-4.

Spaan, J.A.E., Bruschke, A.V.G., Gittenberger-de Groot, A.C., eds.: Coronary circulation. 1987. ISBN 0-89838-978-X.

Visser, C., Kan, G., Meltzer, R., eds.: Echocardiography in coronary artery disease. 1988. ISBN 0-89838-979-8.

Bayés de Luna, A., Betriu, A., Permanyer, G., eds.: Therapeutics in cardiology. 1988. ISBN 0-89838-981-X.

Mirvis, D.M., ed.: Body surface electrocardiographic mapping. 1988. ISBN 0-89838-983-6.

Konstam, M.A., Isner, J.M., eds.: The right ventricle. 1988. ISBN 0-89838-987-9.

Kappagoda, C.T., Greenwood, P.V., eds.: Long-term management of patients after myocardial infarction. 1988. ISBN 0-89838-352-8.

Gaasch, W.H., Levine, H.J., eds.: Chronic aortic regurgitation. 1988. ISBN 0-89838-364-1.

Singal, P.K., ed.: Oxygen radicals in the pathophysiology of heart disease. 1988. ISBN 0-89838-375-7.

Reiber, J.H.C., Serruys, P.W., eds.: New developments in quantitative coronary arteriography. 1988. ISBN 0-89838-377-3.

Morganroth, J., Moore, E.N., eds.: Silent myocardial ischemia. 1988. ISBN 0-89838-380-3.

Ter Keurs, H.E.D.J., Noble, M.I.M., eds.: Starling's law of the heart revisited. 1988. ISBN 0-89838-382-X.

Sperelakis, N., ed.: Physiology and pathophysiology of the heart. 1988. ISBN 0-89838-388-9

De Jong, J.W., ed.: Myocardial energy metabolism. 1988. ISBN 0-89838-394-3.

Hombach, V., Hilger, H.H., Kennedy, H.L., eds.: Electrocardiography and cardiac drug therapy. 1988. ISBN 0-89838-395-1.

Iwata, H., Lombardini, J.B., Segawa, T., eds.: Taurine and the heart. 1988. ISBN 0-89838-396-X.

Rosen, M.R., Palti, Y., eds.: Lethal arrhythmias resulting from myocardial ischemia and infarction. 1988. ISBN 0-89838-401-X.

Iwase, M., Sotobata, I.: Clinical echocardiography. 1989. ISBN 0-89838-0004-1.

Cikes, I., ed.: Echocardiography in cardiac interventions. 1989. ISBN 0-89838-0088-2.

Rapaport, E., ed.: Early interventions in acute myocardial infarction. 1989. ISBN 0-89838-0175-7.

Safar, M.E., Fouad-Tarazi, F., eds.: The heart in hypertension. 1989. ISBN 0-89838-0197-8.

Meerbaum, S, Melzer, R., eds.: Myocardial contrast two-dimensional echocardiography. 1989. ISBN 0-089838-0205-2.

Morganroth, J., Moore, E.N., eds.: Risk/benefit analysis for the use and approval of thrombolytic, antiarrhythmic, and hypolipidemic agents. 1989. ISBN 0-89838-0294-X.

Serruys, P.W., Simon, R., Beatt, K.J., eds.: PTCA – An investigational tool and a non-operative treatment of acute ischemia. 1989. ISBN 0-89838-0346-6.

Ahand, I.S., Wahi, P.I., Dhalla, N.S., eds.: Pathophysiology and pharmacology of heart disease. 1989. ISBN 0-89838-0367-9.